Understanding Medical Terminology

6th edition

Author

Sister Agnes Clare Frenay, SSM, RN, BS in Nr., MS in Nr. Ed.

Professor Emeritus of Nursing
Saint Louis University School of Nursing and
Allied Health Professions
St. Louis, Mo.

Illustrator

Helen M. Smith, RN, BFA, MA, FIAL

Saint Louis University School of Medicine,
St. Louis, Mo.

Published by

The Catholic Hospital Association

St. Louis, Missouri 63104

Contributing Illustrators

Sister Jeanne Derer, SSM, BS, ADA
Sister Susan Scholl, SSM, BS, RN

Sixth Edition

Copyright © 1977
by
The Catholic Hospital Association
St. Louis, Missouri 63104

Second Printing - 1978

Previous editions copyrighted 1958, 1962, 1964, 1969 and 1973

Library of Congress Catalog Card No. 77-73986
ISBN 0-87125-038-1

A. M. D. G.

Dedicated to Christ, the Divine Healer,
and to all those in the health professions
who offer Christ-like service
to the patient

Foreword

The Catholic Hospital Association is happy to have the opportunity to publish the Sixth Edition of UNDERSTANDING MEDICAL TERMINOLOGY. Sister Agnes Clare Frenay, SSM has drawn on her twenty years of teaching experience and her close association with the latest medical developments to produce a highly practical, comprehensive text.

The author's contribution to education and to the health field in particular cannot be overestimated. Her dedication to producing the finest available medical terminology text and updating each edition with the latest information to meet the quickening pace of medical progress has benefited both instructors and students in the allied health field.

Previous editions have been translated into a seven-volume Braille edition by the American Printing House for the Blind in Louisville, Kentucky. Similar transcriptions have been produced by the New York Association for the Blind. The Library of Congress was given permission to transcribe this text into large type in connection with their program for blind persons.

In 1969, in recognition of the author's noteworthy contribution to literature in the health field, the Board of Trustees of The Catholic Hospital Association awarded Sister Agnes Clare a plaque at their annual convention.

The officers and the Executive Board of The Catholic Hospital Association hope that the Sixth Edition will continue to effectively contribute to the ever-increasing needs of education in the health field.

SISTER HELEN KELLEY, DC
President

May 1977

Preface

The sixth edition of UNDERSTANDING MEDICAL TERMINOLOGY is the result of clinical observations supported by concentrated library research over a two year period. The basic content and overall plan of the previous work are retained in the new text, since their practical usefulness has received general recognition. It should be recognized that the tables which consider conditions amenable to surgery merely offer examples of how certain health problems may be solved by surgical intervention. Their purpose is to put into sharp relief medical terms in a manner conducive to the integration of knowledge and the promotion of a better comprehension of definitions.

The health sciences, always in ferment, have assimilated new terms in a wide variety of medical specialties. Much effort has been expended to achieve their clarity of exposition as a means of stimulating sustained interest in the language of medicine. The first chapter continues to be fundamental to the text and should be the focus of attention in teaching and studying medical terminology.

Primary targets of additional terms are cardiovascular disorders in their medical and surgical dimensions, blood components in transfusion therapy, advances in immunology, cytogenetics and nuclear medicine.

A harvest of new medical terms needing clarification of their meaning are reaped from the widening scope of radiology, the impact of computerized tomography on neurosurgical diagnoses and other health fields, ultrasonography and its rapid invasion of the medical specialties, the broadening of virology, parasitology and oncology, all reflecting intense efforts by the medical profession to sustain health.

Bibliographic support is updated and enriched in all chapters. Some areas of current investigation are clarified by pertinent illustrations, such as the modes of ultrasound imaging and the latest method of karyotyping. Since cerebrovascular disease is a common health problem, its illustrations are thought to be of value. Coronary revascularization by saphenous vein graft and internal mammary artery grafts combined demonstrate a trend in current bypass surgery.

As in previous editions individual revised chapters of UNDERSTANDING MEDICAL TERMINOLOGY were submitted to faculty members of *St. Louis University School of Medicine* for preview to insure the correctness of the definitions. Grateful acknowledgement is made to Dr. Vallee L. Willman, Professor of Surgery and Chairman of the Department of Surgery, Dr. Robert M. O'Brien, Professor and Director of Orthopedic Surgery, Dr. Kenneth R. Smith, Professor and Director of Neurosurgery, Dr. Thomas R. Thale, Professor and Chairman of the Department of Psychiatry, Dr. Don C. Weir, Professor of Radiology, Dr. Eugene G. Hamilton, Clinical Professor of Gynecology and Obstetrics, Dr. Stephen F. Bowen, Clinical Professor of Ophthalmology, Dr. Donald J. Mehan, Associate Clinical Professor of Urology, Dr. Charles S. Sherwin, Assistant Clinical Professor of Surgery, Dr. Umit T. Aker, Assistant Clinical Professor of Internal Medicine and Director of Cardiac Catheterization Laboratories, St. Mary's Health Center, and Dr. Lawrence A. Pilla, Assistant Clinical Professor of Radiology.

Recognition and sincere gratitude are extended to Dr. Eugene F. Tucker, Associate Professor of Pathology, St. Louis University and Director of Medical Laboratories, St. Mary's Health Center, and Dr. John A. Gantz, Director of Nuclear

Medicine, St. Mary's Health Center, for their unfailing resourcefulness in assisting in the selection and updating of the terms in their specialties. The expert advice of Dr. William A. Werner, Lung Specialist and Dr. Charles R. Brielmaier, Director of Anesthesiology, St. Mary's Health Center are, likewise, greatly appreciated.

Sister Mary Imelda Pingel, Chairman and Professor of Physical Therapy, and Faculty deserve thanks for sharing their knowledge and experience in editing the chapter of their specialty.

The author's indebtedness to Sister Marylu Stueber for her proficiency in typing the manuscript and unfailing attention to detail in proofreading is indeed great. In addition Sister Jeanne Derer merits grateful acknowledgement for her contributions to the illustrations of the text. The kind volunteer Sister Mary Blanche Kulage who assisted with the proofreading and index is likewise deserving of heartfelt gratitude.

A very sincere thanks is due to Mr. Art Krings of the Universal Printing Company and Florian W. Beuckman of the Typographic Sales, Inc. for their cooperative efforts in seeing the book through the press.

Mr. John Marcus, President of Mathews Book Company, and Mrs. Beverly Parisi, Supervisor for Order and Research Department of this company, deserve recognition and appreciation for their generosity in making the newest medical texts available to update the terminology.

Gratitude is also expressed to Sister Helen Kelley, D.C., President of the Catholic Hospital Association, for publishing the text and to Mrs. Mary Krieger, Director of Publications, for her untiring efforts and support in making the sixth edition a reality.

New copyright permissions were obtained from the American Psychiatric Association for quoting selected definitions of the 4th edition of a *Psychiatric Glossary*; from W. B. Saunders Company for including in the terminology brief statements from the textbook, *The Laboratory in Clinical Medicine* by James A. Halsted, M.D. (ed.) and from Harper & Row Publishers, Inc., for tabulating essential hemodynamic values presented in *Cardiac Diagnosis and Treatment*, 2d ed. by Noble O. Fowler, M.D. (ed.).

UNDERSTANDING MEDICAL TERMINOLOGY in its latest revision should provide a basic reference for those who wish to explore the challenges of medical progress. Its reliability as a text is based within reasonable limits on documentation through intensive library research and consultation with medical experts in the various health fields.

It is anticipated that the text will undergo further transformation in response to the widening perspectives of the health sciences in the future.

SISTER AGNES CLARE FRENAY, SSM

May, 1977

Table of Contents

PART I

TERMS RELATED TO BIOLOGIC DISORDERS

PART II

SUPPLEMENTARY TERMS

List of Tables

List of Illustrations

xv

PART I
TERMS RELATED TO BIOLOGIC DISORDERS

Chapter I
Orientation to Medical Terminology

OBJECTIVES AND VALUES

Medical terminology is the professional language of those who directly or indirectly are engaged in the art of healing. Its strangeness may seem bewildering at first to the average student and its complexity may tax his power of concentration. These difficulties, however, gradually disappear as the student assimilates a working knowledge of the elements of medical terms which enables him to analyze words etymologically and according to their meaning. In the beginning the drudgery of memorizing is somewhat annoying to the novice in the field, but memory work is only a steppingstone to a keener understanding of the professional language. It is obvious that the intellect is constantly engaged in the study of medical terms in various types of mental processes: the analysis of words, their interpretation and, to a moderate degree, the transfer of knowledge, by combining word roots synthetically with prefixes and suffixes.

Since the definitions of terms touch on a number of specialties — medicine, surgery, urology, gynecology, psychiatry, orthopedics, endocrinology, oncology, laboratory diagnosis and others — medical terminology adapts itself easily to the integration and application of knowledge. Professional workers in the health fields, hospital administrators, nurses, medical record administrators, transcriptionists and secretaries, medical and radiologic technologists, physical therapists, respiratory therapists, pharmacists, medical social workers and trial attorneys will find in the subject matter ample material of practical significance for their professional career.

The terms selected (and a selective process is imperative because of the multiplicity of terms) revolve around the human body in health and disease, the one dynamic power of the biologic sciences which never loses its interest value. The time-honored principle to proceed from the normal to the abnormal is realized in the organizational pattern in which anatomic terms form the foundation for diagnostic terms and related operative and symptomatic terms.

Instead of stress on etymologic subtleties and Greek and Latin derivations, emphasis is laid on the meaning of word roots and combining forms because this approach facilitates the acquisition and retention of knowledge.

The primary goal of introducing the student to medical terminology is to help him develop the ability to read and understand the language of medicine. Efforts are directed to promote a knowledge of the elements of medical terms, an understanding of standard medical abbreviations, the ability to spell medical terms, and an appreciation of the logical method found in medical terminology.

BASIC CONCEPTS

The majority of medical terms claim Greek and Latin ancestry. Some have been adopted from modern languages, especially from the German and French. Obviously, the process of coining words by usage continues as time goes on and new scientific advances necessitate verbal expression. Theoretically speaking, word formation should safeguard the purity of language by joining Greek roots to Greek prefixes and suffixes and Latin roots to Latin combining forms. In reality, many medical terms are bilingual in their derivation as, for example, teleradiography which combines the Greek prefix "tele" (distant) with the Latin root "radius" (ray) and Greek root "graphein" (to write) or claustrophobia which joins the Latin root "claustrum" (enclosed space) to the Greek root "phobia" (fear).

1

Concerning the spelling of medical terms, more than one way may be acceptable due to the fact that both the Greek and Latinized spelling of the medical term have been adopted as being correct.   Attempts have been made to give both spellings throughout the text.

The scholar of medical terminology may well be filled with awe when he finds in the writings of Hippocrates (460-370 B.C.) a wealth of terms which are still alive after 2000 years although their meaning may have changed.   Some refer to human anatomy as acromion, apophysis, olecranon, bronchus, thorax, meninges, peritoneum, symphysis and ureter, others bring to mind obstetric concepts as bregma, chorion and lochia, still others reflect a knowledge of diseases and deformities as carcinoma, emphysema, ileus, nephritis, phthisis, kyphosis and lordosis.   One wonders why Aristotle (384-322 B.C.) mentions alopecia, an abnormal baldness and eye conditions as glaucoma, exophthalmos and leukoma.   Was a personal element involved?

It is a worthwhile experience to reach back into antiquity to unravel the intriguing analogies of medical terms.   All sorts of creatures from the animal kingdom have found their way into the language of healing.   The Greek karkinos, crab means carcinoma and the Latin crab, cancer.   Lupus is the Latin word for wolf, coccyx the Greek word for cuckoo.   It is obvious why cochlea (G) refers to a snail and cauda equina (L) to a horse's tail.   However, one is surprised that muscle from the Latin musculus means little mouse and vermis (L) worm when one considers the potential vigor of the former and the vital significance of the latter as a connecting lobe of the cerebellum.

Startling, too, is our semantic indebtedness to the grapevine.   The Greek root staphyle envisions a bunch of grapes and in its combination with cocci reminds of clusters of grapes and berries.   Its Latin partner uva is found in uvea and uvula, both referring to grapes.

The search for the origin of terms stirs our academic interest in the culture of the people who have coined the medical words.   Thus the warlike spirit of the Hellenistic age is reflected in xiphoid, sword; thyroid, shield and thorax, breastplate.   Stapes, stirrup and sella, saddle remind of a horse's trappings, while the ossicles malleus, hammer and incus, anvil depict miniatures of a blacksmith's implements.   Even the names of musical instruments take on medical meanings. Salpinx (G), trumpet and tympanum (L), drum are worthy examples of the intuitive perception of ancient minds.   The study of medical terminology can become indeed a rewarding experience which unveils the character of genius in the medical language.

The pronunciation of medical terms follows no rigid rules.   Flexibility is its outstanding characteristic.   Since authorities do not agree upon any special pronunciation, common usage must prevail.   Even in the same locality and in the same hospital, there will be discrepancies in pronouncing medical terms.   To assist the student in developing the ability to speak the language of medicine, brief discussions of medical subjects have been included in the text for oral reading exercises.

In the process of learning, the cultivation of analyzing medical terms is of primary importance.   It simplifies the assimilation of knowledge and promotes the development of a logical mind.   To analyze means to unloose, to resolve.   The analysis of medical terms is then the systematic breaking up of the term into its component parts — its suffixes, roots and prefixes. This method may convey the meaning in a clear-cut way as, for example:

	Analysis	**Definition**
Appendectomy —	ectomy: removal appendec: appendix	Removal of the appendix

or the meaning may be merely implied requiring a more precise definition as is the case with the term "anemia."   A breakup of this word into the prefix "an" and the root "emia" conveys an exaggerated impression since, in reality, anemia does not refer to a total lack of blood which would be incompatible with life, but merely to a condition characterized by a deficiency of red blood cells and hemoglobin. In other words, a definition explains and interprets a medical term, describing its essential properties in contradistinction to an analysis which breaks up the term in its linguistic elements. The introductory chapter seeks to develop an analytic attitude in the student. By making him aware of the structural design of words and helping him to form the habit of analyzing terms, it lays the foundation for the study of medical terminology. Its mastery will render the understanding of the terms offered in the subsequent chapters comparatively easy.[4]

ELEMENTS OF MEDICAL TERMS

I. Suffixes and Compounding Elements

True suffixes refer to a syllable or syllables denoting a preposition or adverb attached to the end of a word, root, or stem to modify its meaning. Many endings are adjectives or nouns added to a root to form compound words. They may be referred to as combining forms or pseudosuffixes. To simplify learning modifying endings have been classified according to their meanings into diagnostic, operative and symptomatic suffixes and compounding elements.

In analyzing terms it is advisable to begin with the suffix and proceed to the root or root and prefix. This method of approach may reveal the exact definition of the term, or it may convey its applied meaning.

A. Diagnostic Suffixes and Compounding Elements:

Suffix	Term	Analysis	Definition
-cele (G) hernia, tumor, protrusion	cystocele	*kystis:* bladder *kele:* hernia	Hernia of the bladder.
	gastrocele	*gaster:* stomach; —;	Hernia of the stomach.
	hydrocele	*hydor:* water *kele:* tumor	Serous tumor as of testis.
	myelocele	*myelos:* marrow *kele:* protrusion	Protrusion of spinal cord through the vertebrae.
-emia (G) blood	hyperglycemia hyperglycosemia	*hyper:* excessive *glykys:* sweet, sugar *haima:* blood	Abnormally high blood sugar.
	polycythemia	*polys:* many, excessive *kytos:* cell —; —;	Abnormal increase of red blood cells and hemoglobin in the blood.
-ectasis (G) expansion, dilatation	angiectasis	*angeion:* vessel *ektasis:* dilatation	Abnormal dilatation of a blood vessel.
	atelectasis	*ateles:* imperfect; —;	An airless, functionless lung.
	—; neonatorum	—; *neos:* new *natus:* birth, born	Imperfect expansion of lungs at birth.
	bronchiectasis	*bronchos:* bronchus —;	Abnormal dilatation of a bronchus or bronchi.
-iasis (G) condition, formation of, presence of	lithiasis	*lithos:* stone *iasis:* presence of	Formation of stones.
	cholelithiasis	*chole:* bile; —;	Presence of calculi in the gallbladder.
	nephrolithiasis	*nephros:* kidney; —;	Stones present in the kidney.

NOTE: (G) means that the suffix is a Greek derivative, (L) a Latin. The dash and semicolon refer to the suffix which has already been given. In the analysis the Greek and Latin words are used to show the derivation, but the student needs only to learn the English version.

Suffix	Term	Analysis	Definition
-itis (G) inflammation	carditis iritis poliomyelitis	*kardia:* heart *itis:* inflammation *iris:* rainbow, iris *polios:* gray *myelos:* marrow; —;	Inflammation of the heart. Inflammation of the iris. Inflammation of the gray matter of the spinal cord.
-malacia (G) softening	encephalomalacia osteomalacia splenomalacia	*enkephalos:* brain *malakia:* softening *osteon:* bone; —; *splen:* spleen; —;	Softening of the brain. Softening of the bones. Softening of the spleen.
-megaly (G) enlargement	acromegaly hepatomegaly splenomegaly	*akros:* extreme *megas:* large *hepat:* liver; —; *splen:* spleen; —;	Disease marked by enlargement of bones of head and soft part of extremities and face. Enlargement of the liver. Enlargement of the spleen.
-oma (G) tumor	adenoma carcinoma sarcoma	*aden:* gland *oma:* tumor *karkinos:* cancer; —; *sark:* flesh; —;	Glandular tumor. Malignant tumor of epithelial tissue. Malignant tumor of connective tissue.
-osis (G) condition, disease increase	arteriosclerosis dermatosis neurosis	*arteria;* artery *sklerosis:* hardening *derma:* skin *osis:* condition *neuron:* nerve; —;	Hardening of the arteries. Any skin condition. Functional disorder of the nervous system.
-pathy (G) disease	adenopathy myopathy myelopathy	*aden;* gland *pathos:* disease *mys:* muscle; —; *myelos:* marrow; —;	Any glandular disease. Any disease of a muscle. Any pathologic disorder of the spinal cord.
-ptosis (G) falling	blepharoptosis gastroptosis nephroptosis	*blepharon:* eyelid *ptosis:* a falling *gaster:* stomach; —; *nephros:* kidney; —;	Dropping of the eyelid. Downward displacement of the stomach. Downward displacement of the kidney.
-rhexis (G) rupture	angiorrhexis cardiorrhexis hysterorrhexis	*angeion:* vessel *rhexis:* rupture *kardia:* heart; —; *hystera:* uterus; —;	Rupture of a blood vessel or lymphatic. Rupture of the heart. Rupture of the uterus.

B. Operative Suffixes and Compounding Elements:

Suffix	Term	Analysis	Definition
-centesis (G) puncture	paracentesis abdominal para- centesis thoracentesis	*para:* beside *kentesis:* a puncture *abdomen:* belly; —; *thorax:* chest; —;	Puncture of a cavity. Puncture and aspiration of the peritoneal cavity. Aspiration of the pleural cavity.
-ectomy (G) excision	myomectomy oophorectomy tonsillectomy	*mys:* muscle *oma:* tumor *ektome:* excision *oophor:* ovary; —; *tonsilla:* tonsil; —;	Excision of a tumor of the muscle. Removal of an ovary. Removal of tonsils.

Suffix	Term	Analysis	Definition
-desis (G) binding, fixation	arthrodesis	*arthron:* joint *desis:* fixation	Surgical fixation of a joint.
	spondylosyndesis	*spondylos:* vertebra —;	Surgical fixation of the vertebrae.
	tenodesis	*tenon:* tendon; —;	Fixation of a tendon to a bone.
-lithotomy (G) incision for removal of stones	cholelithotomy	*chole:* bile, gall; —;	Incision into gallbladder for removal of stones.
	nephrolithotomy	*nephros:* kidney; —;	Incision into kidney for removal of stones.
	sialolithotomy	*sialon:* saliva	Incision into salivary gland for removal of stones.
-pexy (G) suspension, fixation	hysteropexy	*hystera:* uterus *pexis:* fixation	Abdominal fixation or suspension of the uterus.
	mastopexy	*mastos:* breast; —;	Fixation of a pendulous breast.
	orchiopexy	*orchis:* testis; —;	Fixation of an undescended testis.
-plasty (G) surgical correction, plastic repair of	arthroplasty	*arthron:* joint *plassein:* to form	Reconstruction operation on joint.
	hernioplasty	*hernos:* a young shoot; —;	Plastic repair of hernia.
	proctoplasty	*proktos:* anus, rectum; —;	Surgical repair of rectum.
-rhaphy (G) suture	perineorrhaphy	*perinaion:* perineum *rhaphe:* suture	Suture of a lacerated perineum.
	staphylorrhaphy	*staphyle:* uvula; —;	Suture of a cleft palate.
	trachelorrhaphy	*trachelos:* neck; —;	Suture of a torn cervix uteri.
-scopy (G) inspection, examination	bronchoscopy	*bronchos:* windpipe *skopein:* to examine	Examination of the bronchi with an endoscope.
	cystoscopy	*kystis:* bladder; —;	Inspection of the bladder with a cystoscope.
	esophagoscopy	*oisophagos:* esophagus —;	Endoscopic examination of the esophagus.
-stomy (G) creation of a more or less permanent opening	colostomy	*kolon:* colon; *stoma:* opening	Creation of an opening into the colon through the abdominal wall.
	cystostomy	*kystis:* bladder —;	Creation of an opening into the urinary bladder through the abdomen.
	gastroduoden-ostomy	*gaster:* stomach *duoden:* duodenum	Creation of an opening between stomach and duodenum.
-tomy (G) incision into	antrotomy	*antron:* antrum *tome:* incision	Incision into the antrum of Highmore to establish drainage.
	neurotomy	*neuron:* nerve; —;	Dissection of a nerve.
	thoracotomy	*thorax:* chest; —;	Opening of the chest.
-tripsy (G) crushing, friction	lithotripsy	*lithos:* stone *tripsis:* crushing	Crushing of a calculus in the bladder or urethra.
	phrenicotripsy	*phren:* diaphragm; —;	Crushing of the phrenic nerve.

C. Symptomatic Suffixes and Compounding Elements:

-algia (G) pain	gastralgia	*gaster:* stomach *algos:* pain	Epigastric pain.
	nephralgia	*nephros:* kidney; —;	Renal pain.
	neuralgia	*neuron:* nerve; —;	Lancinating nerve pain.

Suffix	Term	Analysis	Definition
-genic (G) origin	bronchogenic	*bronchos:* windpipe *gennan:* to originate	Originating in the bronchi.
	neurogenic	*neuron:* nerve; —;	Originating in the nerves.
	osteogenic	*osteon:* bone; —;	Originating in the bones.
	pathogenic	*pathos:* disease; —;	Disease producing.
-lysis (G) dissolution, breaking down	hemolysis	*haima:* blood *lysis:* breaking down	A breaking down of red blood cells.
	myolysis	*mys:* muscle; —;	Destruction of muscular tissue.
	neurolysis	*neuron:* nerve; —;	Disintegration of nerve tissue.
-oid (G) like	fibroid	*fibra:* fiber *eidos:* resembling	A tumor of fibrous tissue, resembling fibers.
	lipoid	*lipos:* fat; —;	Fat-like.
	lymphoid	*lympha:* lymph; —;	Resembling lymph.
-osis (G) increase, condition	anisocytosis	*anisos:* unequal *kytos:* cell *osis:* condition	Inequality of size of cells.
	lymphocytosis	*lympha:* lymph; —; —;	Excess of lymph cells.
-penia (G) deficiency, decrease	leukopenia	*leukos:* white *penia:* decrease	Abnormal decrease of leukocytes in the blood.
	neutropenia	*neuter:* neutral; —;	Abnormal decrease of neutrophils in the blood.
-spasm (G) involuntary contractions	chirospasm	*cheir:* hand *spasmos:* spasm or contraction of muscles	A spasm as contraction of the hand. (Writer's cramp)
	dactylospasm	*dactylos:* finger —;	Spasm or cramp in fingers or toes.
	enterospasm	*enteron:* intestine —;	Painful intestinal contractions.

II. Roots

The root stem or main body of a word indicates the organ or part which is modified by a prefix or suffix, or both. Properly, Greek combining forms or roots should be used only with Greek prefixes and suffixes, Latin with Latin. In reality there are many inconsistencies in the word formation of medical terms. A vowel, usually a, i, or o, is often inserted between the combining forms for euphony.

Root	Term	Analysis	Definition
aden- (G) gland	adenectomy	*aden:* gland *ektome:* excision	Excision of a gland.
	adenoma	—; *oma:* tumor	Glandular tumor.
	adenocarcinoma	—; *karkinos:* cancer —;	Malignant tumor of glandular epithelium.
aer- (G) air	aerated	*aer:* air	Filled with air.
	aerobic	*bios:* life	Pertaining to organism which lives only in the presence of air.
	aeroneurosis	—; *neuron:* nerve *osis:* diseased condition	A functional nervous disorder affecting aeroplane flyers.

NOTE: The dash and semicolon refer to the root which has already been given.

Root	Term	Analysis	Definition
angio- (G) vessel	angiotomy	*angeion:* vessel *tome:* a cutting	Dissection of blood vessels.
	angitis or angiitis	—; *itis:* inflammation	Inflammation of the blood vessels or lymphatics.
arth- (G) joint	arthralgia	*arthron:* joint *algos:* pain	Pain in the joints.
	arthritis	—; *itis:* inflammation	Inflammation of the joints.
	arthrology	—; *logos:* study, science	The science of the joints.
blephar- (G) eyelid	blepharedema	*blepharon:* eyelid *oidema:* swelling	Swelling of the eyelids.
	blepharoplasty	—; *plassein:* to form	Plastic operation upon the eyelid.
	blepharoptosis	—; *ptosis:* a falling	Dropping of the upper eyelid.
cardi- (G) heart	cardiac	*kardia:* heart	Pertaining to the heart or esophageal orifice of the stomach.
	phonocardiography	*phono:* sound; —; *graphein:* to write	Graphic recording of heart sounds.
	electrocardiogram	*elektron:* amber; —; *gramma:* writing	A graphic record of the heart beat by an electrometer.
cerebro- (L) brain	cerebral	*cerebrum:* brain	Pertaining to the brain.
	cerebromalacia	—; *malakia:* softening	Softening of the brain.
	cerebrospinal	—; *spina:* a thorn, the backbone	Referring to brain and spinal cord.
cephal- (G) head	cephalad	*kephale:* head *ad:* toward	Toward the head.
	cephalic	—; *ic:* pertaining to	Pertaining to the head.
	cephalitis	—; *itis:* inflammation	Inflammation of the brain.
cerv- (L) neck	cervical	*cervix:* neck *al:* pertaining to	Pertaining to the neck.
	cervicectomy	—; *ektome:* excision	Excision of the neck of the uterus.
	cervicovesical	—; *vesica:* bladder —;	Relating to the cervix uteri and bladder.
cheil, chil- (G) lip	cheilitis	*cheilos:* lip *itis:* inflammation	Inflammation of the lip.
	cheiloplasty	—; *plassein:* to form	Plastic operation of the lip.
	cheilosis	—; *osis:* diseased condition	Morbid condition of the lips due to vitamin B deficiency.
chir- (G) hand	chiromegaly	*cheir:* hand *megas:* large	Abnormal size of the hands, wrists and ankles.
	chiroplasty	—; *plassein:* to form	Plastic surgery on the hand.
	chiropody	—; *pous:* foot	Treatment of conditions of the hands and feet.
chol- (G) bile	cholangitis	*chole:* bile *angeion:* vessel *itis:* inflammation	Inflammation of the bile duct.
	cholecyst	—; *kystis:* bladder, sac	Gallbladder.
	cholecystogram	—; —; *gramma:* mark	A radiogram of the gallbladder.

Root	Term	Analysis	Definition
chondr- (G) cartilage	chondrectomy chondrofibroma chondroma	*chondros:* cartilage *ektome:* excision —; *fibra:* fiber *oma:* tumor —; —;	Excision of a cartilage. A mixed tumor composed of fibrous tissue and cartilage. A cartilaginous tumor.
cost- (L) rib	costochondral costophrenic angle costosternal	*costa:* rib *chondros:* cartilage —; *phren:* diaphragm *angle:* corner —; *sternon:* breast	Pertaining to a rib and its cartilage. The angle formed by the ribs and diaphragm. Referring to the ribs and breast bone.
crani- (G, L) skull	cranial craniotabes craniotomy	*kranion:* skull *al:* pertaining to —; *tabes:* a wasting —; *tome:* incision	Pertaining to the skull. A thinning or atrophy of the skull bones. Surgical opening of skull.
cysto- (G) bladder, sac	cyst cystography cystoscope	*kystis:* bladder, sac —; *graphein:* to write —; *skopein:* to examine	A bladder; any sac containing a liquid. Radiographic examination of the urinary bladder following the introduction of air or opaque solution. Instrument for interior examination of the bladder.
cyt- (G) cell	cytology erythrocyte lymphocyte	*kytos:* cell *logos:* study *erythros:* red *kytos:* cell *lympha:* lymph; —;	The study of cell life. Red blood cell. Lymph cell, a nongranular leukocyte.
dacry- (G) tear	dacryadenitis dacryocele dacryocyst	*dakry:* tear *aden:* gland *itis:* inflammation —; *kele:* hernia —; *kystis:* sac	Inflammation of the lacrimal (tear) gland. Protrusion of the lacrimal sac. The lacrimal sac.
dactyl- (G) finger, toe	dactylitis dactylogram dactylomegaly	*dactylos:* finger *itis:* inflammation —; *gramma:* a mark —; *megas:* large	Chronic disease of bones of fingers or toes in young children. A fingerprint. Abnormal size of fingers and toes.
derm- (G) skin	dermatitis dermal dermopathy	*derma:* skin *itis:* inflammation —; *al:* relating to —; *pathos:* disease	Inflammation of the skin. Relating to the skin. Any skin disease.
encephal- (G) brain	encephalitis encephaloma encephalography	*enkephalos:* brain *itis:* inflammation —; *oma:* tumor —; *graphein:* to write	Inflammation of the brain. Brain tumor. Radiographic examination of head after withdrawal of fluid and replacing it with air.
enter- (G) intestine	enteritis enterocele enterocolitis	*enteron:* intestine *itis:* inflammation —; *kele:* hernia —; *kolon:* colon; —;	Inflammation of the intestines. A hernia of the intestines. Inflammation of intestines and colon.

Root	Term	Analysis	Definition
gastr- (G) stomach	gastrectasis gastroenterostomy gastrointestinal	*gaster:* stomach *ectasis:* dilatation —; *enteron:* intestine *stoma:* opening —; *intestinum:* intestine *al:* pertaining to	Dilatation of the stomach. Formation of a passage between the stomach and the intestine. Pertaining to stomach and intestines.
glyco- (G) sweet	glycemia or gly- cosemia glycosuria	*glykys:* sweet *haima:* blood —; *ouron:* urine	Sugar in blood. Sugar in the urine.
hem, *hemat-* (G) blood	hematemesis hematoma hemophilia	*haima:* blood *emesis:* vomiting —; *oma:* tumor —; *philein:* to love	Vomiting of blood. A blood tumor. Inability of the blood to coagulate.
hepat- (G) liver	hepatic flexure hepatitis hepatolysis	*hepat:* liver *flexura:* a curved part —; *itis:* inflammation —; *lysis:* destruction	The right bend of colon under the liver. Inflammation of the liver. Destruction of liver cells.
hyster- (G) uterus	hysterectomy hysteria hysteropexy	*hystera:* uterus *ektome:* excision —; *ia:* disease of —; *pexis:* fixation	Excision of the uterus. A psychoneurosis marked by emotional instability and somatic symptoms. Abdominal fixation of the uterus or suspension of the uterus.
ile-eile- (L-G) ileum	ileum ileocecal valve ileostomy	*ileum:* ileum —; *caecus:* blind *valva:* one leaf of a double door —; *stoma:* opening	Third part of the small intestines. Two lips or folds at opening between ileum and cecum. Creation of an opening through abdomen into the ileum.
ili- (L) ilium	ilium iliofemoral iliosacral	*ilium:* flank —; *femoralis:* femur —; *sacralis:* sacrum	The wide, upper part of the hip bone. Referring to ilium and femur. Pertaining to ilium and sacrum.
leuk- (G) white	leukemia leukocytosis leukopenia	*leukos:* white *haima:* blood —; *osis:* condition, excess —; *penia:* lack	Disease characterized by an extremely high white count. Excessive increase in number of leukocytes. Abnormal decrease in number of leukocytes.
lip- (G) fat	lipectomy lipemia lipiodol	*lipos:* fat *ektome:* excision —; *haima:* blood —; *iodum:* iodine *oleum:* oil	Excision of fatty tissues. Fat in the blood. An opaque oil used for injection into body cavities for purpose of radiographic examination.
lith- (G) stone	lithiasis lithocystotomy lithoscope	*lithos:* stone *iasis:* presence of —; *kystis:* bladder *tome:* incision —; *skopein:* to examine	Presence of concretions or stones. Incision into bladder to remove calculus or calculi. Instrument for examining stone in bladder.

Root	Term	Analysis	Definition
mening- (G) membrane	meningeal meningitis meningioma meningococcus	*meninx:* membrane *al:* relating to —; *itis:* inflammation —; *oma:* tumor —; *kokkos:* berry	Related to meninges. Inflammation of the membranes of spinal cord and brain. Tumor of the meninges. The microorganism responsible for meningitis.
metr- (G) uterus	metritis metrorrhagia metrorrhexis	*metra:* uterus *itis:* inflammation —; *regnunai:* to burst forth —; *rhexis:* a rupture	Inflammation of the uterine musculature. Bleeding from the uterus. Rupture of the uterus.
myel- (G) marrow	myelitis myelogenous myelosarcoma	*myelos:* marrow *itis:* inflammation —; *gennan:* to produce —; *sark:* flesh	Inflammation of spinal cord or of bone marrow. Originating in marrow. Malignant tumor of the bone marrow.
my- (G) muscle	myitis or myositis myocardium	*mys:* muscle *itis:* inflammation —; *kardia:* heart	Inflammation of a muscle. Heart muscle.
nephr- (G) kidney	nephropexy nephrosclerosis nephrosis	*nephros:* kidney *pexis:* fixation —; *sklerosis:* hardening —; *osis:* condition	Surgical attachment of a floating kidney. Hardening of the kidney. Condition marked by degeneration of renal substance.
ophthalm- (G) eye	ophthalmia —; neonatorum ophthalmology	*ophthalmos:* eye *ia:* disease of —; *neos:* new *natus:* born, birth —; *logos:* study	Severe inflammation of the eye including the conjunctiva. Purulent conjunctivitis in the newborn. Science of the eye and its diseases.
osteo- (G) bone	osteoclasia osteoma osteomalacia	*osteon:* bone *klasis:* a breaking —; *oma:* tumor —; *malakia:* a softening	Surgical fracture of a bone to remedy a deformity. A bony tumor. Softening of the bone.
pneum- (G) lung, air	pneumococcus pneumonia pneumothorax pneumoperitoneum	*pneumon:* lung *kokkos:* berry —; *ia:* disease of *pneumon:* lung *thorax:* chest —; *peritonaion:* peritoneum	Microorganism causing pneumonia and other diseases. Inflammation of the lungs with consolidation and exudation. Introduction of air into the pleural cavity. Introduction of air into the peritoneal cavity.
proct- (G) rectum, anus	proctology proctoscopy proctopexy	*proktos:* rectum *logos:* science —; *skopein:* examine —; *pexis:* fixation	Medical specialty dealing with diseases of the rectum. Instrumental examination of the rectum. Suture of the rectum to some other part.

Root	Term	Analysis	Definition

psycho-
(G)
soul,
mind
	psychiatry
	
	psychoneurosis
	
	psychopathy
		psyche: mind
		iatreia: healing
		—; *neuron:* nerve
		osis: disease or condition
		—; *pathos:* disease
			Medical specialty treating
			  mental and neurotic disorders.
			A functional disorder of mental origin
			  without demonstrable lesion.
			Any mental disease usually related to
			  defective character and personality.

pyel-
(G)
pelvis
	pyelitis
	
	pyelogram
	
	pyelography
		pyelos: pelvis
		itis: inflammation
		—; *gramma:* a mark
		
		—; *graphein:* to write
			Inflammation of the pelvis of the
			  kidney.
			Radiogram of the ureter and
			  renal pelvis.
			Radiography of a renal pelvis and
			  ureter.

pyloro- (G) pylorus, gatekeeper	pylorus pylorostenosis pyloromyotomy	*pyloros:* gatekeeper —; *stenosis:* narrowing —; *mys:* muscle *tome:* a cutting	Orifice between stomach and duodenum. Constriction of pylorus. Incision of the pyloric sphincter to relieve pyloric stenosis.
pyo- (G) pus	pyogenic pyometritis pyonephrosis	*pyon:* pus *genesis:* formation —; *metra:* uterus *itis:* inflammation —; *nephros:* kidney	Pus forming. Purulent inflammation of the uterus. Pus in the renal pelvis.

radi-
(L)
ray
	radioactivity
	
	radiosensitive
	
	radiotherapy
		radius: ray
		activus: acting
		—; *sensitivus:* feeling
		
		—;
		therapeia: treatment
			The ability to emit rays which can
			  penetrate various substances.
			Capable of being destroyed by radio-
			  active substances.
			The use of radiation of any type in
			  treating diseases.

spondyl-
(G)
vertebra
	spondylitis
	
	spondylolisthesis
	
	spondylosyndesis
		spondylos: vertebra
		itis: inflammation
		—; *olisthesis:* a slipping
		
		—; *syndesis:* a binding
		  together
			Inflammation of vertebrae.
			
			Forward dislocation of lumbar
			  vertebrae with pelvic deformity.
			Surgical formation of an ankylosis
			  between vertebrae.

trachel- (G) neck	trachelitis tracheloplasty trachelorrhaphy	*trachelos:* neck *itis:* inflammation —; *plassein:* to form —; *rhaphe:* suture	Inflammation of the cervix uteri. Plastic operation of the cervix uteri. Suturing of a torn cervix uteri.

tubercul-
(L)
tubercle
	tubercle
	
	tubercle bacillus
	tubercular
	tuberculous
	tuberculoma
	tuberculosis
		tuberculum: a little
		  swelling
		—; *bacillus:* rod
		—; *aris:* akin to
		—; *ous:* full of
		—; *oma:* tumor
		—; *osis:* process
			The lesion of tuberculosis: also, a
			  nodular bony prominence.
			Microorganism causing tuberculosis.
			Relating to a bony prominence.
			Affected with tuberculosis.
			A tuberculous abscess or tumor.
			An infectious disease marked by the
			  formation of tubercles in any tissue.

viscer- (L) organ	visceral viscus viscera visceroptosis	*viscus:* organ *al:* pertaining to —; —; —; *ptosis:* a dropping	Pertaining to the internal organs. Organ. Organs. Prolapse of the viscera. Glenard's disease.

III. Prefixes

Among the most frequently used elements in the formation of medical terms are prefixes. A prefix consists of one or two syllables placed before a word to modify its meaning. These syllables are often prepositions or adverbs. Some common prefixes are:

Prefix	Term	Analysis	Definition

ab-
(L)
from,
away from
	abductor
	
	abnormal
	abruptio
	   placentae
		ab: away from
		ductor: that which
		   draws
		—; norma: rule
		—;
		ruptere: break
		placenta: a flat cake
			That which draws away from a common center, as a muscle.
			
			Away from or not correponding to rule.
			A tearing away from or the premature detachment of a normally situated placenta.

a, an (G) without, not	anesthesia apnea asthenia atresia	an: without aesthesis: sensation a: without pnoe: breath —; sthenos: strength —; tresis: a perforation	Loss of sensation. Temporary absence of respiration. Debility, loss of strength. Absence or closure of a normal opening or passage.
ad- (L) adherence, increase, near, toward	adductor adrenal adhesion adnexa	ad: toward ductor: that which draws ad: near ren: kidney ad: to haerere: to stick —; nectere: to tie, to bind	That which draws toward a common center. A ductless gland above the kidney. Abnormal joining of surfaces to each other. Accessory parts; for example, adnexa uteri.
ante- (L) before	anteflexion antenatal antepartum	ante: forward flectere: to bend —; natus: birth —; partum: labor	Forward displacement of an organ; for example, the uterus. Before birth. Before the onset of labor.
anti- (G) against	antisepsis antitoxin antipyretic	anti: against sepsis: putrefaction —; toxikon: poison —; pyretos: fever	The exclusion of putrefactive germs. A protein that defends the body against a toxin. A drug that reduces fever.
bi- (L) two, both, double	biceps —; brachii —; femoris biconvex bilateral bifurcation	bis: two caput: head —; brachii: arm —; femoris: thigh —; convexus: rounded surface —; latus: side —; furca: fork	Two-headed. Muscle of the upper arm having two heads. Muscle of the thigh. Having two convex surfaces as in a lens. affecting both sides. A separation into two branches.
co- con- (L) together, with	congenital defect conjunctiva connective tissue	con: with genitus: born defectus: imperfection —; jungere: to join con: together nectere: to bind	Born with a defect, hereditary. Mucous membrane which lines eyelids. Tissue which connects or binds together.

NOTE: The dash and semicolon refer to the prefix which has already been given.

Prefix	Term	Analysis	Definition
contra- (L) against, opposite	contraception	*contra:* against *concipere:* to conceive	The prevention of conception.
	contraindication	—; *indicare:* to point out	A condition antagonistic to line of treatment.
	contralateral	*contra:* opposite *latus:* side	Affecting the opposite side of the body.
dys (G) bad, difficult, painful	dysentery	*dys:* painful *enteron:* intestine	Inflammation of intestinal mucous membrane accompanied by pain.
	dysmenorrhea	—; *men:* month *rhoia:* a flow	Painful menstruation.
	dyspepsia	*dys:* bad *peptein:* to digest	Imperfect digestion.
	dysphagia	*dys:* difficult *phagein:* to eat	Difficulty in swallowing.
	dysphasia	—; *phasis:* speech	Impairment of speech.
	dyspnea	—; *pnoe:* breathing	Labored or difficult breathing.
	dystocia	—; *tokos:* birth	Difficult labor.
	dysuria	*dys:* painful *ouron:* urine	Painful or difficult urination.
ec- (G) out	ectropion of eyelid cervix uteri	*ek:* out *trepein:* to turn *cervix:* neck *uteri:* of womb	Eversion as the edge of the eyelid or the turning out of the cervical canal of the uterus.
ecto- (G) outside	ectopic pregnancy	*ecto:* outside *topos:* place *prae:* before *natus:* birth	Gestation outside the uterine cavity.
em, en- (G) in	empyema	*em:* in *pyon:* pus	Pus in a body cavity, especially in the pleural cavity.
	encephalopathy	*en;* in *kephale:* head *pathos:* disease	Any disease of the brain.
endo- (G) within	endocardium	*endon:* within *kardia:* heart	Lining membrane of inner surface of the heart.
	endocarditis	—; —; *itis:* inflammation	Inflammation of the endocardium.
	endocrine gland	—; *krinein:* to secrete *glans:* gland	A ductless gland in which forms an internal secretion.
	endocrinology	—; *logos:* science	The science of the endocrines, or ductless glands.
	endometrium	—; *metra:* uterus	The mucous membrane lining the inner surface of the uterus.
	endometritis	—; —; *itis:* inflammation	Inflammation of the endometrium.
	endoscope	—; *skopein:* to examine	Tubular instrument for examining cavities through natural openings.
	endoscopy	—; —;	Inspection of cavities by use of the endoscope.
	endosteum	—; *osteon:* bone	Membrane lining the medullary cavity of long bones.
	endostitis	—; —; *itis:* inflammation	Inflammation of the endosteum.

Prefix	Term	Analysis	Definition
epi- (G) upon, at, in addition to	epidermis epigastrium epiphysis	epi: upon derma: skin —; gaster: stomach epi: at physis: a growing upon	Cuticle or outer layer of the skin. Region over the pit of the stomach. A center of ossification at both extremities of long bones.
ex- (L, G) out, away from, over	exacerbation exeresis exophthalmia exophthalmic goiter expectoration exudate	ex: over acerbus: harsh ex: out eiresis: taking —; ophthalmos: eye —; —; guttur: throat —; pector: chest —; sudare: to sweat	Aggravation of symptoms. Excision of any part. Abnormal protrusion of the eyeballs. A goiter marked by protrusion of the eyeballs. Expulsion of mucus from the lungs. Accumulation of fluid due to inflam- matory condition.
hemi- (G) half	hemiglossectomy hemigastrectomy hemiplegia	hemi: half glossa: tongue ektome: excision —; gaster: stomach —; —; plege: a stroke	Removal of half a tongue. Removal of one-half of the stomach. Paralysis of one-half of the body.
hyper- (G) above, excessive, beyond	hyperacidity hyperadrenalism hypercalcemia hyperemesis gravidarum hyperemia hyperpyrexia hypertension hypertrophy	hyper: excessive acidus: sour —; ad: near ren: kidney ismos: state of —; calx: lime haima: blood —; emesis: vomiting gravida: a pregnant woman —; haima: blood hyper: above pyrexia: fever —; tensio: tension hyper: increased trophe: nourishment	An excess of acid in the stomach. Excess of adrenal secretion. Excess of calcium in the blood. Excessive vomiting during early pregnancy. Congestion. Fever above 106° F. High blood pressure. Increased size of an organ not due to tumor formation.
hypo- (G) beneath, below, deficient	hypochondriac region hypodermic injection hypoglycemia	hypo: beneath chondros: cartilage regio: area —; derma: skin injectus: to throw in hypo: deficient glykys: sugar haima: blood	Part of abdomen beneath the ribs. Injection under the skin. Low blood sugar.
para, par- (G) beside, around, near, abnormal	paracentesis parametrium parametritis paranephritis paranoia	para: beside kentesis: a puncture para: around metra: uterus —; —; itis: inflammation para: beside nephros: kidney, —; para: abnormal nous: mind	Puncture of a cavity with tapping. Fat and connective tissue around the uterus. Inflammation of the parametrium. Inflammation of suprarenal capsules; of connective tissue about the kidney. Mental disease marked by systematized delusions of persecution.

Prefix	Term	Analysis	Definition
(Cont'd)	parathyroid	*para:* beside *thyreos:* shield *eidos:* form	Ductless gland near the thyroid gland.
	parotitis	*par:* near *ot:* ear *itis:* inflammation	Inflammation of the parotid gland.
peri- (G) around, about	pericardium	*peri:* around *kardia:* heart	The double membranous sac enclosing the heart.
	pericarditis	—; —; *itis:* inflammation	Inflammation of the pericardium.
	perimetrium	—; *metra:* womb	Peritoneum covering uterus.
	perimetritis	—; —; *itis:* inflammation	Inflammation of the peritoneum covering of the uterus.
	periosteum	—; *osteon:* bone	The membrane that invests and nourishes the bone.
	periostitis	—; —; *itis:* inflammation	Inflammation of the periosteum.
pre- (L) before, in front of	precancerous	*prae:* before *cancer:* crab	Before the development of carcinoma.
	precordium	—; *cor:* heart	Region over the heart.
	preeclampsia	—; *ek:* out *lampein:* to flash	Eclampsia before delivery. (Eclampsia is a major toxemia during pregnancy.)
	prepatellar bursitis	*prae:* in front of *patella:* kneecap *bursa:* sac *itis:* inflammation	Inflammation of the bursa in front of the patella. (Housemaid's knee.)
	presentation	*praesentatio:* a placing before	Manner of the fetus presenting itself at the cervix.
pro- (L, G) in front of, before, forward	procidentia	*procidentia:* a falling forward	A complete prolapse especially of the uterus.
	prognosis	*pro:* before *gnosis:* a knowing	Prediction of end of disease.
	prolapse	*pro:* forward *lapsus:* slide	A downward displacement of an organ, as the rectum or the uterus.
retro- (L) backward, behind, back of	retroflexion	*retro:* backward *flexio:* a bending	A bending or flexing backward; for example, of the uterus.
	retrogasserian neurotomy	*retro:* back of *gasserian:* pertaining to a ganglion *neuron:* nerve *tome:* incision into	Transection of the posterior root of the retrogasserian ganglion.
	retroperitoneal	*retro:* behind *peritonaion:* peritoneum	Located behind the peritoneum.
	retroversion	*retro:* backward *versio:* a turning	A state of being turned back; for example, of the uterus.
semi- (L) half	semicircular canal	*semi:* half *circulus:* a ring *canal:* a channel	One of the three canals in the labyrinth of the ear.
	semicoma	—; *koma:* lethargy	Mild degree of coma.
	semilunar valves	—; *luna:* moon *valva:* one leaf of a double door	Half-moon shaped valves of the aorta and pulmonary arteries.

Prefix	Term	Analysis	Definition
sub- (L) under, beneath, below	subclavicular	sub: beneath clavicular: a little key	Beneath the clavicle (collar bone).
	subcostal	—; costa: rib	Beneath the ribs.
	subcutaneous	—; cutis: skin	Beneath the skin.
	subinvolution	—; involutio: a turning into	Failure of the uterus to reduce to normal size after childbirth.
	suppuration	sub: under; pur: pus tion: state of	The process of pus formation.
super, supra- (L) above, beyond, superior	supernatant	super: above natare: to float	Floating on surface.
	supraoccipital	—; occiput: back part of the skull	Situated above the occiput.
	suprapubic cystotomy	—; pubis: bone of pelvis kystis: bladder tome: incision	Surgical opening into the bladder from above the symphysis pubis.
	suprarenal	—; ren: kidney al: pertaining to	Adrenal gland above the kidney.
sym, syn- (G) with, along, together, beside	symphysis of pubis	sym: together physis: a growing	Fusion of pubic bones on midline anteriorly.
	synarthrosis	syn: together arthron: joint osis: condition	An immovable joint.
	syndactylism	daktylos: digit, finger ismos: condition	A fusion of two or more fingers or toes; webbing.
trans- (L) across, over	transection	trans: across sectio: cutting	Incision across the long axis; cross section.
	transfusion	—; fusio: a pouring	Injection of the blood of one person into the blood vessels of another.
	transurethral prostatectomy	—; ourethra: urethra prostates: prostate ektome: excision	Excision of the prostate gland through the urethra.
tri- (G) three	tricuspid	tres, tria: three cuspis: a point	Having three cusps or points; tricuspid valve.
	trifacial	—; facialis: facial	Fifth cranial nerve.
	trigone	trigonon: a three-cornered figure	A triangular space, especially that of the lower part of the urinary bladder.

Terms Pertaining to the Body as a Whole

A. Anatomic Division of the Abdomen:*

1. hypochondriac regions (upper lateral regions beneath the ribs) . . . . (1) and (3)
2. epigastric region (region of the pit of the stomach) . . . . (2)
3. lumbar regions (middle lateral regions) . . . . (4) and (6)
4. umbilical region (region of navel) . . . . (5)
5. inguinal regions (lower lateral regions) . . . . (7) and (9)
6. hypogastric region (region below the umbilicus) . . . . (8)

B. Clinical Division of the Abdomen:

1. upper right quadrant . . . . URQ
2. upper left quadrant . . . . ULQ
3. lower right quadrant . . . . LRQ
4. lower left quadrant . . . . LLQ

* See Fig. 1, p. 17.

C. Anatomic Division of the Back:

1. cervical region .... neck
2. thoracic region .... chest
3. lumbar region .... loin
4. sacral region .... sacrum

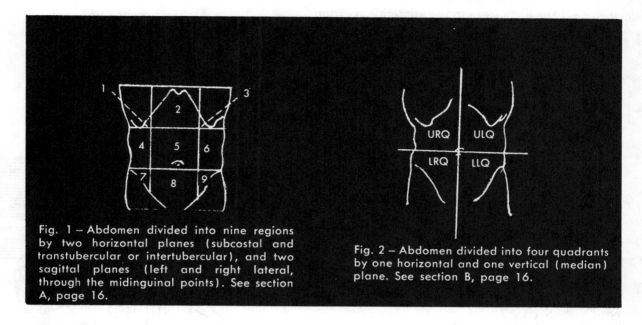

Fig. 1 – Abdomen divided into nine regions by two horizontal planes (subcostal and transtubercular or intertubercular), and two sagittal planes (left and right lateral, through the midinguinal points). See section A, page 16.

Fig. 2 – Abdomen divided into four quadrants by one horizontal and one vertical (median) plane. See section B, page 16.

D. Position and Direction:

1. afferent — conducting toward a structure.
2. anterior or ventral — front of the body (not synonymous in lower limb).
3. central — toward the center.
4. deep — away from the surface.
5. distal or peripheral — away from the beginning of a structure; away from the center.
6. efferent — conducting away from a structure.
7. inferior or caudal — away from the head, situated below another structure.*
8. intermediate — between median and lateral.
9. lateral — toward the side.*
10. medial — toward the median plane.*
11. median — in the middle of a structure.
12. posterior or dorsal — back of the body (not synonymous in lower limb).
13. proximal — toward the beginning of a structure.
14. superficial — near the surface.
15. superior or cephalic — toward the head, situated above another structure.*

E. Planes of the Body:

1. frontal or coronal — vertical plane parallel to the coronal suture of the skull. It divides the body or structure into anterior and posterior portions.
2. horizontal — plane parallel to the horizon.
3. longitudinal — plane parallel to the long axis of the structure.
4. median — lengthwise plane which divides the body or structure into right and left halves.
5. sagittal — any vertical plane parallel to the sagittal suture of the skull and the median plane.
6. transverse — plane at a right angle to the long axis of a structure.

*Refer to F. Anatomic Position

18

F. Anatomic Position:

Anatomists all over the world apply anatomic terms to the body as though it were in what is known as the **anatomic position**. In this position, the body is erect, the eyes look straight to the front, the upper limbs hang at the sides with the palms facing forward, and the lower limbs are parallel with the toes pointing forward. Whether the body lies face upward or downward, or in any other position, the positions and relationships of structure are always described as if the body were in the anatomic position.

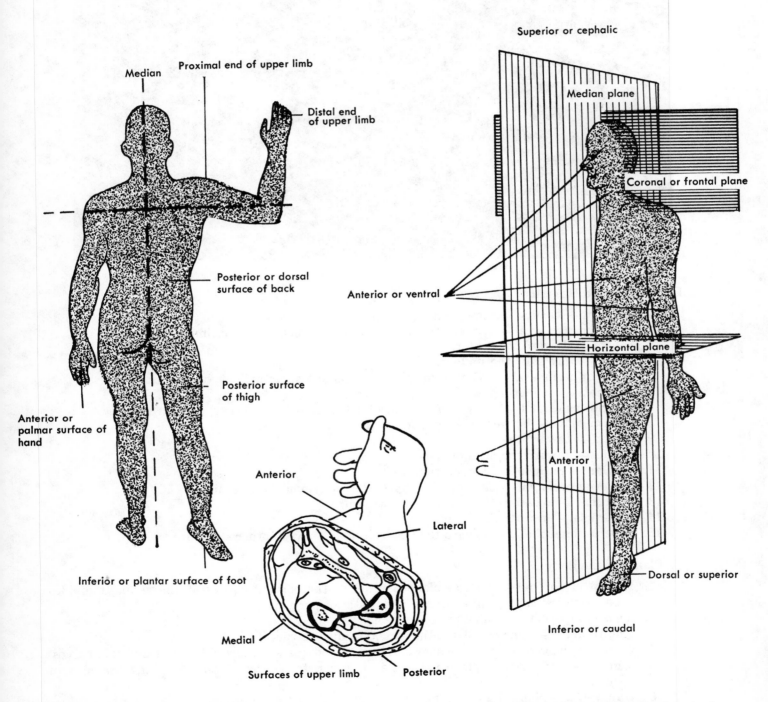

Fig. 3 – Posterior view of body.

Fig. 4 – Directional planes of the body.

REFERENCES AND BIBLIOGRAPHY

1. Blakiston's *Gould Medical Dictionary,* 3rd ed. New York: McGraw-Hill Book Co., 1973.
2. Boucher, Carl O. *Current Clinical Dental Terminology,* 2d ed. St. Louis: The C. V. Mosby Co., 1974.
3. Dorland's *Illustrated Medical Dictionary,* 25th ed. Philadelphia: W. B. Saunders Co., 1974.
4. Stedman's *Medical Dictionary* Illustrated, 23d ed. Baltimore: The Williams & Wilkins Co., 1976.
5. Steen, Edwin. *Medical Abbreviations,* 3d ed. Philadelphia: F. A. Davis Co., 1971.
6. Taber's *Cyclopedic Medical Dictionary,* 12th ed. Philadelphia: F. A. Davis Co., 1973.

Chapter II
Disorders of the Skin and Breast
SKIN

A. Origin of Terms:

1. cutis (L) — skin
2. derma (G) — skin
3. erythema (G) — flush
4. hidros (G) — sweat
5. kelis (G) — stain
6. kerato (G) — horny
7. macula (L) — spot
8. onyx, onych (G) — nail
9. papula (L) — pimple
10. pemphix (G) — blister
11. phyton (G) — plant
12. pigmentum (L) — paint
13. pilus, pili (L) — hair
14. pruritus (L) — itching
15. psora (G) — itch
16. pyon (G) — pus
17. scabo (L) — scratched
18. sebum (L) — tallow
19. squama (L) — scale
20. sudor (L) — sweat
21. tegmen (L) — covering
22. tinea (L) — worm
23. vesica (L) — blister, bladder

B. Anatomic Terms:[33]

1. corium — the true skin or deeper layer containing blood vessels, lymphatics, hair follicles, nerve endings, connective tissue fibers, sweat and sebaceous glands.
2. derma, dermis — synonymous with corium.
3. epidermis — cuticle or outer layer of the skin.
4. epithelium — the layers of cells covering the surfaces of the body, external as well as internal.
5. integument — the skin, composed of the corium and epidermis.
6. pigment — a coloring substance.
7. pilosebaceous — pertaining to hair and oil glands.
8. sebaceous glands — oil glands of the skin.
9. sebum — oily substance secreted by sebaceous glands.
10. subcutaneous tissue — a layer of loose, connective tissue containing fat.
11. sudoriferous glands — sweat glands.

C. Diagnostic Terms:

1. acne — any inflammatory condition of the sebaceous glands.[33]   The more common forms are:
   a. acne albida — white nodules or milia on face.
   b. acne papulosa — papular lesions.
   c. acne rosacea, simple rosacea — condition characterized by thickened skin especially on the nose, due to hypertrophy of sebaceous glands.
   d. acne vulgaris — a common form of acne, marked by papules, pustules and comedones.[42]
2. albinism — a congenital lack of normal skin pigment.
3. alopecia — loss of hair, baldness.
4. angioedema, angioneurotic edema, Quincke's edema — diffuse swelling of the loose tissues of the face, eyelids, lips, tongue, larynx, gastrointestinal tract, others.[10]
5. atopic skin disorders — allergic skin conditions such as angioedema, urticaria, atopic drug reactions and food allergy in atopic dermatitis. Atopy or allergy tends to be of the familial type.[10, 12]
6. burn — the effect of exposure to heat, chemicals, electricity or sunshine.
   a. first degree burn — redness or hyperemia involving superficial layers of skin.

    b. second degree — blisters or vesication involving deeper layers of skin.

    c. third degree burn — destruction involving any tissue below the skin.

7. callositas, keratosis — a circumscribed thickening and hypertrophy of the horny cells of the epidermis.

8. carbuncle — a circumscribed inflammation of the skin and deeper tissues causing necrosis and suppuration.

9. cellulitis — inflammation of skin and subcutaneous tissue with or without formation of pus.

10. decubitus ulcer, bedsore, pressure sore — an ulcer which develops in an area where the skin covers a bony prominence and is damaged by continuous pressure, impoverished circulation and nutrition.[42, 48, 50]

11. dermatitis — inflammation of the skin. Some common forms are:

    a. contact dermatitis, dermatitis venenata — inflammatory reaction to an irritant or a sensitizer; for example, poison ivy, ragweed, metal, chemical, rubber, others.[10, 12, 33, 52]

    b. exfoliative dermatitis — exfoliation or scaling off of dead skin associated with crust formation, generalized redness and edema.[42]

    c. dermatitis medicamentosa — drug eruption. Macular, urticarial, vesicular, bullous, pustular or hemorrhagic lesions may occur.[33, 42]

12. dermatophytosis — superficial fungus infection (mycosis) which is readily transmitted from person to person, attacks the skin, nails and hair, thrives in moisture and is caused by dermatophytes:

    a. Epidermophyton — fungus infects the skin.

    b. Microsporum — fungus is found in the skin and hair.

    c. Trichophyton — fungus attacks the skin, nails and hair.[7, 33, 45]

13. dermatophytosis of foot, epidermophytosis, tinea pedis, athlete's foot — parasitic or fungal infection, chiefly affecting the skin between the toes associated with intense itching, sogginess, fissures, small blisters and scaling of skin.[42]

14. eczema — cutaneous inflammatory condition producing red, papular and vesicular lesions, crusts and scales.

15. epidermolysis — the epidermis being loosely attached to the corium, tends to exfoliate and form blisters.[41]

16. epidermolysis bullosa, acantholysis bullosa, Goldschneider's disease — a hereditary condition characterized by dissolution of the layers of the skin and blister formation in response to slight irritation.[41]

17. gangrene — a form of necrosis or putrefaction of tissue.

    a. diabetic gangrene — associated with diabetes mellitus.

    b. embolic gangrene — caused by circulatory obstruction due to embolus.

    c. gas gangrene — due to infection with bacillus Welchii, an anaerobic microorganism.

18. leukoderma — white patches of skin due to local absence of pigment.

19. lichen planus — inflammatory condition of skin and mucous membrane characterized by small, flat papules that appear shiny, dry and violet in color. Linear, anular and irregular patches are found on neck, wrists and thighs.[7, 42]

20. lupus vulgaris — a type of cutaneous tuberculosis, marked by reddish-brown patches in which tiny nodules are embedded.

21. melanoderma — abnormal brown or black pigmentation of the skin.

22. onychia — inflammation of the nail bed.

23. paronychia — infected skin around the nail.

24. pediculosis — infestation with lice.

25. pemphigus — skin disease characterized by the appearance of crops of bullae of various sizes.[26, 28, 42, 52]

26. pilonidal cyst — an epidermal inclusion cyst of the sacral area, usually a teratomatous (hair containing) cyst which may become infected and undergo suppuration.[48]

27. psoriasis — eruption appearing in circular patches of various sizes, showing a definite line of demarcation. Remissions and exacerbations are common.[42]

28. pyoderma — bacterial infection affecting

    a. the skin

(1) impetigo contagiosa — infectious skin disease characterized by discrete vesicles which change to pustules and crusts, appear in crops usually on the face and are caused by staphylococci and streptococci.[42]

(2) pyoderma faciale — cyanotic or reddish erythema associated with deep or superficial cystic lesions or abscesses.

  b. pilosebaceous apparatus (hair and oil glands) causing

(1) furunculosis — purulent infection of hair follicles usually by *Staphylococcus aureus* which may result in necrosis of hair follicles and formation of furunculoid abscesses.[42]

(2) staphylococcic folliculitis — intradermal pustules surrounding hair follicles, usually due to *Staphylococcus aureus*.[42]

29. rhinophyma — red, large, nodular hypertrophic masses around the tip and wings of the nose, seen in men past 40 years of age.[7]

30. scabies — contagious skin condition caused by the mite *Sarcoptes scabiei* which lays her eggs in burrows under the skin causing an intensely pruritic, vesicular eruption between the fingers, folds of axillae, buttocks, under the breasts and other areas.[21, 42]

31. steatoma — sebaceous cyst.

32. tinea — any fungal skin disease, frequently due to ring worms.

  a. tinea barbae, tinea sycosis — ringworm of beard.

  b. tinea capitis, tinea tonsurans — ringworm of scalp, forming circular bold patches, seen chiefly in school boys.

  c. tinea corporis, tinea circinata — ringworm of body, usually noted for ring-shaped eruption, scaling, vesiculation and itching. It is transmitted by animal contact.

  d. tinea pedis — athlete's foot.

  e. tinea unguinum, onychomycosis — ringworm of nails, especially toe nails causing thickening and scaling under the nail plate.[42, 45]

33. tumors of the skin — new growths of the skin (See Part II — Chapter on Oncology).

  a. basal cell epithelioma, basal cell carcinoma — slowly growing tumor made up of pearly or waxy looking nodules surrounding a central depression which is prone to ulcerate and bleed. The rolled border of the tumor is characteristic. Since it rarely or never metastasizes its malignant nature is questionable.[16, 33, 43, 48]

  b. keloid — a new growth of scar tissue.[33]

  c. keratocanthoma — rapidly growing nodule arising from the epidermis and containing a horn filled crater, usually a benign lesion.[40]

  d. nevus, mole, birthmark — congenital pigmentation of a circumscribed area of the skin.

  e. seborrheic keratosis, basal cell papilloma — a benign, superficial, epithelial tumor, a few or hundreds in number, light tan to black in color depending on melanin content, characterized by horny overgrowth (hyperkeratosis), primarily occurring in the middle aged and elderly.[33, 48]

  f. squamous cell epithelioma — a malignant epithelial tumor which tends to ulcerate and form crusts. It develops in areas of chronic irritation such as scars from burns or leukoplakic lesions.[41, 48]

34. ulcer — a break in the skin or mucous membrane resulting from varicose veins, trauma or other causes.

35. urticaria, hives, nettle rash — skin eruption of pale or reddish wheals, usually associated with intense itching. May occur as an acute self-limited episode due to food allergy, drug reaction or emotional stress or in chronic form as a characteristic feature of rheumatic and connective tissue disorders.[12, 42]

D. Operative Terms:

1. cryosurgery of skin — freezing the skin with liquid nitrogen or solid carbon dioxide in order to destroy the lesion.[51, 55]

2. curettage of skin — removal of superficial lesions with a skin curette.[43]

3. dermabrasion — surgical removal of nevi or scars using sandpaper or other abrasives.[3]

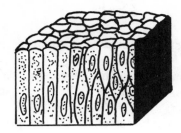

A. Simple, columnar epithelium
(three-dimensional view)

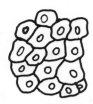

B. Simple, columnar epithelium
(surface view)

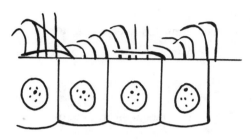

C. Ciliated epithelium

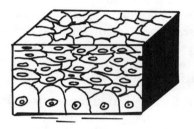

D. Stratified squamous epithelium

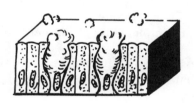

E. Goblet cells

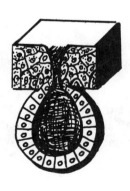

F. Simple alveolar glands

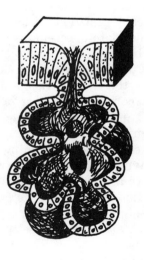

G. Compound alveolar glands

Fig. 5 — Various types of simple epithelium (A, B, C, D) and various types of glands (E, F, G).

23

4. electrodesiccation — the use of short, high frequency electric sparks for drying cells and tissue.
5. electrosurgical excision of burn — excision of full-thickness burn using the electrosurgical unit at the level of the fascia. The procedure leaves a dry fascial bed for immediate grafting.[31]
6. fulguration of skin — the use of long, high frequency electric sparks for destroying tissue.
7. incision and drainage of infected skin lesion.
8. Linton flap procedure — operation for stasis dermatitis and ulceration refractory to simpler method. All incompetent communicating veins are ligated and divided to relieve ambulatory venous hypertension in superficial veins. This prevents progression of dermatitis, ulceration and pigmentation of overlying skin in the lower limb.[11]
9. local excision of skin lesion.
10. plastic operation on skin — surgical correction of defect.
11. skin grafting — transfer of skin from a normal area to cover denuded areas. A dermatome may be used to obtain these skin transplants.

E. Symptomatic Terms:

1. anular, formerly annular — ring-shaped.
2. café au lait spots — light brown flat spots, variable in shape and size, seen in neurofibromatosis (von Recklinghausen's disease).[52]
3. chloasma — patches of brown or yellowish pigmentation on skin otherwise normal.
4. cicatrix of skin — a scar left by a healed wound.
5. cicatrization — healing by scar formation.
6. comedo (pl. comedones), blackhead — excretory duct of skin plugged by discolored sebum.
7. confluent — lesions joined or run together.
8. depigmentation — partial or complete loss of pigment; occurs in albinism, atrophic skin and scars.
9. dermatographism, dermographia — skin writing. Urticarial wheals appear where skin was marked by pencil or blunt instrument.[12]
10. discoid — shaped like a disc.
11. discrete — lesions are disconnected, separate from one another.
12. ecchymosis (pl. ecchymoses) — purple spot or bruise due to seepage of blood into the skin.
13. eczematoid, eczematous — eczema-like inflammatory lesion which tends to thicken, to become scaly, vesicular, crusty, or weeping.
14. eruption — a rash or skin lesion.
15. erythema — diffuse redness of skin.
16. excoriation — linear break of skin or scratch mark due to surface trauma.
17. granulation — a method of repair or healing following loss of tissue or pyogenic infection.
18. guttate — droplike.
19. keratotic — pertaining to a horny thickening.
20. hyperpigmentation — the presence of an abnormal amount of pigment in the skin seen in a considerable number of systemic diseases such as adrenal insufficiency, acromegaly, and others. In the familial progressive type of hyperpigmentation patches of excessive pigmentation enlarge in size with increasing age.[52]
21. intertriginous — between two folds of skin.
22. macule — discolored patch or spot on the skin.
23. milia (sing. milium) — tiny white nodules appearing on skin, frequently below the eyes.
24. moniliform — beaded.
25. multiform — several forms of the skin lesions.
26. papule — a pimple.
27. petechiae — pin size hemorrhagic spots in the skin.
28. proliferation — process of rapid reproduction or similar cells.
29. pustule — a small elevation of the skin containing pus or lymph.
30. seborrheal, seborrheic — pertaining to seborrhea, an oversecretion of sebaceous glands.

31. serpiginous — creeping in a snakelike manner.
32. vesication, vesiculation — formation of blisters.

BREASTS

A. Origin of Terms:

1. areola (L) — a small area or space
2. grapho (G) — to write
3. lac (L) — milk
4. mamma (L) — breast
5. mastos (G) — breast
6. thele (G) — nipple
7. therme (G) — heat
8. xeros (G) — dry

B. Anatomical Terms:

1. areola — area of pigmented skin surrounding the nipple. It becomes dark during pregnancy and remains so thereafter.
2. mammary gland — glandular tissue of the breast composed of 15 to 20 compound alveolar lobes, each connected with the nipple by a lactiferous duct.
3. papilla mammae — the nipple.

C. Diagnostic Terms:

1. abscess of breast, mammary abscess — a localized collection of pus of mammary tissue.
2. amastia — absence of a breast.
3. athelia — absence of a breast nipple.
4. breast cancer — malignant mammary tumor, a painless or painful mass which may be associated with skin and muscle attachment, discharge, crusting and retraction of nipple, changes in contour of affected breast and metastases to regional lymph nodes.[5, 32, 46, 53]
   a. carcinoma of breast — malignant tumor usually arising from ductal epithelium of mammary gland.
   b. sarcoma of breast — rare, nonepithelial, malignant mammary tumor, e.g., cystosarcoma and fibrosarcoma.
5. cystic disease of breast — the most common breast lesion composed of gross cysts that may be accompanied by microscopic cysts. Haagensen distinguishes 4 types:
   a. galactoceles, cysts containing inspissated milk.
   b. cysts formed in duct ectasia (dilated duct).
   c. cysts due to fat necrosis caused by trauma.
   d. cysts related to intraductal papilloma.[18]
6. fissure of nipple — a deep furrow in nipple.
7. hyperplasia of breast, hypermastia — abnormally large breast, usually pendulous and sagging.
8. hypoplasia of breast, hypomastia — abnormally small breast.
   a. unilateral hypomastia — one breast underdeveloped the other normal or overdeveloped. This results in mammary asymmetry and disfigurement.
   b. bilateral hypomastia — both breasts are abnormally small.
9. occlusion of lactiferous ducts — blockage of lumen of milk-conveying ducts.
10. Paget's disease of nipple — cancer directly beneath the nipple, seen in elderly women. Areola, nipple and surrounding skin may be weeping and eczematoid.[46, 53]
11. thelitis — inflammation of the nipple.

D. Operative Terms:

1. biopsy of breast — excision of small piece of mammary tissue for diagnostic evaluation.
   a. biopsy of apex of axilla — method of detecting axillary lymph node metastasis.
   b. biopsy of internal mammary node — method of detecting internal mammary node metastasis.[9, 17]
2. mammaplasty, mammoplasty, mastoplasty — surgical reconstruction of the breast.[18]

    a. augmentation mammaplasty — implantation of a retromammary prosthesis for an underdeveloped breast.[4, 24, 49]

    b. reduction mammaplasty — repair of an overdeveloped, pendulous breast by partial removal of the mammary gland and fixation of the breast to its normal position.[1, 22, 23, 34, 44]

    c. Strömbeck's mammaplasty — surgical reduction of the breast using a double pedicled flap to protect the nipple and preserve the dermis and its blood supply followed by reconstruction of breast.[35]

3. mastectomy, mammectomy — removal of a breast.

    a. radical mastectomy — removal of an entire breast including axillary dissection and surgical division of pectoralis major and minor muscles.[47]

    b. simple mastectomy — removal of a breast without dissection of axillary lymph nodes.

    c. subcutaneous mastectomy — below-the-skin removal of benign lesion of the mammary gland and subcutaneous reconstruction of the breast by implanting a prosthesis.[20, 27, 37, 38]

4. mastopexy — surgical fixation of a pendulous breast.

5. mastotomy — incision and drainage of a breast abscess.

E. Symptomatic Terms:

1. mastalgia, mastodynia — breast pain occurring in premenstrual period, mastitis, mammary cancer and other disorders.

2. peau d'orange — skin simulating orange peel; seen in inflammatory breast cancer.

3. skin retraction — dimpling and puckering of skin due to benign or malignant lesions underneath.

RADIOLOGY

A. General Terms:

1. fluorescence — the property of becoming luminous through the influence of x-rays or other agents.

2. fluoroscopy — direct x-ray examination using a fluoroscopic screen in a darkened room.

3. laminograms, planigrams, polytomes, tomograms — body section radiograms; x-ray pictures of a thin layer of body tissue of varying depths without interference with the intervening structures.

4. radiogram, roentgenogram, skiagram (skia (G) shadow) — picture made on a photographic film by means of x-rays.

5. radiography, roentgenography, skiagraphy, — the making of x-ray photographs.

6. radiologist — a physician who uses roentgen, radium and other forms of radiant energy for diagnostic and therapeutic purposes.

7. radiology — the study or science concerned with the use of various forms of radiant energy in the diagnosis and treatment of disease.

8. radium — a radioactive substance used in treating certain diseases.

9. radon — a heavy radioactive gas which is given off in the disintegration of radium.

10. roentgenography — the use of x-rays in the production of an image on a photographic film.

11. roentgenologist — a physician who uses x-rays in the diagnosis and treatment of disease.

12. roentgen rays, x-rays — a form of radiant energy capable of penetrating solid and opaque objects.

B. Terms Related to Diagnostic Radiology:

1. mammography, Egan technique — soft tissue mammary radiography based on varying degrees of absorption of the x-ray beam by fatty, fibroglandular and cancerous tissue in the breast in decreasing order of translucency.

2. mammograms, Egan technique — three radiographic views of the breast which outline:

    a. benign lesions, nodules or cysts well circumscribed usually surrounded by a thin halo of radiolucent fat.

b. malignant lesions, spicular, ragged irregular in shape and poorly circumscribed, frequently associated with thickening and retraction of skin, nipple deformity, axillary lymph node involvement, microcalcifications and venous congestion. Since the presence of fat serves to identify lesions no radiopaque substance is injected into the lactiferous ducts. As a result the breast is not distorted and pathologic conditions are clearly delineated. Mammography may also be used in screening studies of asymptomatic women and in postmastectomy follow-up examinations.[6, 15, 54]

3. senography — an improved method of soft tissue mammary radiography using a Senograph, a special apparatus for contrast and detail in the detection of breast cancer.

4. thermography — the recording of infrared radiations of the skin as a cancer detection tool. Black or dark areas of the thermogram register abnormally increased skin temperature which may be indicative of the presence of a malignant lesion.[2, 6, 15, 25, 57]

5. xeroradiography of breast — an x-ray method of obtaining images of breast structures on selenium-coated metal plates.[6, 14, 15]

C. Terms Related to Therapeutic Radiology:

1. laser radiation — an intensely strong, narrow beam of light that may be used to destroy selected skin lesions. Laser means light amplification by the stimulated emission of radiation.[8, 16]

2. radiation therapy in carcinoma of the breast — treatment of value:
    a. in selected inoperable cases for palliation.
    b. as an adjunct to surgery: preoperative irradiation and as postoperative therapy following radical mastectomy to enhance the cure rate and survival.[39]
    c. for postoperative recurrence of lesion.
    d. in the management of metastatic bone involvement
    Radical surgery is the treatment of choice for carcinoma of the breast, since it is not possible to eradicate the disease by radiation therapy. However, there is sufficient clinical evidence that irradiation has brought about five year cures in patients treated for inoperable lesions.[19]

3. radium therapy — treatment of pathologic conditions with radium which continually emits radiation at a constant rate regardless of environmental conditions.

4. superficial x-ray therapy — radiation therapy used for surface lesions; for example, selected skin conditions and tumors.

CLINICAL LABORATORY

A. General Terms:

1. allergen, allergin, sensitizer — substance which produces various allergic manifestations; for example, skin reactions.[10, 12]

2. allergy — hypersensitivity to a particular substance. Eczema, urticaria, dermatitis due to drugs or roentgen-rays are forms of allergic conditions.[12]

3. desensitization — process of abating allergic manifestations and making a person susceptible to a substance of therapeutic value by repeatedly giving him small doses of it.[12]

4. eosinophilia — abnormal increase of eosinophils in differential white count present in skin diseases such as pemphigus or certain forms of dermatitis.

5. hapten — an incomplete allergen.[12]

6. sensitivity — state of being sensitive.

7. sensitization — process of being sensitized.

B. Terms Related to Laboratory Diagnosis:

1. frozen section — microscopic study of slides made from fresh tissue of lesion. It is valuable for rapid diagnosis while patient is on operating room table to determine the need for conservative surgery, should the tissue section show a benign lesion, or for radical surgery, should a malignant lesion be found.

2. incisional biopsy — tissue of lesion obtained for pathologic verification. This procedure is indicated when the tumor mass is very large. Otherwise excisional biopsy is the method of choice.
3. skin tests for hypersensitivity — small amount of specific protein is scratched or injected into the skin to determine the protein causing food allergy or other morbid conditions.
4. SMA profile — sequential multiple analyses profile or broad laboratory screening.

ABBREVIATIONS

A. General:

CC — chief complaint
cc — cubic centimeter
Derm. — dermatology
Dx — diagnosis
FH — family history
FS — frozen section
H — hypodermic

MH — marital history
PH — past history
PI — present illness
Rx — take
STD — skin test dose
Subcu. — subcutaneous
TPR — temperature, pulse and respiration
ung. — ointment

B. Coding Systems, Nomenclature, Others:

CPHA — Commission on Professional and Hospital Activities

H-ICDA — *Hospital Adaptation of ICDA*

ICD — International Classification of Diseases

ICDA — *International Classification of Diseases Adapted* (official)

ICD-9-CM — *International Classification of Diseases, 9th Revision Clinical Modification**

INI — *International Nursing Index*

ISBN — International Standard Book Number

MSH — Medical Subject Headings

NLM — *National Library of Medicine*

SNDA — *Standard Nomenclature of Diseases and Operations*

C. Nursing Organizations:

AACN — American Association of Critical Care Nurses
ANA — American Nurses Association
ANC — US Army Nurse Corps
ANF — American Nurses Foundation
BHDP — Baccalaureate and Higher Degree Programs

CPNP — Council of Practical Nursing Programs
ICN — International Council of Nursing
NLN — National League for Nursing
NNC — US Navy Nurse Corps
VNA — Visiting Nurse Association

D. Other Paramedical Organizations:

AAPA — American Academy of Physicians Assistants
AART — American Association for Respiratory Therapy
ADA — American Dietetic Association
AMRS — American Medical Record Association

APAP — Association of Physician Assistant Programs
APTA — American Physical Therapy Association
ASHP — American Society of Hospital Pharmacists
ASRT — American Society of Radiologic Technologists

---

*The new classification will be put into effect January 1, 1979 to promote uniform, comparable statistics for an international exchange of health data and epidemiologic research.

E. Health Organizations:[36]

ACS— American Cancer Society
AHA — American Hospital Association
AMA — American Medical Association
APHA — American Public Health
    Association
ARC — American Red Cross
CDC — Center for Disease Control
CHHA — Council of Home Health
    Agencies
CHS — Community Health Service
HEW — Department of Health,
    Education and Welfare

NIH — US National Institute of Health
NHI — National Health Insurance
NSC — National Safety Council
OCDM — US Office of Civil and Defense
    Mobilization
PAHO — Pan American Health Organization
USPC — US Peace Corps
USPHS — US Public Health Service
VA — US Veteran Administration
WHO — World Health Organization

ORAL READING PRACTICE

Pemphigus

There are several forms of **dermatitis** in which a **bullous eruption** develops but they are distinguished from true bullous diseases by a short duration and good prognosis.[28]

The term **pemphigus**, derived from the Greek **pemphix**, "blister", points up the chief characteristic of **pemphigus vulgaris**, namely, the formation of blisters. These **blebs** arise suddenly on apparently normal or slightly **erythematous** skin and form oval-shaped or round blisters containing clear **serum**. The blisters tend to be **flaccid** and to break easily. The **epidermis** becomes detached leaving increasingly larger areas of **denudation**. The **Nicholsky** sign is always positive. It is obtained by pressing on the skin with the finger tip. The epidermis then slides off and a raw surface remains. The **denuded** areas are slow in healing and constitute a continuous threat of infection.

Pemphigus has been compared with a serious burn, but, in reality, the trauma of a burn is a single occasion and the lesion is frequently localized. On the other hand, the injury inflicted upon the skin by numerous crops of **bullae** followed by widespread denudation presents a still **more** serious problem than that of many a burn. The blisters vary in size from a few **millimeters** in diameter to ten **centimeters**. New lesions develop while old ones disappear. Since the crops arise rapidly, often overnight, and old lesions heal slowly, the areas of denudation are extensive. Eventually, crusts form over the raw surface. If **pyogenic bacteria** get beneath these crusts, foul-smelling pus collects and increases the patient's physical distress. There is no scarring; only a **hyperpigmented** lesion remains after healing. The formation of bullae in the **oral cavity** is particularly painful. Blebs about 5 millimeters in diameter are scattered over the **buccal mucosa.** They appear spontaneously, rupture and leave new **ulcers** which inflict much pain. Blebs may also occur on other **orificial mucous membranes.**

The etiology of pemphigus is still unknown. Some authorities believe that it is metabolic in nature or caused by **bacterial** or **viral** infections; however, no theory has yielded convincing evidence.

The common type of pemphigus is a chronic, recurrent disease, afflicting only adults. Acute **exacerbations** may be followed by brief or prolonged periods of remission. As a rule, pemphigus vulgaris lasts from several months to years. Untreated, it is a fatal disease, but with the judicious use of **Cortisone** the **prognosis** is favorable.[26, 28, 42, 52]

Table 1

SOME CONDITIONS OF THE SKIN AND BREAST AMENABLE TO SURGERY

Organs Involved	Diagnoses	Operations	Operative Procedures
Skin	Seborrheic keratoses	Epidermal curettage[a]	Lesions frozen with ethyl chloride and curetted
	Basal cell carcinoma — small lesion	Curettage Electrodesiccation	Lesion and all extensions removed with skin curette Remaining cells destroyed by surgical diathermy
Skin	Basal cell carcinoma — small lesion	Cryosurgery of skin lesion[b]	Freezing with cryosurgical spray or by insertion of microthermocouple
Skin Sebaceous glands Hair follicles Nail bed Nail fold	Infected steatoma Furuncle or carbuncle of hair follicles Onychia, paronychia Infected ingrowing toe nail	Incision and drainage of glands of skin; of hair follicles; of nail bed or fold	Surgical opening of infected sebaceous glands, etc. to induce drainage
Subcutaneous areolar tissue	Cellulitis of forearm	Incision and drainage of subcutaneous areolar tissue	Surgical opening of infected area and insertion of drain
Skin, subcutaneous tissue	Dermoid of skin Lipoma of subcutaneous tissue	Local excision of dermoid or lipoma	Removal of benign neoplasm
Skin	Cicatrix of skin due to burn (Structures beneath skin undamaged)	Excision of cicatricial skin lesion Use of split-thickness or full thickness skin graft	Removal of excess scar tissue and replacement by covering area with either half or full thickness of the skin removed by a knife or dermatome
Skin Subcutaneous tissue	Thermal burn injury	Electrosurgical excision of full thickness burn	Burned skin and subcutaneous tissue removed by electrosurgery at level of fascia Immediate skin grafting of dry fascial bed
Skin of neck, chin or cheek	Contracture from scar of old burns or injuries	Reconstruction operation *First stage:* Preparation of pedicle or Gillies' tube flap *Second stage:* Excision of scar Coverage of denuded area with pedicle *Third stage:* Removal of pedicle	Skin and subcutaneous tissue from donor area raised and pedicle tubed Removal of deep scar, distal end of pedicle severed and sutured into defect with pedicle still attached Pedicle opened and returned to donor area
Skin of axilla	Cicatricial contracture of axilla	Z-plasty	Defect corrected by using sliding flaps of skin
Breast	Abscess of breast due to *Staphylococcus aureus* or other infectious agents	Mastotomy with drainage	Surgical opening and evacuation of abscess Insertion of drain

Organs Involved	Diagnoses	Operations	Operative Procedures
Breast	Carcinoma of breast	Radical mastectomy	Removal of breast, pectoral muscles and lymph nodes
Breast	Overdevelopment of breast (pendulous breast)	Mastopexy	Fixation of a pendulous breast
Breast	Unilateral hypomastia	Augmentation mammaplasty of underdeveloped breast	Implantation of a Cronin silicone prosthesis in a retromammary pocket
	Hypermastia of contralateral breast	Reduction mammaplasty of overdeveloped breast	Partial excision of mammary tissue High fixation of breast
Breast	Cystic disease of breast — benign lesions	Subcutaneous mastectomy[c]	Excision of cystic mammary gland below the skin Subcutaneous reconstruction by implanting a prosthesis

[a]A. N. Domonkos. *Andrews' Diseases of the Skin — Clinical Dermatology*, 6th ed. Philadelphia: W. B. Saunders Co., 1971, p. 967.

[b]L. M. Vistnes *et al.* An evaluation of cryosurgery for basal cell carcinoma. *Plastic and Reconstructive Surgery*, 55:71-75, January, 1975.

[c]F. B. Kern *et al.* Subcutaneous mastectomy and reconstruction in large breasts. *Plastic and Reconstructive Surgery*, 54:648-650, December, 1974.

REFERENCES AND BIBLIOGRAPHY

1. Carlsen, L. *et al.* A variation of the Biesenberger technique of reduction mammoplasty. *Plastic and Reconstructive Surgery*, 55: 653-656, June, 1975.
2. Cary, J. *et al.* Thermal evaluation of breast disease using local cooling. *Radiology*, 115: 73-77, April, 1975.
3. Clabaugh, W. A. Tattoo removal by superficial dermabrasion. *Plastic and Reconstructive Surgery*, 55: 401-405, April, 1975.
4. Courtiss, E. H. Selection of alternatives in augmentation mammoplasty. *Plastic and Reconstructive Surgery*, 54: 552-557, November, 1974.
5. Dall'Olmo, C. A. Lobular carcinoma of the breast in situ. *Archives of Surgery*, 110: 537-542, May, 1975.
6. Dodd, G. D. and Goldman, A. M. Mammography, xeroradiography and thermography in the diagnosis of breast cancer. In Holland, James F. and Frei, Emil III, *Cancer Medicine.* Philadelphia: Lea & Febiger, 1973, pp. 356-378.
7. Domonkos, A. N. Lichen planus — Pyoderma — Rhinophyma. *Andrews' Diseases of the Skin — Clinical Dermatology*, 6th ed. Philadelphia: W. B. Saunders Co., 1971, pp. 239-240 and 266-267.
8. _____. Laser radiation. *Ibid.*, pp. 967-968.
9. Egan, R. L. Breast biopsy priority: Cancer versus benign preoperative masses. *Cancer*, 35: 612-617, March, 1975.
10. Ellis, E. F. Allergic disorders. In Vaughan, Victor C. III and McKay, R. James. *Nelson Textbook of Pediatrics*, 10th ed. Philadelphia: W. B. Saunders Co., 1975, pp. 492-521.
11. Field, Paul. The role of the Linton flap procedure in the management of stasis dermatitis and ulceration in the lower limb. *Surgery*, 70: 920-926, December, 1971.
12. Fisher, Alexander A. *Contact Dermatitis*, 2d ed. Philadelphia: Lea & Febiger, 1973, pp. 21-26.
13. Fleming, I. D. *et al.* Skin cancer in black patients. *Cancer*, 35: 600-605, March, 1975.
14. Frankl, G. *et al.* Xeroradiographic detection of occult breast cancer. *Cancer*, 35: 542-548, February, 1975.
15. Gershon-Cohon, J. *et al.* Modalities in breast cancer detection: Xeroradiography, mammography, thermography and mammometry. *Cancer*, 24: 1226-1230, December, 1969.
16. Goldman, L. *et al.* Laser treatment of basal cell epithelioma injected with magnetic iron particles. *Archives of Dermatology*, 110: 751-752, November, 1974.
17. Goldman, W. P. Triple biopsy for carcinoma of the breast: A clinical study of 200 cases. *Surgery*, 70: 628-634, October, 1971.
18. Haagensen, C. D. Cystic disease of the breast. In *Diseases of the Breast*, 2d ed. Philadelphia: W. B. Saunders Co., 1971, pp. 155-156.
19. _____. The radiotherapy of breast carcinoma. *Ibid.*, pp. 734-753.
20. Hartley, J. H. *et al.* Subcutaneous mastectomy. *Plastic and Reconstructive Surgery*, 56: 5-8, July, 1975.
21. Hejazi, N. *et al.* Scabies. *Archives of Dermatology*, 111: 37-39, January, 1975.

32

22. Herman, S. *et al.* Revisional surgery after reduction mammoplasty. *Plastic and Reconstructive Surgery,* 55: 422-427, April, 1975.

23. Hoffman, G. W. *et al.* Reduction mammoplasty. *Southern Medical Journal,* 64: 1106-1111, September, 1971.

24. Huger, W. E. Avoidable pitfalls in augmentation mammoplasty. *Southern Medical Journal,* 68: 703-710, June, 1975.

25. Isard, H. J. Breast thermography — The mammatherm. *Radiologic Clinics of North America,* 12: 167-188, April, 1974.

26. Jordan, R. E. Pemphigus and bullous pemphigoid. In Conn, Howard F. *Current Therapy.* Philadelphia: W. B. Saunders Co., 1974, pp. 635-637.

27. Kern, F. B. *et al.* Subcutaneous mastectomy and reconstruction in large breasts. *Plastic and Reconstructive Surgery,* 54: 648-650, December, 1974.

28. Krain, L. S. Pemphigus. *Archives of Dermatology,* 110: 862-865, December, 1974.

29. Lambert, A. Primary closure of radical mastectomy. *Archives of Surgery,* 110: 843-844, July, 1975.

30. Lever, Walter F. and Schauburg — Lever, Gundula. *Histopathology of the Skin,* 5th ed. Philadelphia: J. B. Lippincott Co., 1975.

31. Lewis, R. L. *et al.* Electrosurgical excision of full-thickness burn. *Archives of Surgery,* 110: 191-197, February, 1975.

32. Lynch, H. T. *et al.* Familial breast cancer in a normal population. *Cancer,* 34: 2080-2086, December, 1974.

33. Mescon, H. *et al.* The skin. In Robbins, Stanley L. *Pathologic Basis of Disease.* Philadelphia: W. B. Saunders Co., 1974, pp. 1374-1419.

34. Meyer, R. *et al.* Reduction mammoplasty with an L-shaped suture line. *Plastic and Reconstructive Surgery,* 55: 139-148, February, 1975.

35. Müller, F. E. Late results of Strömbeck's mammoplasty. *Plastic and Reconstructive Surgery,* 54: 664-666, December, 1974.

36. *Nursing Outlook,* 14: 83, December, 1966.

37. Pennesi, V. R., *et al.* The incidence of obscure carcinoma in subcutaneous mastectomy — Results of a national survey. *Plastic and Reconstructive Surgery,* 56: 9-12, July, 1975.

38. Perras, C. *et al.* Subcutaneous mastectomy. *American Journal of Nursing,* 73: 1568-1570, September, 1973.

39. Potter, J. F. Preoperative irradiation and surgery for certain cancers. *Cancer,* 35: 84-90, January, 1975.

40. Rapaport, J. Giant keratocanthoma. *Archives of Dermatology,* 111: 73-75, January, 1975.

41. Reed, W. B. *et al.* Epidermolysis bullosa dystrophica with epidermal neoplasms. *Archives of Dermatology,* 110: 894-902, December, 1974.

42. Rees, B. Skin and appendages. In Krupp, Marcus A. and Chatton, Milton, *Current Medical Diagnosis and Treatment,* 15th ed. Los Altos, California: Lange Medical Publications, 1976, pp. 32-74.

43. Reymann, F. Multiple basal cell carcinoma of the skin. *Archives of Dermatology,* 111: 877-879, July, 1975.

44. Ribeiro, L. A new technique for reduction mammoplasty. *Plastic and Reconstructive Surgery,* 55: 330-334, March, 1975.

45. Rice, A. K. Common skin infections in school children. *American Journal of Nursing,* 73: 1905-1909, November, 1973.

46. Rush, B. F. Breast. In Schwartz, Seymour I. (ed.). *Principles of Surgery,* 2nd ed. New York: McGraw-Hill Book Co., 1974, pp. 527-554.

47. Scanlon, E. F. Modified radical mastectomy. *Cancer,* 35: 710-713, March, 1975.

48. Schwartz, Seymour I. Skin and subcutaneous tissue. In *Principles of Surgery,* 2d ed. New York: McGraw-Hill Book Co., 1974, pp. 513-526.

49. Snyder, G. B. Planning an augmentation mammoplasty. *Plastic and Reconstructive Surgery,* 54: 132-141, August, 1974.

50. Stellar, Stanley *et al.* Carbon dioxide laser debridement of decubitus ulcers. *Annals of Surgery,* 179: 230-237, February, 1974.

51. Vistnes, L. M. *et al.* An evaluation of cryosurgery for basal cell carcinoma. *Plastic and Reconstructive Surgery,* 55: 71-75, January, 1975.

52. Wheeler, C. E. Certain cutaneous diseases with significant systemic manifestations. In Beeson, Paul B. and McDermott, Walsh. *Textbook of Medicine,* 14th ed. Philadelphia: W. B. Saunders Co., 1975, pp. 1846-1862.

53. Wilson, J. L. Diseases of the breast. In Krupp, Marcus A. and Chatton, Milton. *Current Medical Diagnosis and Treatment,* 15th ed. Los Altos, California: Lange Medical Publications, 1976, pp. 399-414.

54. Wolfe, J. N. Mammography. *Radiologic Clinics of North America,* 12: 189-203, April, 1974.

55. Wooldridge, W. E. *et al.* Treatment of skin cancer by cryosurgery. *Missouri Medicine,* 72: 28-34, January, 1975.

56. Zackin, Henry *et al.* Prevention of postoperative shifting of mammary prostheses. *Plastic and Reconstructive Surgery,* 55: 713, June, 1975.

57. Ziskin, M. C. Computer diagnosis of breast thermograms. *Radiology,* 115: 341-347, May, 1975.

Chapter III

Musculoskeletal Disorders

BONES

A. Origin of Terms:

1. calcaneus (L) — heel bone
2. cancellus (L) — lattice
3. coxa (L) — hip bone
4. diploë (G) — fold
5. femur (L) — thigh
6. genu (L) — knee
7. ischion (G) — hip
8. lacuna (L) — lake
9. medulla (L) — marrow
10. myelos (G) — marrow
11. os (pl. ossa) (L) — bone
12. osteon (G) — bone
13. pes, ped (L) — foot
14. physis (G) — growth
15. pelvis (L) — basin
16. planta (L) — sole
17. pod, podo (G) — foot
18. sternon (G) — breast bone
19. trochanter (G) — runner
20. xiphoid (G) — sword

B. Anatomic Terms:[27]

1. bone, osseous tissue — the hardest type of connective tissue which provides a supporting framework for the body.
2. bone marrow, medulla — soft, central part of bone.
   a. red marrow — fills cancellous bone and manufactures red blood cells and hemoglobin.
   b. yellow marrow — fills the medullary cavity and contains fat cells.
3. cancellous bone — spongy bone composed of a loose latticework of bony trabeculae and bone marrow within the interspace.
4. compact bone, cortex of bone — solid bone rich in calcium.
5. diaphysis — shaft of long bone.
6. diploë — spongy bone between the two tables of the skull.
7. endosteum — membrane lining the walls of the medullary cavity.
8. epiphysis (pl. epiphyses) — extremity of long bones and center of ossification for growing bone.
9. matrix of bone — collagenous fibers and a ground substance in which calcium is deposited.
10. medullary cavity — marrow-filled cavity within the shaft of long bones.
11. metaphysis — enlarged part of the shaft near the epiphysis of a long bone.
12. ossification — bone formation.
13. osteoblasts — bone forming cells.
14. osteoclasts — bone absorbing cells.
15. osteocytes — bone cells lying in lacunae within intercellular substance.
16. osteoid — calcifiable osseous tissue, yet uncalcified.
17. periosteum — outer covering of bone.
18. trabeculae — slender spicules or anastomosing bars of spongy bone.
19. trochanter — bony prominence of the upper extremity of the femur below the femoral neck.
   a. major or greater trochanter — large bony projection located externally and laterally between femoral neck and shaft.
   b. minor or lesser trochanter — conical bony prominence located medially and laterally at the junction of the femoral neck and shaft.

C. Diagnostic Terms:

1. bone cyst — a fluid containing bone lesion.
   a. aneursymal bone cyst — a solitary vascular lesion which usually arises from medullary or cancellous structures, affects the ends of the shaft and pushes outward

34

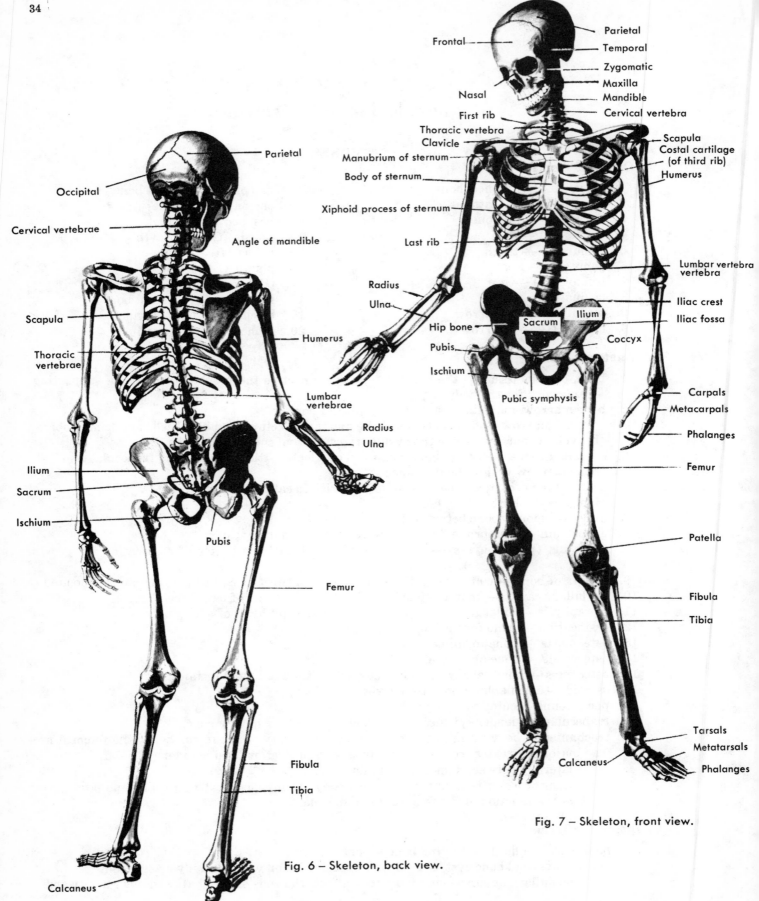

Parietal

Occipital

Cervical vertebrae

Scapula

Thoracic vertebrae

Ilium

Sacrum

Ischium

Angle of mandible

Humerus

Lumbar vertebrae

Radius

Ulna

Pubis

Femur

Fibula

Tibia

Calcaneus

Fig. 6 – Skeleton, back view.

Frontal

Parietal

Temporal

Zygomatic

Maxilla

Mandible

Nasal

Cervical vertebra

First rib

Thoracic vertebra

Clavicle

Scapula

Manubrium of sternum

Costal cartilage (of third rib)

Body of sternum

Humerus

Xiphoid process of sternum

Last rib

Lumbar vertebra vertebra

Radius

Ulna

Iliac crest

Iliac fossa

Hip bone

Ilium

Sacrum

Pubis

Coccyx

Ischium

Pubic symphysis

Carpals

Metacarpals

Phalanges

Femur

Patella

Fibula

Tibia

Tarsals

Metatarsals

Calcaneus

Phalanges

Fig. 7 – Skeleton, front view.

eroding soft and osseous tissue.   Other sites are the spine and scapula.
When the cyst bursts hemorrhage may be severe.[2]

    b. solitary bone cyst — disorder of growing skeleton consisting of a capsule-like cyst wall lined with soft tissue and filled with fluid.   It occurs at the end of shafts, ribs, clavicle, mandible, pubic bone and heel.[2]

2. cervical rib — a supernumerary rib attached to a cervical vertebra.

3. coxa plana — flattening of head of femur.

4. coxa valga — widening of angle between the shaft and neck of femur.

5. coxa vara — diminishing of angle between the shaft and neck of femur.

6. deformity of bone — congenital or acquired abnormality of bone resulting in disfigurement.

7. epiphysitis, acute — inflammatory process of the epiphyseal region of a long bone, marked by tenderness and pain of the joint.

8. epiphysiolysis, slipped epiphysis — a loosening or separation of the epiphysis from the shaft, usually a slipping of the upper femoral epiphysis.   There is eversion of the limb resulting in displacement and limping.[2, 49]

9. epulis — a fibrous tumor arising from the gum.

10. Ewing's sarcoma — malignant new growth originating in the shaft of long bones and spreading through the periosteum into soft tissues.   Metastases occur early.   Femur, tibia, humerus, fibula and pelvic bones are frequently involved.[3, 68]

11. exostosis (pl. exostoses) — bone tumor, osteoma, a benign osseous growth.

12. fibrosarcoma of bone — malignant tumor derived from bone marrow, metaphysis or periosteum and found on femur, humerus and jaw bones.[3, 38]

13. fibrous dysplasia of bone, Albright's syndrome — metabolic bone disease characterized by rapid resorption of bone and fibrous replacement of marrow, distortion of one or several bones, brownish pigmentation of the skin, and precocious puberty in girls.[1, 45, 74]

14. fracture — a broken bone.   Long bone fractures are frequently associated with nerve injury.

    a. nonpenetrating or closed fracture — no external wound present.

    b. penetrating or open fracture — an external wound communicating with the fracture.
Fractures may be:

      (1) capillary — hairlike line of break.

      (2) comminuted — bone splintered into small fragments.

      (3) complicated — broken bone injuring adjacent structure, e.g. fractured rib piercing the lung.

      (4) compound — an open wound leading down to the fracture.

      (5) depressed — broken bone inwards as in certain skull fractures.

      (6) greenstick — incomplete break which may be associated with bowing of shaft.

      (7) impacted — broken fragment wedged into other bony fragment.

      (8) pathologic — a spontaneous fracture due to bone destruction in certain diseases: cancer, syphilis, osteomalacia, osteoporosis, others.

      (9) simple — uncomplicated fracture, no open wound.

    (10) transverse — break across the bone.   For example: Colles fracture — transverse fracture of radius above the wrist with displacement of the hand.[72]

15. fracture of hip — a break in upper end of femur.[57]   The two main types are:

    a. femoral neck fracture — bone broken through the neck of the femur.[11, 17, 61]

    b. trochanteric fracture — bone broken below, around or between the greater or lesser trochanters.[22, 47, 57, 78]

16. genu valgum — knock knee.

17. genu varum — bowleg; deformity involving either tibia alone, or femur, tibia and fibula; seen in rickets and corrected by high doses of vitamin D.

18. giant cell tumor, benign — osteolytic tumor containing numerous giant cells.   It arises at the epiphysis and does not interfere with joint motion until late.   It may undergo malignant transformation or recur after removal.   It is questionable if it should be considered an entity.[3, 83]

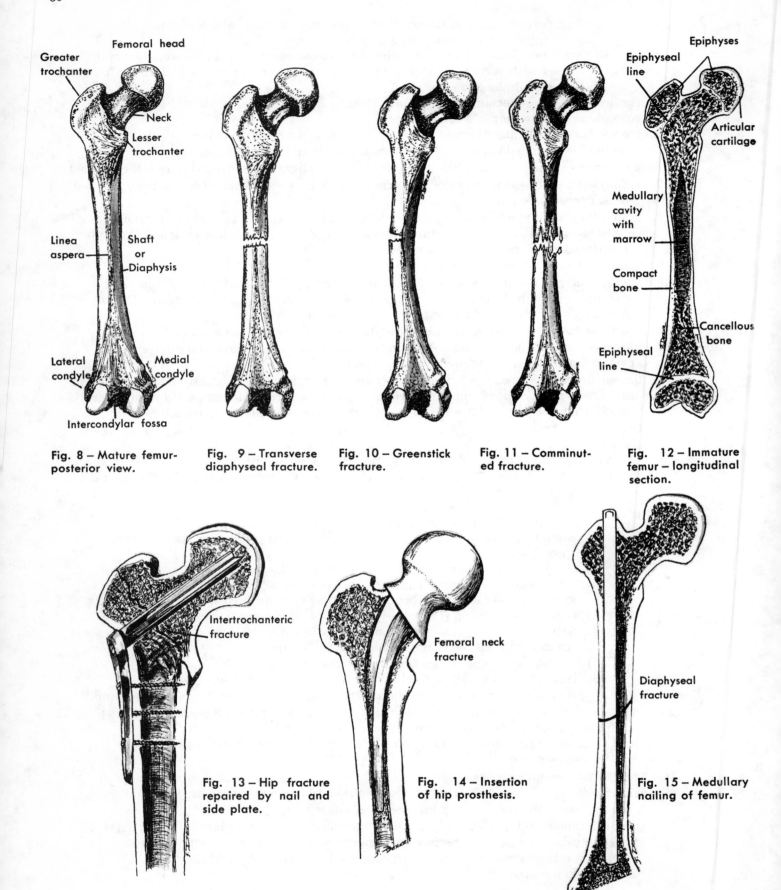

Fig. 8 – Mature femur-posterior view.

Fig. 9 – Transverse diaphyseal fracture.

Fig. 10 – Greenstick fracture.

Fig. 11 – Comminut-ed fracture.

Fig. 12 – Immature femur – longitudinal section.

Fig. 13 – Hip fracture repaired by nail and side plate.

Fig. 14 – Insertion of hip prosthesis.

Fig. 15 – Medullary nailing of femur.

19. myeloma, plasmacytoma — malignant neoplasm derived from plasma cells and usually associated with abnormal protein metabolism. It may occur as
    a. multiple myeloma — a malignant type of widespread bone destruction with gradual replacement of cancellous bone by neoplasm seen in age groups above 50 years old and as
    b. solitary myeloma — single lesion found in any location but most frequently in vertebral column. Back pain is severe.[3]
20. osteitis — inflammation of bone.
21. osteitis deformans, Paget's disease of bone — slowly progressive disease occurring in advanced age, characterized by extensive bone destruction, followed almost immediately by abnormal bone repair of the weakened, deossified skeleton which yields deformities and pathologic fractures.[2, 45, 73]
22. osteoblastoma — a benign lesion, thought by Aegerter to be a "collection of reparative bone reactions", typically found in the spine where it may cause cord compression and paraplegia.[3, 52, 76]
23. osteochondritis deformans juvenile, coxa plana, Legg-Calvé-Perthes disease — self-limited disease in children, age 4-10; characterized by flattening of the femoral head resulting in limping and restricted motion.[24]
24. osteoclasia, osteolysis — resorption and destruction of osseous tissue.
25. osteoclastoma — a true tumor, usually occurring in the young after closure of the epiphysis and involving the femur, tibia, radius and phalanges of the hands and feet. It erodes the cortex from within and causes cortical expansion. If complicated by an aneurysmal bone cyst, the osteoclastoma grows rapidly and becomes very destructive.[3]
26. osteogenic sarcoma — highly malignant, vascular tumor usually involving the upper shaft of long bones, the pelvis or knee. Metastases are common and life-threatening.[3, 40, 59]
27. osteoid osteoma — a benign, small, very painful tumor, found in almost any bone of the skeleton but most frequently in the lower extremities.[3, 40, 43, 79]
28. osteoma — benign osseous tumor usually of facial and frontal bones. Headache and seizures may be due to intracranial osteomas.[3]
29. osteomalacia — softening of bone caused by deficiency in calcium or phosphorus or both, needed for ossification of mature bone in adults. In children the primary cause is lack of vitamin D and sunlight necessary for the normal absorption of the vitamin.[4, 35, 45]
30. osteomyelitis — inflammation of the bone and bone marrow. Infective agents may be pyogenic bacteria, Brucella, Salmonella or other organisms.[40]
31. osteoporosis, porous bone — disorder of protein metabolism characterized by diffuse decrease of bone density and marked increase in porosity which are most pronounced in the spine and pelvis.[3, 35, 45]
32. renal (azotemic) osteodystrophy — bone disorder due to defective mineralization complicating chronic renal failure.[4, 35]
33. rickets, rachitis — calcium and vitamin D deficiency of early childhood which leads to demineralizaton of bones and deformities.
34. sequestrum — dead bone separated from surrounding tissue.
35. supernumerary bone — extra bone.
36. vitamin D refractory rickets, familial hypophosphatemia — a relatively common type of rickets in which abnormal phosphate loss and deficient mineralization are associated with renal tubule insufficiency.[4, 35]
37. whiplash injury of neck — compression of cervical spine involving the bones, joints and intervertebral disks. It is due to a sudden throwing forward and then backward of the head, usually caused by car accident when the collision is from the rear.

D. Operative Terms:

1. amputation — partial or complete removal of limb for crushing injury, intractable pain, gangrene, vascular obstruction or uncontrollable infection.[82]
2. bone grafting, transplantation of bone — insertion of a bone graft.[46]

a. autografting or autotransplantation of bone — removal of bone from one site and implanting it at another site to promote bone union, replace destroyed bone or immobilize joint in surgical fusion.

b. homografting or homotransplantation of bone — surgical use of bone from bone bank obtained from amputations, ostectomies or rib resections of nonmalignant, noninfectious cases.

3. epiphyseal arrest — surgical procedure for retarding growth at the epiphysis by equalizing length of lower extremities.

4. epiphyseal stapling — temporary arrest of epiphyseal growth by stapling the epiphysis to control leg length discrepancy.[49]

5. epiphysiodesis — implanting bone grafts across the epiphyseal plate to secure immobilization of epiphysis. Operation is done for slipped femoral epiphysis following insertion of metal pins.

6. exostectomy — removal of a benign bone tumor (exostosis), e.g. a bunion (hallux valgus).

7. ostectomy — excision of a bone.

8. osteoclasis — surgical refracture of a bone in case of malunion of broken parts.

9. osteoplasty — reconstruction or repair of a bone.

10. osteotomy — surgical division or section of a bone.

11. replantation of an extremity — restorative surgery of an accidentally amputated limb to its functional capacity including

   a. restoration of circulation by anastomoses of blood vessels.

   b. internal fixation of diaphyseal fracture of bone by intramedullary nail.

   c. repair of nerves and tendons.

   d. debridement of devitalized tissue.

   e. closure by suturing undamaged soft tissue of dismembered limb to stump.

   f. split-thickness grafts for denuded skin areas.[60]

12. sequestrectomy — surgical removal of a piece of dead bone.

13. surgical correction of fracture — this may be achieved by

   a. closed reduction — manipulation and application of cast, or application of splint or traction apparatus in selected cases when the fractured ends are not in alignment.

   b. open reduction and internal fixation — manipulation and

      (1) insertion of plate and screws.

      (2) insertion of medullary nail for diaphyseal fractures (shaft of long bones) ; extraction of nail after bone union.[58]

      (3) insertion of a nail with a side plate such as a Jewett nail for trochanteric or femoral neck fractures.[11, 22, 47, 57, 61, 78]

      (4) insertion of a hip prosthesis, Fred Thompson or Austin Moore type, in selected femoral neck fractures. Occasionally prostheses are used for severe fractures of the upper or lower end of the humerus.[7, 17, 57, 61]

   c. simple immobilization — application of a cast or splint when the fractured ends are in apposition.

14. surgical correction of facial defects :[12, 21, 36, 44]

   a. bone grafting of hemimandibular defects.

   b. bone graft reconstruction following hemimandibulectomies.

   c. craniofacial osteotomies for correction of facial anomalies.

E. Symptomatic Terms:

1. callus — substance growing between ends of fractured bone and converted into osseous tissue in the process of repair.

2. crepitation — grating sound made by movement of fractured bones.

3. decalcification — the removal of lime salts, especially from bone.

4. demineralization — deficiency or loss of bone minerals which occurs in osteoporosis, osteomalacia, cancer or other disorders.

5. necrosis of bone — devitalization of osseous tissue; formation of dead bone.

   a. aseptic — without infection.

    b. avascular — from deprivation of blood supply due to fracture, loss of periosteum, exposure to radioactive substances, or other causes.

    c. ischemic — same as avascular necrosis of bone.[57]

6. nidus — focal point from which a pathologic lesion develops.
7. ostealgia, osteodynia — bone pain.
8. osteophyte — bony outgrowth or osseous excrescence.
9. phantom limb pain — painful sensation felt by amputee as if the limb were still intact, probably of central origin.
10. sequestration — process of bone necrosis resulting in dead bone.

JOINTS, BURSAE, CARTILAGES, LIGAMENTS

A. Origin of Terms:

1. ankyle (G) — stiff joint
2. arthron (G) — joint
3. bursa (L) — purse, sac
4. cartilage (L) — gristle
5. cavus (L) — hollow
6. chondros (G) — gristle
7. condylos (G) — knuckle
8. cubitus (L) — elbow
9. hallux (L) — great toe
10. kyphos (G) — hump
11. ligament (L) — that which ties
12. lordosis (G) — bending backbone
13. luxatio (L) — to dislocate
14. malleus (L) — hammer
15. mandibulum (L) — lower jaw bone
16. meniskos (G) — crescent
17. pes, pedes (L) — foot, feet
18. planus (L) — flat
19. scolios (G) — curved
20. spondylos (G) — vertebra
21. talus (L) — heel, ankle
22. taliped (L) — club footed

B. Anatomic Terms:

1. acetabulum — cup-shaped socket on the external surface of the innominate bone in which the head of the femur lies.
2. articulation — joint.
   a. cartilaginous joint — bones united by fibrocartilage or hyaline cartilage.
   b. fibrous joint — bones united by fibrous tissue.
   c. synovial joint, diarthrodial joint — bones united by a joint capsule and ligaments. Cartilage covers the articular surface of the bones. The joint capsule is composed of a fibrous layer lined by synovial membrane.
3. bursa (pl. bursae) — connective tissue sac containing lubricating fluid, sometimes synovia.
4. intervertebral disc — fibrocartilage between the bodies of the vertebrae composed of
   a. anulus* fibrosus — an outer fibrous ring encircling the nucleus pulposus.
   b. nucleus pulposus — an inner gelatinous mass.
5. ligaments — fibrous, connective tissue bands uniting articular ends of bones.
6. meniscus — fibrocartilage found in certain joints.
7. synovial membrane — inner lining of a joint capsule secreting synovia.
8. volar — pertaining to the palm of the hand or sole of the foot.

C. Diagnostic Terms:

1. ankylosis — stiff joint.
2. arthritis — inflammation of joints.
   a. atrophic or rheumatoid arthritis which produces constitutional symptoms in addition to painful, inflammatory, multiple joint involvement.[5, 18, 23]
   b. gouty arthritis — metabolic disorder, usually involving one joint (monarticular). Urate crystals are highly increased and found in various tissues. Pain is relieved by colchicine. *Look out for Kidney Stones. Calcium deposits*

---

* Spelling of anulus according to *Nomina Anatomica*, 1964, p. 67.

c. infectious arthritis, pyogenic arthritis, septic arthritis —
   (1) acute infectious arthritis — acute inflammatory process affecting synovial and subchondrial tissues and causing articular destruction. It is usually due to pyogenic cocci such as gonococci, meningococci, pneumococci, staphylococci and streptococci.[23]
   (2) chronic infectious arthritis — persistent infection of joint causing pain, swelling, restricted joint motion and deformity.[23]
d. hypertrophic arthritis, osteoarthritis — a degenerative condition of cartilage and enlargement of bone at the joint margins, occurring particularly in older persons. It often affects the terminal phalanges, knees, hips and spine and results in contractures, deformities and stiffness of affected joints.[15, 23]
e. Marie Strümpell arthritis, ankylosing spondylitis — painful inflammatory joint disease characterized by progressive stiffening of the spine caused by fusion of vertebral bodies.[18, 75]
f. traumatic arthritis — a group of disorders resulting from single or repetitive trauma to joints:
   (1) acute synovitis, traumatic synovitis — this may be due to a single episode of articular trauma to the synovial membrane of a joint and may be associated with hemarthrosis and sprains. The articular cartilage is intact.
   (2) disruptive trauma of joint — the major supporting structures have ruptured and the articular cartilage is damaged. Meniscal tears, intraarticular fractures and severe sprains may be present.
   (3) posttraumatic osteoarthritis — residual damage from disruptive trauma may lead to restricted mobility, deformity and articular instability.
   (4) repetitive articular trauma — a chronic arthritis of the affected joints may develop due to occupational hazards or sports.
   (5) other types of trauma — arthropathy may develop following decompression, radiation, frostbite or the like.
      Medicolegal problems may arise when there is an aggravation of pre-existing arthritis and the causal relationship between the traumatic episode and joint affections is veiled.[66, 80]

3. arthropathy — any disease of the joints.
4. Baker's cyst — synovial fluid-filled lesion found in muscles, other tissues or near a joint in advanced osteoarthritis.[5]
5. bursitis — inflammation of a bursa.
6. chondritis — inflammation of a cartilage.
7. chondroblastoma — benign, vascular, cartilaginous tumor arising from the epiphysis of a long bone.[32]
8. chondrocalcinosis, pseudogout — acute, recurrent joint disease affecting the cartilaginous structures of large joints especially the knee. Synovial fluid contains calcium pyrophosphates.[5, 18]
9. chondroma — benign neoplasm arising from cartilage.
10. chondrosarcoma — malignant tumor derived from cartilage.
11. coxarthrosis — a hip joint; trophic degeneration of hip joint.[18]
12. destructive coxopathy — painful disability of hip joint associated with nocturnal distress of inflammatory type. Joint motion is moderately impaired.
13. dislocation — displacement of a bone from its natural position in a joint.
14. fibrositis, muscular rheumatism, periarthritis, periarticular fibrositis — rheumatoid condition affecting the muscles and tissues around the joints.[18]
15. hallux malleus — hammer toe.
16. hallux valgus — deflection of great toe to outer side of foot and subsequent development of bony prominence.[77]
17. hallux varus — deflection of great toe to inner side of foot.
18. hemarthrosis — bloody effusion in a joint cavity. It is prone to occur in hemophiliacs.[5, 18]
19. herniated intervertebral disc, herniated nucleus pulposus — tear of anulus fibrosus followed

by protrusion of the nucleus pulposus, compression of nerve root, back pain with or without sciatic radiation and paresthesias (pricking or numbness) of calf or foot. The rupture usually occurs in the lumbar, sacral and cervical regions of the spine.

20. internal derangement of knee joint — term refers to various joint lesions which interfere with motion (locking, snapping, buckling) due to atrophy of thigh muscles, tenderness or pain and joint swelling. Some leading causes are tears of menisci, ligaments, patellar or quadriceps tendons, loose bodies, fracture or chondromalacia of patellae.

21. kyphosis — hunchback; abnormal posterior curvature of thoracic spine.

22. lordosis — hollow-back; anterior convexity of lower spine.

23. painful shoulder, cervicobrachial pain syndromes — articular or extra-articular disorders characterized by tenderness, moderate to agonizing pain and limitation of motion in the shoulder girdle, neck and arm. All or some of these symptoms are present in

a. adhesive capsulitis, adhesive bursitis, frozen shoulder, periarthritis of the shoulder joint — adhesions within the bursa, articular tendosynovitis and calcareous deposits causing stiffness and atrophic changes.[18, 40]

b. carpal tunnel syndrome — painful condition resulting from a compression of the median nerve within the carpal tunnel as evidenced by a flattening or circular constriction of the nerve. Tingling, aching or burning pain in fingers, radiating to forearm and shoulder may be constant or episodic and aggravated by strenuous manual activity.[18, 40, 64]

c. cervical spondylosis, cervical disk disease — degenerative disorder of cervical disk, characterized by progressive thinning of the joint cartilage, spinal cord and nerve root compression resulting from extrusion of the nucleus pulposus and subsequent pain radiating to the back of the neck and head, shoulder and arm.[40]

d. epicondylalgia, epicondylitis, tennis elbow — pain syndrome primarily affecting the lateral and median regions of the elbow and radiating to the upper arm and forearm. It is accentuated by repetitive grasping.[18, 40]

e. hand-shoulder syndrome — peculiar clinical entity in which pain radiates from shoulder to finger tips. The patient spontaneously immobilizes the affected extremity which leads to atrophy and edema of the hand. Later overactivity of sympathetic nerves results in a sweaty, cold, painful hand followed by stiffness and fibrosis of joints. Syndrome may occur in myocardial ischemia, following myocardial infarction and infrequently in bronchogenic carcinoma.[18, 40]

f. supraclavicular nerve entrapment syndrome — compression of middle branch of supraclavicular nerve at its passage through the bone canal in the clavicle causing pain and numbness. Neuralgia can be relieved by decompression of the nerve.[28]

g. supraspinatus syndrome — disorder caused by adhesions, calcium deposits or tears in rotator cuff resulting in a painful shoulder, limited motion, muscle atrophy and spasm.

24. skeletal dysplasias — disturbances of bone growth, congenital or inherited, most severe if present in early infancy, less harmful if developing in adult life, causing progressive destruction of osseous tissue as a result of chondroid and osteoid abnormalities.[1] Examples are:

a. dysplasias due to impaired chondroid production — probably a metabolic defect of the maturation of chondroblasts (immature cartilage cells).

(1) achondroplasia — congenital, hereditary abnormality of chondroblastic cell growth at the epiphyses and subsequent development of a peculiar dwarfism.

(2) osteochondromatosis, hereditary multiple exostoses — osteochromas or bony outgrowths from the ends of cortical bone which may be associated with deformities of the knee, wrist, elbow and long bones or other defects.[1]

b. dysplasias due to impaired osteoid production — a group of developmental abnormalities characterized by the presence of either insufficient, excessive or immature osteoid.[1] Examples are:

(1) osteogenesis imperfecta, brittle bones — an inherited connective tissue disorder affecting the skeleton and occurring as

(a) osteogenesis imperfecta congenita — a severe form which develops prenatally and may be fatal in infancy.[13]

(b) osteogenesis imperfecta tarda — a moderately severe form which develops in childhood.[8]

Clinical features include fragility of bones, fracture proneness at an early age, multiple pathologic fractures, deformities of long bones, excessive digital laxity, white or blue sclerae, deafness, a peculiar squeaky voice and crackling laugh.[1, 8, 13, 40]

(2) osteopetrosis, marble bones, Albers-Schönberg disease — a rare congenital bone disorder thought to be due to a persistence of primitive chondro-osteoid which interferes with its replacement by mature bone.   Since osteoid formation is insufficient, the bones are fracture-prone, marble and chalk-like.[1]

25. Reiter's syndrome — a triad of inflammatory states: urethritis (nongonococcal), conjunctivitis and arthritis, probably due to chlamydial or mycoplasmal infection.[18, 23]

26. scoliosis — lateral spinal curvature.[43, 50, 70]

27. spondylitis — inflammation of one or several vertebrae.[5, 23, 75]

28. spondylolisthesis — forward slipping of a lumbar vertebra on the adjacent vertebra below, usually associated with pelvic deformity.[34, 53, 85]

29. spondylosis — ankylosis of vertebrae; also any degenerative lesion of the spine.[51]

30. sprain — injury to joint with tearing of tendons and ligaments.

31. Still's disease — painful rheumatoid arthritis in children associated with retarded growth, glandular and splenic enlargement.[18]

32. subluxation — incomplete dislocation.

33. synovioma — a highly malignant fibroblastic sarcoma, apparently originating in periarticular structures and occurring in older children and young adults.   It also presents in a benign form.[5, 18]

34. talipes — clubfoot:

    a. equinus — forefoot touches ground; walking on toes.

    b. planus — arch broken; entire sole rests on ground.

    c. valgus — foot everted; inner side of sole touches ground.

    d. varus — foot inverted; outer side of sole rests on ground.

35. vertebral injuries — trauma to the spine resulting in compression fractures of the vertebrae, fractures and dislocations or flexion fractures of the spine associated with minimal spinal cord damage.

D. Operative Terms:

1. arthroclasia — surgical breaking of a stiff joint.

2. arthrodesis, artificial ankylosis — surgical fixation of a joint to immobilize the joint.

3. arthrolysis — freeing the joint from fibrous bands or excess cartilage to restore its mobility.

4. arthroplasty — surgical repair of a joint.   The hip, knee, elbow and temporomandibular joints are best suited for reconstruction.

    a. arthroplasties of the hip joint.

      (1) Charnley low-friction arthroplasty — a total hip arthroplasty or total hip replacement for rheumatoid arthritis or any type of destructive hip disease. The prosthesis has two components: (1) an acetabular cup or socket of high density polyethylene and (2) a femoral component of vitallium or stainless steel consisting of a small femoral head for low friction which lodges in the socket and a prosthetic stem embedded in the intramedullary canal of the femur. Acrylic cement is used to seat the acetabular cup and prosthetic stem.   The cement provides rigid fixation and stability.[9, 14, 16, 19, 33, 41, 57]   A few of the many modifications of Charnley total hip replacement are those of Müller[33], Harris[34], Mc Kee-Farrar[20] and Ring.[19]

      (2) Colonna capsular arthroplasty — operation for congenital dislocation of the hip. This procedure retains the gliding mechanism between the displaced head of the femur and its capsule.   The acetabulum is usually deepened and enlarged.[30]

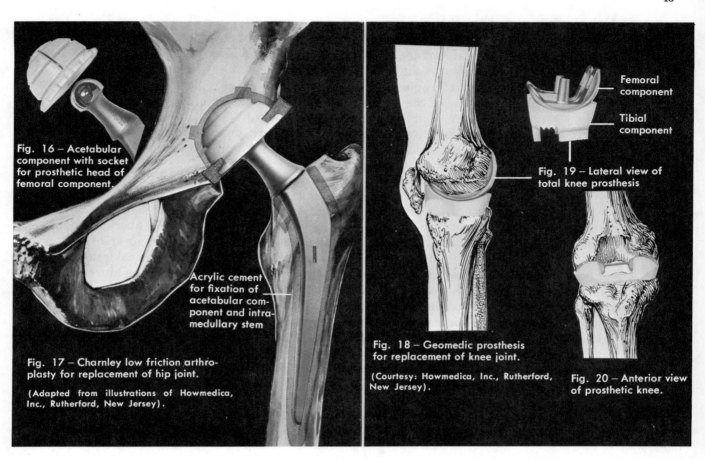

Fig. 16 – Acetabular component with socket for prosthetic head of femoral component.

Fig. 17 – Charnley low friction arthroplasty for replacement of hip joint.

(Adapted from illustrations of Howmedica, Inc., Rutherford, New Jersey).

Acrylic cement for fixation of acetabular component and intramedullary stem

Femoral component

Tibial component

Fig. 19 – Lateral view of total knee prosthesis

Fig. 18 – Geomedic prosthesis for replacement of knee joint.

(Courtesy: Howmedica, Inc., Rutherford, New Jersey).

Fig. 20 – Anterior view of prosthetic knee.

(3) Moore or Thompson prosthetic arthroplasty — surgical repair of arthritic hip including amputation of head and neck of femur, acetabular remodeling and reconstruction and seating of prosthesis in femoral shaft and acetabulum.[25]

(4) vitallium mold arthroplasty — molding a joint and interposing a nonirritating substance between bony surfaces to improve joint function and lessen pain in rheumatoid arthritis and bony or fibrous ankylosis. Interposition of material between joint surfaces such as autogenous fascia or inert metal (vitallium) also prevents recurrence of ankylosis.[25]

b. arthroplasties of the knee.

(1) compartmental total knee arthroplasty — reconstruction of the articulating surfaces limited to the affected compartment of the knee joint and correction of deformities in the presence of intact ligaments providing joint stability.[29]

(2) geomedic (or geometric) total knee arthroplasty — removal of sufficient bone and insertion of femoral and tibial components of the geomedic prosthesis for total knee replacement.[29, 57, 69]   See Figs. 18, 19 and 20.

(3) patellofemoral joint replacement — conservative surgical procedure in which a minimum of diseased bone is removed, a knee implant for resurfacing the patellofemoral joint is inserted and any interference with patellar ligaments avoided to safeguard joint stability.

(4) polycentric total knee arthroplasty — replacement of the involved articulating surfaces of the tibial plateaus and femoral condyles to relieve pain and restore joint motion and stability.[29, 57]

(5) Walldius arthroplasty — salvage operation for severe pain and instability of the knee joint in rheumatoid arthritis using a vitallium hinge prosthesis (Walldius) with 10 centimeter stems. Insertion of the prosthesis is done by the anterior transverse approach with retention of the knee cap and usually without acrylic cement since it fails to achieve joint stabilization.[65]

   c. arthroplasties of the shoulder.

     (1) partial shoulder arthroplasty, hemireplacement of shoulder — replacement of the articular surface of the humeral head by a Neer prosthesis in the presence of an intact rotator cuff and glenoid cavity.

     (2) total shoulder arthroplasty, total glenohumeral joint replacement — replacement of both the head of the humerus and the glenoid fossa in the presence of a massive tear or other defect in the rotator cuff.[48]

Indications for surgical intervention are disabling rheumatoid arthritis or osteoarthritis with a painful shoulder and limited joint motion which remain uncontrolled by conservative treatment.[37, 48, 54, 62]

   d. arthroplasty of temporomandibular joint — surgical breaking of a stiff joint to relieve disabling ankylosis caused by rheumatic, degenerative, infectious or traumatic arthritis.   The mandibular condyle is resected and remodeled.[66]

5. arthroscopy — endoscopic examination of the magnified joint, enhanced by fiberoptic light transmission and provision for joint irrigation to relieve pain from injury or arthritis. The procedure is primarily indicated in the detection of articular and meniscal lesions or other internal derangements of the knee.   Its usefulness in evaluating the hip, ankle, shoulder and elbow joints needs to be established.[39]

6. arthrotomy — surgical opening of a joint.

7. bunionectomy, surgical correction of valgus deformity — removal of bony prominence (bunion) from medial aspect of first metatarsal head.

8. chondrectomy — removal of a cartilage.

9. chondroplasty — plastic repair of a cartilage.

10. Harrington instrumentation and fusion — operation for correcting scoliosis and spondylolisthesis.   Metal rods and hooks are directly implanted on the spine.   Articular fusion is achieved by inserting bone grafts from the ilium.[10, 34]

11. synovectomy — partial or total removal of a synovial membrane lining of a joint capsule.

E. Symptomatic Terms:

1. arthralgia, arthrodynia — joint pain.

2. capsular laceration — tear of a joint capsule.

3. crepitus, articular — the grating of joints.

4. detachment of cartilage — separation of cartilaginous material from a joint.   Loose bodies limit motion.

5. effusion, hemorrhagic — bleeding into synovial sac.

6. effusion, synovial — an overproduction of joint fluid.

7. Heberden's nodes — hard nodules at the distal phalangeal joints of the fingers in osteoarthritis.

8. lipping — liplike bony growths at the joints in osteoarthritis; for example: the marginal lipping of the acetabular rim and head of the femur in degenerative hip disease.

9. lumbago — dull, aching pain in the lumbar region of back.

10. rheumatoid nodules — subcutaneous nodules located over bony prominences, e.g. elbow or back of heel.   They exert pressure and are present in advanced rheumatoid arthritis.

11. spur — projection from a bone.

12. tophus, pl. tophi — deposit of urate crystals in subcutaneous tissue near a joint.

DIAPHRAGM, MUSCLES, TENDONS

A. Origin of Terms:

1. fascia (L) — band

2. leios (G) — smooth

3. myo- (G) — muscle

4. phragm (G) — fence, wall

5. rhabdo- (G) — rod, striated

6. tendo-, teno- (G) — tendon

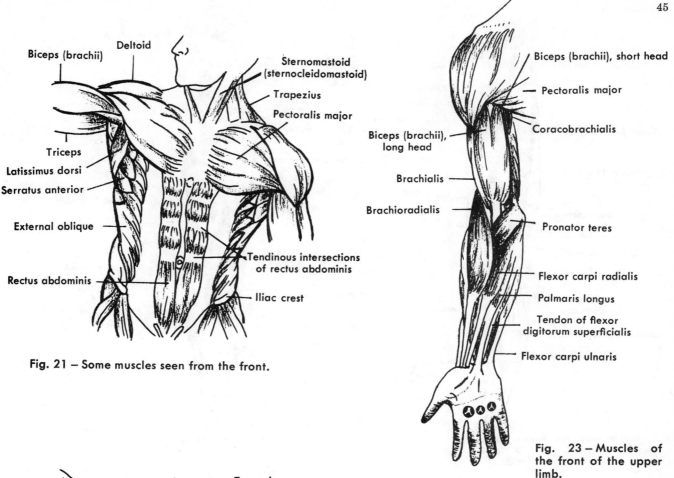

Fig. 21 – Some muscles seen from the front.

Fig. 23 – Muscles of the front of the upper limb.

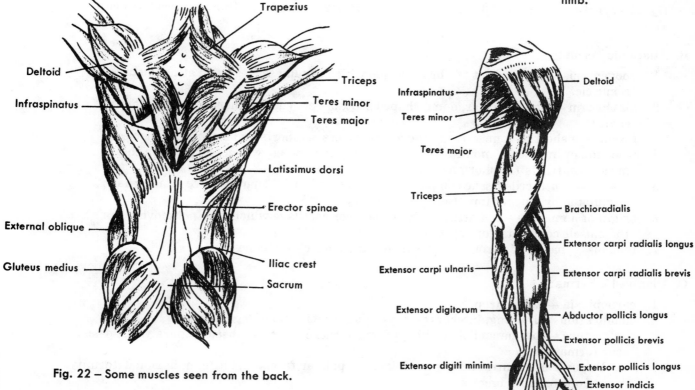

Fig. 22 – Some muscles seen from the back.

Fig. 24 – Muscles of the back of the upper limb.

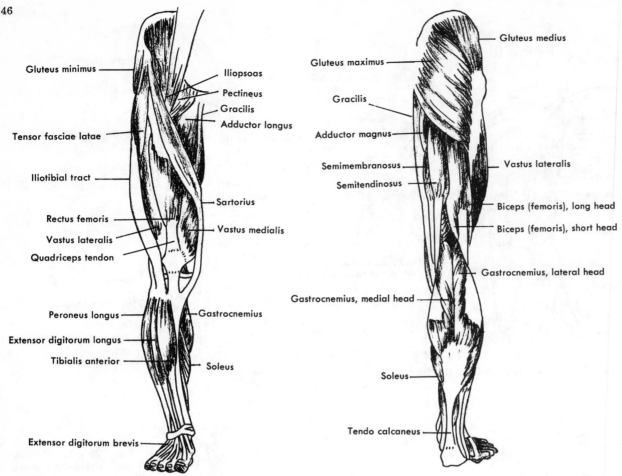

Fig. 25 — Muscles of the front of the lower limb.

Fig. 26 — Muscles of the back of the lower limb.

B. Anatomic Terms:

1. aponeurosis — a flat sheet of fibrous tissue which usually serves as an attachment for a muscle.
2. diaphragm — the muscular, dome-shaped septum between the thoracic and abdominal cavities.
3. fascia — a sheet of connective tissue which covers, supports and separates muscles.
4. insertion of muscle — end attached to the bone or cartilage which moves when the muscle contracts (or shortens).
5. muscle — contractile tissue composed of units that have the power to contract when stimulated by a nerve impulse.
6. origin of a muscle — end attached to the bone or cartilage which does not move when the muscle contracts (or shortens).
7. tendons — bands of fibrous tissue which attach muscles to bones.

C. Diagnostic Terms:

1. carpoptosia — wrist drop.
2. claudication — limping, intermittent type due to ischemia of leg muscles.
3. contracture — permanent shortening of one or more muscles caused by paralysis, spasm or scar formation.
   a. Dupuytren's contracture — shrinkage of palmar fascia resulting in flexion deformity of one or more fingers.
   b. Volkmann's contracture — flexion deformity of wrist and fingers which may be due to circulatory interference by a tight cast.

4. disuse atrophy — muscle wasting caused by immobilization.
5. fascitis, fasciitis — inflammation of the fascia.[26]
6. graphospasm — writer's cramp.
7. hiatus hernia, diaphragmatic hernia — protrusion of an abdominal organ, usually a portion of the stomach through the esophageal opening of the diaphragm.
8. leiomyoma — benign, smooth muscle tumor.
9. muscular dystrophy — progressive disease of unknown etiology, marked in infants by enlarged calves, waddling gait, sway back and winged shoulders. As the disease advances there is extensive wasting of muscles and development of bizarre deformities.
10. myasthenia gravis — chronic neuromuscular disorder, characterized by weakness, usually first manifested in ocular muscles resulting in bilateral ptosis of eye lids and sleepy appearance. The myasthenic facies is apathetic and expressionless. There may be involvement of the muscles of speech, mastication and swallowing. When the chest muscles are affected, dyspnea may develop. Infrequently weakness of the legs interferes with walking. Symptoms fluctuate in severity ranging from exacerbations to remissions.
11. myoma — benign muscular tumor.
12. myosarcoma — malignant muscular tumor.
13. myositis — inflammatory process of muscles.
14. paralysis — loss of sensation and voluntary movements, either temporary or permanent.
    a. flaccid — lower motor neuron involvement.
    b. spastic — upper motor neuron involvement.
15. polymyositis — a primary myopathy characterized by muscle weakness in pelvic and shoulder girdles, distal lower and upper extremities, muscle pain or tenderness. It may be associated with connective tissue disease.
16. rhabdomyoma — a striated muscle tumor.
17. tenosynovitis, tendosynovitis — inflammation of a tendon and its synovial sheath.
18. torticollis, wryneck — contraction of a sternocleidomastoid muscle, drawing the head to one side and causing asymmetry of face; may be congenital or acquired.

D. Operative Terms:

1. myoplasty — surgical repair of a muscle; for example, by free muscle graft or pedicle graft.
2. myorrhaphy — suture of a muscle.
3. myotasis — stretching of a muscle.
4. tenodesis — suture of end of tendon to skeletal attachment (tendon torn at point of insertion).
5. tenoplasty, tendoplasty — surgical repair of a tendon.
6. tenosynovectomy — resection or removal of a tendon sheath.

E. Symptomatic Terms:

1. clonic spasm — rapid, repeated, muscular contractions.
2. cramp — prolonged, intense spasm of one muscle.
3. hyperkinesia — purposeless, excessive, involuntary movements.
4. hypotonia — reduced muscle tension associated with muscular atrophy.
5. rigidity, rigor — stiffness, muscular hardness.
6. tonic spasm — excessive, prolonged, muscular contractions.
7. tremors — oscillating, rhythmic movements of muscle groups.

RADIOLOGY

A. Terms Related to Diagnostic Radiology:[14, 29, 84]

1. air arthrogram, pneumoarthrogram — air injection into a joint for radiographic evaluation. For example it is possible to outline the menisci of the knee and visualize major tears and displacements of large tears.

2. arthrography — contrast study of joints, an aid in establishing the diagnosis and giving guidance to the modality of treatment of joint disorders.
   a. knee arthrogram — double contrast x-ray study of the knee for evaluating the menisci and articular cartilage. The arthrogram delineates a torn meniscus, abnormality of the patellar mechanism, chondromalacia or derangement of the knee joint.[42]
   b. shoulder arthrogram — radiographic study of shoulder joint to determine the cause of shoulder pain such as recurrent dislocation or subluxation of the shoulder, rotator cuff tears or anterior abnormalities of the rotator cuff, soft tissue injuries or anterior capsular derangement.[55]
   c. wrist arthrogram — radiographic study of the radiocarpal and distal radioulnar joints to demonstrate traumatic injury or a difficult wrist ganglion which may be associated with carpal tunnel syndrome.[55]
3. scanogram — a radiogram of a structure of the body using special technique for accurate measurements of its length. Scanograms are made to determine the length of the medullary canal before medullary fixation is attempted. The selection of the medullary nail depends on scanographic findings.
4. scanography — a method of x-ray examination for accurate measurement of the length of structures of the body usually of the long bones. It is used to determine leg length discrepancy.
5. stereoradiography, stereoroentgenography, stereoskiagraphy (stereo (G) - solid) — obtaining an x-ray picture from two similar positions to give the object seen an appearance of relief, depth and solidity.
6. tomography of skeleton — body section radiography for the diagnosis of bone disorders. Extraneous structures overlying the region under study are blurred enabling the tomograms to clearly demonstrate osteolytic and inflammatory lesions, exquisite detail of joint derangements, erosions and ischemic necrosis which cannot be seen on the conventional radiogram.[56]
7. xeroradiography (xeros (G) - dry) — the taking of a radiogram by using a selenium coated plate and developing it without liquid chemicals.

B. Terms Related to Therapeutic Radiology:

1. radiation necrosis of bone — bone destruction by ionizing radiation or radioactive substances.
2. radiotherapy — radiant energy used in the treatment of disease. Radiotherapy combined with chemotherapy is used in the treatment of metastatic sarcoma to relieve bone pain. In Ewing's sarcoma local irradiation of the primary site together with systemic antineoplastic drugs as treatment has lengthened the period of survival and made complete tumor eradication a probability.[67, 71]
3. radiosensitive — capable of responding to irradiation.
4. radioresistant — incapable of receiving benefit from irradiation.

CLINICAL LABORATORY

A. Terms Related to Blood Chemistry:

1. serum calcium determination — a function test of the parathyroids which produce parathormone. This hormone is concerned with the regulation of the calcium content of the blood. Calcium is important in bone production.
2. serum phosphorus determination — a test designed to obtain the concentration of phosphorus in blood serum. Calcium phosphate is found in the bones and teeth.

B. Terms Related to Urine Studies:

1. Bence-Jones protein — a peculiar type of protein molecule which is excreted in the urine in the majority of cases of multiple myeloma, amyloidosis and in certain bone tumors.[63]
2. determination of calcium in urine and feces — these tests are concerned with the calcium balance in the body.

3. normal calcium balance — in health the calcium intake exceeds the calcium excretion of urine and feces together.

C. Terms Related to the Specific Diagnosis of Joint Disease.

1. F-II latex fixation test — serologic test for the detection of the rheumatoid factor (RF).
2. serum uric acid determination — abnormal increase in serum uric acid usually indicative of gouty arthritis or gout.
3. synovial fluid studies — examination of joint fluid to aid in the diagnostic and prognostic evaluation of joint disease by demonstrating the severity of the inflammatory process of synovial tissue. In most cases the synovial fluid is obtained by aspirating the suprapatellar space of the knee joint. The examination includes:
   a. appearance and consistency of joint fluid.
   b. culture of synovial fluid to detect the presence or absence of infective agent.
   c. cytology of joint fluid: red and white cell counts, differential count, identification of crystals such as urate crystals.[64]

Table 2

SERUM CALCIUM AND SERUM PHOSPHORUS IN BONE DISEASES

Serum	Normal Values[a]	Increased Values	Decreased Values
Calcium Adults Children Infants	Method of Clark - Collip 9.5-11.0 mg/dl .... or 4.7-5.5 mEq/L 10.0-11.5 mg/dl .... or 5.0-5.8 mEq/L 10.5-12.0 mg/dl .... or 5.2-6.0 mEq/L	Multiple myeloma Metastases to bone	Renal osteodystrophy Osteomalacia
Phosphorus Adults Children Infants	Colorimeter Method of Bodansky 2.5- 4.0 mg/dl .... 4.5- 5.5 mg/dl .... 5.5- 6.5 mg/dl	Renal osteodystrophy	Rickets Osteomalacia

a Cf. Opal E. Hepler. *Manual of Clinical Laboratory Methods*, 4th ed. Springfield, Illinois: Charles C. Thomas, 1955, pp. 305-309. The abbreviation **mEq/L** refers to milliequivalents per liter.

Table 3

CALCIUM IN URINE AND FECES IN BONE DISEASES

Calcium	Normal Values[a] Method of Wang	Increased Values	Decreased Values
Urine	50-300 mg per 24 hour specimen (Range of 0.2 to 4.6 mg per kg)	Metastases to bone Multiple myeloma Paget's disease	Osteomalacia Renal osteodystrophy Rickets
Feces	0.4-0.8 gm in 24 hrs. depending on Ca intake Average of 70% of total Ca excreted by body	....	Osteomalacia ....

a *Ibid.*, pp. 305-307.

ABBREVIATIONS

A. General:

ASS — anterior superior spine
AP — anteroposterior
Ca — calcium, cancer
CDH — congenital dislocation of
    the hip
C_1 — first cervical vertebra
C_2 — second cervical vertebra
DIP — distal interphalangeal (joint)
D_1 — first dorsal vertebra
D_2 — second dorsal vertebra
EMG — electromyogram
Fx — fracture
IDK — internal derangement of the
    knee
IM — intramuscular
IS — intercostal space

LCP — Legg-Calvé-Perthes (disease)
LIF — left iliac fossa
LLE — left lower extremity
LOM — limitation of motion
L_1 — first lumbar vertebra
L_2 — second lumbar vertebra
LUE — left upper extremity
MP — metacarpal-phalangeal
MSL — midsternal line
Ortho — orthopedics
PIP — proximal interphalangeal (joint)
RIF — right iliac fossa
RLE — right lower extremity
ROM — range of motion
RUE — right upper extremity

B. Amputations and Prostheses:

AE — above the elbow
AK — above the knee
BE — below the elbow
BK — below the knee
HD — hip disarticulation
HP — hemipelvectomy
KB — knee bearing

KD — knee disarticulation
PTB — patellar tendon bearing
    (prosthesis)
SACH — solid ankle cushion heel
    (foot prosthesis)
SD — shoulder disarticulation
THR — total hip replacement
TKR — total knee replacement

C. Organizations:

MDAA — Muscular Dystrophy
    Association of America, Inc.

NSCCA — National Society for
    Crippled Children and Adults

ORAL READING PRACTICE

Paget's Disease of Bone

When in 1877 Sir James Paget described the disease which now bears his name, he erroneously called it osteitis deformans considering it a form of chronic **inflammatory** affection of osseous tissue.   Paget's disease is a peculiar bone disorder with an insidious onset, **asymptomatic** early phase, a plateau of apparent stationary involvement, perhaps lasting years, followed by progressive disease and complications which may terminate life.   Its **etiology** is unknown.   It is not a metabolic disturbance since it primarily attacks bones under pressure of weight bearing, leaving those of the upper body relatively untouched.   An exception is the skull which shows radiologic evidence of **osteoporosis circumscripta,** so termed because **osteoporotic** changes are limited to a circumscribed area.

The incidence of Paget's disease of bone is highest in advancing years and greater in males than in females.   It is a rather common affliction amounting to three percent in the age group past forty.

The pathologic characteristics comprise concurrent processes of **osteoclastic** and **osteoblastic** activity resulting in marked bone destruction and rapid bone repair, architectural abnormality of new bone, increased **vascularity** and **fibrosis.**   Instead of normal resorption and replacement of bone, metabolic processes are disorganized and irregular. New bone may undergo osteolysis as soon as it is formed. Osteoblasts produce coarse, distorted **trabeculae** which **anastomose** in a peculiar fashion exhibiting a mosaic design.

In the skull **osteolytic** (osteoclastic) activity predominates. A lesion of **decalcification** forms, particularly in the outer **cranial** table. It is termed **osteoporosis circumscripta.** Gradually dense areas resembling tufts of cotton appear in the **rarefied** lesion and the **demarcation** between **diploë,** the two cranial tables, becomes indistinct.

The patient's **contour** portrays the influence of pathologic, skeletal changes in advanced Paget's disease. His spine is **kyphotic,** stature shortened, position crouched and abdomen pendulous. The **anterolateral** bowing of his legs results in a waddling, slow gait. The face appears small compared to the protruding skull, which characteristically shows **bitemporal** enlargement.

Pain develops with progressive bone involvement and varies from a mild dull ache to intermittent or persistent **ostealgia.** Fractures occur frequently, heal readily and are the most common complication of Paget's disease. They may be occasioned by trivial incidents such as tripping on stairs or turning in bed.

The patient with Paget's disease, immobilized because of fracture or intercurrent disease, is likely to develop **hypercalciuria, renal calculi** and **hypercalcemia.** Since bone repair is markedly decreased during immobilization, **osteoporosis** of disuse becomes a problematic issue. Bone destruction persists unabated, thus liberating an excessive amount of calcium which is spilled into urine instead of being **deposited** in bone. This may lead to **nephrolithiasis** and serious **sequelae.** If the kidneys are unable to handle the high surplus of calcium, hypercalcemia is prone to develop. It is signalled by dryness of mouth and nose, nausea and vomiting. Untreated, the **prognosis** may be fatal.

Malignant degeneration of diseased bone is a constant threat. Whenever **osteogenic sarcoma, fibrosarcoma** or malignant **osteoclastoma** develop, the patient has probably reached the terminal phase of his life. **Palliative** measures must be instituted to bring relief of ostealgia and other distressing symptoms.[2, 45, 73]

Table 4

SOME ORTHOPEDIC CONDITIONS AMENABLE TO SURGERY

Organs Involved	Diagnoses	Operations	Procedures
Rib	Supernumerary rib	Costectomy	Removal of rib
Shoulder	Chronic tendinitis	Partial acromionectomy	Removal of outer edge of acromion
Shoulder	Calcified deposits in rotator cuff	Curettment of rotator cuff	Split deltoid approach and scraping of cuff to remove deposits
Shoulder	Severe rheumatoid arthritis of shoulder — or Advanced glenohumeral osteoarthritis Massive tear in rotator cuff	Total shoulder arthroplasty (total glenohumeral joint replacement)	Detachment of deltoid from clavicle and anterior acromion Division of subscapularis Preparation of medullary canal Excision of head of humerus and insertion of revised humeral prosthesis Glenoid component anchored with acrylic cement Meticulous repair of deltoid and scapularis tendon[a]
Humerus	Osteomyelitis of humerus	Osteotomy with curettage and drainage	Surgical opening of bone, scraping of medullary canal and insertion of drain

Organs Involved	Diagnoses	Operations	Procedures
Humerus	Sequestrum	Sequestrectomy and saucerization	Excision of dead bone and removal of infected or foreign matter, scar and granulation tissue
Ulna Radius	Crushing injury with loss of blood supply to hand and wrist	Amputation of forearm	Removal of forearm below elbow
		Biceps cineplasty for operating prosthetic device	Construction of skin tunnel through biceps muscle; tunneled muscle to move artificial hand
Hand Wrist joint	Traumatic severence of hand Disarticulation at wrist joint	Replantation of hand Internal fixation with Kirschner wires	First wire passed through carpus and up the medullary cavity of radius Second wire crossed from base of 5th metacarpal through cortex of radius Repair of vessels and tendons
Carpal tunnel Transverse carpal ligament Median nerve	Carpal tunnel syndrome	Surgical division and partial excision of transverse carpal ligament Synovectomy of flexor synovialis	Complete section and partial removal of carpal ligament Removal of thickened synovial membrane to decompress the median nerve
Spine	Scoliosis	Harrington's operation instrumentation and fusion for correction of scoliosis	Implantation of metal rods and hooks directly on the spine followed by fusion to provide distractive and compressive forces of spinal curve
Spine	Spondylolisthesis	Modified Hibbs arthrodesis of spine	Excision of cartilage from articular facets, packing bone chips into joint spaces; iliac bone grafting
Hip joint	Early degenerative arthritis	High femoral osteotomy	Incision through upper end of femur usually in subtrochanteric region Medial displacement of distal femur resulting in change in weight bearing position of femoral head[a]
Hip joint	Degenerative arthritis	Vitallium mold arthroplasty Austin Moore or Fred Thompson arthroplasty	Reconstruction of femoral head and placement of deep cup over head Replacement of femoral head with hip prosthesis
Hip joint	Advanced rheumatoid arthritis and ankylosing spondylitis of hip — or Advanced osteoarthritis	Charnley low-friction arthroplasty for total hip replacement	Lateral oblique incision to expose upper end of femoral shaft Dislocation of hip and removal of femoral head and neck and of destructive joint lesions Insertion of small femoral head and stem in shaft Cement used for seating the acetabular cup and prosthetic stem to provide rigid fixation[a, b]

Organs Involved	Diagnoses	Operations	Procedures
Hip joint	Congenital dislocation of hip	Colonna capsular arthroplasty	*First stage* Hamstring stretching and surgical division of adductor tendon *Second stage* Reconstruction of acetabulum Placement of capsule-covered femoral head into reconstructed acetabulum
Femur	Slipped femoral epiphysis	Trochanteric osteotomy	Section of femur, abduction and internal rotation of distal fragment, blade-plate fixation
Femur	Fracture of femoral neck	Excision of femoral head and insertion of hip prosthesis Fred Thompson or Austin Moore type Internal fixation by insertion of Smith-Petersen nail	Removal of femoral head and most of neck — replacement by metal prosthesis Three flanged nail driven over guide wire through femoral neck and head, guide wire removed
Femur	Intertrochanteric fracture of femur	Internal fixation by insertion of hip nail Jewett type or Neufeld type or Key type or Holt type	Nail driven over guide wire through femoral neck and into head of femur, side plate fixed to shaft with screws
Femur	Transverse diaphyseal fracture of femur	Internal fixation by insertion of intramedullary nail Küntscher type or Lottes type	Medullary nail driven over guide wire into medullary cavity occupying the entire canal
Knee	Recurrent dislocation of patella	Hauser operation	Medial and distal transplantation of tibial tubercle and its patellar tendonᶜ
Knee	Chondromalacia of patella	Patellaplasty Complete patellectomy	Partial resection and plastic repair of patella Removal of patella
Knees	Genu valgum	Stapling operation	Oblique skin incision Stapling the medial femoral condyles
Tibia Fibula Foot	Crushing injury and uncontrollable infection of distal portion of lower extremity	Below-knee amputation	Incision of skin flaps Division of anterolateral muscles Ligation of blood vessels Removal of leg and stump closure Application of rigid elastic plaster dressing and prosthetic unit

Organs Involved	Diagnoses	Operations	Procedures
Foot	Hallus valgus deformity	Keller operation	Resection of proximal half of first phalanx of great toe Excision of bony prominence
Anterior cruciate ligament	Tear of anterior cruciate ligament, separation of anterior attachment	Reconstruction of torn anterior cruciate ligament	Repair of ligament by restoring the anterior attachment
Quadriceps tendon	Old rupture of quadriceps tendon	Repair of old rupture of quadriceps tendon-application of cast	Approximation of tendon ends with heavy braided silk sutures; cast applied with knee extension
Tendon Achilles or Tendon calcaneus	Abnormal shortening of tendon calcaneus	Tenoplasty with lengthening of tendon calcaneus	Surgical repair of tendon
Synovium Tendon sheath	Synovioma highly malignant fibroblastic sarcoma of ankle of foot	Radical removal of malignant synovioma Regional lymph node dissection — or Amputation of the affected limb	Wide excision of neoplasm Removal of lymph nodes Removal of foot and lymph nodes
Sternocleido-mastoid muscle	Torticollis, congenital	Brown and McDowell excision of sternocleidomastoid muscle Tenotomy of upper and lower end of sternocleidomastoid muscle or both ends	Abnormal muscle freed from underlying structures and excised Muscle lengthened by division of one or both ends allowing shortened muscle to retract
Flexor muscles of hip	Hip flexion contracture in spastic cerebral palsy	Myotomies for release of spastic hip flexor muscles	Surgical division of all taut flexor muscles of hip

a Robert M. O'Brien, M.D. Personal communications.

b L. P. Brady. Charnley low friction arthroplasty. *Clinical Orthopaedics and Related Research*, 118: 7-9, July-August, 1976.

c M. Stewart. Dislocations. In Crenshaw, A. H. (ed.). *Campbell's Operative Orthopaedics*, 5th ed. St. Louis: The C. V. Mosby Company, 1971, p. 451.

REFERENCES AND BIBLIOGRAPHY

1. Aegerter, Ernest and Kirkpatrick, John. The skeletal dysplasias. In *Orthopedic Diseases*, 4th ed. Philadelphia: W. B. Saunders Co., 1975, pp. 87-200.

2. _____. Miscellaneous diseases of the skeleton. *Ibid.*, pp. 407-458.

3. _____. Tumors and tumor-like processes. *Ibid.*, pp. 461-620.

4. _____. Metabolic diseases of bone. *Ibid.*, pp. 331-375.

5. _____. Diseases of joints and muscles — Soft part tumors. *Ibid.*, pp. 623-775.

6. Aglietti, P. *et al.* A new patella prosthesis design and application. *Clinical Orthopaedics and Related Research*, 107: 175-187, March-April, 1975.

7. Albright, J. P. *et al.* Treatment for fixation complications: Femoral neck fractures. *Archives of Surgery*, 110: 30-36, January, 1975.

8. Albright, J. P. *et al.* Osteogenesis imperfecta tarda — The morphology of rib biopsies. *Clinical Orthopaedics and Related Research*, 108: 204-213, May, 1975.

9. Amstutz, H. C. *et al.* Total joint replacement for ankylosed hips. *Journal of Bone and Joint Surgery*, 57-A: 619-625, July, 1975.

10. Armstrong, G. W. D. A transverse loading system applied to a modified Harrington instrumentation. *Clinical Orthopaedics and Related Research*, 108: 70-75, May, 1975.

11. Askin, S. R. *et al.* Femoral neck fractures in young adults. *Clinical Orthopaedics and Related Research*, 114: 259-264, January-February, 1976.

12. Bakamjian, V. Y. Use of temporal muscle flap for reconstruction after orbito-maxillary resections for cancer. *Plastic and Reconstructive Surgery*, 56: 171-177, August, 1975.

13. Bauze, R. J. *et al.* A new look at osteogenesis imperfecta. *Journal of Bone and Joint Surgery*, 57-B: 2-12, February, 1975.

14. Brady, L. P. Charnley low friction arthroplasty. *Clinical Orthopaedics and Related Research*, 118: 7-9, July-August, 1976.

15. Cameron, H. U. *et al.* Observations on osteoarthritis of the hip joint. *Clinical Orthopaedics and Related Research*, 108: 31-40, May, 1975.

16. Carbanela, M. E. Total hip replacement arthroplasty. *Geriatrics*, 31: 61-66, March, 1976.

17. Carnesale, P. G. *et al.* Primary prosthetic replacement for femoral neck fractures. *Archives of Surgery*, 110: 27-29, January, 1975.

18. Christian, C. L. Diseases of the joints. In Beeson, P. B. and McDermott, W. (eds.). *Textbook of Medicine*, 14th ed. Philadelphia: W. B. Saunders Co., 1975, pp. 150-163.

19. Convery, F. R. *et al.* The relative safety of polymethylmethacrylate. A controlled clinical study of randomly selected patients treated with Charnley and Ring total hip replacements. *Journal of Bone and Joint Surgery*, 57-A: 57-64, January, 1975.

20. Dandy, D. J. *et al.* The management of local complications of total hip replacement by the McKee-Farrar technique. *Journal of Bone and Joint Surgery*, 57-B: 30-35, February, 1975.

21. Dingman, R. O. *et al.* Surgical corrections of lesions of the temporomandibular joints. *Plastic and Reconstructive Surgery*, 55: 335-340, March, 1975.

22. Ecker, M. L. *et al.* The treatment of trochanteric hip fractures using a compression screw. *Journal of Bone and Joint Surgery*, 57-A: 23-27, January, 1975.

23. Engleman, E. P. *et al.* Arthritis and allied rheumatic disorders. In Krupp, Marcus A. and Chatton, Milton. *Current Medical Diagnosis and Treatment*, 15th ed. Los Altos, California: Lange Medical Publications, 1976, pp. 477-501.

24. Ferguson, A. B. The pathology of Legg-Perthes disease and its comparison with aseptic necrosis. *Clinical Orthopaedics and Related Research*, 106: 7-18, January-February, 1975.

25. Freedman, M. T. Radiologic aspects of femoral head replacements and cup mold arthroplasties. *Radiologic Clinics of North America*, 13: 45-56, April, 1975.

26. Furey, G. J. Plantar fasciitis. The painful heel syndrome. *Journal of Bone and Joint Surgery*, 57-A: 672-673, July, 1975.

27. Gardner, E. *et al.* Anatomy — A Regional Study of Human Structure, 3rd. ed. Philadelphia: W. B. Saunders Co., 1969.

28. Gelberman, R. H. *et al.* Supraclavicular nerve-entrapment syndrome. *Journal of Bone and Joint Surgery*, 57-A: 119, January, 1975.

29. Gilula, L. A. *et al.* Radiology of recently developed total knee prostheses. *Radiologic Clinics of North America*, 13: 57-66, April, 1975.

30. Gold, R. H. *et al.* Surgical procedures for congenital dislocations of the hip. *Radiologic Clinics of North America*, 13: 123-137, April, 1975.

31. Goldberg, V. M. *et al.* Osteoid osteoma of the hip in children. *Clinical Orthopaedics and Related Research*, 106: 41-47, January-February, 1975.

32. Green, P. *et al.* Benign chondroblastoma. Case report with pulmonary metastasis. *Journal of Bone and Joint Surgery*, 57-A: 418-420, April, 1975.

33. Hamilton, L. R. *et al.* Experience with total hip replacement at Ochsner Clinic. *Southern Medical Journal*, 68: 575-579, May, 1975.

34. Harrington, P. R. *et al.* Spinal instrumentation in the treatment of spondylolisthesis. *Clinical Orthopaedics and Related Research*, 117: 157-163, June, 1976.

35. Heaney, R. P. The osteoporoses — The osteomalacias — Renal osteodystrophy. In Beeson, B. P. and McDermott, W. (eds.). *Textbook of Medicine*, 14th ed. Philadelphia: W. B. Saunders Co., 1975, pp. 1826-1835.

36. Hinderer, U. T. Malar implants for improvement of the facial appearance. *Plastic and Reconstructive Surgery*, 56: 157-165, August, 1975.

37. Hughes, M. and Neer, C. S. Glenohumeral joint replacement and postoperative rehabilitation. *Physical Therapy*, 55: 850-858, August, 1975.

38. Huvos, A. G. Primary fibrosarcoma of bone — A clinicopathologic study of 130 patients. *Cancer*, 35: 837-847, March, 1975.

39. Jackson, R. W. *et al.* Arthroscopy of the knee. *Clinical Orthopaedics and Related Research*, 107: 87-92, March-April, 1975.

40. Jergesen, F. H. Bone and joint diseases. In Krupp, Marcus A. and Chatton, Milton. *Current Medical Diagnosis and Treatment*, 15th ed. Los Altos, California: Lange Medical Publications, 1976, pp. 502-520.

41. Johnson, C. F. *et al.* Preventing emboli after total hip replacement. *American Journal of Nursing*, 75: 804-806, May, 1975.

42. Kaye, J. J. *et al.* Arthrography of the knee. *Clinical Orthopaedics and Related Research*, 107: 73-80, March-April, 1975.

43. Keim, H. A. *et al.* Osteoid osteoma as a cause of scoliosis. *Journal of Bone and Joint Surgery*, 57-A: 159-163, March, 1975.

44. Kiehn, C. L. *et al.* Surgical correction of lesions of the temporomandibular joints. *Plastic and Reconstructive Surgery*, 55: 484-486, April, 1975.

45. Kolb, F. O. Metabolic bone diseases — Nonmetabolic bone disease. In Krupp, Marcus A. and Chatton, Milton. *Current Medical Diagnosis and Treatment*, 15th ed. Los Altos, California: Lange Medical Publications, 1976, pp. 679-686.

46. Langer, F. *et al.* The immunogenicity of fresh and frozen allogeneic bone. *Journal of Bone and Joint Surgery*, 57-A: 216-220, March, 1975.

47. Laros, G. S. Current views of hip fracture — Intertrochanteric fractures. *Archives of Surgery*, 110: 18-19 and 37-40, January, 1975.

48. Linscheid, R. L. *et al.* Total shoulder arthroplasty. *Geriatrics*, 31: 64-69, April, 1976.

49. Loyd, R. D. *et al.* Acute slipped capital femoral epiphysis. *Southern Medical Journal*, 68: 857-862, July, 1975.

56

50. Mac Ewen, D. *et al.* Acute neurological complications in the treatment of scoliosis. A report of the Scoliosis Research Society. *Journal of Bone and Joint Surgery*, 57-A: 404-408, April, 1975.

51. Macnab, I. Cervical spondylosis. *Clinical Orthopaedics and Related Research*, 109: 69-77, June, 1975.

52. Marsh, B. W. *et al.* Benign osteoblastoma: Range of manifestations. *Journal of Bone and Joint Surgery*, 57-A: 1-9, January, 1975.

53. Nachemson, A. *et al.* Syposium — spondylolisthesis. *Clinical Orthopaedics and Related Research*, 117: 2-178, June, 1976.

54. Neer, C. S. Replacement arthroplasty for glenohumeral osteoarthritis. *Journal of Bone and Joint Surgery*, 56-A: 1-13, January, 1974.

55. Nelson, C. L. *et al.* Upper extremity arthrography. *Clinical Orthopaedics and Related Research*, 107: 62-72, March-April, 1975.

56. Norman, A. The use of tomography in the diagnosis of skeletal disorders. *Clinical Orthopaedics and Related Research*, 107: 139-145, March-April, 1975.

57. O'Brien, Robert M. M.D. Personal communications.

58. Oh, I. *et al.* Closed intramedullary nailing for ununited femoral shaft fractures. *Clinical Orthopaedics and Related Research*, 106: 206-215, January-February, 1975.

59. Ohno, T. *et al.* Osteogenic sarcoma — A study of one hundred and thirty cases. *Journal of Bone and Joint Surgery*, 57-A: 397-404, April, 1975.

60. Paletta, F. X. Replantation of the amputated extremity. *Annals of Surgery*, 168: 720-727, October, 1968.

61. Pankovich, A. M. Primary internal fixation of femoral neck fractures. *Archives of Surgery*, 110: 20-26, January, 1975.

62. Paradis, D. K. and Ferlic, D. C. Shoulder arthroplasty in rheumatoid arthritis. *Physical Therapy*, 55: 157-159, February, 1975.

63. Perry, M. C. *et al.* The clinical significance of Bence Jones proteinuria. *Mayo Clinic Proceedings*, 50: 234-238, May, 1975.

64. Phalen, G. S. The carpal-tunnel syndrome. Seventeen years' experience in diagnosis and treatment of 654 hands. *Journal of Bone and Joint Surgery*, 48-A: 211-228, March, 1966.

65. Phillips, H. *et al.* The Walldius hinge arthroplasty. *Journal of Bone and Joint Surgery*, 57-B: 59-62, February, 1975.

66. Pinals, R. S. Traumatic arthritis and allied conditions. In Hollander, Joseph L. and Mc Carty, Daniel J. *Arthritis and Allied Conditions*, 8th ed. Philadelphia: Lea & Febiger, 1972, pp. 1391-1410.

67. Pomeroy, T. C. Combined modality therapy of Ewing's sarcoma. *Cancer*, 35: 36-47, January, 1975.

68. Pritchard, D. J. *et al.* Ewing's sarcoma. *Journal of Bone and Joint Surgery*, 57-A: 10-16, January, 1975.

69. Reckling, F. W. Performance analysis of an ex vivo geomedic total knee prosthesis. *Journal of Bone and Joint Surgery*, 57-A: 108-112, January, 1975.

70. Robbins, P. *et al.* Scoliosis in Marfan's syndrome. Its characteristics and results of treatment in thirty-four patients. *Journal of Bone and Joint Surgery*, 57-A: 358-367, April, 1975.

71. Rosen, G. *et al.* Combination chemotherapy and radiation therapy in the treatment of metastatic osteogenic sarcoma. *Cancer*, 35: 622-630, March, 1975.

72. Sarmiento, A. *et al.* Colles' fractures. Functional bracing in supination. *Journal of Bone and Joint Surgery*, 57-A: 311-317, April, 1975.

73. Saville, P. D. Paget's disease of bone: Osteitis deformans. In Beeson, P. B. and McDermott, W. (eds.). *Textbook of Medicine*, 14th ed. Philadelphia: W. B. Saunders Co., 1975, pp. 1841-1843.

74. _____. Fibrous dysplasia. *Ibid.*, p. 1843.

75. Schaller, J. G. *et al.* Juvenile rheumatoid arthritis — Ankylosing spondylitis. In Vaughan, Victor C. III and McKay, R. James. *Nelson Textbook of Pediatrics*. Philadelphia: W. B. Saunders Co. 1975, pp. 522-532.

76. Seki, T. *et al.* Malignant transformation of benign osteoblastoma. A case report. *Journal of Bone and Joint Surgery*, 57-A: 424-426, April, 1975.

77. Shapiro, F. *et al.* The Mitchell distal metatarsal osteotomy in the treatment of hallux valgus. *Clinical Orthopaedics and Related Research*, 107: 225-231, March-April, 1975.

78. Shelton, M. L. Subtrochanteric fractures of the femur. *Archives of Surgery*, 110: 41-48, January, 1975.

79. Sim, F. H. *et al.* Osteoid osteoma: Diagnostic problems. *Journal of Bone and Joint Surgery*, 57-A: 154-159, March, 1975.

80. Sprague, B. L. Proximal interphalangeal joint injuries and their initial treatment. *Journal of Trauma*, 15: 380-385, May, 1975.

81. Staudt, A. R. Femur replacement. *American Journal of Nursing*, 75: 1346-1348, August, 1975.

82. Tooms, R. E. Amputations. In Crenshaw, A. H. *Campbell's Operative Orthopaedics*. St. Louis: The C. V. Mosby Co., 1971, pp. 885-889.

83. Tornberg, D. N. *et al.* Multicentric giant-cell tumors in the long bones. A case report. *Journal of Bone and Joint Surgery*, 57-A: 420-422, April, 1975.

84. Weir, Don C. Roentgenographic signs of cervical injury. *Clinical Orthopaedics and Related Research*, 109: 9-17, June, 1975.

85. Wiltse, L. L. *et al.* Fatigue fracture: The basic lesion in isthmic spondylolisthesis. *Journal of Bone and Joint Surgery*, 57-A: 17-22, January, 1975.

Chapter IV
Neurologic and Psychiatric Disorders
NERVES

A. Origin of Terms:

1. axon (G) — axis
2. dendron (G) — tree
3. ganglion (G) — knot
4. lemma (G) — sheath
5. nucleus (L) — little kernel
6. plexus (L) — braid
7. radicle (L) — root
8. synapse (G) — clasp

B. Anatomic Terms:

1. nerve — a collection of many nerve fibers.
   a. cranial nerves — 12 pairs of nerves made up of either motor or sensory fibers or both.
   b. spinal nerves — 31 pairs of mixed nerves.
2. nerve cell, neuron — basic component of nerve tissue consisting of a cell body or neuron body and one or more processes. The neuron is the anatomic unit of the central nervous system.
   a. structure of neurons[16, 17]
      (1) axon, axone — slender process of a neuron body arising from specialized protoplasm known as axon hill. It contains many neurofibrils but **no** Nissl bodies.
      (2) cell body — neuron body composed of a nucleus embedded in cytoplasm which contains neurofibrils, Nissl bodies, mitochondria and others. The cell body maintains the nutrition of the whole neuron.
      (3) dendrite, dendron — a protoplasmic extension from the cell body forming an irregular knobby process, which is wide at the base and narrows down rapidly. Dendrites greatly increase the cell body's receptive surface.
      (4) effector — organ of response which reacts to the impulse, for example, a muscle or a gland.
      (5) ganglion (pl. ganglia) — a collection of neural cell bodies lying outside the central nervous system.
      (6) myelin sheath — protective covering of axons, composed of lipids and protein and interrupted by constrictions, the nodes of Ranvier.
      (7) neurilemma, neurolemma, sheath of Schwann — a thin, cellular membrane covering the axis cylinder of a non-medullated nerve fiber or enclosing the myelin sheath of a medullated nerve fiber of **peripheral nerves.**
      (8) neurofibrils — delicate threads found in the cell bodies and processes of neurons.
      (9) Nissl bodies — RNA (ribose nucleic acid) granules present in the cell bodies of neurons.
      (10) receptor — end organ which responds to various stimuli (pain, touch, and others) and converts them into nervous impulses.[16, 17]
   b. classification according to function
      (1) afferent neurons — conduct impulses from receptor to central nervous system.
      (2) association, intercalated or internuncial neurons — located within the central nervous system; transmit impulses between neurons.
      (3) efferent neurons — conduct impulses away from the central nervous system to the effector organ.[16, 17]
3. nerve fiber — the axon with its sheaths.
4. plexus (pl. plexuses) of spinal nerves — a network of nerve fibers. For example:
   a. brachial plexus — an intermingling of the 5th through 8th cervical and the 1st thoracic nerves which supply the upper limb.
   b. sacral plexus — an intermingling of the 4th and 5th lumbar and first four sacral nerves which help to supply the lower limb.

5. roots of spinal nerves — they attach the nerves to the spinal cord.
   a. ventral (anterior) root — composed of efferent fibers and has no ganglion.
   b. dorsal (posterior) root — composed of afferent fibers and has a small ganglion.
6. synapse — the point of contact between the axon of one neuron and a dendrite or cell body of another neuron.[16, 17]

C. Diagnostic Terms:

1. Bell's palsy — a functional disorder of the seventh cranial nerve which may result in a unilateral paralysis of facial muscles, and distortion of taste perception. Etiology is unknown.
2. causalgia — posttraumatic paroxysms of unbearable peripheral nerve pain of a burning quality aggravated by heat, slight friction, anxiety and emotion. It appears to be stimulated by efferent sympathetic nerve impulses.[86, 47]
3. Guillain-Barré syndrome, acute idiopathic polyneuropathy — widespread disorder of the peripheral motor nerves, characterized by progressive flaccid paralysis of an ascending type associated with sensory disturbances. When the chest muscles and diaphragm become affected, respiratory difficulties arise. Cranial nerve involvement, particularly that of the facial nerve, may develop last in the course of the disease, or it may be the initial pathology followed by motor impairment of a descending type.[25, 64]
4. herniated nucleus pulposus, herniated intervertebral disc — tear in posterior joint capsule and bulging of portions of intervertebral disc resulting in nerve root irritation and compression followed by sciatic pain and paresthesias and occasionally by paresis or paralysis.[101]
5. neurilemoma, neurilemmoma* — usually a benign, encapsulated, solitary tumor, produced by the proliferation of Schwann cells. It may originate from a sympathetic, peripheral or cranial nerve.[57]
6. neuroma — a tumor of tissue found in nervous system; obsolete term, a more specific designation is preferable, e.g.:
   a. ganglioneuroma — true neuroma.
   b. pseudoneuroma, amputation neuroma — false neuroma or traumatic neuroma.
7. polyneuritis, polyneuropathy — widespread neural lesions due to nutritional deficiencies especially of vitamin B complex. The chief symptoms are pain and paresthesia.[25]
8. radiculitis — any involvement of the spinal nerve roots due to either infection, toxins, trauma, protrusion of intervertebral disk or degenerative diseases.
9. sciatic neuritis, sciatica — a very painful involvement of the sciatic nerve.
10. trigeminal neuralgia, trifacial neuralgia, tic douloureux — paroxysms of lancinating pain of one or more areas innervated by the fifth cranial nerve.[111]
11. trigeminal neurinoma — rare, benign tumor of the trigeminal nerve characterized by mild pain or paresthesia, diminished corneal reflex and weakness of muscles of mastication.

D. Operative Terms:

1. ganglionectomy — excision of a ganglion
2. neuroanastomosis — surgical communication between nerve fibers.
3. neurectomy — excision of a nerve or lesion of a nerve, for example, a solitary neuroma.[97]
4. neurolysis — freeing a nerve from adhesions. In peripheral nerve surgery, dissection is best achieved by use of the Zeiss microscope with 6 to 10 times magnification.[45]
5. neuroplasty — plastic repair of a nerve.
6. neurorrhaphy — suture of an injured nerve.
7. neurotomy — transection of a nerve.[97]
8. supraorbital and supratrochlear neurectomy — surgical procedure for tic douloureux when the first division of the trigeminal nerve causes pain in the area above the eye socket (orbit).[46, 111]

---

* Also — neurolemoma, neurolemmoma.

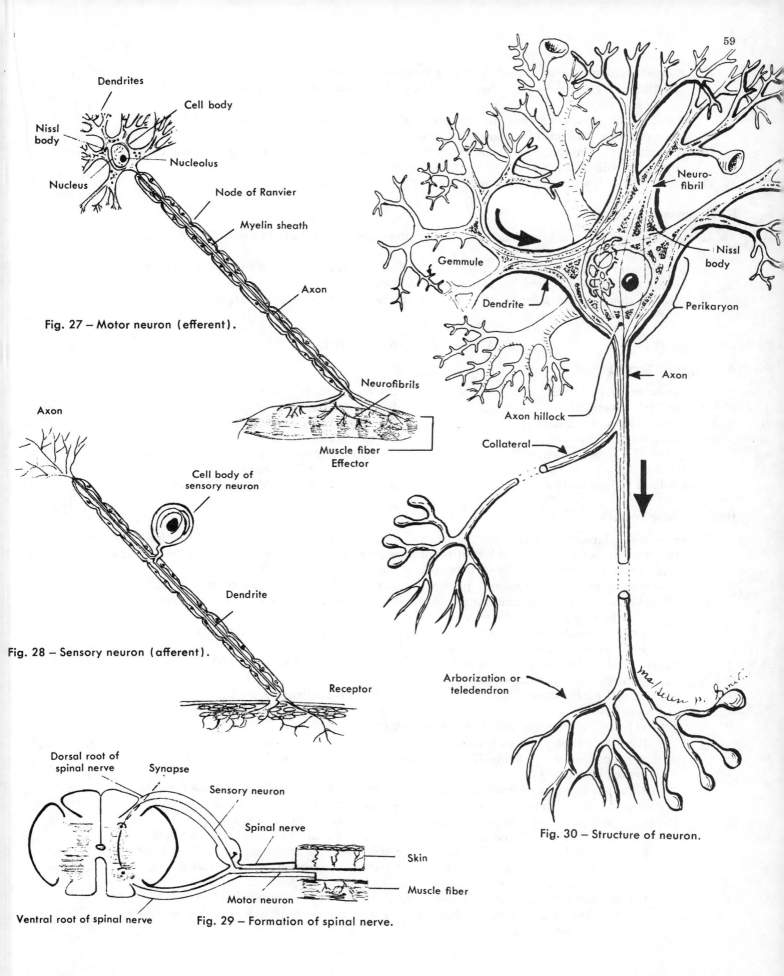

59

Dendrites

Cell body

Nissl body

Nucleolus

Nucleus

Node of Ranvier

Myelin sheath

Axon

Fig. 27 — Motor neuron (efferent).

Neurofibrils

Muscle fiber
Effector

Axon

Cell body of
sensory neuron

Dendrite

Fig. 28 — Sensory neuron (afferent).

Receptor

Neuro-
fibril

Gemmule

Dendrite

Nissl body

Perikaryon

Axon

Axon hillock

Collateral

Arborization or
teledendron

Fig. 30 — Structure of neuron.

Dorsal root of
spinal nerve

Synapse

Sensory neuron

Spinal nerve

Skin

Muscle fiber

Ventral root of spinal nerve

Motor neuron

Fig. 29 — Formation of spinal nerve.

9. sympathectomy — excision of part of a sympathetic nerve.
   a. thoracic ganglionectomy for causalgia or Raynaud's disease affecting the upper extremities.
   b. lumbar ganglionectomy for causalgia, Raynaud's disease and thromboangiitis obliterans affecting the lower extremities.
10. trigeminal decompression — compression of ganglion and root of trigeminal complex with dry cottonoid to relieve pain in tic douloureux.[47]
11. vagotomy — transection of a vagus nerve.

E. Symptomatic Terms:

1. aural vertigo — episodic attacks of severe dizziness due to lesion in ear (labyrinthine lesion).
2. paroxysmal pain — sudden, recurrent or periodic attack of pain as in tic douloureux.
3. tactile stimulation — evoking a response by touch.
4. trigger area — point from which the pain starts as in trigeminal neuralgia.

BRAIN AND SPINAL CORD

A. Origin of Terms:

1. cerebrum (L) — brain
2. cord (G) — string
3. cortex (L) — rind, bark
4. encephalon (G) — brain
5. gyrus (L) — convolution
6. lamina (L) — thin plate
7. medulla (L) — marrow
8. meninges (G) — membranes
9. myelo- (G) — marrow
10. occiput (L) — back of head
11. pons (L) — bridge
12. spina (L) — thorn
13. thalamo- (G) — chamber
14. ventricle (L) — little belly or cavity

B. Anatomic Terms:

1. brain, encephalon[16] — major part of central nervous system. It is divided into the forebrain or prosencephalon, midbrain or mesencephalon and hindbrain or rhombencephalon and comprises the following structural and functional components.
   a. cerebellum — second largest part of the brain which serves as a reflex center for the coordination of muscular movements. It is divisible into two hemispheres and a median portion, the vermis.
   b. cerebrum — the largest part of the brain which is divided into two hemispheres by a deep groove, the longitudinal fissure.[16, 17]
   c. cerebral cortex — the surface of the cerebrum composed of gray matter and arranged in folds known as convolutions or gyri.
   d. cerebral localization — definite regions of the cerebral cortex performing special functions:
      (1) the motor areas which influence voluntary muscular activity.
      (2) the sensory areas where sensations reach the conscious level.
   e. corpus callosum — a bridgelike structure of white fibers which joins the two hemispheres.[16, 17]
2. brain stem — upward continuation of cervical cord which consists of numerous bundles of nerve fibers and nuclei. Its structural components include the following:
   a. diencephalon, interbrain — small but important part of forebrain comprising
      (1) epithalamus — area including several nuclei and the pineal body or epiphysis.
      (2) hypothalamus — small mass below the thalamus containing nuclei and fibers. It is an integrating center for the autonomic nervous system and through its relation to the hypophysis for the endocrine system.
      (3) metathalamus — area of the lateral and medial geniculate bodies.
      (4) subthalamus — a mass of nuclei and fibers important in regulating muscular activities.

(5) thalamus — a mass of nuclei situated on either side of the third ventricle. It is the great sensory relay station.[16, 17]

b. medulla oblongata, myelencephalon, marrow brain — extends from upper cervical cord to pons; contains vital centers regulating heart action, vasomotor activity, respiration, deglutition and vomiting.

c. mesencephalon, midbrain — extends from pons below to forebrain above and is composed of nuclei and bundles of fibers.

d. pons — part of metencephalon (afterbrain) composed of bundles of fibers and nuclei which are located between the medulla and midbrain.

3. meninges — covering membranes of the brain and the spinal cord.

a. dura mater — serves as outer protective coat and is composed of strong fibrous tissue.

b. arachnoid — is the middle layer and consists of thin meshwork. The subarachnoid space contains cerebrospinal fluid.[16, 17]

c. pia mater — dips down between the convolutions and adheres closely to the brain.

4. nucleus (pl. nuclei) — a group of nerve cells within the central nervous system.

a. basal nuclei, formerly basal ganglia — masses of nerve cells deeply embedded in the white matter of the forebrain, for example, the lentiform nucleus.

5. ventricles and aqueduct

a. lateral ventricles — fluid-filled spaces, one in each cerebral hemisphere.

b. third ventricle — a fluid-filled space beneath the corpus callosum.

c. cerebral aqueduct — a narrow canal which connects the third and fourth ventricles.

d. fourth ventricle — an expansion of the central canal of the medulla oblongata. The ventricles contain cerebrospinal fluid which is formed by the capillaries of the choroid plexuses. The fluid seeps from the third ventricle into the cerebral aqueduct and fourth ventricle and from there into the central canal. It reaches the subarachnoid space through openings in the roof of the fourth ventricle and circulates around the cord and brain in this space, thus providing a water-cushion and shock absorber for the delicate nerve tissue.[16, 17]

6. spinal cord — portion of central nervous system located in the vertebral canal and giving rise to 31 pairs of spinal nerves. It extends from the foramen magnum to the second lumbar vertebra and is composed of white substance which surrounds the inner gray matter of the cord. Several lengthwise grooves demarcate the white matter into long columns. The deepest groove is the anterior median fissure which, together with the posterior median septum, almost separates the cord into two equal halves.

The **white matter** consists of myelinated fibers arranged in longitudinal bundles and grouped into 3 columns, the anterior, lateral and posterior funiculi. Afferent white fibers form the ascending nerve tracts which carry impulses from the cord to the brain. Efferent white fibers represent descending nerve tracts which bring messages from the brain to the cord.

The **gray matter** is H-shaped in cross-section and consists mainly of cell bodies. The anterior horn contains motor cells from which the motor fibers of the peripheral neurons arise. Sensory relay neurons are located in the posterior horn.[16, 17]

C. Diagnostic Terms:

1. amyotrophic lateral sclerosis — degenerative disease of the lateral motor tracts of the spinal cord causing widespread muscle wasting, weakness, fasciculations and usually a mild degree of spastic paralysis of lower extremities.[17, 76, 83]

2. anencephalia, anencephalus — absence of brain.

3. brain abscess — localized lesion of suppuration within the brain, generally secondary to ear infection, sinusitis or other infections.[12, 17]

4. brain tumor, intracranial tumor — benign or malignant space-occupying brain lesion.

a. adnexal tumor — derived from pineal body or choroid plexus. It may compress the aqueduct and cause obstructive hydrocephalus or exert pressure on the hypothalamus and be associated with diabetes insipidus or precocious puberty.

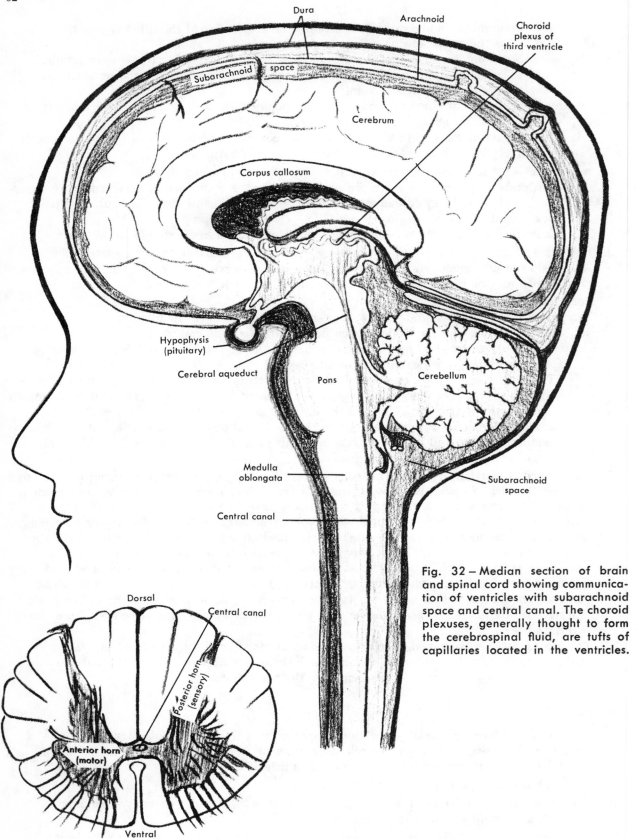

Dura

Arachnoid

Choroid plexus of third ventricle

Subarachnoid space

Cerebrum

Corpus callosum

Hypophysis (pituitary)

Cerebral aqueduct

Pons

Cerebellum

Medulla oblongata

Central canal

Subarachnoid space

Fig. 32 — Median section of brain and spinal cord showing communication of ventricles with subarachnoid space and central canal. The choroid plexuses, generally thought to form the cerebrospinal fluid, are tufts of capillaries located in the ventricles.

Dorsal

Central canal

Posterior horn (sensory)

Anterior horn (motor)

Ventral

Fig. 31 — Transverse section of spinal cord at level of origin of third lumbar nerve.

b. congenital tumor — a slowly growing, highly invasive tumor; e.g., a dermoid or teratoma.

c. medulloblastoma — a highly malignant cerebellar tumor which metastasizes freely to the subarachnoid space, cerebrum and cord.

d. meningeal tumor — neoplasm arising from the covering membranes of the brain or cord.   The meningioma may cause compression and distortion of the brain.

e. metastatic tumor — most primary tumors may metastasize to the brain, especially breast and lung tumors.

f. pituitary tumor — arises from anterior pituitary (adenohypophysis) and may compress the normal portion of the pituitary, the hypothalamus and optic chiasm.

g. primary brain tumors — comprise a large number of intracranial tumors, especially, the gliomas which contain malignant glial cells.   Some neoplasms of the glioma group are presented:

   (1) astrocytoma — a slowly growing tumor containing astrocytes that infiltrate widely into neighboring brain tissue and may undergo cystic degeneration.

   (2) ependymoma — tumor arises from the lining of the ventricular wall, is highly malignant and invasive.

   (3) glioblastoma multiforme — the most malignant glioma, rapidly growing, causing edema and necrosis of brain tissue.

   (4) oligodendroglioma — similar to astrocytoma in behavior, different in histologic structure.[17, 35, 103, 108]

5. cerebral concussion — transient state of unconsciousness following head injury immediately as a result of damage to the brain stem.[48]

6. cerebral palsy — condition characterized by paralysis, incoordination and other aberrations of motor or sensory functions due to pathology of the brain.[71, 97]

7. cerebrovascular disease — any disorder in which one or more of the cerebral blood vessels have undergone pathologic changes.[25, 33, 67, 70]

a. cerebral aneurysm, intracranial aneurysm — dilation of an artery of the brain resulting in a thinning and weakening of the arterial wall.   Common locations are the internal carotid and middle cerebral arteries.   Rupture and hemorrhage may occur and cause serious brain damage.[9, 33]

b. cerebral arteriovenous malformation — structural vascular defect, generally found in young patients with recurrent subarachnoid hemorrhage and epilepsy.[21, 70]

c. cerebral atherosclerosis — a primary degeneration of the intima by atheromatous plaques (lipid deposits) usually located in the basilar artery, the middle and posterior cerebral arteries, and at the branching of the internal carotids.   The subsequent narrowing of the vessels may lead to inadequate oxygenation and nutrition of the brain by the reduced cerebral circulation.   Brain softening, neural atrophy, and senile plaques add further damage and predispose to physical and mental deterioration.[9, 60, 67, 70]

d. cerebral embolism — sudden occlusion of a cerebral blood vessel by a circulatory embolus composed of air bubble, blood clot, fat cells or bacteria.[67]

e. cerebral infarction — local necrosis of brain tissue due to loss of blood supply in vascular obstruction.[33, 67, 70]

f. cerebral ischemia — anemia of the brain resulting from diminished cerebral blood flow. Some important causes are circulatory obstruction of the intra- or extracranial arteries by atheroma, thrombus or embolus, severe hypotension, arteritis or stenosis of an artery.   Recurrent ischemic episodes are thought to signal impending stroke.[5]

g. cerebral thrombosis — formation of a thrombus within an intracranial artery leading to its occlusion and subsequent necrosis of the area supplied by the thrombosed vessel.[33, 67, 70]

h. cerebrovascular accident, stroke, apoplexy — neurologic disorder caused by pathologic changes in the extracranial or intracranial blood vessels, primarily by atherosclerosis, thrombosis, embolic episodes, hemorrhage or by arterial hypertension.   Cerebral infarction or necrosis of brain tissue may occur in the affected lesion.[33, 99]   The completed stroke, usually recognized by a rather sudden loss of consciousness and other marked neurologic insult, is **preceded** by

(1) transient ischemic attacks — symptoms of minor brain damage evidenced by numbness, unilateral weakness, visual deficits, motor disability and the like. They last from minutes to hours.   A complete return to the pre-attack status may occur or there may be residual damage.[25, 33, 99]

(2) progressive stroke — neurologic manifestations are persistent and become more serious, signalling impending stroke.[9, 20, 33, 67, 99]

i. cerebrovascular insufficiency syndrome — clinical evidence of minor brain damage: numbness, motor weakness, slurred speech, others; may develop from pathologic changes of the intracranial vessels, especially the anterior, middle and posterior cerebral arteries.[20]   More frequently it is caused by extracranial vascular obstruction leading to cerebral ischemia as seen in the

(1) internal carotid syndrome, internal carotid stenosis, internal carotid ischemia — stenotic lesion usually resulting from atheromatous process near the bifurcation of the common carotid artery.   It may cause contralateral hemiparesis or hemiplegia, speech difficulties, visual defects and others.[25, 33, 67]

(2) subclavian steal syndrome, proximal subclavian stenosis, skeletal muscle ischemia of arm — syndrome due to impaired blood flow to the basilar artery or brachiocephalic trunk near the origin of the vertebral artery.   The decreased vascular pressure beyond the occluded segment initiates retrograde flow in the vertebral artery and siphons the blood away from the brain.   This stealing of blood which reduces the cerebral circulation thus causing neurologic deficit, is demanded by the muscles for exercise of the affected arm.   The low or absent blood pressure and pulse on the site of the subclavian occlusion in contrast to those markedly higher of the unaffected arm are diagnostic evidence.[25, 33, 70]

(3) vertebrobasilar syndrome, vertebral artery stenosis or basilar artery stenosis, vertebrobasilar ischemia — syndrome manifests cerebellar involvement: vertigo, disequilibrium, ataxia and cranial nerve damage, facial paralysis, motor and sensory disturbances, and others.[25, 33]

j. intracranial hematoma — local mass of extravasated blood which formed subsequent to intracranial hemorrhage.   Chronic lesions may become encapsulated.   Epidural and subdural hematomas, located above or below the dura mater, are usually due to head injury.[4, 78, 103]

k. intracranial hemorrhage — rupture of a vessel beneath the skull with seepage of blood into the brain coverings or substance.   It may be caused by head injury, stroke or ruptured aneurysm.   Brain damage depends on the location and extent of the lesion involved.[4, 54, 70, 103]

l. subarachnoid hemorrhage — bleeding into the subarachnoid space which in some cases is associated with excruciating headache, convulsions and coma.   It is due to head injury or ruptured intracranial aneurysm.[4, 17, 85]

8. chorea — nervous disorder characterized by bizarre, abrupt, involuntary movements.
   a. Huntington's chorea, adult chorea — hereditary form with onset in adult life, involvement of basal ganglia and cortex, choreiform movements and mental decline.
   b. Sydenham's chorea, juvenile chorea — disorder of childhood and adolescence with insidious onset of jerky movements usually occurring during rheumatic fever.[17, 106]

9. encephalitis lethargica — inflammation of the brain marked by somnolence and ocular paralysis.   It is caused by a filtrable virus.

10. encephalocele — protrusion of some brain substance through a fissure of the skull.

11. epilepsy — convulsive disorder consisting of recurrent seizures and impaired consciousness.[1, 17, 42]

12. Friedreich's ataxia — familial disease, seen in the young.   Involvement of cerebellum, pyramidal tracts and peripheral nerves result in sensory impairment, unsteady gait,

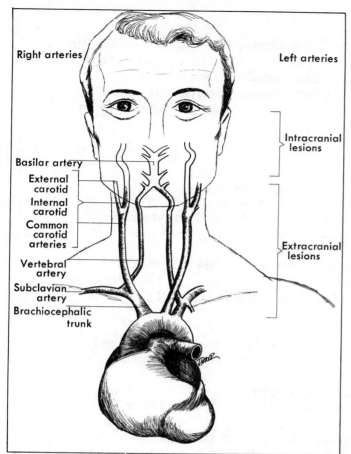

Fig. 33 — Location of extracranial or intracranial vascular lesions in cerebrovascular disease.

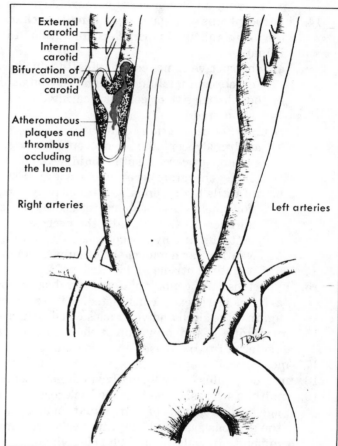

Fig. 34 — Occlusive lesion at the bifurcation of the common carotid artery extending into the internal carotid artery.

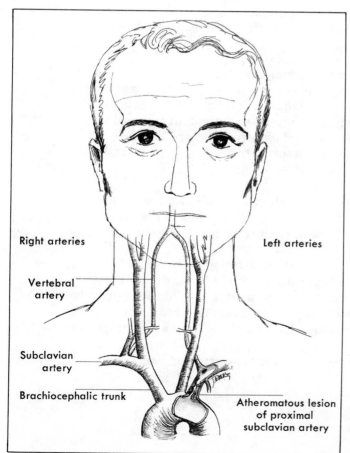

Fig. 35 — Subclavian steal syndrome. Proximal left subclavian artery stenosed by atheroma resulting in impoverished blood supply to the arm. The cerebral circulation is altered to relieve ischemia of the arm muscles during exercise.

contractures and deformities such as lordosis and high arching feet with toes cocking up. Optic atrophy and myocardial disease may occur.[87]

13. head injury, craniocerebral trauma — injury to the head, usually associated with a fractured skull and affecting directly or indirectly and at varying degree one or more cerebral centers. The severity and extent of brain damage is usually, but not exclusively indicated by
    a. state of consciousness
    b. intracranial pressure
    c. respiratory exchange
    d. circulatory ability to supply the brain with oxygen and nutrients
    e. prevention or control of cerebral hemorrhage, edema and infection.[17, 40, 48, 78]

14. hydrocephalus — a pathologic condition characterized by a dilatation of the ventricles of the brain and an abnormal accumulation of intraventricular cerebrospinal fluid.[21]
    It may be
    a. obstructive or noncommunicating due to an interference with the circulation of the cerebrospinal fluid through the ventricular system.
    b. nonobstructive or communicating due to an interference in absorption of cerebro-spinal fluid.
    Some other distinctions comprise:
    a. adult hydrocephalus, hydrocephalus *ex vacuo* — a rare type in which the increased volume of cerebrospinal fluid develops as a compensatory response to brain atrophy in degenerative cerebral disease.[13, 35, 97]
    b. infantile hydrocephalus — relatively common form which occurs before closure of fontanelles and is characterized by increasing cranial enlargement and prominent forehead. Occasionally the process is arrested.[97]
    c. posttraumatic hydrocephalus — type due to head injury which may result in ventricular hemorrhage or subarachnoid bleeding and blockage of the aqueduct and fourth ventricle by blood clot.[4]

15. hypertensive encephalopathy — cerebral vasoconstriction and edema. The cerebral arteries are greatly constricted. The swollen, pale and anemic brain is compressed against the skull and ventricles causing increased intracranial pressure.

16. meningitis — inflammation of the meninges resulting from infectious agents such as bacteria, fungi, viruses or other causes.

17. meningocele — protrusion of the meninges through a cranial fissure.

18. microcephalus — abnormally small head sometimes associated with idiocy.

19. multiple sclerosis, disseminated sclerosis — slowly progressive disease, striking the 20-40 age group. Areas of demyelination and scar tissue plaques are scattered throughout the nervous system disrupting nerve transmission. Numbness, fatigability, clumsiness, difficulty in walking and blurring vision may be followed by severe incoordination, spasticity, paralysis, incontinence, scanning speech, intention tremor, nystagmus and blindness.[17, 25, 87, 101]

20. myelitis — inflammation of the spinal cord.

21. neurofibromatosis, von Recklinghausen's disease — hereditary disorder of the nervous system in which multiple neurofibromas and café-au-lait spots are found on the skin. The tumors are usually asymptomatic and rarely cause compression of the spinal cord or sensory nerve damage.

22. paralysis agitans, Parkinson's disease — slowly progressive neurologic disorder of middle life, primarily affecting the nuclei of the brain stem. Rigidity, slow movements, tremors, masklike facies and a monotonous voice are clinical findings. Characteristically festination is present. The patient's body is stooped forward; his steps are short, shuffling along with increasing pace, once locomotion has started. His gait is propulsive or retropulsive.[1, 17, 25]

23. poliomyelitis — viral disease with lesions in the central nervous system and varying symptomology.[105]
    forms:

a. asymptomatic, nonparalytic poliomyelitis — abortive type devoid of symptoms referable to the central nervous system.

b. paralytic poliomyelitis.

   (1) bulbar poliomyelitis — involvement of cranial nerve nuclei; particularly the respiratory center in the medulla. It is the most serious type of poliomyelitis causing respiratory paralysis.

   (2) spinal paralytic poliomyelitis — usually an involvement of anterior horn cells of the spinal cord resulting in characteristic stiffness of the neck and spine, tightness of the hamstring muscles followed by paralysis of lower extremities. It presents the classical form of poliomyelitis.[105]

24. spina bifida — congenital defect consisting in the absence of a vertebral arch of the spinal column. It may cause a

a. meningocele — protrusion of the meninges through the defect in the spinal column.

b. meningomyelocele — herniation of the cord and meninges through the defect of the vertebral column.

c. syringomyelocele — protrusion of cord and meninges through defect in spine. Cord tissue is a thin-walled sac filled with fluid from the central canal.

25. spinal cord injury — trauma to cord produced by fracture or dislocation of spine may cause irreversible damage and disability.[101]

a. compression of cervical cord — complete transverse compression of cervical cord may cause lifelong quadriplegia (paralysis of arms and legs) and loss of sphincter control or be fatal due to phrenic nerve injury and subsequent respiratory paralysis.

b. compression of thoracic or lumbar cord — pressure on this area may cause paraplegia (paralysis below the waist) and sphincter disturbances.[87, 108]

Compression of spinal cord may also be due to cord tumor and herniated intervertebral disc affecting the spinal nerve root of the lesion.[87, 101]

26. subacute sclerosing panencephalitis (SSPE), Dawson's encephalitis — uncommon form of inflammation of the brain occurring between 4 to 20 years of age. Three stages are recognized:

a. behavioral disorders at the onset

b. mental deterioration, myoclonic jerkings and convulsive seizures as the disease progresses

c. stupor, dementia, rigidity, blindness and coma in the terminal phase.[30, 38]

27. tabes dorsalis, locomotor ataxia — syphilis of the central nervous system clinically recognized by peculiar gait.

D. Operative Terms:

1. carotid artery ligation — tying a carotid artery in its cervical portion (neck) or using a Selverstone or Crutchfield clamp to gradually occlude the blood flow in the extracranial portions of the common or internal carotid artery.[92]

2. carotid endarterectomy — removal of plaques or the intimal lining of a carotid artery in occlusive cerebrovascular disease. This removal may be carried out at the carotid bifurcation and followed by a reconstruction of an internal carotid artery with a Dacron graft.[49, 92, 97]

3. carotid reconstruction operation — repair of carotid artery with a graft or bypass.[92]

4. cingulumotomy — cingulum destruction by stereotaxic surgery with positioning of electrodes in target area. Operation is done under radiographic guidance for relief of psychogenic pain, manic depressive reactions and other disorders.[50, 97]

5. cordectomy — removal of portion of the spinal cord to convert a spastic paraplegia to a flaccid paraplegia. This enhances rehabilitation.

6. cordotomy, chordotomy — section of a nerve fiber tract (usually the spinothalamic tract) within the cord for relief of pain.

a. percutaneous cordotomy — surgical interruption of the pain fibers in the high cervical cord by means of percutaneous electric needle. This is done under biplane radiographic control.[92, 97]

b. selective cordotomy — palliative surgery for obtaining sensory loss in local pain region, as in arm, leg or trunk.

7. craniectomy — removal of part of skull bone; a method of approach to the brain.

8. craniotomy — opening of skull. Burr or trephine openings into the skull are made in order to prepare a bone flap. This osteoplastic flap is separated from the skull during brain surgery and replaced when the skull is closed. Osteoplastic craniotomy is a common method of approach to the brain.[92]

9. cryoneurosurgery — the operative use of cold in the destruction of neurosurgical lesions.

10. decompression of
    a. brain — removal of a piece of skull bone, usually in the subtemporal region with opening of the dura mater to relieve intracranial pressure.
    b. spinal cord — removal of bone fragments, hematoma or lesion to relieve pressure on cord.[92]

11. drainage of meninges for abscess or hematoma — evacuation of subarachnoid or subdural space.

12. excision of brain lesion — complete removal if lesion does not encroach on vital centers.

13. laminectomy — excision of one or more laminae of vertebrae; method of approach to spinal cord.

14. microneurosurgery — use of the surgical binocular microscope which provides a powerful light source, up to 25 times magnification and a clear stereoscopic view of the brain. Microsurgical techniques and dissection are employed for
    a. acoustic tumors
    b. cerebral aneurysms
    c. pituitary tumors
    d. spinal cord tumors and other neurosurgical procedures.[45, 82, 97]

15. operations for parkinsonism — surgical procedures directed toward the destruction of areas of basal nuclei presumably affected by the disease.
    a. pallidotomy, formerly pallidectomy — surgical interruption of nerve pathways coming from globus pallidus to relieve intractable tremor and rigidity. Division of nerve fibers is usually achieved by use of electrocautery or chemical solution. Cryogenic agents, ultrasonic waves and stereotaxic techniques may be employed.[1, 92]
    b. thalamotomy formerly thalamectomy — partial destruction of thalamus for relief of tremors and rigidity. The stereotaxic instrument is applied to the skull. By means of radiographic visualization the target area is located and lesions are created by electrolytic, chemical, ultrasonic or cryogenic methods.[1, 50, 92, 97]

16. stereotaxic neurosurgery — operative procedure that uses three dimensional measurement for precisely locating the neurosurgical target area in
    a. acromegaly
    b. cerebral aneurysm
    c. diabetic retinopathy
    d. manic depressive reactions
    e. Parkinson's disease
    f. psychogenic pain
    g. temporal lobe epilepsy.[1, 50, 73, 97]

17. stereotaxy — the use of stereotaxic instrument fixed onto the skull with screws like a scaffold. From this a probe, containing either a chemical, electric or cryogenic agent, is introduced through a burr opening into the target area of the brain.[50, 73, 92, 97]

18. surgical shunts for hydrocephalus — detour channels, surgically created to relieve an accumulation of cerebrospinal fluid in the brain.[13]
    a. ventriculoatrial or ventriculocaval shunt — insertion of Holter, Pudenz or Hakim valve to channel the cerebrospinal fluid from the lateral ventricle to either an atrium or the superior vena cava via the jugular vein. This operation is performed for communicating hydrocephalus.[34, 51, 92, 97]
    b. ventriculocisternostomy, Torkildsen operation — surgical procedure for obstructive

hydrocephalus. A catheter is used to shunt the fluid from a ventricle to the cisterna magna.[51, 92]

   c. ventriculoperitoneal shunt — detour channel shunting the cerebrospinal fluid from the enlarged ventricular system into the peritoneal cavity.[97]

19. tractotomy — section of a nerve fiber tract within the brain stem for relief of intractable pain.

20. trephination — cutting a circular opening or boring a hole into skull; a method of approach to the brain.[92]

E. Symptomatic Terms:

1. analgesia — loss of normal sense of pain.
2. anesthesia — loss of sensation; may be associated with unconsciousness.
3. aphasia — difficulty with the use or understanding of words due to lesions in association areas.
    a. motor aphasia — verbal comprehension intact, but patient unable to use the muscles which coordinate speech.
    b. sensory aphasia — inability to comprehend the spoken word if auditory word center is affected and the written word if the visual word center is involved. The patient will not understand the spoken or written word if there is an involvement of both centers.
4. ataxia — motor incoordination.
5. aura — patient's awareness of pending epileptic seizure.
6. cerebrospinal otorrhea — escape of cerebrospinal fluid from the ear following craniocerebral trauma. It is due to a fistulous communication between the ventricular system or subarachnoid space and the ear.[48]
7. cerebrospinal rhinorrhea — escape of cerebrospinal fluid from the nose following craniocerebral trauma. It is due to a fistulous passage leading from the ventricular system or subarachnoid space to the nose.[48]
8. coma — state of unconsciousness or deep stupor.
9. convulsion — paroxysms of involuntary muscular contractions and relaxations.[42]
10. diplegia — paralysis on both sides of body.
11. dysarthria — incoordination of speech muscles affecting articulation.
12. dyskinesia — abnormal involuntary movement and body posture due to brain lesion.
    a. athetosis — slow, wormlike, writhing movement especially in hands and fingers.
    b. ballism — violent, flinging, shaking or jerking movements of extremities.
    c. chorea — quick, explosive, purposeless movements.
    d. dystonia — abnormal posture from twisting movements usually of limbs and trunk.
13. euphoria — a sense of well-being associated with mild elation.
14. fasciculation — involuntary twitchings of groups of muscle fibers.
15. festination — quick, shuffling steps; accelerated gait seen in Parkinson disease.[1, 17]
16. hemiparesis — slight degree of paralysis of one side of body.
17. hemiplegia — paralysis affecting one side of body.
18. hyperesthesia — increased sensibility to sensory stimuli.
19. intention tremor — trembling when attempting voluntary movement.
20. nystagmus — constant movements of the eyeballs as seen in the brain damage and disorders of vestibular apparatus.[98]
21. paraparesis — slight paralysis of lower limbs.
22. paraplegia — paralysis of lower limbs and at varying degrees of lower trunk.
23. paresis — partial paralysis.
24. paresthesia — abnormal sensation, heightened sensory response to stimuli.
25. scanning speech — hesitant, slow speech, pronouncing words in syllables.[25, 26]
26. syncope — fainting.
27. tic — involuntary, purposeless contractions of muscle groups as twitching of facial muscles, eye blinking or shrugging of shoulder.

PSYCHIATRIC DISORDERS

A. Origin of Terms:

1. analysis (G) — dissolving
2. catatonia (G) — low tension
3. dement (L) — unsound mind
4. dynamo (G) — power
5. hallucinate (L) — to wander in mind
6. mania (G) — madness
7. ment (L) — mind
8. phren (G) — mind
9. psyche (G) — soul, mind
10. psychedelic (G) — mind-manifesting
11. schizo (G) — split
12. soma (G) — body

B. General Terms:

1. commitment — legal consignment of a mentally unsound or defective individual to an institution.
2. descriptive psychiatry — system of psychiatry which implies the study of clinical patterns, symptoms and classification.
3. dynamic psychiatry — the study of emotional processes, their origins, and the mental mechanisms. Implies the study of the active, energy-laden and changing factors in human behavior and their motivation. Dynamic principles convey the concepts of change, of evolution, and progression or regression.[3]
4. ego — in psychoanalytic theory, one of the three major divisions in the model of the psychic apparatus, the others being the id and superego. The ego represents the sum of certain mental mechanisms, such as perception and memory, and specific defensive mechanisms. The ego serves to mediate between the demands of primitive instinctual drives (the id), of internalized parental and social prohibitions (the superego), and of reality. The compromises between these forces achieved by the ego tend to resolve intrapsychic conflict and serve an adaptive and executive function. As used in psychiatry, the term should not be confused with its common usage in the sense of "self-love" or "selfishness."[3, 69]
5. extrasensory perception (ESP) — perception without recourse to the conventional use of any of the five physical senses. It is the same as effective sensory projection.[3]
6. mental health — a state of being, relative rather than absolute, in which a person has effected a reasonably satisfactory integration of his instinctual drives. His integration is acceptable to himself and to his social milieu as reflected in his interpersonal relationships, his level of satisfaction in living, his actual achievement, his flexibility, and the level of maturity he has attained.[3]
7. orthopsychiatry — an approach to the study and treatment of human behavior that involves the collaborative effort of psychiatry, psychology, psychiatric social work, and other behavioral, medical and social sciences in the study and treatment of human behavior in the clinical setting. Emphasis is placed on preventive techniques to promote healthy emotional growth and development, particularly of children.[3]
8. psychiatry — the medical science which deals with the origin, diagnosis, prevention, and treatment of mental and emotional disorders.[3]
9. psychodynamics — a predictive science which recognizes unconscious drives in human behavior.
10. psychometry — psychologic measurement or testing of mental processes and potentials including psychopathologic variants.
11. surrogate — a substitute person. In its psychiatric meaning the patient may emotionally respond to a person, e.g. an authority figure, as he did to a parent.[102]
12. telepathy — the communication of thought from one person to another without the intervention of physical means; not generally accepted as scientifically valid.[3]

C. Diagnostic Terms:

1. depression — a common psychiatric disorder manifested by morbid sadness, melancholy, feelings of dejection, guilt, loneliness and hopelessness; impaired thinking, concentration

and decisiveness and diminished interest in work and recreation.   A depression may also be a symptom or syndrome.[2, 9, 10]
  a. manic-depressive illness — a major affective disorder characterized by unusual mood swings from normal to deep depression or alternating high and low spirits with intermittent remissions.[9, 10, 52, 94]
    Recognized are a
    (1) bipolar type — both manic and depressive phases are present at variable duration.
    (2) unipolar type — the patient experiences recurrent episodes of depression or less frequently recurrent manic attacks.[93]
  b. psychotic depressive reaction — a depressive psychosis attributed to an internal conflict or a painful event such as the death of a loved one.   Reality testing is impaired.[93]
2. mental retardation, mental deficiency — abnormally low intellectual functioning from birth or childhood associated with impairment of maturation, social adjustment and learning ability.   There are five degrees of retardation:
  a. borderline mental retardation _____IQ 68-83
  b. mild mental retardation _____IQ 52-67
  c. moderate mental retardation _____IQ 36-51
  d. severe mental retardation _____IQ 20-35
  e. profound mental retardation _____IQ under 20.
  Clinical subcategories of mental retardation include those related to
    (1) maternal infection, intoxication and trauma
    (2) disorders of metabolism, growth and nutrition
    (3) chromosomal abnormality
    (4) psychologic environmental deprivation and others.
3. neuroses, sing. neurosis — disorders in which the dominant trait is anxiety.   They may be expressed directly or controlled unconsciously by psychologic mechanisms.   There is no distortion of reality or personality disorganization.   Some neuroses are presented:
  a. anxiety neurosis — overconcern bordering on panic usually associated with somatic manifestations.
  b. hysteric neurosis — involuntary functional disorder or psychogenic loss, initiated by emotionally charged situation relevant of underlying conflict.
    (1) conversion type — disorder of special senses or voluntary nervous system characterized by loss of sight, hearing, smell, feeling of pain, and associated with ataxia (muscular incoordination) and paralysis.   The patient seems indifferent about his symptoms which bring relief from unpleasant obligations.[18, 102]
    (2) dissociative type — hysteric neurosis in which the patient's identity or state of consciousness is altered as evidenced by symptoms of amnesia, multiple personality, fugue and somnambulism.[102]
      (a) fugue — personality dissociation characterized by amnesia and involving actual physical flight from the customary environment or field of conflict.[3, 102]
      (b) others.
  c. neurasthenic neurosis, neurasthenia — chronic fatigability, weakness and exhaustion causing genuine distress.   No secondary gain is sought by patient.[18]
  d. traumatic neurosis — any functional nervous condition which follows an accidental physical injury or psychologic shock.[10, 18, 69, 102, 104, 110]
4. organic brain syndrome — syndrome characterized by impairment of orientation, memory, mental functioning related to comprehension, learning and acquisition of knowledge, defective judgment, shallowness of affect and emotional instability.   Functional brain tissue is impaired at varying degree.   The syndrome may be acute or chronic, reversible or irreversible, and related to the patient's basic personality pattern, interpersonal relations and conflicts, as well as environmental factors.[18]

5. personality disorder — condition marked by maladaptive behavior pattern that is deeply
   ingrained in the personality. Some examples are
   a. alcoholic addiction — physiologic dependence on alcohol as evidenced by appearance
      of withdrawal symptoms when alcohol is withheld. An irresistible craving for
      intoxicating beverages and loss of self-control are dominant behavior problems of the
      alcoholic.[22, 36, 69, 93]
   b. drug dependence — addiction to or dependence on opiates, synthetic analgesics,
      barbiturates, psychostimulants, hallucinogens and others. Habitual use is necessary
      for diagnosis. Withdrawal symptoms may be absent.[10, 22, 36, 89, 93]
   Other personality disorders are:
   c. antisocial personality — personality disorder characterized by a persistent refusal to
      follow the norms of society.[102]
   d. cyclothymic personality — individual manifesting mood swings from elation to
      depression.
   e. inadequate personality — individual unable to respond to intellectual, emotional,
      social and physical demands in a satisfactory manner.
   f. schizoid personality — individual being oversensitive, shy, seclusive, unsociable,
      eccentric and autistic; apparently detached in conflict situation.[18, 93]
6. psychophysiologic disorder — any disorder representing the visceral expression of or
   functional response to emotion, for example: irritable colon, mucous colitis, heartburn,
   hyperventilation.[69, 93]
7. psychosis, pl. psychoses — a major mental illness in which the patient's intellectual
   functioning is impaired to a degree that he cannot meet the ordinary demands of life and
   exhibits abnormal patterns of thought, feeling and action.[18]
8. psychoses associated with organic brain syndrome:
   a. acute alcoholic intoxication — disorder comprises a variety of acute brain syndromes
      caused by alcohol such as delirium tremens, alcoholic hallucinosis, others.[36]
   b. Korsakov's psychosis — a chronic brain syndrome associated with a prolonged use
      of alcohol. Clinical features are peripheral neuropathy, disorientation, impaired
      memory and confabulation.[36, 93]
   c. presenile dementia — cortical brain syndrome in age group below sixty.
   d. psychosis with brain trauma — psychosis developing after head injury. If it occurs
      in childhood, mental retardation is a common sequel.
   e. psychosis with cerebral arteriosclerosis — condition similar to presenile and senile
      psychosis. Arterial occlusion of brain vessels may result in physical and mental
      deterioration.
   f. pychosis with cerebrovascular disturbance — common circulatory disorder usually
      associated with cerebral thrombosis, embolism or hemorrhage.
   g. senile dementia — a chronic organic brain syndrome due to brain atrophy in the
      aging process resulting in physical and mental deterioration at various degrees.[18]
9. schizophrenia — severe mental disorder of psychotic depth marked by disturbances
   in behavior, mood, and ability to think. Altered concept formation may lead to a
   distortion of reality, delusions and hallucinations which tend to be self-protective.
   Emotional disharmony and bizarre regressive behavior are frequently present.[11]
   The American Psychiatric Association distinguishes 11 types, some of which
   are given here:
   a. catatonic type — marked disturbance in activity with either generalized
      inhibition (mutism, stupor, negativism, waxy appearance) or by excessive
      motor activity and excitement. Gross personality disorganization is a
      prominent feature.
   b. hebephrenic type — shallow inappropriate emotions, disorganized thinking,
      unpredictable childish behavior and mannerisms, indicative of gross personality
      disorganization.
   c. latent type — prepsychotic or borderline schizophrenia with definite symptoms
      but no schizophrenic episode.

d. paranoid type — schizophrenia in which grandiose or persecutory delusions are dominant characteristics. They are usually associated with hostility, aggressiveness and hallucinations.[11, 18, 69, 80, 84]

D. Terms Related to Shock Therapy:

Several types of shock therapy are employed in psychiatric treatment:
1. electroconvulsive or electroshock treatment — the use of electric current to cause unconsciousness and/or initiate convulsions.[66]
2. electronarcosis — narcoticlike state produced as therapeutic measure.
3. electrostimulation — avoidance of convulsive seizures when using electric current.
4. insulin coma therapy — inducing hypoglycemic reaction by the administration of large doses of insulin.[66]
5. subcoma insulin therapy — producing drowsiness or somnolence by insulin injection, but no coma.

E. Terms Related to Psychotherapy:

Psychotherapy may be defined as treatment of emotional and personality problems by psychologic means. The following terms refer to psychotherapeutic techniques.
1. abreaction — an expressive form of psychotherapy which encourages a reliving of repressed emotional stress situations in a therapeutic setting. It releases painful emotions and increases insight.[102]
2. activity therapy — program of activities prescribed for patients on the basis of psychologic understanding of their specific needs. Types of therapy are:
   a. bibliotherapy
   b. educational therapy
   c. music therapy
   d. occupational therapy
   e. recreational therapy
3. behavior therapy — a therapeutic approach which attempts to bring about direct change by helping the individual to unlearn maladaptive and destructive behavior and to enhance his abilities for socially acceptable and productive behavior.[10]
4. biofeedback — provision of information to the subject based on one or more of his physiologic processes, such as brainwave activity or blood pressure, often as an essential element of visceral learning.[3]
5. group psychotherapy — a method of psychotherapy applied to a group. Group leaders help patients to gain insight into their emotional difficulties and conflicts, to understand their causes and to translate their defensive reactions into acceptable behavior.[66, 104]
6. hypnosis — a state of semiconscious suggestibility. Through verbal suggestion the patient's attention is withdrawn from other stimuli and focused on the therapist's procedure. Under hypnosis symptoms are made to disappear. Posthypnotic suggestion is important.
7. milieu therapy — the utilization of a modified and controlled environment in the treatment of mental disease.[24]
8. narcoanalysis — psychotherapy is offered under the influence of drugs.
9. persuasion — a form of psychotherapy which utilizes reasoning and moralizing discussions to change faulty attitudes.
10. play therapy — psychotherapeutic approach to children who tend to reveal their hidden resentments, feelings and frustrations in play. An analytic therapist uses his interpretations of play as a guide to treatment.
11. pschyoanalysis — a type of insight therapy developed by Sigmund Freud. Psychoanalytic treatment seeks to influence behavior by bringing into awareness unconscious emotional conflicts in an effort to overcome them.[69, 182]
12. rational-emotive therapy — a humanistic type of psychotherapy, highly cognitive and empirical, based on the assertion that man's rational or irrational beliefs about his own person influence his actions and outlook on life. By recognizing and changing his irrational beliefs man gains control over his emotional life and recovers his mental health.[32]
13. supportive psychotherapy — therapeutic efforts directed toward a strengthening of the

patient's ego in order to reduce anxiety.   The real problem remains unsolved and may become acute again at a crucial moment.

14. transactional analysis — a type of insight therapy developed by Eric Berne.   It seeks to understand the psychologic interaction between patient and therapist.[3, 102]

15. transference — a patient's unconscious reaction to a psychiatrist which is a repetition of an early childhood relationship to a parent, sibling or other.   The psychiatrist utilizes the transfer situation to gain insight into the patient's disturbing emotional conflicts and to plan his psychotherapy accordingly.[69, 102]

F. Terms Related to Psychopharmacology:

1. antianxiety agents — drugs which exhibit a central calming effect.   They are used in the treatment of mild to moderate anxiety.

2. antidepressants — psychic energizers which relieve despondency, tension, fatigue and mental depression.

3. antipsychotic agents — drugs used in treating psychoses and controlling excitation of central nervous system.[66]

4. ataractics — tranquilizing agents widely used in psychiatric disorders such as agitation, aggressive outbursts, psychomotor overactivity and the like.   They are the same as antianxiety agents.

5. hallucinogens — chemical agents producing hallucinations, disturbed thought processes and depersonalization in normal persons.

6. psychedelics — drugs which apparently expand consciousness and enlarge vision.[55]

7. psychopharmacology — science dealing with drugs that affect the emotions.

8. psychotogens — drugs producing psychotic behavior.

G. Symptomatic Terms:

1. aggression — forceful, self-assertive, attacking action, verbal, physical or symbolic.

2. agitation — chronic restlessness, important psychomotor reaction of emotional stress.

3. ambivalence — opposing drives or emotions; for example, love and hatred for the same person.

4. amnesia — a loss of memory, pathologic in nature.

5. anaclitic — leaning on; refers to dependence of infant on mother, abnormal later in life.

6. autism — a form of thinking which seeks to satisfy unfulfilled desires but completely disregards reality factors.

7. blocking — a sudden interruption in the stream of thought.

8. body image — the conscious and unconscious picture a person has of his own body at any moment.   The conscious and unconscious images may differ from each other.[3]

9. catalepsy — diminished responsiveness usually characterized by trance-like states.   May occur in organic or psychologic disorders or under hypnosis.[3]

10. catharsis — a wholesome emotional release by talking about one's problems or repressed feelings.

11. circumstantiality — the inclusion of numerous details in conversation before the essential idea is expressed.

12. compulsion — a powerful drive to perform ritualistic acts e.g. handwashing.

13. confabulation — fabrication of stories in response to questions about situations or events that are not recalled.[3]

14. cyclothymic — refers to mood swings out of proportion to stimuli.

15. delirium — syndrome characterized by clouding of consciousness, incoherence of ideas, mental confusion, bewilderment, hallucinations and illusions.[65]

16. delusions — false beliefs resulting from unconscious needs and maintained irrespective of contrary evidence.
    a. delusions of grandeur — exaggerated ideas about one's position and importance.
    b. delusions of persecution — false ideas that one is the target of persecution.

c. delusions of reference — erroneous assumption that casual, unrelated remarks are directed to oneself.[80]

17. dementia — an irreversible impairment of cognitive intellectual capacities.[102]
18. depersonalization — loss of sense of one's own identity.
19. dissocial behavior — the term refers to individuals who are not classifiable as antisocial personalities but who follow more or less criminal pursuits, such as racketeers, dishonest gamblers, prostitutes and dope peddlers; formerly called sociopathic personalities.[3, 18]
20. empathy — an objective insight into the feelings of another person in contrast to sympathy which is subjective and emotional.
21. hallucinations — false sensory perceptions without actual external stimulation.
22. illusions — falsely interpreted sensory perceptions.
23. incoherence in speech — illogic flow of ideas which is difficult to comprehend by the hearer.
24. libido — a psychoanalytic term denoting the psychic drive that energizes living.
25. malingering — a conscious simulation of illness used to avoid an unpleasant situation or for personal gain.[3]
26. mental mechanism — term refers to a number of intrapsychic processes primarily functioning on an unconscious level such as most of the defense mechanisms. Thinking, memory and perception are included.[3, 69]
    a. compensation — an individual's striving to make up for deficiencies.
    b. conversion — emotional conflict expressed in somatic symptoms.
    c. denial — reality factors denied in an effort to resolve emotional conflict.[69]
    d. displacement — tension reducing mechanism in which an emotional response is transferred from its real source to a more acceptable substitute.[69]
    e. dissociation — a group of ideas, memories and feelings which have escaped from normal consciousness and the control of the individual.[69]
    f. identification — unconscious imitation of another.
    g. projection — mental mechanism by which unacceptable desires are disowned and attributed to another.[69]
    h. regression — an anxiety evading mechanism, a readoption of immature patterns of thought, behavior and emotional responses.[69]
    i. repression — a common mechanism which excludes unacceptable desires, impulses and thoughts from conscious awareness.[69]
    j. sublimation — the channelling of undesirable impulses and drives away from their primitive objectives into activities of a higher order. This defense mechanism is nonpathogenic.[3, 69]
27. obsession — persistent thought which the individual knows is unrealistic.
28. phobia — any morbid fear.
29. sensory deprivation — experience of being cut off from usual external stimuli and the opportunity for perception. May occur in various ways such as through loss of hearing or eyesight, by solitary confinement, by travelling in space. May lead to disorganized thinking, depression, panic, delusions and hallucinations.[3]
30. somnambulism — sleep walking, writing or performing other acts automatically in a somnolent state without remembering the fact on awakening.

RADIOLOGY

A. Terms Related to Diagnostic Radiology:

1. cerebral angiography — a method of demonstrating the cervical and cerebral blood vessels by taking a series of radiograms during the injection of a contrast medium. Extracranial atheromatous occlusions of the carotid, vertebral and subclavian arteries producing cerebrovascular insufficiency can be readily detected and are surgically correctable. A radiographic visualization of the intracranial vasculature may be of diagnostic value in locating space-occupying lesions, brain tumors, cerebral aneurysms, embolism and thrombosis. Various techniques have been devised.[33, 60, 75, 99]

    a. aortic arch catheterization, thoracic aortography — this procedure includes a percutaneous puncture with insertion of a catheter, its retrograde advancement into the aortic arch usually by the transfemoral route and an arterial injection of a contrast medium for each of the serial angiograms. In occlusive disease or tortuosity of the iliacs a brachial, axillary, or subclavian artery may be used. The procedure demonstrates the site and extent of vascular occlusions and of collateral blood vessels and permits the determination of the regional circulation time.[33, 75, 99]

    b. vertebrobasilar angiography — a visualization of the vertebral arteries is achieved in various ways. For example: a right vertebral artery can be identified by introducing a contrast medium into the brachiocephalic trunk via a percutaneous puncture of the right subclavian artery followed by a series of angiograms.[33] The procedure is primarily used in the detection of subarachnoid hemorrhage and subtentorial abnormalities.[99]

2. discography — a diagnostic aid in the detection of herniated lumbar or cervical intervertebral discs. A contrast medium is directly injected into the disc and followed by radiograms of the spine.

3. myelography — the injection of a radiopaque substance into the subarachnoid space either by lumbar or cisternal puncture. This permits the observation of its rise and fall in the spinal canal with the fluoroscope when the position of the patient is changed.[91]

4. ventriculography — the introduction of air into the ventricular system following the removal of cerebral fluid. This procedure permits radiographic examination of the brain.[79]

B. Terms Related to Special Radiographic Techniques:

1. angiotomography, angioautomography — section angiograms for visualization of selected cerebral blood vessels. For example:
    a. vertebral arteriogram — angiogram of value in demonstrating arterial aneurysm.
    b. vertebral venogram — angiogram useful in visualizing brain stem glioma or other pathologic disorders.[81]

2. computed tomography (CT) of the brain, ACTA technique — a radiologic method using an automatic computerized transverse axial (ACTA) tomographic scanner for establishing a diagnosis. The patient's head is placed in the center of the scanning ring and the x-ray beam is directed to scan the brain from 180 different angles. Multiple profiles of x-ray transmission reflect variations in tissue absorption. The ACTA technique readily distinguishes between white and gray matter, fissures, gyri and ventricles and visualizes hydrocephalus, cerebral hematomas, tumors, infarcts, aneurysms, cerebral atrophy, metastasis and arteriovenous malformation. Since ACTA scanning is not encumbered by a water medium it can be used for the radiologic study of virtually every body organ.[27, 41, 90, 100]

3. computed tomography (CT) of the brain, EMI technique — a radiographic study of the intracranial contents using an EMI scanner built by England's Corporation EMI Limited. Diagnostic evidence is provided by scanning the brain 180 times at various angles with a narrow x-ray beam. Contiguous slices show differential tissue absorption which is calculated by a computer and presented in a series of images of the cerebral structures. This method offers a rich source of anatomic and pathologic information, particularly in regard to primary and metastatic tumors of the brain. A limiting and undesirable feature is the need of a water medium in performing the procedure.[6, 74, 100]

4. magnification cerebral angiography — enlargement technique for enhancement of vascular detail and optimal visualization of abnormalities such as aneurysms, cerebrovascular disease, arteriovenous malformations, gliomas and others.[63]

5. subtraction cerebral angiography — technique used as a complement to magnification of angiogram. The procedure includes the making of a
    a. base angiogram — a radiographic image without using a contrast medium.
    b. diapositive — a photographic contact print showing a reversal of image relationships: white to black. It is superimposed on an angiogram of the radiographic series.

c. subtraction image — angiogram shows improved visualization due to removal of overlying bone and contrast medium that would otherwise obscure the vascular detail.[63]

C. Basic Terms Related to Diagnostic Ultrasound:

1. contact scanning — contact of ultrasound with skin while scanning by means of a coupling agent such as a soluble aqueous gel.[7, 79]
2. coupling agent — agent needed to keep the ultrasound transducer in contact with the skin.
3. crystal — component of transducer which sends out vibrations producing sound.
4. density — mass per unit of volume.
5. diagnostic presentation:
   a. modes — methods of display or imaging:
      (1) A-mode — amplitude modulation which portrays echoes as vertical spikes and reflects the height of the spike in proportion to the strength of the echoes. The transducer remains stationary.[7, 23, 79]
      (2) B-mode — brightness modulation which depicts echoes on a linear trace as dots differing in size and intensity relative to the strength of the echoes. Two methods are used:
         (a) B-mode in time motion (TM) — the transducer remains in a fixed position while used to reflect echoes of a moving structure.
         (b) B-mode, B scan, ultrasonography — the transducer is guided across the body region under study, producing a transectional, bidimensional image of the structures.[23, 79]
      (3) M-mode — motion modulation which displays the changing pattern in echoes with the transducer in fixed position and the trace moving sideways.[7, 79]

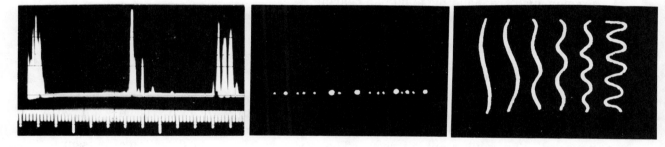

Fig. 36 — A-mode . . . amplitude . . . spikes; B-mode . . . brightness . . . dots; M-mode or T-mode (TM) . . . time motion representing 3 methods of ultrasound imaging. The B and M modes are schematic.

   b. Doppler ultrasound — continuous ultrasonography, concerned with the change in the frequency of sound waves which are reflected from a pulsating target or circulating blood in a vessel and are transmitted as audible sounds.[23, 79]
6. echography — reflected ultrasound imaging.[7] Related terms are:
   a. anechoic, sonolucent — echo-free, nonproductive of echoes.
   b. echogenic — echo-producing, productive of echoes.
   c. echogenicity — ability to produce echoes.
   d. echogram — a graphic record of reflected ultrasound imaging.
   e. echographic signs:
      (1) attenuation sign — a decrease in reflective sound or echoes in solid tissue used to differentiate solid from cystic fluid-filled lesions.
      (2) posterior echo accumulation sign — an indication of the fluid-filled cystic nature of an anechoic pattern.[79]
7. frequency — number of cycles per second.[79]
8. grey scale ultrasound — an ultrasound image containing various shades of grey rather than only black and white. A grey scale image contains more complete information since echoes of the intermediate strength are recorded.[79]

9. Hertz (Hz) — a unit of frequency equivalent to one cycle per second.[7]
10. impedence — product of the density and velocity of a material.
11. megaHertz — 1,000,000 Hertz or one million cycles per second.
    (1 Hz = 1 cycle per second.)
12. noninvasive — without entering the body or any surface with an instrument, tube, needle etc., including contrast material.[79]
13. reflection — the return of an echo from a surface, the strength of return being related to impedence.[79]
14. scan, ultrasound — any procedure which moves the sonic beam and is simultaneously followed by the trace.[7]
15. sonic — pertaining to the audible range; sound is heard by the human ear.
    a. subsonic — below the audible range; sound is too weak to be heard.
    b. ultrasonic — above the audible range.
16. strength of echo — sensitivity of sound beam capable of delineating differences in tissue density with minute precision.[7]
17. transducer, ultrasonic — electronic instrument which converts electric energy into mechanical energy.[7]
18. ultrasonic scan — any procedure which moves the sonic beam and is simultaneously followed by a trace.
19. ultrasonography, diagnostic — the recording of ultrasonic waves as they pass through deep structures of different density in order to locate pathologic lesions.
    a. reflective ultrasound — use of echoes reflected from tissues.
    b. transmission ultrasound — use of ultrasound after passage through areas of interest in the body.[79]
20. ultrasound, ultrasonic — referring to sound beams of frequencies over 20,000 cycles per second which are inaudible to human hearing.
21. velocity — product of frequency times wave length ($V = f\lambda$).
22. wave length — distance between one given point and the next similar point of a wave measured in the direction of propagation.[79]

D. Terms Related to Diagnostic Ultrasound of the Brain:

1. echoencephalography — a rapid determination of intracranial midline displacements using ultrasonic pulse echo techniques. As soon as the density of the brain tissue is altered, a pulse beam of high frequency sound, emitted by the transmitter, will echo back and be recorded on an oscillographic screen. The procedure aids in the detection of pressure-producing and space-occupying brain lesions, cerebrovascular disease, seizure disorder, hydrocephalus, mental retardation and brain death.[68, 91]
2. ultrasonography (Doppler) in supraorbital region — blood flow measurements by the transmission of a sound wave of ultrasonic frequency.[33, 100]
    a. **Normal blood flow** — the direction of the blood flow is from the ophthalmic artery into the supraorbital artery and over some ramifications into the external carotid artery.
    b. **Retrograde blood flow** — a reversal of the blood flow occurs in occlusion of the internal carotid artery and is detectable by ultrasonography.[33]

E. Terms Related to Therapeutic Radiology:

1. radioresistant neoplasms — tumors composed of cells which cannot be destroyed by radiotherapy without producing irreversible damage to the surrounding normal structures; for example, many brain tumors are radioresistant.*
2. radiotherapy for intracranial tumors — postoperative irradiation, an effective treatment tool, after the removal of low-grade astrocytomas and medulloblastomas. Limited or no benefit is obtained from radiotherapy for intracranial metastasis of primary breast cancer.[8, 26]

---

*Don C. Weir, M.D. Personal communications.

CLINICAL LABORATORY

A. Terms Related to Cerebrospinal Fluid Studies:

1. collection of cerebrospinal fluid —
    a. cisternal puncture — removal of cerebrospinal fluid from the cisterna magna, for example, in case of blocking of central canal of spinal cord.
    b. lumbar puncture — needle puncture of subarachnoid space of the lumbar cord used in determining cerebrospinal fluid (CSF) pressure and removing CSF for diagnostic evaluation or other purposes.
    c. ventricular puncture — removal of ventricular fluid, rarely done on adults except for ventriculography, but a common procedure for infants with open fontanels.
2. examination of cerebrospinal fluid (CSF)
    a. chemical analysis of CSF: chloride, protein, glucose, bilirubin, others.
    b. cytology of spinal fluid — cell count and differential leukocyte count of spinal fluid.
    c. Lange colloidal gold test — test for cerebrospinal fluid. The curve obtained aids in the differential diagnosis of disorders of the nervous system.
    d. Queckenstedt test — diagnostic maneuver consisting in compression of one or both jugular veins which normally results in a quick, brief rise of pressure of the cerebrospinal fluid. In blockage of vertebral canal, the rise in CSF is minimal or absent.
    e. turbidity of spinal fluid — cloudy appearance due to the presence of microorganisms, granules or flaky material in spinal fluid.
    f. VDRL of spinal fluid — qualitative and quantitative tests for neurosyphilis.
    g. xantochromic — canary yellow. Xantochromic spinal fluid may occur in cerebral hematoma, subarachnoid hemorrhage, toxoplasmosis, abscesses and tumors.[53, 61]

B. Terms Related to Special Diagnostic Procedures:

1. electroencephalography — the tracing or recording of the electric current generated in the cerebral cortex by brain waves. Marked irregularities indicate pathologic conditions such as epilepsy, brain tumors, scars and other disorders. The procedure is an aid to medical diagnosis and treatment.
2. electronystagmography — electric stimulation of the eyeball to induce nystagmus for the recording of eye movements in nystagmus.[91, 98]
3. facial thermography — a photographic measurement of skin temperatures of the face. In a controlled environment the skin temperatures reflect variations in blood flow. The central portion of the supraorbital region is the only skin area of the face which receives its blood supply from the terminal branches of the internal carotid artery. In severe stenosis of the internal carotid artery the decreased blood flow lowers the skin temperature in the medial supraorbital region. The cool area is detectable by a thermogram.[23, 33]
4. rheoencephalography — graphic registration of the changes in conductivity of nerve tissue caused by vascular factors.[97]

C. Terms Related to Psychometric Tests:[10, 12]

1. intelligence tests — devices set up to determine an individual's native intellectual ability including the level of his functioning in various areas. The following tests have been widely accepted.
    a. Stanford-Binet — shows range of mental ability by age. It is assumed that mental growth stops at the age of fifteen.
    b. Wechsler Adult Intelligence Scale — a verbal and a performance test designed to measure the intellectual capacity of adults at different age levels.
    c. Wechsler Intelligence Scale for Children — test devised primarily to classify children according to their intellectual abilities.[12]

2. projective tests — methods employed to uncover a subject's unconscious attitudes, needs and relationships to others. When taking a test, the subject projects the pattern of his own psychological life and thus reveals the underlying dynamics of his personality structure. Of value are the following:
   a. Minnesota Multiphasic Personality Inventory — affords insight into various phases of the patient's personality.[95]
   b. Rorschach Personality Test — attempts to detect conscious or unconscious personality traits and conflicts through eliciting the individual's associations to a set of ink blots.
   c. Thematic Apperception Test — uses twenty pictures to stimulate projective expression of personality traits.[12]

D. Terms Related to Neurologic Examination:[91]

1. Babinski reflex — extension of the great toe with or without plantar flexion of other toes when examiner strokes the sole. A positive Babinski suggests organic disease of the pyramidal tracts.
2. Brudzinski sign — when head is passively flexed on chest, the patient draws up legs reflexly. This occurs in meningeal irritation and meningitis.
3. carotid compression test — evaluation of cerebral blood flow by compressing the carotid arteries digitally. This may lead to the detection of cerebrovascular insufficiency. An irritable carotid sinus reflex is evoked by unilateral compression.
4. Kernig sign — when the patient is supine and his thigh is flexed upon the abdomen, he is unable to extend the leg. This sign is present in meningeal irritation and meningitis.
5. Romberg sign — inability of ataxics to stand steady with their eyes closed and feet together.

E. Terms Related to Miscellaneous Tests:[109]

1. barbiturate serum concentration — Method of Schreiner
   Potentially fatal level of intoxication with
   a. most short acting barbiturates .... 3.5 mg/dl
   b. phenobarbital approximately .... 8.0 mg/dl.
2. ethanol blood concentration
   mild to moderate intoxication .... 80-200 mg/dl
   marked intoxication .... 250-400 mg/dl
   severe intoxication .... above 400 mg/dl.

ABBREVIATIONS

A. General:

ANS — autonomic nervous system
AESP — applied extrasensory projection
CA — chronologic age
CBF — cerebral blood flow
CBS — chronic brain syndrome
CNS — central nervous system
cps — number of cycles per second
CP — cerebral palsy
CR — conditioned reflex
CS — conditioned stimulus
CS — completed stroke
CSF — cerebrospinal fluid
CVA — cerebrovascular accident
CVD — cerebrovascular disease

DCR — direct cortical response
DSM — Diagnostic and Statistical Manual of Mental Disorders
DT — delirium tremens
ECT — electroconvulsive therapy
EEG — electroencephalogram
ESP — effective sensory projection extrasensory perception
Ej — elbow jerk
EST — electric shock therapy
ICT — insulin coma therapy
IQ — intelligence quotient
Kj — knee jerk
LP — lumbar puncture
LSD — lysergic acid diethylamide

MAO — monoamine oxidase
MS — multiple sclerosis
NREM — no rapid eye movements
(sleep)
OBS — organic brain syndrome
PEG — pneumoencephalogram
PNS — peripheral nervous system

REM — rapid eye movements
(deep sleep)
SLE — St. Louis encephalitis
SNS — sympathetic nervous system
SR — stimulus response
TIA — transient ischemic attack
TIA-IR — transient ischemic attack —
incomplete recovery
UCR — unconditioned reflex

B. Tests

CAT — Child's Apperception
Test
ITPA — Illinois Test of Psycho-
linguistic Ability
MMPI — Minnesota Multiphasic
Personality Inventory
TAT — Thematic Apperception
Test

WAIS — Wechsler Adult
Intelligence Scale
WISC — Wechsler Intelligence
Scale for Children
WPPSI — Wechsler Preschool and
Primary Scale of
Intelligence

C. Organizations:

AA — Alcoholics Anonymous
ABPN — American Board of
Psychiatry and
Neurology
ADA-MHA — Alcohol, Drug Abuse
and Mental Health
Administration
APA — American Psychiatric
Association

CMHC — Community Mental Health
Center
MHA — Mental Health Associa-
tion
NAMH — National Association
of Mental Health
NARC — National Association for
Retarded Children
NIMH — US National Institute for
Mental Health

D. Ultrasound:

A-mode — amplitude modu-
lation
B-mode — brightness modu-
lation
f — frequency
Hz — Hertz

mHz — megaHertz
M-mode — motion modulation
TM — time motion
TP — time position
V — velocity
λ — wave length

ORAL READING PRACTICE

Drug Abuse and Dependence — Major Psychiatric Problem

The multiphasic causes that made modern society receptive to the degrading influence of addicting drugs are linked with scientific progress which facilitates their production and distribution.   Another dimension is the **psychosocial milieu** of many adult users who seek to drown their problems, relieve their depression and recapture happiness in a dream world.[58]   In teenagers and adolescents peer pressure, a craving for excitement and revolt against legal restrictions are dominant incentives of drug abuse.[44]   Children, trusting and vulnerable, easily fall prey to the allurements of peddlers.   Still worse the neonate who has become drug addicted in his **intrauterine** existence because of his maternal heritage, begins life physiologically damaged, **icteric, hypoxic** and **neuralgic,** suffering the pangs of withdrawal symptoms.

The essential components of drug addiction are tolerance, physical dependence and psychologic dependence or habituation.

Tolerance refers to the diminishing effect of the drug after continuous use. Consequently, the addict will take increasingly larger doses to attain the desired pleasurable effect and comfort provided by the drug.

Physical dependence reveals an altered physiologic state resulting from the frequent administration of the drug over a predictable period of time.[10, 36] If the drug is withheld, the abstinence syndrome develops.

Psychologic dependence or habituation is manifested by an irresistible craving compelling the addict to use the drug as an escape measure from unpleasant situations and a psychologic crutch for a new lease on life.[36]

Drugs commonly causing dependence in this country are **narcotics**: opium, morphine, heroin, dilaudid; **sedative-hypnotics**: barbiturates, meprobamate, diazepam, glutethimide; **stimulants**: amphetamines, cocaine and many other drugs. **Hallucinogens** also known as psychedelics or psychotogens are high risk agents because of their unpredictable effect and psychosis-inducing properties.[10, 19, 56, 89]

Since 1950 the problem of **heroin addiction** among teenagers and adolescents has become acute in the large metropolitan areas. Heroin users begin snuffing the potent narcotic, then take it subcutaneously and finally intravenously. The high, pleasurable feeling of early heroin use is followed by episodes of low feeling and depression as drug dependence develops and the addict experiences the torments of withdrawal symptoms.[36, 56] To escape these torments he feels compelled to increase his heroin supply irrespective of morality and the law. The stage is set for crime.[31, 43, 58, 59]

Various degrees of **abstinence phenomena** develop in narcotic dependence beginning with restlessness, craving for the drug and anxiety. This is followed on the second level by restless sleep, yawning, **rhinorrhea, lacrimation** and **diaphoresis**. As dependence increases **pupillary** changes, diminished **reactivity** to light, **anorexia**, gooseflesh, muscular twitching and **arthralgia** mark the third level of the abstinence syndrome. The climax is reached when extreme restlessness, insomnia, fever, **tachycardia**, hypertension, **hyperpnea** appear and diarrhea, nausea and vomiting result in marked weight loss indicating widespread **cardiovascular, respiratory** and **gastrointestinal** involvement.[36, 57]

Marijuana's legal control has been a debatable issue since it does not seem to cause psychic dependence. However there is overwhelming evidence that marijuana can become the vehicle of contact with the subculture of drug users who disseminate the **illicit drug scene**.[77, 88] Experimentation with more harmful drugs: **psychedelics, amphetamines** and **heroin**, so often observed in habitual users, makes marijuana smoking an extremely dangerous habit.

Research indicates that psychedelics do not stimulate physical or psychologic dependence.[55] Tolerance to mescaline evolves slower than that of psilocybin. Psychedelics are usually taken in small dosage **orally**, once or twice, rarely over a prolonged period. Their adverse effects are multiple. They trigger **transient psychosis** in normal individuals, create ecstatic dreamlike states in some, agitation, anxiety and depression in others driving them to commit suicide. Psychedelics produce **erratic behavior, visual hallucinations, delusions, panic, distortions** of time and space which may last days and weeks after taking a single dose.[55] Users of these drugs are the emotionally unstable or immature, the borderline schizophrenic and deeply depressed.[10, 14, 19, 22, 36, 39, 43, 44, 57, 58, 89]

Table 5

SOME CONDITIONS AMENABLE TO NEUROSURGERY

Organs Involved	Diagnoses	Operations	Operative Procedures
Brain Carotid arteries	Cerebrovascular insufficiency due to atherosclerotic plaque at the bifurcation of the common carotid artery	Carotid endarterectomy of extracranial lesion	Incision to expose the obstructive plaque Peeling out the lesion Arterectomy closed by suturing a Dacron patch into it to widen the artery

Organs Involved	Diagnoses	Operations	Operative Procedures
Brain Internal carotid artery Middle cerebral artery	Massive thrombotic occlusion of internal carotid artery with embolization of middle cerebral artery causing cerebral ischemia	Microsurgical anastomosis of temporal artery to middle cerebral artery[a]	Craniectomy or osteoplastic flap Use of operating microscope Creation of a surgical union of the temporal artery and patent segment of middle cerebral artery to support the circulation[a]
Brain Meningeal artery	Rupture of middle meningeal artery Epidural hemorrhage Epidural hematoma	Surgical exploration of subtemporal region Removal of epidural hematoma	Drilling exploratory burr holes Burr hole enlarged for exposure of hematoma Removal of epidural hematoma by suction
Brain Subarachnoid space	Subarachnoid hemorrhage from ruptured aneurysm of internal carotid artery	Ligation of carotid artery[b] Intracranial clipping or ligation of aneurysm	Tying the carotid artery in the neck Applying a clip or ligature to the aneurysmal sac[b]
Brain Subdural space	Subdural hematoma of the brain	Drainage of subdural space Craniotomy and excision of hematoma	Evacuation of the clot through trephine opening in the skull Surgical opening of the skull and removal of subdural hematoma
Brain Dura mater	Craniocerebral injury: open depressed fracture with dural laceration	Decompression, suture of dura mater	Elevation of depressed fracture and repair of dural laceration
Brain Meninges	Meningioma, benign	Craniotomy with excision of meningioma	Opening into skull, osteoplastic flap, removal of tumor
Brain Glial tissue	Primary malignant glioma	Craniotomy with resection of tumor	Opening into skull, osteoplastic flap, removal of tumor
Brain Choroid plexus Ventricles	Obstructive, noncommunicating hydrocephalus Nonobstructive communicating hydrocephalus	Ventriculocisternostomy, Torkildsen procedure Ventriculocaval shunt Insertion of Holter or Pudenz valve[b]	Shunting cerebrospinal fluid from third ventricle to the cisterna magna by means of plastic catheter Shunting the cerebrospinal fluid from the lateral ventricle to the superior vena cava via the jugular vein by the insertion of a one-way valve
Brain Hypophysis	Pituitary tumor Hyperpituitarism	Stereotaxic cryo-hypophysectomy[c]	Diamond drill dissection of anterior wall of sella turcica using the surgical microscope Accurate placement of cryoprobes for destruction of hypophysis and tumor
Brain Basal nuclei	Paralysis agitans or Parkinson's disease	Stereotaxic thalamotomy[b]	Introduction of radiofrequency electrode through burr hole Electrode carried to the surgical target by stereotaxic instrument Destruction of ventrolateral nucleus of thalamus[b]

Organs Involved	Diagnoses	Operations	Operative Procedures
Brain Trigeminal nerve	Trigeminal neuralgia (Tic douloureux)	Retrogasserian neurotomy	Transection of sensory root of trigeminal nerve
Brain Vestibulocochlear nerve	Acoustic neurilemmoma	Suboccipital craniectomy Microneurosurgical excision of acoustic tumor[d]	Excision of portion of skull, transmeatal approach Removal of acoustic tumor from internal auditory canal by microdissection[d]
Spinal cord	Intractable pain due to any cause	Cordotomy Percutaneous high cervical cordo- tomy[b]	Transection of pain tracts in spinal cord Stereotaxic method used for locating and interrupting the spinothalamic tract in the cervical cord[b]
Spinal cord Ganglia	Intractable pain in extremity due to Causalgia Raynaud's disease Buerger's disease	Sympathectomy	Removal of sympathetic chain and ganglia
Spinal cord Subarachnoid space	Intractable pain in malignant disease	Alcohol injection as nerve block	Injection of alcohol into sub- arachnoid space
Lumbar spinal cord Sensory nerve roots	Intractable pain of posterior spinal nerve roots at lumbar level	Posterior lumbar rhizotomy	Section of posterior spinal nerve roots in lumbar region
Spinal cord Sensory nerve roots	Intractable pain due to herniated nucleus pulposus	Laminectomy Excision of herniated nucleus pulposus[b]	Removal of laminae of vertebrae concerned and lesion[b]

[a]Kenneth R. Smith, M.D. Personal communications.
[b]Edmund A. Smolik, M.D. Personal communications.
[c]C. B. Wilson. Stereotaxic hypophysectomy. In Youmans, Julian (ed.). *Neurological Surgery*, Vol. III. Philadelphia: W. B. Saunders Co., 1973, pp. 1908-1914.
[d]R. W. Rand. Acoustic neuromas. In Youmans, Julian (ed.). *Neurological Surgery*, Vol. III. Philadelphia: W. B. Saunders Co., 1973, pp. 1432-1465.

REFERENCES AND BIBLIOGRAPHY

1. Adams, J. E. Parkinson's disease — epilepsy. In Dunphy, J. Engelbert and Way, Lawrence W. *Current Surgical Diagnosis and Treatment.* 2d ed. Los Altos, California: Lange Medical Publications, 1975, pp. 776-777.
2. Ahmadi, P. M. *et al.* Depressive syndrome induced by oral contraceptives. *Diseases of the Nervous System,* 37: 406-408, July, 1976.
3. *A Psychiatric Glossary,* 4th ed. Washington, D.C.: American Psychiatric Association, 1975. *Verbatim,* with permission.
4. Astrom, K. E. *et al.* Traumatic diseases of the brain. In Wintrobe, Maxwell M. (ed.). *Harrison's Principles of Internal Medicine,* 7th ed. New York: McGraw-Hill Book Co., 1974, pp. 1780-1790.
5. Austin, George M. (ed.). *Microsurgical Anastomoses for Cerebral Ischemia.* Springfield, Illinois: Charles C. Thomas, 1976.
6. Baker, H. L. *et al.* Early experience with the EMI Scanner for study of the brain. *Radiology,* 116: 327-333, August, 1975.
7. Barnett, Ellis and Morley, Patricia. *Abdominal Echography.* London: Butterworths & Co., 1974, pp. 2-132.
8. Bloom, H. J. G. Combined modality therapy for intracranial tumors. *Cancer,* 35: 111-120, January, 1975.
9. Bondurant, W. W. Depression and manic depres-

sion. In Conn, Howard F. *Current Therapy 1976*. Philadelphia: W. B. Saunders Co., 1976, pp. 839-845.

10. Brophy, J. J. Psychiatric disorders. In Krupp, Marcus A. and Chatton, Milton J. *Current Medical Diagnosis and Treatment*, 15th ed. Los Altos, California: Lange Medical Publications, 1976, pp. 594-644.

11. Cancro, R. Schizophrenia. In Conn, Howard F. *Current Therapy 1976*. Philadelphia: W. B. Saunders Co., 1976, pp. 845-849.

12. Carr, A. C. Psychological testing of intelligence and personality. In Freedman, Alfred M., Kaplan, Harold I., Sadock, Benjamin J. *Comprehensive Textbook of Psychiatry*, 2d ed., Vol I. Baltimore: Williams & Wilkins Co., 1975, pp. 736-757.

13. Cassidy, F. M. Adult hydrocephalus. *American Journal of Nursing*, 72: 494-497, March, 1972.

14. Chappel, J. N. Methadone and chemotherapy in drug addiction. *Journal of American Medical Association*, 228: 725-728, May 6, 1974.

15. Chase, T. N. *et al.* Huntington's chorea. *Archives of Neurology*, 26: 282-284, March, 1972.

16. Chusid, Joseph G. Central nervous system. In *Correlative Neuroanatomy and Functional Neurology*, 16th ed. Los Altos, California: Lange Medical Publications, 1976, pp. 1-70.

17. Chusid, J. G. Nervous system. In Krupp, Marcus A. and Chatton, Milton J. *Current Medical Diagnosis and Treatment*, 15th ed. Los Altos, California: Lange Medical Publications, 1976, pp. 553-593.

18. Committee on Nomenclature and Statistics of the American Psychiatric Association. *Diagnostic and Statistical Manual of Mental Illness*, 2d ed. Washington, D.C.: American Psychiatric Association, 1968.

19. Condon, A. and Roland, A. Drug abuse jargon. *American Journal of Nursing*, 71: 1738-1739, September, 1971.

20. Cooley, Denton A. Cerebrovascular insufficiency syndromes and their surgical treatment. *Hospital Medicine*, 8: 20-25, September, 1965.

21. Cronquist, S. *et al.* Hydrocephalus and congestive heart failure caused by intracranial arteriovenous malformations in infants. *Journal of Neurosurgery*, 36: 249-254, March, 1972.

22. Crowley, T. J. *et al.* Drug and alcohol abuse among psychiatric admissions: A multidrug clinical-toxicologic study. *Archives of General Psychiatry*, 30: 13-20, January, 1974.

23. Curcio, B. M. Ultrasonography and thermography. In Merrill, Vinita. *Atlas of Roentgenographic Positions and Standard Radiologic Procedures*, 4th ed., Vol III. St. Louis: The C. V. Mosby Co., 1975, pp. 946-959.

24. Daniels, R. S. Milieu therapy. In Freedman, Alfred, Kaplan, Harold, Sadock, Benjamin. *Comprehensive Textbook of Psychiatry*, 2d ed., Vol. II. Baltimore: Williams & Wilkins Co., 1975, pp. 1990-1994.

25. De Jong, Russell N. and Sugar, Oscar (eds.). Congenital disorders — Tumors. *Neurology and Neurosurgery 1976*. Chicago: Year Book Medical Publishers Inc., 1976, pp. 347-450.

26. Deutsch, M. *et al.* Radiotherapy for intracranial metastases. *Cancer*, 34: 1607-1611, November, 1974.

27. DiChiro, G. Computerized axial tomography in syringomyelia. *New England Journal of Medicine*, 292: 13-16, January 2, 1975.

28. DiChiro, G. *et al.* Spinal descent of cerebrospinal fluid in man. *Neurology*, 26: 1-8, January, 1976.

29. Dix, M. R. Episodic vertigo. In Conn, Howard F. *Current Therapy 1976*. Philadelphia: W. B. Saunders Co., 1976, pp. 695-700.

30. Dubois-Dalcq, M. *et al.* Subacute sclerosing panencephalitis. *Archives of Neurology*, 31: 355-363, December, 1974.

31. DuPont, R. L. and Katon, R. N. Development of a Heroin-Addiction Treatment Program. *Journal of American Medical Association*, 216: 1320-1324, May 24, 1971.

32. Ellis, Albert. *Humanistic Psychotherapy*. New York: Julian Press, Inc., 1973.

33. Fields, Wm. S. Aortocranial occlusive vascular disease (stroke). *Clinical Symposia*, 26: 3-31, September, 1974.

34. Fischer, E. G. Ventriculo-direct atrial shunts. *Journal of Neurosurgery*, 36: 438-440, April, 1972.

35. Fishman, R. A. Intracranial tumors and states causing increased intracranial pressure. In Beeson, P. B. and McDermott, W. (eds.). *Textbook of Medicine*, 14th ed. Philadelphia: W. B. Saunders Co., 1975, pp. 734-741.

36. Freedman, Alfred M., Kaplan, Harold I. and Sadock, Benjamin J. Drug dependence. *Comprehensive Textbook of Psychiatry*, Vol. II. 2d ed. Baltimore: Williams and Wilkins Co., 1975, pp. 1298-1348.

37. Friedman, A. P. Headache. In Conn, Howard F. *Current Therapy 1976*. Philadelphia: W. B. Saunders Co., 1976, pp. 692-695.

38. Furr, S. C. Subacute sclerosing panencephalitis. *American Journal of Nursing*, 72: 93-95, Jan., 1972.

39. Galanter, M. *et al.* Marijuana and social behavior. *Archives of General Psychiatry*, 30: 518-521, April, 1974.

40. Galbraith, J. G. Craniocerebral trauma. In Conn, Howard F. *Current Therapy 1976*. Philadelphia: W. B. Saunders Co., 1976, pp. 724-727.

41. Gargano, R. P. *et al.* Transverse axial tomography of the spine. *Neuroradiology*, 6: 254-258, January, 1974.

42. Glaser, G. H. The epilepsies. In Beeson, P. B. and McDermott, W. (eds.). *Textbook of Medicine*, 14th ed. Philadelphia: W. B. Saunders Co., 1975, pp. 723-734.

43. Goldstein, A. Heroin addiction. *Archives of General Psychiatry*, 33: 353-358, March, 1976.

44. Greenblatt, D. J. *et al.* Drug abuse and the emergency room physician. *American Journal of Psychiatry*, 131: 559-562, May, 1974.

45. Gurdjian, E. Stephens and Thomas, M. L. Use of microsurgery in neurolysis. In *Operative Neurosurgery*, 3rd ed. Baltimore: The Williams and Wilkins Co., 1970, p. 582.

46. ———. Supraorbital and supratrochlear neurectomy and avulsion. *Ibid.*, pp. 188-189.

47. ———. Trigeminal decompression. *Ibid.*, pp. 192-194.

48. ———. Head injury, skull fracture, concussion, others. *Ibid.*, pp. 235-289.

49. ———. Endarterectomy of carotid bifurcation —

86

Teflon graft reconstruction of internal carotid artery. *Ibid.,* pp. 306-309.

50. _____. Stereotaxis — Cingulotomy, fornicotomy, thalamotomy, amygdalotomy. *Ibid.,* pp. 216-219.

51. _____. Surgical treatment of hydrocephalus — Ventriculocisternal intubation — Ventriculocaval shunt — Insertion of Holter valve. *Ibid.,* pp. 199-210.

52. Hays, P. Manic-depressive psychoses. *Archives of General Psychiatry,* 33: 1187-1188, October, 1976.

53. Hepler, Opal E. *Manual of Clinical Laboratory Method,* 4th ed. Springfield, Illinois: Charles C. Thomas, Publisher, 1955, pp. 150-157.

54. Huckman, M. J. *et al.* Intracerebral hemorrhage. In Newton, T. H. and Potts, D. G. (eds.). *Radiology of the Skull and Brain Angiography,* Vol. II, Book 4. St. Louis: The C. V. Mosby Co., 1974.

55. Hunt, H. T. Psychedelic model of altered states of consciousness. *Archives of General Psychiatry,* 33: 867-876, July, 1976.

56. Kales, A. *et al.* Chronic hypnotic drug use: Ineffectiveness, drug withdrawal and dependence. *Journal of American Medical Association,* 227: 513-517, February, 1974.

57. Kaufman, R. E. *et al.* Overdose treatment: Addict folklore and medical reality. *Journal of American Medical Association,* 227: 411-413, January 28, 1974.

58. Khantzian, E. J. *et al.* Heroin use as an attempt to cope: Clinical observations. *American Journal of Psychiatry,* 131: 160-164, February, 1974.

59. Kilcoyne, M. *et al.* Nephrotic syndrome in heroin addicts. *The Lancet,* 1: 17-20, January 1, 1972.

60. Kilgore, B. B. *et al.* Arterial occlusive disease in adults. In Newton, Thomas H. and Potts, D. Gordon (eds.). *Radiology of the Skull and Brain,* Vol. II, Book 4. St. Louis: The C. V. Mosby Co., 1974, pp. 2310-2343.

61. Krentz, M. J. and Dyken, P. R. Cerebrospinal fluid cytomorphology — sedimentation vs. filtration. *Archives of Neurology,* 26: 253-257, March, 1972.

62. Kurland, H. D. Treatment of headache pain with autoacupressure. *Diseases of the Nervous System,* 36: 127-129, March, 1976.

63. Leeds, N. E. Image enhancement with magnification and subtraction. *Radiologic Clinics of North America,* 12: 241-256, August, 1974.

64. Lichtenfield, P. Autonomic dysfunction in the Guillain-Barré syndrome. *American Journal of Medicine,* 50: 772-780, June, 1971.

65. Lowy, F. H. Delirium. In Conn, Howard F. *Current Therapy 1976.* Philadelphia: W. B. Saunders Co., 1976, pp. 837-839.

66. May, P. A. Schizophrenia. In Freedman, Alfred, Kaplan, Harold, Sadock, Benjamin J. *Comprehensive Textbook of Psychiatry,* 2d ed., Vol. I. Baltimore: Williams & Wilkins Co., 1975, pp. 955-982.

67. McCormick, William F. and Schochet, Sidney S. *Atlas of Cerebrovascular Disease.* Philadelphia: W. B. Saunders Co., 1976, pp. 107-250.

68. McKinney, W. M. Echoencephalography. In King, Donald L. (ed.). *Diagnostic Ultrasound.* St. Louis: The C. V. Mosby Co., 1974, pp. 52-71.

69. Meissner, W. W. *et al.* Theories of personality and psychopathology — Classical psychoanalysis. In Freedman, Alfred M., Kaplan, Harold I., Sadock,

Benjamin J. *Comprehensive Textbook of Psychiatry,* 2d ed., Vol. I. Baltimore: Williams & Wilkins Co., 1975, pp. 482-573.

70. Miller, Fisher C. Cerebrovascular diseases. In Wintrobe, Maxwell M. (ed.). *Harrison's Principles of Internal Medicine,* 7th ed. New York: McGraw-Hill Co., 1974, pp. 1743-1780.

71. Molnar, G. E. Cerebral palsy. *Archives of Physical Medicine and Rehabilitation,* 57: 153-158, April, 1976.

72. Murray, M. Analytic and behavioral approaches to symptoms. *American Journal of Psychotherapy,* 30: 561-570, October, 1976.

73. Hashhold, B. S. Stereotactic neurosurgery. In Sabiston, David C. (ed.). *Davis-Christopher Textbook of Surgery.* Philadelphia: W. B. Saunders Co., 1972, pp. 1324-1327.

74. New, Paul F. J. *et al.* Computed tomography with the EMI scanner in the diagnosis of primary and metastatic intracranial neoplasms. *Radiology,* 114: 75-88, January, 1975.

75. Newton T. H. *et al.* Techniques of catheter cerebral angiography. In Newton, Thomas H. and Potts, D. Gordon, (eds.). *Radiology of the Skull and Brain,* Vol. II, Book 4. St. Louis: The C. V. Mosby Co., 1974, pp. 920-938.

76. Oshiro, L. S. *et al.* Virus-like particles in muscle from a patient with amyotrophic lateral sclerosis. *Neurology,* 26: 57-60, January, 1976.

77. Pack, A. T. *et al.* Quitting marijuana. *Diseases of the Nervous System,* 37: 205-209, April, 1976.

78. Perkins, R. K. Craniocerebral trauma. *Current Surgical Diagnosis and Treatment,* 2d ed. Los Altos, California: Lange Medical Publications, 1975, pp. 746-751.

79. Pilla, Lawrence A., M.D. Personal communications.

80. Polatin, P. Psychiatric disorders: paranoid states. In Freedman, Alfred M., Kaplan, Harold I., Sadock, Benjamin J. *Comprehensive Textbook of Psychiatry,* 2d ed., Vol. I. Baltimore: Williams & Wilkins Co., 1975, pp. 992-1002.

81. Poole, G. J. *et al.* Angiotomography. In Newton, Thomas H. and Potts, D. Gordon, (eds.). *Radiology of the Skull and Brain,* Vol. II, Book 1. St. Louis: The C. V. Mosby Co., 1974, pp. 981-1001.

82. Rand, R. W. Microneurosurgery for aneurysm of the vertebral-basilar artery system. *Journal of Neurosurgery,* 27: 330-332, October, 1967.

83. Richardson, E. P. *et al.* Degenerative diseases of the nervous system. In Wintrobe, Maxwell M. (ed.). *Harrison's Principles of Internal Medicine,* 7th ed. New York: McGraw-Hill Book Co., 1974, pp. 1833-1848.

84. Rieder, R. O. *et al.* The offspring of schizophrenics. *Archives of General Psychiatry,* 32: 200-211, February, 1975.

85. Robinson, J. L. *et al.* Subarachnoid hemorrhage in pregnancy. *Journal of Neurosurgery,* 36: 27-33, January, 1972.

86. Rogers, C. R. Client-centered psychotherapy. In Freedman, Alfred M. *et al. Comprehensive Textbook of Psychiatry,* Vol. II, 2d ed. Baltimore: The Williams & Wilkins Co., 1975, pp. 1831-1842.

87. Sabra, F. *et al.* Diseases of the spinal cord. In Wintrobe, Maxwell M. (ed.). *Harrison's Principles of Internal Medicine*, 7th ed. New York: McGraw-Hill Book Co., 1974, pp. 1737-1743.

88. Salzman, Carl *et al.* Marijuana and hostility. *American Journal of Psychiatry*, 133: 1029-1033, September, 1976.

89. Sata, L. S. *et al.* Narcotic addiction. In Conn, Howard F. *Current Therapy 1976*. Philadelphia: W. B. Saunders Co., 1976, pp. 832-835.

90. Schellinger, D. *et al.* Early clinical experience with the ACTA scanner. *Radiology*, 114: 257-262, February, 1975.

91. Schmidt, R. P. Neurologic diagnostic procedures. In Beeson, P. B. and McDermott, W. (eds.). *Textbook of Medicine*, 14th ed. Philadelphia: W. B. Saunders Co., 1975, pp. 630-634.

92. Smolik, Edmund A., M.D. Personal communications.

93. Solomon, Philip and Patch, Vernon D. (eds.). *Psychiatry*, 3rd ed. Los Altos, California: Lange Medical Publications, 1974, pp. 169-340.

94. Spalt, L. *et al.* Suicide: an epidemiologic study. *Diseases of the Nervous System*, 33: 23-29, January, 1972.

95. Spitzer, R. L. Psychiatric rating scales. In Freedman, Alfred, Kaplan, Harold, Sadock, Benjamin. *Comprehensive Textbook of Psychiatry*, 2d ed., Vol. II. Baltimore: Williams & Wilkins Co., 1975, pp. 2015-2031.

96. *Stedman's Medical Dictionary*, 23rd ed. Baltimore: The Williams & Wilkins Co., 1976, p. 1230.

97. Sugar, Oscar, DeJong, Russell N. *Neurology and Neurosurgery*, 1976, pp. 267-485.

98. *Symposium of Neuro-Ophthalmology Transactions of the New Orleans Academy of Ophthalmology*. St. Louis: The C. V. Mosby Co., 1976.

99. Taveras, Juan and Wood, Ernest H. Cerebral angiography. *Diagnostic Neuroradiology*, 2d ed., Vol. II. Baltimore: Williams & Wilkins Co., 1976, pp. 543-985.

100. _____. Computerized x-ray tomography (CT brain scan). *Ibid.*, pp. 997-1020.

101. _____. Diseases of spinal cord. *Ibid.*, pp. 1091-1249.

102. Thale, Thomas R., M.D. Personal communications.

103. Tucker, Eugene F., M.D. Personal communications.

104. Valko, R. J. Group therapy for patients with hysteria. *Diseases of the Nervous System*, 37: 484-489, September, 1976.

105. Weinstein, L. Poliomyelitis. In Wintrobe, Maxwell M. (ed.). *Harrison's Principles of Internal Medicine*, 7th ed. New York: McGraw-Hill Book Co., 1974, pp. 950-956.

106. Weitzman, D. O. Chorea in Huntington's disease. *Diseases of the Nervous System*, 37: 264-268, May, 1976.

107. Wetzel, R. D. Hopelessness, depression and suicide intent. *Archives of General Psychiatry*, 33: 1069-1073, September, 1976.

108. Wilson, C. B. Spinal trauma — Brain tumors. In Dunphy, J. Englebert and Way, Lawrence W. *Current Surgical Diagnosis and Treatment*, 2d ed. Los Altos, California: Lange Medical Publications, 1975, pp. 752-761.

109. Wintrobe, Maxwell M. (ed.) *Harrison's Principles of Internal Medicine*, 7th ed. New York: McGraw-Hill Book Co., 1974, pp. 2039-2044.

110. Woolsey, R. M. Hysteria: 1875-1975. *Diseases of the Nervous System*, 37: 379-385, July, 1976.

111. Young, R. F. Trigeminal and glossopharyngeal neuralgia. In Conn, Howard F. (ed.). *Current Therapy 1976*. Philadelphia: W. B. Saunders Co., 1976, pp. 712-714.

Chapter V
Cardiovascular Disorders

HEART AND CORONARY ARTERIES

A. Origin of Terms:

1. cardia (G) — heart
2. cardium (L) — heart
3. cor (L) — heart
4. corona (G) — crown
5. cuspid (L) — point, cusp
6. luna (L) — moon

B. Anatomic Terms:[106, 114]

1. cavities of the heart — the four heart chambers.
   a. atria (sing. atrium) — the two chambers which form the base of the heart and receive the venous blood.
   b. ventricles — the two chambers which lie anteriorly to the atria and propel blood into arteries.
2. conduction system of the heart — neuromuscular tissue specialized for the conduction of electric impulses. (Components arranged in order of function instead of alphabetic order.)[148]
   a. sinoatrial node, sinus node (SA node) — node situated in the wall of the right atrium. It is the pacemaker of the heart since it transmits impulses to both atria stimulating them to contract simultaneously.[23]
   b. atrioventricular node (AV node) — node found in the septum of the heart near the junction of the atria and ventricles. It relays impulses from the atria to the atrioventricular bundle.[148]
   c. atrioventricular bundle, bundle of His — a bundle of specialized neuromuscular tissue within the atrioventricular septum transmitting impulses from the AV node to the Purkinje fibers.[148]
   d. Purkinje fibers — cardiac muscle fibers of the conduction system which ramify beneath the endocardium and deliver impulses to the ventricular myocardium initiating contraction of the ventricles.[148]
3. heart wall and covering
   a. endocardium — interior lining of the heart wall.
   b. myocardium — the heart muscle.
   c. myocardial sinusoids — endothelium-lined spaces lying between the myocardial muscle fibers and enabling the ventricular myocardium to absorb blood in a sponge-like manner.
   d. pericardium — covering of the heart, composed of a fibrous and serous pericardium. The former fits loosely around the heart. The latter consists of a visceral layer or epicardium which adheres closely to the myocardium and a parietal layer which lines the inner surface of the fibrous pericardium. The pericardial cavity is a narrow space between the parietal and visceral layers. It contains a minimal amount of serum that serves as a lubricant.
4. orifices and valves of the heart and great vessels.
   a. atrioventricular orifices and valves — openings and cuspid valves between atria and ventricles.
      (1) mitral valve, bicuspid valve — valve between left atrium and left ventricle It contains two endothelial folds or cusps which come together when the ventricle contracts.
      (2) tricuspid valve — three endothelial folds or cusps which guard the right atrioventricular orifice.

    b. foramen ovale — opening between the two atria in fetal life. It normally closes after birth.

    c. semilunar valves — half moon-shaped flaps within the aorta and pulmonary trunk which prevent the blood from flowing back into the ventricles.[106, 114]

  5. sinuses, arteries and nerves:

    a. aortic sinuses, sinuses of Valsalva — 3 dilated spaces of the root of the aorta, related to the 3 cusps of the aortic valve.

    b. coronary arteries — branches of the ascending aorta arising from the right and left aortic sinuses. The blood vessels with their branches supply the heart muscle and form numerous anastomoses of small arteries and precapillaries. In the event of a sudden occlusion of a major coronary artery these anastomotic channels may not be able to provide adequate collateral circulation. But if a major coronary artery is slowly occluded, these channels may enlarge and maintain a sufficient blood supply to the heart muscle.[106, 114]

    c. coronary sinus — a short, broad vessel into which most of the veins of the heart empty. It, in turn, empties into the right atrium.[148]

    d. internal thoracic arteries, internal mammary arteries — blood vessels, usually arising from the subclavian arteries and passing downward on either side of the sternum. They are approximately the same caliber as the coronary arteries. They can be surgically relocated from the chest wall to a coronary artery distal to an obstructing lesion to revascularize the heart muscle.[148]

    e. parasympathetic fibers — preganglionic fibers which reach the heart via the vagus nerve. Ganglia in the heart have postganglionic fibers distributed to both the atria and ventricles. Impulses slow the heart and depress contractions.

    f. sympathetic fibers carried by the cervical and thoracic cardiac nerves to the heart muscle — fibers involved in control of the heart rate and the force of its contraction. Afferent fibers join the vagus nerve to aid in regulation of blood volume and heart rate.[114, 148]

C. Diagnostic Terms:

  1. aneurysm — a dilatation or bulging out of the wall of the heart, aorta or any other artery. Thrombi may form in the sac, break off and lead to embolism. Aneurysm may rupture. Ventricular aneurysms are usually complications of coronary atherosclerosis and myocardial infarction.[1, 68, 85, 87]

  2. angina pectoris

    a. classic angina pectoris — syndrome characterized by short attacks of substernal precordial pain which radiates to the left shoulder and arm. It is provoked by exertion and relieved by rest. Electrocardiographic (ECG) findings may show atrioventricular or intraventricular defects of conduction, nonspecific ST-T changes, an old myocardial scar or other abnormalties. About 30% of ECG studies are likely to be normal.[107, 125]

    b. unstable angina pectoris — angina in which the chest pain is more prolonged and severe than in classic angina and remains unrelieved by rest and nitroglycerine. There is electrographic evidence of myocardial ischemia, but infarction or necrosis are absent in the early phase. A favorable prognosis depends on the evolution of the collateral circulation to compensate for the impoverished blood flow of the myocardium or on revascularization surgery which has been reported to be about 80% successful. Untreated many patients eventually develop myocardial infarction and die.[131, 141]

    c. variant angina, Prinzmetal's angina — anginal chest pain at rest, prone to occur on awakening and tending to be cyclic in nature. It is usually associated with

      (1) transient S-T segment elevations or other electrographic abnormalities

      (2) spasm of the proximal right coronary artery, identified by coronary arteriography and otherwise essentially normal arteries. The spasm is

intermittent and correlates with the symptoms and electrographic findings.[54, 59, 82, 148]

3. anomalies, congenital — gross structural defects of the heart or great intrathoracic vessels arising during fetal development.

 a. atrial septal defect — abnormality resulting in a shunting of oxygenated blood from the left into the right atrium.   There are wide variations of atrial septal defects in size, position and shape.   Shunting is minimal when the defect is small.   A persistent foramen ovale is one of the septal defects which may be encountered.[93, 102, 123, 143]

 b. cor triatriatum — a heart with 3 atrial chambers due to an obstructing membrane that partitions the left atrium, thus impeding the pulmonary venous circulation causing pulmonary venous congestion, hypertension and congestive heart failure.[90, 137, 140]

 c. cor triloculare — a heart composed of 3 chambers resulting from the absence of the interatrial or interventricular septum.[107]

 d. isolated pulmonic stenosis, pure pulmonary stenosis — a narrowing of the pulmonary valve or of the infundibulum associated with an intact ventricular septum.   The stenotic defect causes pulmonary outflow tract obstruction.   (Infundibulum is the cone-shaped area of the right ventricle from which the pulmonary artery begins.)

 e. patent ductus arteriosus — persistence of communication between pulmonary artery and aorta after birth.   In normal infants the closure of the ductus takes place during the first six weeks of life.

 f. tetralogy of Fallot — a complex of congenital defects usually considered as having four parts:

  (1) ventricular septal defect — a malformation of the septum of the ventricles.

  (2) pulmonic stenosis — same as isolated type except that involvement is associated with other defects.

  (3) dextroposition of the aorta — a transposition of the aorta to the right.

  (4) hypertrophy of the right ventricle — increased size of the ventricle, nature's way of compensating for the added load imposed by the defects.   The first two are essential parts of the complex.

 g. ventricular septal defect — anomaly existing in various forms, for example:

  (1) isolated absence of the ventricular septum, partial or total — occasionally multiple.

  (2) defect associated with other anomalies.[93, 102, 117, 123, 140, 143, 148]

4. cardiac arrest — cessation of effective heart action, usually caused by asystole or ventricular fibrillation.

5. cardiac arrhythmias, cardiac dysrhythmias — irregularities of heart action including disturbances of rate, rhythm and conduction either related or unrelated to other cardiac disease, supraventricular (atrial) or ventricular.   Some major arrhythmias which seriously interfere with cardiac or circulatory efficiency are presented.[41, 67, 126, 148]

 a. atrial arrhythmias — disorders of rhythm having their origin in the SA node. They may be provoked by ischemia, drug toxicity or atrial distention.   If uncontrolled, atrial arrhythmias may become life threatening.[83, 148]

  (1) atrial fibrillation — extremely rapid, vermicular, ineffectual contractions of the atria resulting in irregularity of rhythm in the ventricles.   The atrial rate is 350 per minute or more.

  (2) atrial flutter — rapid, regular cardiac action of 250-350 beats per minute usually occurring in paroxysms, which are more prolonged than atrial tachycardia.   The atrial impulse may produce a rapid ventricular rate or result in an atrioventricular block of varying degree (e.g. 2:1, 3:1 or 4:1)

  (3) paroxysmal atrial tachycardia (PAT) — rapid, regular contractions of the atria initiated by an irritable center within the atrium outside the sinoatrial node.   Rate is about 160-200.   Ventricular contractions are in 1:1 ratio with

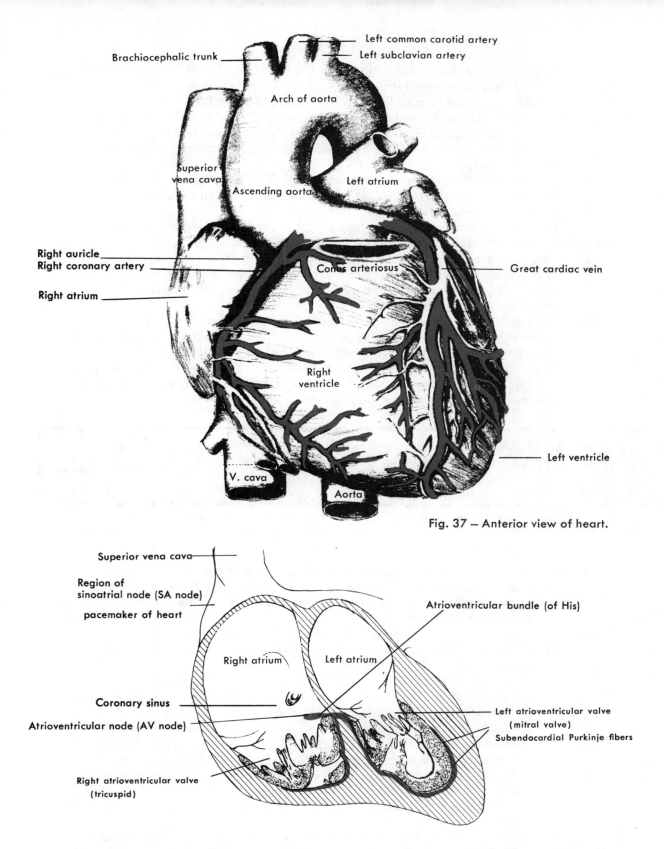

Fig. 37 — Anterior view of heart.

Fig. 38 — Schematic diagram of conduction system of heart. Impulses pass from sinoatrial node through both atria stimulating them to contract. The atrioventricular node is thereby activated, and transmits impulses to the atrioventricular bundle and its right and left limbs, resulting in the contraction of both ventricles.

atrial contractions.   This arrhythmia (PAT) is practically indistinguishable from nodal paroxysmal tachycardia.   The patient may encounter a sudden forceful thump and subsequent attack of palpitation.

  b. atrioventricular nodal arrhythmias — disorders arising in the atrioventricular node.[83]

      (1) atrioventricular nodal rhythm — pacemaker function assumed by AV node in response to sustained failure of sinoatrial node to send impulses to the atrioventricular node.

      (2) premature atrioventricular nodal contractions (PNC) — arrhythmia due to irritation of the atrioventricular node which produces an ectopic stimulus and subsequent premature nodal contractions.[83]

Frequent recurrence of PNC's may signal progressive myocardial infarction.

  c. ventricular arrhythmias — disorders of rhythm arising within the ventricles.

      (1) premature ventricular contractions (PVC) — the most common disturbance of rhythm, frequently an index of myocardial damage and anoxia.   If more than 6 PVC's per minute occur, ventricular efficiency may be seriously impaired.

      (2) ventricular tachycardia — disorder heralding a high degree of irritability frequently associated with myocardial infarction.   The irritable center within the ventricular wall produces a rapid ventricular rate which may change to ventricular fibrillation or ventricular standstill.   The rate is 150-250 or more and the rhythm slightly irregular.   Sudden dizziness, precordial pain, dyspnea and weakness are common complaints.[83]

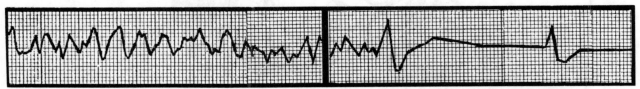

Fig. 39 — Ventricular fibrillation: life-threatening arrhythmia.

Fig. 40 — Terminal ventricular fibrillation and ventricular standstill — the dying heart.

      (3) ventricular fibrillation — extremely rapid, nonsynchronous contractions of ventricular muscle bundles, irregularities in rhythm and force resulting in no ejection of blood from the fibrillating ventricles.   It may terminate in ventricular standstill.[148]

  d. conduction disturbances — abnormalities in the cardiac conduction system.[23, 127]

      (1) atrioventricular block — delay or obstruction of impulses arising above or within the atrioventricular node.[127]

         (a) first degree heart block — prolongation of atrioventricular conduction time, delay of impulses on their ventricular pathway.   Possible causes: increased vagal tone, myocardial ischemia, drug toxicity.[32]

         (b) second degree or partial heart block — type one, benign form — blockage of one atrial beat after 6 to 8 conducted beats and dropping of respective ventricular beat (Wenckebach pause) ; type two, serious form — not all impulses are transmitted to the bundle of His by the atrioventricular node resulting in various ratios (2:1, 3:1, 4:1, other) of atrial contractions to ventricular contractions.   Wrist pulse is 40-50 beats per minute.[27, 32]

         (c) third degree or complete block — no atrial impulses are transmitted to the bundle of His by the atrioventricular node.   Wrist pulse is 30 to 40 beats per minute as a result of beats initiated within the conduction mechanism of the ventricle.[148]

      (2) bundle branch block — obstruction of the wave of excitation in either branch of the atrioventricular bundle.

(3) hemiblock — term referring to electrographic patterns that precede or coexist bundle branch blocks or are precursors of A-V conduction abnormalities.[19]

(4) Stokes-Adams syndrome — cardiac standstill which occurs with certain forms of heart block, causes syncope and possible fatal convulsions.

(5) Wolff-Parkinson-White syndrome — a congenital disorder of atrioventricular conduction which may be associated with recurrent paroxysmal tachycardia, atrial flutter or other ectopic rhythms.[29, 45, 127]

6. cardiac tamponade, pericardial tamponade — compression of the heart by effusion or hemorrhage in the pericardium which may seriously obstruct the venous inflow to the heart, raise the venous pressure, reduce the cardiac output, cause hypotension, distention of the neck veins and orthopnea.[108, 128]

7. cardiopulmonary arrest — heart-lung arrest due to sudden and unexpected cessation of respiration and functional circulation.[107]

8. congestive heart failure — condition in which the heart is unable to pump adequate amounts of blood to tissues and organs. This is generally due to diseases of the heart causing low cardiac output. It can result from other conditions (anemia, hyperthyroidism) in which the demand for blood is greater than normal and the heart fails despite high cardiac output.
   a. left-sided heart failure — failure of the left ventricle precipitated by serious coronary, hypertensive or valvular heart disease. Except in mitral stenosis it produces variable degrees of left ventricular dilatation followed by pulmonary congestion and edema, salt and water retention, scanty urinary output, cerebral hypoxia and coma.
   b. right-sided heart failure — failure of the right ventricle characterized by venous congestion of portal system with ascites and enlargement of liver and spleen.
   In advanced disease left and right-sided congestive heart failure coexist.[106, 107, 119, 128, 148]

9. coronary atherosclerosis — chronic disorder characterized by the presence of lipid deposits which form fibrous fatty plaques within the intima and inner media of the coronary arteries.[103, 116, 125]

10. coronary atherosclerotic heart disease — the most common heart condition. Progressive thickening of the intima of the coronary arteries leads to occlusion, caused by narrowing of the lumen and intravascular clotting.[31, 107, 116, 125]

11. cor pulmonale — heart-lung disease characterized by right ventricular hypertrophy due to pulmonary disorders which seriously impair ventilatory function and result in pulmonary hypertension.
    a. acute form — caused by massive pulmonary embolism occurring within hours.
    b. chronic form — caused by diffuse pulmonary fibrosis, obstructive emphysema or obstructive vascular disease developing within months.[107]

12. Ebstein's anomaly — tricuspid insufficiency due to a spiral-like attachment of a valve leaflet of the tricuspid resulting in atrial enlargement, defective ventricular filling, right-to-left shunting, other impairments and variable clinical manifestations as dyspnea, cyanosis, clubbing of fingers, precordial thrill, systolic or diastolic mumurs.[110]

13. endocarditis, bacterial — acute or subacute disease of the lining of the heart and especially valve leaflets. It is caused by infective organisms which enter the blood stream and initiate a bacteremia clinically recognized by fever, fatigue, heart murmurs, splenomegaly, embolic episodes and areas of infarction.[108, 124]

14. Libman-Sacks endocarditis — condition characterized by verrucose lesions found in the endocardium of patients with terminal disseminated lupus erythematosus.[108]

15. ischemic heart disease — cardiac disease in which the prominent feature is a markedly reduced blood supply to the heart muscle, generally due to coronary atherosclerosis. The resultant myocardial ischemia may produce myocardial infarction, heart failure or angina pectoris.[25, 107, 116, 148]

16. myocardial disease, primary:
    a. myocarditis — inflammation of the heart muscle which may result in myocardial fibrosis, followed by cardiac enlargement and congestive heart failure.

b. myocardosis — condition characterized by cardiac dilatation, congestive failure and embolization.[25, 128]

17. myocardial disease, secondary:
   heart disease associated with noninfectious systemic disease such as
   a. amyloidosis
   b. carcinoidosis
   c. collagen diseases
   d. endocrinopathy
   e. sarcoidosis
   f. systemic muscular and neurologic disorders.[25, 108, 119, 128]

18. myocardial infarction, acute — clinical syndrome manifested by persistent, usually intense cardiac pain, unrelated to exertion and often constrictive in nature followed by diaphoresis, pallor, hypotension, dyspnea, faintness, nausea and vomiting. The underlying disease is usually coronary atherosclerosis which progressed to coronary thrombosis and occlusion and resulted in a sudden curtailment of blood supply to the heart muscle and myocardial ischemia.
   a. inferior wall infarction, diaphragmatc infarction — infarction due to occlusion of right coronary artery.
   b. lateral wall infarction — infarction resulting from occlusion of diagonal branch of left anterior descending artery or of left circumflex artery.
   c. posterior wall infarction — infarction precipitated by occlusive lesions of right coronary artery or circumflex coronary artery branch.[23, 25, 51, 69, 128]

19. pericarditis — inflammation of the covering membranes of the heart. Its distinctive feature is pericardial friction rub, a transitory, scratchy or leathery sound elicited on auscultation.
   a. constrictive pericarditis, chronic — disorder characterized by a rigid, thickened pericardium which prevents adequate filling of the ventricles and may lead to congestive heart failure.
   b. purulent pericarditis — disease caused by pyogenic bacteria which may be associated with purulent, pericardial effusion.[121, 128]

20. rheumatic heart disease — involvement of the heart occurring in the course of rheumatic fever and attacking the myocardium, pericardium and endocardium with the valvular endocardium as the site of predilection.[107, 118, 124, 143]

21. valvar heart disease, chronic — disorder referring to any permanent organic deformity of one or more valves. Stenosis of the valve tends to increase the cardiac work load and precipitate cardiac failure.
   a. aortic stenosis — reduction in the valve orifice interfering with the emptying of the left ventricle.
   b. mitral stenosis — a very common sequela of rheumatic fever, marked by the development of minute vegetations and thrombi which narrow the orifice of the valve leaflets. Calcifications form as the disease progresses.
   c. tricuspid stenosis — defect associated with mitral stenosis. It reduces the valve to a small triangular opening which causes resistance in the flow of blood from the right atrium to the right ventricle and leads to congestion of the lungs and liver.[87, 118, 124]

D. Operative Terms:

1. biopsy of pericardium — excision of a small piece of pericardial tissue for microscopic study.
2. cardiac biopsy — excision of tissue from the heart for the purpose of diagnosing various disease states. This can be done at the time of the operation or by means of a biotome adapted to an intracardiac catheter. Under fluoroscopic control the biotome is passed through the right saphenous vein to the right atrium and right ventricle for biopsy. Tissue studies aid in the evaluation of the patient's condition prior to cardiovascular surgery.[148]
3. cardiac massage, open — emergency thoracotomy and manual compression of the heart, 40-60 times a minute, in an attempt to force blood from the ventricles into the aorta and pulmonary artery.

4. cardiac transplantation, heart transplantation — removal of a human cadaver heart for implantation into a recipient who is in irreversible cardiac failure. The procedure includes a median sternotomy, cannulation of vena cavae, cardiopulmonary bypass, surgical divisions of the ascending aorta, main pulmonary artery and atria, the excision of donor and recipient hearts and implantation of donor heart by atrial and vascular anastomoses to recipient.[28, 148]

5. correction of congenital septal defects:
   a. atrial septal defect — closure of defect under direct vision using cardiopulmonary bypass with or without hypothermia.
   b. ventricular septal defect — repair of defect by
      (1) direct suture or
      (2) use of ventricular patch such as Ivalon pledget.
      Extracorporeal circulation with or without hypothermia is employed.[24, 120, 135, 140]

6. correction of patent ductus arteriosus —
   a. catheter closure of ductus — under fluoroscopic control a catheter is percutaneously placed into the femoral artery and advanced across the ductus through the right heart. A closure plug is rammed into the ductus. No thoracotomy is needed. This method has been employed infrequently.[135, 136, 140, 148]
   b. complete division of patent ductus — the ductus is divided and the pulmonic and aortic ends are closed separately by suture.[148]

7. correction of transposition of the great vessels.
   a. Blalock-Hanlon operation — surgical creation of an atrial septal defect as a palliative method which provides increased intracardiac mixing of the oxygenated and unoxygenated blood.
   b. Mustard operation — surgical revision of the atrial septum, transposing the venous return to match the transposed outflow tracts.
   c. Rashkind operation, atrioseptostomy by balloon catheter — surgical creation of an atrial septal defect for palliation.[14, 55, 58, 140, 148]

8. mitral commissurotomy — separation of the stenotic valve at points of fusion.[132]

9. myocardial revascularization — operative procedure which supplies the ischemic heart muscle with systemic arterial blood. Various techniques are used, for example:
   a. aortocoronary artery bypass — revascularization of the heart muscle by attaching autogenous saphenous vein grafts (SVG) to the ascending aorta and the coronary arteries distal to the occlusions. Vascular obstructions are thus bypassed and adequate blood flow to the heart is immediately restored. Since coronary atherosclerosis frequently involves several vessels, multiple grafts are often employed to safeguard permanent circulatory efficiency.[71, 78, 89, 100, 130, 148]
   b. internal mammary-coronary artery anastomoses — cardiac revascularization by joining internal mammary artery grafts (IMAG) to one or more coronary arteries to bypass occlusive lesions and relieve myocardial ischemia. Since IMA grafts have proven to be highly patent and stable, they are successfully used when recurrence of disabling angina due to graft closure or progressive coronary atherosclerosis necessitates reoperative revascularization.[9, 46, 52, 61, 71, 72, 89] Unstable angina may be effectively treated with venous autografts or internal mammary artery autografts or both.*[9, 47, 61, 130] The use of freeze-preserved saphenous vein allografts or soft flexible catheter stents in aortocoronary bypass needs further evaluation.[75, 138]

10. pericardiectomy — incision and partial dissection of the pericardium to relieve the heart from constricting fibrous adhesions.

11. pulmonary banding — operation performed on infants who are unable to withstand a complete correction of an interventricular septal defect. The pulmonary artery is partially tied off to diminish the amount of blood to the lung.[140]

12. tetralogy of Fallot — the following operations may be performed:
    a. shunting procedures, anastomoses of left subclavian and pulmonary artery and aorta.

_____

*See Fig. 41 and Fig. 42, p. 96

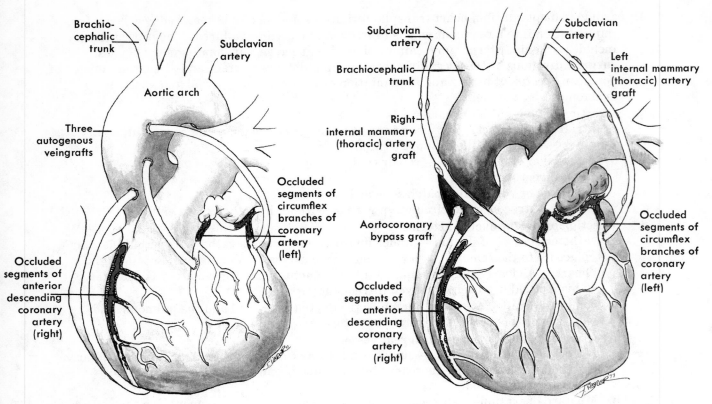

Fig. 41 — Direct myocardial revascularization by triple aortocoronary artery bypass using autogenous vein grafts.

Fig. 42 — A combination of aortocoronary and internal mammary artery bypass grafts for myocardial revascularization.

    b. correction of pulmonary stenosis by valvotomy or valvoplasty.

    c. direct vision cardiac surgery, removal of pulmonic obstruction and repair of interventricular defect using hypothermia and heart-lung machine, or machine alone.[135, 140, 148]

13. valve replacement surgery — removal of incompetent or stenotic valve and its replacement with a

    a. normal cadaver valve or stented heterograft. Valve leakage, stenosis or shrinkage lead to functional failure.[87, 133]

    b. prosthetic valve such as cloth-covered Starr-Edwards prosthesis or low-profile Teflon disc Beall prosthesis. Thromboemboli, infection and regurgitation are dreaded complications.[12, 18, 39]

14. valvotomy — incision into a valve.

    a. mitral valvotomy — splitting the two commissures (areas of fusion) of the mitral valve to widen its opening.

    b. pulmonary valvotomy — incising the valve of the pulmonary artery to improve the pulmonary circulation.

15. ventricular aneurysmectomy — excision of aneurysm which may harbor large ventricular thrombi, decreasing the pumping efficiency of the heart.[148] The procedure is usually combined with coronary revascularization using saphenous vein bypass grafts.[73, 85, 87]

E. Terms Related to Specific Procedures:

1. automation — the use of mechanical, hydraulic, pneumatic, electric and electronic devices to perform automatic measurements and control functions.

2. cardiac monitor — an electronic device which applied to a patient reveals the electric activity of the heart by visual and auditory signals and thereby permits the immediate detection of dangerous arrhythmias.

3. **cardiac pacing, physiologic** — a normal response to myocardial stimulation initiated at the sinoatrial node followed by atrial contractions, activation of the atrioventricular node, spread of the impulse through the bundle of His and subsequent contractions of the ventricles.

4. **cardiac pacing, electronic** — substitution of normal cardiac pacing in Stokes-Adams syndrome, ventricular standstill, certain dysrhythmias as tachyarrhythmias and myocardial infarction (controversial issue).

   a. **pacemakers in use:**

   (1) an external cardiac pacemaker — an electronic device for stimulating the ventricles through the closed chest wall in cardiac standstill.

   (2) an implantable cardiac pacemaker for temporary or permanent use — an electronic device achieving myocardial stimulation by means of epicardial or endocardial, unipolar or bipolar electrodes. Recent technical improvements are reduced size of pulse generator and prolonged pacemaker life due to rechargeability.[19, 22, 23, 57, 74]

   b. **types of pacing:**

   (1) demand pacing — impulse is fired by pacemaker according to patient's need. If QRS complex fails to occur within a given period, pacing impulse is triggered. If QRS complex develops within a certain interval, pacing impulse is withheld.[19, 21, 23, 127]

   (2) fixed-rate pacing — impulse is generated at a predetermined rate irrespective of intrinsic cardiac rhythm.

   (3) synchronized pacing — impulse is fired synchronously with the P wave of the patient. One electrode is placed in the atrium, the other in the ventricle. Since the atria are stimulated to pour their entire contents into both ventricles, cardiac function is almost normal and synchronous. A drawback is that a thoracotomy may be needed for a stable epicardial insertion of the atrial electrode.

   c. **methods of pacing:**

   (1) epicardial pacing — asynchronous or synchronous pacing in response to impulses of electrodes firmly attached to the epicardium and a pulse generator concealed in a subcutaneous pocket.

   (2) transthoracic pacing — ventricular stimulation achieved by electrodes inserted through the chest wall into the ventricle. A battery-powered pacer serves as a power source. Since pacing can be quickly initiated, transthoracic pacing is an effective emergency measure for resuscitating patients in cardiac arrest.

   (3) transvenous pacing — an electrode catheter introduced into the heart through the jugular or other suitable vein, its tip lodged in the right ventricular apex and the battery case located in a subcutaneous pouch below the clavicle. The rate is fixed, usually 75 impulses per minute. No thoracotomy is required. Transvenous pacing may be used temporarily for myocardial stimulation to control bradycardia and prevent ventricular standstill.[19, 21, 22, 23, 127]

5. **cardiopulmonary bypass** — a mechanism for diverting the blood around the heart and lungs for the purpose of providing inflow occlusion to the heart. This enables the surgeon to operate on a bloodless heart muscle under direct vision.

6. **cardiopulmonary resuscitation** — heart-lung revival achieved by establishing a patent airway and restoring respiratory and circulatory functions by drugs, electric myocardial stimulation, closed or open chest cardiac compression.

7. **cardioversion** — direct current (DC) countershock applied to the chest to convert abnormal rhythms to normal sinus rhythm.[99, 148]

8. **coronary artery perfusion** — introduction of blood into the coronary arteries by catheters during procedures in which the root of the aorta is opened.[148]

9. **countershock** — use of an external electronic defibrillator to terminate the disorderly electric activity within the heart that provokes the arrhythmia. In ventricular fibrillation a brief high voltage shock abruptly stops the chaotic twitching of the

ventricular muscle fibers.   If effective the natural cardiac pacemaker regains control and restores normal contractions.

10. defibrillator — mechanical device for applying electric shock to the closed chest or to the open heart to terminate abnormal cardiac rhythms.

11. diastolic augmentation procedure — a circulatory assistive technique in which a balloon, placed in the aorta, is inflated during diastole and collapsed during systole (phase-shift). This reduces the pressure against which the heart pumps yet increases diastolic pressure and thus favorably influences coronary flow.[148]

12. direct current defibrillation — countershock by a capacitor discharge defibrillator (DC type) instead of alternating current of the old type defibrillator (AC type).

13. elective cardiac arrest, cold anoxic arrest — standstill of the heart induced by cross-clamping the aorta and cardiac cooling.   The temperature may be lowered by perfusing the coronary arteries with a cold solution, instilling a coolant into the pericardial sac or applying ice to the myocardium.   Cold anoxic arrest provides a motionless, dry operative field conducive to aortic valve surgery and repair of congenital defects.[148]

14. electromagnetic flowmetry — measurement of blood flow by electromagnetic technique, useful as a diagnostic adjunct to cardiac catheterization and vascular surgery, especially by measuring flow in shunts, bypass grafts and anastomoses.   There is convincing evidence that intraoperative blood flow measurements can predict the fate of aortocoronary artery bypass grafts.[7, 8, 52, 76, 148]

15. exhaled-air ventilation — artificial respiration using the mouth-to-mouth, mouth to nose or mouth-to-tracheal stoma method to restore ventilatory lung function.

16. external arteriovenous (AV) shunt — procedure used to facilitate access to the patient's circulation by cannulation of blood vessels for prolonged hemodialysis.   One piece of Silestic tubing is inserted into an artery, the other into an adjacent vein.   They are then brought on top of the skin and connected with each other by a removable Teflon connector.

17. external cardiac compression — the application of rhythmic pressure (60 times per minute) over the lower sternum to compress the heart and produce artificial circulation.

18. extracorporeal circulation — blood circulating outside of the body, a form of cardiopulmonary bypass.   It may be achieved by using a heart-lung machine.

19. heart-lung machine — apparatus used to substitute for cardiopulmonary function.   It permits a direct vision approach to cardiac lesions requiring corrective surgery.   Venous blood returning to the heart is not allowed to enter the right atrium, but is sucked away by two tubes, one in each of the main veins.   It is then pumped into an artificial lung. After this the oxygen laden blood enters a reservoir, passes through filters and is pumped to the patient's arterial sytem.   Many different types of heart-lung machines are now in use.

20. hemodilution — reduction of normal red cell mass of the blood and its subsequent oxygen content.   It may be due to injury, hemorrhage or blood dyscrasias or therapeutically used as in cardiovascular surgery to prime the pump oxygenator system.
    a. extreme hemodilution — total washout achieved by removing most of the blood and replacing it with colloid electrolyte solution which maintains a normal circulating volume and colloid osmotic pressure of plasma.[84, 130]
    b. moderate hemodilution — induced dilution of the normal blood which keeps the volume of the packed red cells (VPRC) above 20 per cent and may be used as prime in cardiopulmonary bypass and in treating shock, polycythemia and high viscosity disorders[84, 130]

21. hyperbaric oxygenation, hyperbaroxia — the clinical use of elevated atmospheric pressure produced in a hyperbaric chamber.   Its principal effects are increased oxygenation and oxygen tension.   Hyperbaroxia is thought to be of value in some instances of cardiac surgery and the treatment of cardiogenic shock due to acute myocardial infarction.[148]

22. induced hypothermia — artificial reduction of the body temperature in an effort to lower the metabolic requirements of the patient.   He is then better able to tolerate the interruption of cardiac inflow.

23. intra-aortic balloon counterpulsation — a method of circulatory assistance for left

ventricular power failure and cardiogenic shock refractory to adrenergic stimulation. A balloon catheter is inserted in the femoral artery and advanced to the descending thoracic aorta. Circulatory assistance is provided by diastolic counterpulsation which is monitored by electrocardiographic recordings. Similar procedures have gained acceptance.[88]

24. medical electronics — the use of electronics in medical areas. Electronics refers to the action of charged electric particles in any medium: solid, liquid or gas.

25. normothermia — environmental temperature that maintains body temperature and metabolic requirements at normal levels. In current cardiovascular surgery, normothermia is usually preferred to induced hypothermia.

26. oscillation — a movement to and fro.

27. oscillometer — instrument for measuring any kind of oscillations; for example, those related to blood pressure.

28. oxymetry — measuring the amount of oxygen in a series of blood samples either chemically or by reading cuvette oxymeters of the samples obtained through a catheter from each heart chamber or vessel.[113]

29. perfusion in intracardiac surgery — method of providing oxygenated blood to the body by a heart-lung machine while interrupting the circulation through the heart.

30. precordial shock — electric treatment of arrhythmias.
   a. elective procedure for converting certain tachyarrhythmias to normal rhythm. It is known as cardioversion.
   b. emergency procedure for controlling ventricular fibrillation. It is usually referred to as defibrillation.[83]

31. pulmonary wedge pressure (PWP) — measurement of filling pressure of the left heart using an open ended catheter wedged into a small pulmonary artery. A Swan-Ganz catheter is one such device. The procedure aids in differentiating congestive heart failure, allergic drug response or fat embolism.[144, 148]

32. sphygmomanometer — instrument measuring blood pressure.

33. stethoscope — instrument for listening to sounds within the body.

34. Swan-Ganz pulmonary artery catheterization — insertion of balloon tipped catheter by subclavian venipuncture in order to catheterize the pulmonary artery and achieve hemodynamic monitoring of critically ill patients.[6]

35. synchronized direct current (DC) countershock — electric shock producing cardioversion by the use of a synchronized capacitator. The synchronizer is contraindicated in ventricular fibrillation.

36. transducer, medical use — a transforming device which transmits energy from a patient to a monitoring machine.

37. treadmill exercise tolerance — stress test for evaluating the ability of the coronary circulation to meet the metabolic demands of an increasing exercise load. The patient is subjected to graded exercise on the treadmill or bicycle ergometer until his electrocardiogram shows ischemic changes.[13, 50, 81]

38. two-step exercise test, Master's test — exercise test of coronary reserve. Within 1½ minutes the patient goes up and down 2 steps, 9 inches high, 15 to 25 times. A postexercise electrocardiogram is taken at once. If it is negative a 3 minute double two-step test is performed. As soon as the patient experiences pain the exercise is discontinued.[101]

39. Valsalva maneuver — effective treatment for paroxysmal atrial tachycardia and similar disorders. The patient is instructed to inhale deeply, hold his breath and then strain down forcefully while slowly counting for 10 seconds. The Valsalva maneuver is also used as a test for cardiac reserve.[28]

F. Symptomatic Terms:

1. anasarca — massive edema with serous effusion especially in the right pleural and peritoneal cavities. It occurs in right heart failure and systemic congestion.

2. Aschoff bodies — nodular lesions of the myocardium, pathognomonic (characteristic) of rheumatic disease.
3. asystole — cardiac standstill, no contractions of the heart.
4. bradycardia — slow heart action.
5. cardiac edema — retention of water and sodium in congestive heart failure due to circulatory impairment.
6. cardiac syncope — fainting associated with marked sudden decrease in cardiac output.
7. cardiogenic shock — syndrome related to cardiovascular disease, primarily to myocardial infarction, cardiac tamponade, massive pulmonary embolism or others. It is clinically characterized by mental torpor, reduction of blood pressure and pulse pressure, tachycardia, pallor, cold, clammy skin and signs of congestive heart failure.[144]
8. carotid sinus syncope, vasopressor type — fainting or clouded consciousness without change in heart rate. It is due to hyperirritability of the carotid sinus or local disease.
9. ischemia — reduced blood supply to an organ usually due to arterial narrowing or occlusion in advanced atherosclerosis.
   a. cerebral ischemia — local anemia in the brain.
   b. myocardial ischemia — inadequate blood supply to the heart muscle.
10. murmur — blowing sound heard on auscultation.
11. palpitation — subjective awareness of skipping, pounding or racing heart beats.
12. postinfarction (Dressler's) syndrome — syndrome developing within the first week or weeks after myocardial infarction. It exhibits the clinical features of a benign form of pericarditis with or without effusion.[66]
13. sinus rhythm — normal cardiac rhythm initiated at the sinoatrial node.
14. systole — rhythmic contractions of the heart particularly those of the ventricles which pump the blood through the body.
15. tachycardia — rapid heart action.

ARTERIES, CAPILLARIES, VEINS

A. Origin of Terms:

1. angio (G) — vessel
2. artery (G) — air duct
3. diastole (G) — expansion
4. hemangio- (G) — blood vessel
5. phleb- (G) — vein
6. pulsus (L) — stroke, beat
7. systole (G) — contraction
8. thrombos (G) — clot
9. varix (L) — swollen vein
10. vena (L) — vein

B. Anatomic Terms:[5, 102, 114]

1. aorta — the main artery of the trunk.
2. blood pressure
   a. systolic — the force exerted by the blood against the arterial walls at the end of the contraction of the left ventricle.
   b. diastolic — the force exerted by the blood against the arterial walls at the end of the relaxation of the left ventricle.
3. coats of arteries:
   a. tunica externa, adventitia — outer coat.
   b. tunica media — middle coat.
   c. tunica intima — inner coat.

C. Diagnostic Terms:

1. acute limb ischemia — a sudden catastrophic interruption of the blood flow to an extremity demanding emergency surgery to save the limb and the life of the patient, particularly if he is debilitated and advanced in years. Vascular disorders such as acute arterial embolization and the deposition of atheromatous plaques associated with bleeding and a

relatively rapid thrombus formation precipitate the occlusive event. The limb is waxy pale, cold, painful or insensitive to touch and exhibits rigidity or deep muscle tenderness.

2. aneurysm of aorta — dilatation of a weakened part of the wall of the vessel.
   a. dissecting type — progressive splitting of middle coat which may involve the entire circumference of the aorta. When pulsating blood is driven between the media and intima, the tear may rapidly extend the whole length of the aorta causing excruciating, ripping pain. A cystic medial necrosis with excess mucoid material is a frequent pathologic finding.
   b. fusiform type — tubular swelling of the walls of the aorta involving the three coats and circumference.
   c. sacculated type — saclike bulging of a weakened part of the aorta formed by the middle and outer coats.[33, 105]

3. aortic arch syndrome, pulseless disease, Takayasu's syndrome — group of disorders characterized by occlusion of vessels of the arch of the aorta associated with extremely weak or absent pulses, low blood pressure in upper extremities and diminished circulation to the brain that may result in neurologic deficit.[104, 143, 148]

4. aortic atresia — congenital absence of normal valvar opening in aorta. Heart failure develops within days.[124]

5. aortic stenosis — congenital or acquired narrowing of valvar opening into aorta.[143]

6. aortoiliac disease, Leriche's syndrome — gradual thrombosis of terminal aorta near the bifurcation and extending to the iliac arteries. Claudication and trophic changes may be present.[34]

7. arteriosclerosis — degenerative, vascular disorder characterized by a thickening and loss of elasticity of arterial walls. It assumes 3 distinctive morphologic forms.
   a. atherosclerosis — the most common form in which an intimal plaque or atheroma is produced by focal lipid deposits. In the beginning the atheroma is soft and pasty. With time the plaque may undergo fibrosis and calcification or it may ulcerate into the arterial lumen. Ulcerated plaques are prone to cause mural thrombosis and eventually arterial occlusion. Arteriosclerosis and atherosclerosis are frequently used as synonyms.
   b. arteriolosclerosis — a vascular disorder which affects the small arteries and arterioles and seems to be secondary to hypertension.
   c. Mönckeberg's medial calcific sclerosis, medial calcinosis — a vascular disorder in which ring-like calcifications occur in the media of muscular arteries. It is clinically of little importance since the medial lesions fail to encroach on the arterial lumen.[34, 103, 116]

8. arteriosclerosis obliterans — arterial obstruction of extremities, particularly affecting the lower limbs and causing ischemia.[34]

9. carotid occlusive disease — extracranial and/or intracranial vascular disorder usually due to atheromatous lesions which obstruct carotid arteries and if progressive may lead to reduced blood flow in the brain, transient ischemic attacks, cerebrovascular insufficiency and stroke.[34, 149]

10. coarctation of aorta — constriction of a segment of the aorta.[123]

11. dilatation of aorta — abnormal enlargement of the aorta.

12. embolism — a "throwing in"; blocking of a blood vessel by a clot or other substance brought to its place by the circulating blood.

13. hypertension — a pathologic elevation of the blood pressure, according to WHO (World Health Organization) consistently exceeding 160/95 mmHg.[107, 115, 125]

14. hypertensive vascular disease — sustained high blood pressure associated with cardio-vascular, renal and retinal changes.[107, 125]

15. peripheral arterial insufficiency of extremities — impaired circulation to the extremities, particularly to the lower limbs. It is characterized by claudication, coldness, pallor, trophic changes, ulceration and gangrene in the involved extremity.[10]

16. peripheral vascular disease — any disorder directly affecting the arteries, veins and lymphatics except those of the heart.

17. phlebitis — inflammation of the veins.

18. phlebosclerosis — a hardening of the walls of the veins.

19. Raynaud's disease — painful vascular disorder characterized by peripheral spasms of the digital arterioles of the fingers and toes which may result in gangrene.

20. rupture of an aneurysm — a break in the weakened vascular wall of an aneurysm associated with hemorrhage.

21. subclavian steal syndrome — a symptom complex of cerebrovascular insufficiency, usually due to segmental atheromatous occlusion of the subclavian artery proximal to the vertebral artery. Since the circulation through the vertebral artery is reversed, the subclavian is said "to steal" cerebral blood. A delay in the arrival time of the radial pulse on the affected side is diagnostic of reversed vertebral artery flow. A localized murmur and a difference in brachial blood pressure are common manifestations. The patient may experience dizziness, vertigo, light headedness, tinnitus, blurred vision, headache and ataxia.[5] _Staggering gait_

22. thoracic outlet syndromes — neurovascular compression syndromes affecting the structures of the thoracic outlet. Offending lesions are detected by angiography. Included are:
    a. cervical rib and scalenus anticus syndrome — a cutoff or torsion of subclavian artery may be present.
    b. scalenus anticus and pectoralis minor syndrome — a cutoff or torsion of subclavian artery and a compression or thrombosis of axillary veins may be demonstrated by angiography.
    c. scalenus anticus syndrome and tightness of costoclavicular space — a ridge-like compression of subclavian artery and venous compression or thrombosis may produce the syndrome.[142]

23. thromboangiitis obliterans, Buerger's disease — inflammatory, obstructive disease involving primarily the peripheral blood vessels of the lower extremities.[34, 104]

24. thrombophlebitis — inflammatory reaction of the walls of veins to infection, associated with intravascular clotting.[105]

25. thrombosis — formation of blood clots in a blood vessel, leading to circulatory obstruction.[62, 122]

26. varicose veins, varicosity — condition of having distended and tortuous veins, most commonly present in lower extremities.[36, 105]

D. Operative Terms:

1. anastomosis of blood vessels — end-to-end union of two different blood vessels or two segments of same blood vessel after excision of lesion.

2. anastomosis for aortic coarctation — joining the aortic segments end-to-end after removal of constricted region or joining the left subclavian to the descending aorta if former method is not feasible.[30]

3. aneurysmectomy — removal of an aneurysm.

4. aneurysm, resection of — excision of aneurysm and repair of arterial defect by insertion of homograft or prosthesis.[150]

5. aortic aneurysm resection, abdominal — clamping of aorta and iliac arteries, opening of the aneurysm, removal of thrombus and reconstruction by means of a preclotted knitted dacron graft.[148]

6. aortofemoral bypass grafting — procedure of choice for aortoiliac occlusive (Leriche) disease consisting in appropriate vascular clamping and graft anastomoses, usually end-to-side, below and above the obstructed segments to bypass circulatory occlusions. The formation of collateral vessels may maintain the circulation in graft failure.[60, 150]

7. aortoiliac replacement grafting — excision of occluded segments of the aorta and iliac arteries followed by graft replacement. Graft failure is life-threatening.[5, 60]
8. arterial homograft — arteries obtained at autopsies under aseptic technic and preserved by freezing, dry freezing or chemicals in a blood vessel bank. They are used for replacing the excised segments of an artery.
9. bypass graft, autogenous — implantation of an autograft, usually a segment of a saphenous vein to bypass a vascular obstruction such as occlusive lesions of the coronary, femoropopliteal or carotid-subclavian arteries. The occluded vascular segment is left in place. Circulatory efficiency is usually restored.[5, 8]
10. embolectomy — emboli may be excised directly or removed by retrograde method via femoral arteries by balloon catheter. With balloon deflated Fogarty catheter is inserted into a vein where embolus is located. When in proper position, the balloon is inflated. By withdrawing the catheter the clot is pulled through the incision to the body surface.[53]
11. endarterectomy — removal of the inner coat (intima) of an artery for occlusive vascular disease.
12. femoropopliteal arterial reconstruction — bypass surgery for restoring the circulation in femoral artery occlusion. The saphenous vein is removed from the knee to the saphenofemoral junction and the obstruction is bypassed by an autogenous graft of the saphenous vein.[7, 77]
13. femorotibial bypass grafting — autogenous graft of reversed saphenous vein or reversed cephalic vein placed from common femoral artery to posterior or anterior tibial artery to bypass the obstructed arterial segment.[56, 134]
14. phleborrhaphy — suture of a vein.
15. phlebotomy — opening of a vein; for example, to reduce high red count in polycythemia vera by bloodletting.
16. shunt for portal hypertension — method of diverting a large volume of blood from the hypertensive portal system into the normal systemic venous circulation. This operation prevents hemorrhages from esophageal varices which result from portal hypertension.[150] (See Chapter VIII — Digestive Disorders)
17. subclavian steal syndrome operations:
    a. carotid-subclavian anastomosis — joining the carotid and subclavian arteries to improve cerebral blood flow.
    b. carotid-subclavian bypass graft — implanting an autograft in carotid and subclavian arteries to bypass the occluded segment of the subclavian artery.
    c. subclavian-subclavian bypass — inserting a knitted preclotted Dacron graft and anastomosing one end of the graft with the right and the other end with the left subclavian artery thus creating a crossover bypass of the occluded arterial segment.[5, 8, 40]
18. thrombectomy — removal of a thrombus; for example, from an occluded portal vein.
19. vein stripping — surgical procedure to relieve varicosity.[150]
20. venesection — incision into a vein.

E. **Symptomatic Terms:**
1. acrocyanosis — bluish discoloration of finger tips and toes.[35]
2. angiospasm, vasospasm — involuntary contractions of the muscular coats of blood vessels; spasm of blood vessels.
3. claudication — limping.
    a. lower extremity claudication — inadequate blood supply associated with cramping pains in the calf muscles. It is usually relieved by rest, thus being intermittent.[148]
    b. upper extremity claudication, brachial claudication — inadequate blood supply to an arm causing intermittent or persistent cramping pain.
4. extravasation — escape of fluid; serum, lymph or blood into the adjacent tissues.
5. digital — referring to fingers and toes.
6. digital blanching — fingers and toes becoming pallid due to vasospasm of digital arterioles; seen in Raynaud's disease.

7. ischemia — local anemia of an organ or part resulting from circulatory obstruction or vasospasm.

sudden onset 8. paroxysmal digital cyanosis — attacks of cyanosis caused by the interruption of blood flow in palmar and plantar arteries.

9. pedal circulation — circulation in the foot.

10. pulse — contractions of an artery which can be felt by a finger.
   a. bigeminal pulse — coupled beats.
   b. Corrigan or water hammer pulse — strong, jerky beat followed by a sharp decline and collapse of beat.
   c. dicrotic pulse — arterial beat with weak secondary wave which may be mistaken for two beats.

11. pulse deficit — difference between apical heart rate and radial pulse rate, found in cardiac disease.

12. shock — complex syndrome affecting the various body systems due to the inability of cells to metabolize oxygen and needed substrates normally. Classification according to
   a. etiology:
      (1) cardiogenic shock — phenomenon caused by decreased cardiac output as in myocardial infarction, serious injury or cardiac surgery
      (2) hypovolemic shock — syndrome due to markedly decreased blood volume
      (3) septic shock — serious state resulting from infections, septicemia or bacteremia
      (4) other kinds.
   b. onset:
      (1) early shock — initial arteriolar or venous constriction, accelerated contractability of the heart, hyperventilation, other effects.
      (2) late shock — life-threatening impairment of cellular metabolism causing advanced hypovolemia, intravascular clotting and respiratory failure.[144]

13. vasoconstriction — a narrowing of the vascular lumen, resulting in decreased blood supply.[35]

14. vasodepression — collapse due to vasomotor depression.

15. vasodilatation — a widening of the vascular lumen, increasing the blood supply to a part.[35]

16. vasomotor — referring to nerves which control the muscular contractions of blood vessels.

RADIOLOGY

A. Terms Related to the Diagnostic Radiology of Blood Vessels:

1. aortography — injection of opaque solution for x-ray examination of the aorta.
   a. abdominal aortogram — injection of opaque solution into the abdominal aorta through a catheter which is introduced through the femoral artery or a needle puncture of the aorta in the lumbar region.[2]
   b. thoracic aortogram — injection of opaque solution into the ascending aorta per catheter, retrogradely introduced either through femoral or axillary arteries or by a cutdown of the brachial artery.[2, 147]

2. arteriography — radiographic examination of arteries following the injection of a contrast medium.

3. femoral arteriogram — radiographic examination of the femoral and popliteal arteries after the injection of a contrast medium. A few seconds later serial films are made to detect the presence and extent of occlusive vascular disease.[34, 70]

4. percutaneous splenoportography — radiologic study of directional blood flow patterns in portal hpertension. After the injection of 40 ml of 50% Hypaque into the spleen, radiograms are taken at intervals to visualize the splenic and portal veins. The demonstration of collateral blood flow, an opaque coronary vein and short gastric veins are predictive of bleeding, especially from gastroesophageal varices. The procedure is combined with taking spleen pressures. Their elevation adds further evidence of pending hemorrhage.[147]

5. splenoportogram — a radiologic image of the portal circulation obtained by injecting radiopaque material into the spleen. Splenoportograms can also be obtained on venous phase following splenic arteriography.[2]

6. venography — radiographic examination of veins following the injection of an opaque solution.[147]

B. Terms Related to the Diagnostic Radiology of the Heart and Blood Vessels:

1. angiocardiography
   a. peripheral angiocardiography — injection of contrast medium into the basilic or cephalic veins of the arm for examining the chambers of the heart and pulmonary circulation.[2]
   b. selective angiocardiography — injection of contrast material through a catheter placed into the chamber or vessel of interest.[2]
   c. selective retrograde aortography and left ventriculography — retrograde aortic catheterization for passing a radiopaque catheter across the aortic valve into the left ventricle. The correct position of the catheter is ascertained either by fluoroscopic or television guidance or radiogram. This method discloses ventricular septal defects, aneurysms, mitral and aortic regurgitation and other pathology.[43, 48, 94]
   d. selective right ventricular angiography — visualization of the anatomic structures involved in tetralogy of Fallot, transposition of the great vessels, patent ductus arteriosus and similar conditions.
   e. successive angiocardiograms — serial films taken at accurately recorded intervals. They reveal the time and sequence of filling of the great vessels and chambers of the heart as well as their position, size and configuration.[43, 48, 68, 94]

2. angiocardiographic filming techniques.
   a. angiocardiography with large films — technique using regular x-ray films with rapid film changers of 2 to 12 films per second. Rapid filming of heart and vessels may be either single plane or biplane.
   b. cineangiocardiography — technique of recording radiographic image of the heart and great blood vessels on a motion picture film.[2]
   This complex procedure combines cardiac catheterization and selective angiocardiography. Under fluoroscopic guidance the cardiac catheter is maneuvered through the heart chambers and pulmonary artery. An image amplifier visualizes the cardiovascular structures. The frame speed of the motion picture camera ranges from a few frames up to 200 frames. Both cineangiographic and large film techniques require a power injector with or without timing devices.[2, 43, 48, 94]

3. angiocardiographic injection techniques — injection of contrast media via catheter or needle using a suitable pressure injector.
   a. standard injection of opaque substance — injection with automatic high pressure injector irrespective of the time in the cardiac cycle.[2]
   b. time injection of contrast material — technique in which beginning of the injection may be triggered by electronic timing devices at any point in the cardiac cycle, using the electrocardiogram as a reference. It can be limited to the duration of either systole or diastole depending on the lesion of opacified chamber of interest, such as a systolic injection into the atrium and a diastolic injection into the ventricle.[2]

4. cardiac fluoroscopy — x-ray examination of the heart using a fluoroscope, preferably an image intensifier coupled with closed-circuit TV which permits visualization of fine details because of contrast and increased brightness, useful in delineating cardiac motion and intracardiac calcifications.[2]

5. cardiac series with barium swallow — the patient drinks a barium solution while fluoroscopic and radiographic examinations are performed to reveal abnormalities of the cardiac outline and esophageal displacement.[2]

6. cardiac tomography — sectional radiography of the heart.

7. radiokymography — the use of roentgen rays for recording the pulsations of the cardiac borders.[113]

C. Terms Related to Diagnostic Ultrasound of Cardiovascular Disorders:

1. Doppler ultrasonic flowmetry — ultrasound techniques for obtaining phasic, continuous and instantaneous measurement of velocity (speed) of blood flow in various cardiovascular disorders, especially in aortic valvar disease and venous thrombosis.   It is the method of choice for assessing vascular patency, incompetence, or occlusion.[26, 91]
2. echoaortography — ultrasonic study of the aorta.
    a. B-mode imaging — ultrasound technique for detecting atheromatous lesions, calcifications or aneurysms of the aorta.   A thrombus may produce fine echoes, a dissecting aneurysm thin linear echoes, advanced calcifications, strong echoes.[11]
    b. grey scale imaging — echographic method for detecting abdominal aortic aneurysm and measuring the vascular lumen distinct from the thrombus that transmits denser internal echoes than the lumen.[42]
    c. echography of aortic root — screening technique for assessing bicuspid aortic valve, a congenital defect which predisposes to serious aortic disorders.   The normal aortic valve has 3 cusps.[79]
3. echocardiography — graphic recording of ultrasound waves reflected from the heart for the purpose of
    a. studying the development of mitral stenosis from the onset of rheumatic heart disease
    b. determining the severity of mitral stenosis
    c. appraising the leaflet motion after mitral valvotomy[17, 80, 113]
    d. testing the functional capacity of the prosthetic valves following surgical valve replacement
    e. reflecting the left ventricular outflow tract and aortic valve[79, 96]
    f. delineating pericardial effusion and pericardial absence[92, 113]
    g. aiding in the diagnosis of congenital and acquired heart disease.[37, 38, 92]

CLINICAL LABORATORY

A. Terms Related to Selected Tests in Cardiovascular Conditions:

1. antistreptolysin-O titer — a diagnostic aid for rheumatic fever which may be used as screening test in statewide programs.[118]
2. atherogenic index (pl. indices) — determination of serum lipoproteins by ultracentrifugal analysis as a possible aid in the detection of factors causing atherosclerosis.[129]
3. blood culture — method of isolating the causative microorganisms in specific infectious diseases by placing blood withdrawn from a vein on or in suitable culture media.   It is of value in establishing the diagnosis of bacterial endocarditis.
4. cardiac index — cardiac output in relation to body size, useful in assessing the cardiovascular status, particularly after open heart surgery.[113, 139, 148]
5. central venous pressure (CVP) — measurement of pressure within the superior vena cava reflecting the pressure of the right atrium and expressed in centimeters of water pressure. CVP provides some index of the adequacy of the pumping action of the heart and of the blood volume in the vessels.
    Normal values — usually CVP _____ 5-8 cm of water
    Increase indicative of overload of right heart in congestive heart failure.
    Decrease suggestive of reduced blood volume and need of fluid replacement.[144]
6. C-reactive protein antiserum — nonspecific test for tissue breakdown and disseminated inflammatory conditons.   It is often used to follow the clinical course of the disease. Results are usually positive in rheumatic fever and carditis, rheumatoid arthritis, arteriosclerotic heart disease with myocardial infarction, Hodgkin's disease, widespread invasive malignancies and infections.[113]

7. erythrocyte sedimentation rate — speed with which red blood cells settle when mixed with anticoagulant.
   Normal values — Wintrobe and Landsberg's method
   Men _____ 0- 9 mm
   Women and girls _____ 0-20 mm
   Increase in coronary thrombosis, rheumatic fever, rheumatoid arthritis, pericarditis, tuberculosis and others.[113]

8. isoenzyme — distinct molecular fraction of a certain enzyme found in various tissues and separated by electrophoresis of serum. Of clinical significance are cardiac isoenzymes released into the serum in myocardial injury:
   a. creatine phosphokinase isoenzyme, CPK-2 (CPK-MB) — a more specific test for myocardial infarction than the serum enzyme CPK. The rise of CPK-2 activity parallels that of CPK and the isoenzyme has usually disappeared from the serum within 48 hours. Other isoenzymes are CPK-1 (CPK-BB) found in serious disorders of the central nervous system and CPK-3 (CPK-MM) present in angina pectoris, skeletal muscle and normal sera.[95, 113, 129]
   b. lactic dehydrogenase isoenzymes, LDH-1, LDH-2 — both fractions prove to be useful indicators of myocardial infarction. LDH-5 activity is abnormally high in liver disease.[113, 129]

9. serum enzymes of the heart muscle:
   a. creatine phosphokinase (CPK) — enzyme released into the blood following injury to the heart muscle or skeletal muscles.
   b. glutamic oxalacetic transaminase (GOT) — enzyme widely distributed in body tissues but found in its highest concentration in the heart muscle and liver.
   c. lactic dehydrogenase (LDH) — enzyme primarily found in the heart muscle, skeletal muscles and kidneys, also in cerebrospinal fluid, serum and serous effusion.

10. serum enzyme tests in myocardial infarction (MI) — determination based on the principle that high levels of enzyme activity reflect the evolution and extent of damage to the heart muscle. Since the enzymes are also present in other organs, the tests are nonspecific.
    a. serum creatine phosphokinase (SCPK) — determination of serum CPK activity, a useful test due to the early CPK rise after myocardial infarction and the absence of the enzyme from the liver and blood cells. Since CPK appears in skeletal muscle, muscular dystrophy of Duchenne may have to be ruled out. CPK levels are increased in acute lung disease.[113, 129]
    b. serum glutamic oxalacetic transaminase (SGOT) — valuable diagnostic aid in myocardial infarction. Highly elevated GOT levels usually suggest massive heart damage and poor prognosis. They tend to be absent in coronary insufficiency and angina pectoris. GOT activity may also be increased in congestive heart failure with infarcts, tachyarrhythmias, pericarditis, pulmonary infarction or embolism and liver disease.[113, 129]

Table 6

APPROXIMATE SERUM ENZYME ACTIVITY AFTER MYOCARDIAL INFARCTION

Serum Enzyme	Activity[a]			Normal Values[b] (30°C)
	Onset	Peak	Return to Normal	
CPK	2- 3 hrs	24- 36 hrs	2- 3 days	0- 50 mIU/ml[c]
GOT	6-12 hrs	24- 48 hrs	4- 7 days	0- 19 mIU/ml
LDH	12-24 hrs	72-120 hrs	12-14 days	0-300 mIU/ml

[a]James A. Halsted (ed.) *The Laboratory in Clinical Medicine.* Philadelphia: W. B. Saunders Co., 1976, pp. 281-283 (With permission).

[b]Paul B. Beeson and Walsh Mc Dermott (eds.) *Textbook of Medicine,* 14th ed. Philadelphia: W. B. Saunders Co., 1975, pp. 1886-1887.

[c]mIU/ml means milliInternational Units per milliliter.

c. serum lactic dehydrogenase (SLDH) — determination of LDH activity in serum, useful test because of late enzyme rise and its prolonged elevation. A disadvantage is its lack of specificity resulting from enzyme release into red blood cells, liver, lung and skeletal muscle.[113, 129]

Table 6 compares the occurrence of the characteristic rise, maximal elevation and decline to normal levels of the chief enzymes released into the serum after myocardial injury.

B. Terms Related to Cardiac Catheterization and Coronary Artery Catheterization:

1. cardiac catheterization, **right side** — a procedure of diagnostic value in detecting various cardiac defects and diseases. A radiopaque cardiac catheter is inserted into an accessible vein and passed into the heart and pulmonary artery. Various technics may be employed. If the basilic or the cephalic vein is used as a starting point, the catheter passes through the innominate vein and superior vena cava into the right atrium, right ventricle and pulmonary artery. If the saphenous vein is used, the catheter enters the heart through the inferior vena cava and traces its course through the cardiac chambers and pulmonary artery. Oxygen saturation of the blood in the chambers and the pressure recorded therein determine the defect within the heart, if present. Different indicator techniques aid in the detection and quantitation of shunts. Oxygen data or dye curves may be used for calculation of cardiac output. Although right cardiac catheterization is of great diagnostic value in certain heart lesions it is incomplete if cineangiography does not accompany the hemodynamic data.[2, 86, 113]

2. cardiac catheterization, **left side** — there are several ways of accomplishing the objectives of obtaining pressures and blood samples in the left side of the heart.

    a. catheterization of the left atrium
        (1) suprasternal or Radner method — inserting a needle behind the suprasternal notch and directing it downward into the left atrium. The pulmonary artery, aorta and left ventricle can be entered by the same method.
        (2) transseptal or Ross method — inserting a long needle through a catheter up to the right atrium and then pushing the needle out the catheter and puncturing the atrial septum at the foramen ovale.[64, 86, 94, 113]
        Modifications of this method are:
            (a) Brockenbrough technique — the cardiac catheter itself is slipped over the needle into the left atrium following transseptal puncture with the needle in the catheter.[2]
            (b) Shirey technique — the cardiac catheter is passed retrogradely through the brachial artery cutdown into the aorta, left ventricle and left atrium.[2]
        In the Radner method only the pressures may be recorded; in the Brockenbrough or Shirey technique, cineangiograms may be obtained by injection of opaque media through the catheter.[2]

    b. cardiac catheterization of left ventricle
        (1) direct puncture of left ventricle — use of a small gauge needle either through the apex, Brock technique, or through subxiphoid approach, Lehman technique.[2]
        (2) retrograde method — femoral or arm approach using a percutaneous or cutdown technique respectively.[2]

3. cardiac pressures — pressures created by the force of the contraction within the heart chambers upon the circulating blood.

4. hemodynamics — a study of blood circulation and blood pressure.

5. oscilloscope — an instrument for displaying electric signals as those made by blood pressure, electrocardiogram, heart sounds or other electric signals upon a cathode ray tube monitoring screen.[2]

6. selective catheterization of the coronary arteries
    a. Judkins technique — technique uses percutaneous puncture of femoral artery and introduction of 3 different-shaped catheters in succession for catheterization of left and right coronary arteries and left ventricular cineangiography.[2, 48, 94, 113]

Table 7

INTRACARDIAC PRESSURES

Internal Structures (Individual supine)	Normal Hemodynamic Values[a]	
	Average mmHg	Range mmHg
Right atrium	2.8	1- 5
Right ventricle		
systolic	25.0	17- 32
end-diastolic	4.0	1- 7
Pulmonary artery		
systolic	25.0	17- 32
diastolic	9.0	4- 13
mean	15.0	9- 19
Left atrium	8.0	2- 12
Left ventricle		
systolic	130.0	90-140
end-diastolic	8.0	5- 12
Brachial artery		
systolic	130.0	90-140
diastolic	70.0	60- 90

[a]Normal values of intracardiac pressures according to Noble O. Fowler, M.D., (ed.). *Cardiac Diagnosis and Treatment*, 2d ed. New York: Harper & Row, Publishers, 1976, p. 12 (With permission).

Under fluoroscopic or television guidance a catheter is introduced into the common femoral artery and advanced via aortic arch to the coronary orifice. Catheter manipulation differs for selective left and right coronary artery catheterization. Following contrast injection rapid direct serial radiography and cinephotofluorography provide coronary visualization thereby revealing the presence and extent of occlusive arterial heart disease.[86]

b. Sones technique — technique uses approach through the brachial artery following cutdown. A single catheter is inserted for the catheterization of both coronary arteries and left ventricular cineangiography.[2, 86]

Selective catheterization of the coronary arteries is done according to an accepted technique:

(1) to assess the potential need for heart surgery in angina pectoris
(2) to evaluate operative results
    (a) the extent of revascularization following the Vineberg procedure
    (b) the patency of aortocoronary saphenous vein grafts or internal mammary artery grafts following bypass surgery
(3) to detect progression of coronary atherosclerotic heart disease leading to graft closure.[94]

C. Terms Related to Special Recordings of Heart Action:

1. apexcardiogram (ACG) — recording low frequency vibrations of the precordium when a transducer is placed against the chest wall. The graphic record of the movements reflects the apex beat of the heart.[113]
2. ballistocardiography — electrographic recording of bodily movements during the cardiac cycle.[43, 113]
3. bipolar lead — lead with 2 electrodes, one negative and one positive.[23]
4. electrocardiography — graphic recording of the electric waves of the cardiac cycle or spread of excitation throughout the heart. It is an invaluable diagnostic aid in the detection of arrhythmias and myocardial damage. The meaning of the waves is:

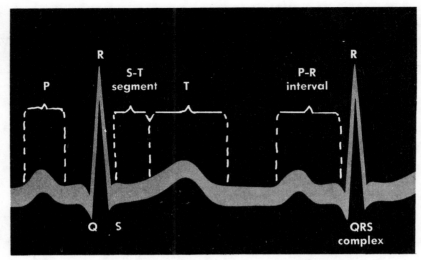

Fig. 43 — Normal electrocardiographic cycle (Adapted from Disorders of the Heart Beat by American Heart Association).

a. P wave — wave reflects the contraction of the atria.
b. PR interval — period in which the impulse passes through the atria and AV node, normally 0.16-0.20 seconds.
c. QRS complex — waves represent ventricular excitation or depolarization of the ventricular myocardium, normally 0.12 seconds.[163, 112]
d. Q wave — downward deflection and beginning of the complex.
e. R wave — large upward wave.
f. S wave — second large downward deflection and end of the QRS complex.
g. ST segment — the interval between the completion of depolarization and recovery of ventricular muscle fibers. The segment may be depressed or elevated in myocardial injury.
h. T wave — recovery phase following the contraction. Inversion of the T wave usually reflects injury or ischemia of the heart muscle.[23, 83, 113]

5. electrocardiography (ECG) — some techniques:
   a. ambulatory electrographic (Holter) monitoring — continuous ECG recording of an ambulatory high risk patient for early assessment and treatment of cardiac ischemia and ventricular arrhythmias or evaluation of response to activity or artificial pacemaker.[66, 111, 113, 145]
   b. His bundle electrography (HBE) — combined atrial and ventricular ECG, showing the spread of the electric current throughout the heart muscle and separating conduction into two distinct subdivisions:
      (1) PH interval — onset of P wave to His bundle activation or conduction time through both atria.
      (2) HR interval — His bundle activation to onset of QRS complex termed ventricular activation.[3, 23, 113]
   c. intracardiac electrography (IE) — adjunct to standard surface ECG using recordings by electrode catheters, percutaneously introduced into the heart via femoral or other suitable veins to assess arrhythmias and conduction disturbances.[49]
6. electrokymography — recording of the movements of the heart and great vessels by an electrokymograph.[113]
7. kinetocardiography, precordial cardiography — a method of recording vibrations of the chest wall produced by heart action.[113]
8. phonocardiography — graphic recording of heart sounds, usually on an oscilloscope for quick scanning or upon a tape recorder for a permanent record.[113]

9. phonocardiography, intracardiac — sound tracing recorded from within the cardiac chambers through a phonocatheter which has a microphone at the tip. Method seeks to detect minor defects not revealed by cardiac catheterization.

10. plethysmography — instrumental recording of variations in size of a part or organ caused by fluctuations in the size of the vascular bed.

11. pulse analysis — use of special transducer for recording of
    a. carotid pulse — an initial abrupt rise corresponding to opening of aortic valve, subsequent brief tidal wave and decline with closing of aortic valve and a gradual return to the baseline.[113]
    b. jugular venous pulse — an accurate reflection of right atrial activity recording waves of atrial systole, the filling of the right ventricle and tricuspid function.[113]

12. vectorcardiography — a graphic recording of the direction and magnitude of the instantaneous electric forces of the heart from a cathode ray tube. A polaroid photographic camera is frequently used.[2]

ABBREVIATIONS

ACG — angiocardiography, apexcardiogram
AHA — American Heart Association
ASD — atrial septal defect
ASHD — arteriosclerotic heart disease
ASO — arteriosclerosis obliterans
AV — atrioventricular, arteriovenous
BBB — bundle branch block
BP — blood pressure
CCA — circumflex coronary artery
CCCR — closed chest cardiopulmonary resuscitation
CCU — coronary care unit
CHD — coronary heart disease
CHF — congestive heart failure
CPB — cardiopulmonary bypass
CPK — creatine phosphokinase
CPR — cardiopulmonary resuscitation
CRP — C-reactive protein
CVA — cerebrovascular accident
CVD — cardiovascular disease
CVP — central venous pressure
DM — diastolic murmur
ECG — electrocardiogram
EKG — electrocardiogram
ESR — erythrocyte sedimentation rate
Hg — mercury
HLR — heart-lung resuscitation
HVD — hypertensive vascular disease
IABP — intra-aortic balloon pump
IASD — interatrial septal defect
IMAG — internal mammary artery graft
IVC — inferior vena cava
IVSD — interventricular septal defect
LA — left atrium
LAD — left anterior descending (coronary artery)

LD — lactic dehydrogenase
LHF — left heart failure
LV — left ventricle
LVH — left ventricular hypertrophy
M — murmurs
MI — myocardial infarction
mm Hg — millimeters of mercury
MS — mitral stenosis
PA — pulmonary artery
PAC — premature atrial contractions
PAT — paroxysmal atrial tachycardia
PDA — patent ductus arteriosus
PPS — postperfusion syndrome
PVC — premature ventricular contractions
PWP — pulmonary wedge pressure
RA — right atrium
RCA — right coronary artery
RF — rheumatic fever
RHF — right heart failure
RV — right ventricle
RVH — right ventricular hypertrophy
SA — sinoatrial (node)
SBE — subacute bacterial endocarditis
SGOT — serum glutamic oxalacetic transaminase
SGPT — serum glutamic pyruvic transaminase
SLD — serum lactic dehydrogenase
SR — sedimentation rate
SVC — superior vena cava
SVG — sapheneous vein graft
TIA — transient ischemic attack
VC — vena cava
VCG — vectorcardiogram
VHD — valvar heart disease
VSD — ventricular septal defect
WPW — Wolff-Parkinson-White (syndrome)

ORAL READING PRACTICE

Coarctation of the Aorta

Coarctation of the aorta is one of the most interesting **congenital cardiovascular** defects amenable to surgery. It consists of a constriction of a segment of the aorta and occurs in two types. The first type is a rare condition in which the aortic obstruction is located proximal to the **ductus arteriosus.** The **lumen** of the **aorta** is atretic or completely blocked so that the impairment of the systemic circulation presents a grave problem. This defect is incompatible with life and the child dies in infancy if corrective surgery cannot be performed.

The other type of coarctation is a common form which yields to surgical intervention. There may be either a narrowing or a complete **stenosis** of the **aortic lumen distal** to the left **subclavian** artery and to the insertion of the ductus. The latter is generally **ligamentous** and **obliterated.** The aorta near the constriction appears to be normal in size, but its major proximate branches are generally enlarged. The **intercostal** arteries distal to the obstruction, likewise, show an increase in size. The constriction of the aorta is usually limited to a short segment and permits a fair life expectancy, if not associated with other cardiovascular defects.

The outstanding diagnostic characteristic of aortic coarctation is a high blood pressure in the arms and a low blood pressure with a barely perceptible pulse in the legs. The differential diagnosis hinges on this disparity of the blood pressure in the extremities and the diminished or absent **femoral** pulse. Since the oxygenated blood reaches the systemic circulation, the patient's color remains normal. Hypertension may lead to **cerebrovascular** accident. In addition infection presents a constant threat to the **debilitated** patient since nutritional deficiency may accompany the impoverished systemic circulation.

When a short aortic segment is constricted, the clinical symptoms are absent or so minimal that they may escape notice, especially in childhood. In adolescence, symptoms of **fatigability,** decreased exercise tolerance, **epistaxis, syncope** and coldness of the feet tend to develop and cause varying degrees of disability. In untreated cases the life span rarely exceeds the fourth decade. Death may ensue from **rupture** of the aorta, **bacterial endocarditis** or **congestive** heart failure.

Efforts to relieve coarctation involve one of the most daring operations on the great vessels of the cardiovascular system. The optimum age for surgical correction is within the second decade of life according to Gross and between the ages of six and twelve years according to Hufnagel. During this period the aorta has a high degree of elasticity, works with facility, shows little or no evidence of **degenerative** changes and is in good condition for making a sizeable anastomosis.

The surgical procedure consists of the removal of the constricted region and an end-to-end anastomosis of the aortic segments. Where no surgical communication of the aortic segments can be created, the left subclavian artery may be joined to the descending aorta. Suitable bypass grafts may be implanted for complex or recurrent coarctations of the aorta.

Postoperatively, progress is spectacular. The blood pressure in upper and lower extremities equalizes, the femoral artery pulsation is present almost immediately and the circulation is markedly improved. The most dreaded complications are infection of the suture line resulting in leakage or dissolution of the anastomosis.[30, 117, 123, 140, 143]

Table 8

SOME CARDIOVASCULAR CONDITIONS AMENABLE TO SURGERY

Organs Involved	Diagnoses	Operations	Procedures
Heart Pulmonary artery Aorta	Patent ductus arteriosus	Complete division of ductus arteriosus	Obliteration of ductus by dividing ductus and suturing the cut ends

Organs Involved	Diagnoses	Operations	Procedures

Heart
Pulmonary
   artery
Aorta
	Complete transposition
	  of the pulmonary
	  artery and of the aorta
		Blalock-Hanlon
		  operation
		Closed heart surgery
			Right thoracotomy and exposure
			  of interatrial groove.
			Occlusion of vessels, application
			  of Satinsky-type clamp,
			  section of both atria
			Removal of segment and portion
			  of septum

Heart
Atria
Septum
	Interatrial septal defect	Repair of interatrial
		  septal defect
		Open method under
		  direct vision
			Interatrial septal defect closed by
			  direct suture or patch
			Extracorporeal circulation

Heart
Ventricles
Septum
	Congenital heart disease
	Interventricular septal
	  defect with pulmonary
	  hypertension
		Banding of pulmonary
		  artery
			Pulmonary artery constricted with
			  umbilical tape in instances
			  where direct closure is contra-
			  indicated

Heart
Ventricles
Septum
	Interventricular septal
	  defect
		Open cardiotomy and re-
		  pair of interventricular
		  defect under direct
		  vision
			Incision into right ventricle and
			  exposure of defect
			Repair with suture or ventricular
			  patch
			Extracorporeal circulation with
			  or without hypothermia

Heart
Ventricles
Pulmonary artery
	Tetralogy of Fallot
	  1. ventricular defect
	  2. pulmonic stenosis
	  3. dextroposition of
	     aorta
	  4. hypertrophy of right
	     ventricle
		Shunting operations
		  Blalock's method
		  Potts-Smith's method
		
		Brock's operation
		Total correction of
		  Tetralogy of Fallot
		Open heart surgery
			Joining right or left subclavian
			  to pulmonary artery
			Anastomosis between pulmonary
			  artery and aorta
			Removal of pulmonic obstruction
			Defects totally repaired using
			  suture closure or patch for
			  closure
			Infundibulum resected to correct
			  pulmonary stenosis
			Cardiopulmonary bypass with or
			  without hypothermia

Heart
Atria
Ventricles
	Atherosclerotic,
	  heart disease
	Adams-Stokes syndrome
	  atrioventricular block
		Insertion of transvenous
		  endocardial pacemaker
			Catheter electrode
			  passed through incision in
			  jugular vein and lodged in apex
			  of right ventricle
			Subcutaneous tunnel and
			  pocket constructed
			Catheter electrode fastened
			  to pacemaker
			Pacemaker inserted into pocket

Heart
Left ventricle
	Ventricular aneurysm
	Left heart failure
		Ventricular aneurysm-
		  ectomy
		Open heart surgery
			Transverse sternotomy with
			  bilateral thoracotomy; heart
			  opened
			Removal of aneurysm, its sac and
			  related thrombus
			Reconstruction of left ventricle
			  and closure of heart
			Extracorporeal circulation with
			  or without hypothermia

Heart
Right atrium
	Myxoma of right atrium
	  with progressive right
	  heart failure
		Atriotomy with excision
		  of primary cardiac
		  tumor
		Open heart surgery
			Right atrium opened and myxoma
			  removed
			Use of cardiopulmonary bypass
			  with or without hypothermia

Organs Involved	*Diagnoses*	*Operations*	*Procedures*
Heart Pericardium	Constrictive pericarditis Adherent pericardium	Pericardiectomy Pericardiolysis	Partial removal of pericardium Breaking up of adhesions

Heart
Myocardium
Coronary
  arteries
	Obstructive coronary
	  artery disease with
	  myocardial ischemia
	  and angina pectoris
		Myocardial revascu-
		  larization by
		  aortocoronary
		  bypass with
		  autogenous grafts
		  of saphenous vein
		Open heart surgery
			Surgical creation of new ostium
			  in ascending aorta and new
			  openings into vessels of the
			  aortic arch for implanting the
			  proximal ends of the vein grafts
			Anastomoses of distal ends of
			  grafts with coronary arteries to
			  bypass occlusive lesions
			Extracorporeal circulation with
			  or without hypothermia

Heart
Myocardium
Coronary
  arteries
	Progression of
	  coronary athero-
	  sclerotic heart
	  disease with
	  graft closure
	  and recurrence
	  of disabling
	  angina pectoris
		Reoperative
		  revascularization
		  by internal
		  mammary-coronary
		  artery anastomoses
			Median sternotomy
			Pericardium opened
			Circulatory support as needed
			Internal mammary artery grafts
			  implanted in coronary branches
			  to bypass occlusions
			Pump oxygenator primed with
			  colloid electrolyte solution
			Moderate hemodilution with
			  or without hypothermia

Heart	Far advanced occlusive
	  coronary artery
	  disease, diffuse
	  myocardial damage,
	  irreversible left
	  ventricular failure
		Median sternotomy
		Cardiac homotrans-
		  plantation
			Sternal split incision
			Simultaneous division of aorta,
			  pulmonary artery and atria
			  followed by excision of donor
			  and recipient hearts
			Implantation of donor heart by
			  atrial and vascular anastomoses
			  to recipient heart
			Extracorporeal circulation with
			  or without hypothermia

Heart
Pulmonary valve
	Pulmonic valvar
	  stenosis
		Pulmonary valvotomy
		Closed method or
		Open heart surgery
			Division and dilation of valve
			Extracorporeal circulation if
			  open method used

Heart
Mitral valve
	Mitral stenosis due to
	  rheumatic carditis
	Combined mitral stenosis
	  and mitral insufficiency
		Mitral commissurotomy
		
		Mitral valvoplasty
			Separation of commissure of
			  stenotic valve
			Suture or plastic repair of valve;
			  use of prosthesis

Heart
Aortic valve
Mitral valve
	Aortic stenosis and
	  insufficiency
	Mitral stenosis and in-
	  sufficiency due to
	  rheumatic heart
	  disease
		Excision and replacement
		  of aortic valve and
		  mitral valve with
		  Starr-Edwards aortic
		  and mitral prostheses
			Removal of calcified cusps of aortic
			  valve and seating of aortic
			  prosthesis
			Total removal of calcified mitral
			  valve and insertion of mitral
			  valve prosthesis
			Extracorporeal circulation,
			  coronary artery perfusion
			  and hypothermia

Aorta	Dissecting aneurysm of
	  thoracic aorta
		Resection of aneurysm
		Replacement with a
		  plastic prosthesis
			Aneurysm removed and defect
			  bridged with prosthesis

Organs Involved	Diagnoses	Operations	Procedures
Aorta	Atherosclerotic aortoiliac occlusion	Aortoiliac endarterectomy	Incision into left external iliac artery and removal of plaque Dissection of segmentally obstructed portion of intima of 1. common iliac arteries near bifurcation of aorta and 2. terminal aorta
Aorta	Aortic coarctation	Excision of coarctation Aortic anastomosis	Removal of constricted area and joining cut ends together with suture
Artery	Subclavian steal syndrome	Subclavian-subclavian crossover bypass graft	Extrathoracic approach Subclavian artery crossclamped Dacron graft anastomosed to vessel and tunneled subcutaneously in tissues of anterior neck Second anastomosis performed
	Left-sided proximal subclavian obstruction	Carotid-subclavian bypass graft	Supraclavicular approach Restoration of blood supply to the brachiocephalic region by using an autogenous saphenous vein graft
Artery	Occlusive femoropopliteal disease due to atherosclerotic lesions Pregangrenous state	Femoropopliteal arterial reconstruction by the use of reversed autogenous vein graft	Removal of the saphenous vein from knee to saphenofemoral junction Vein reversed and attached to patent vessel by end-to-end anastomosis bypassing the obstruction
Artery	Embolus in femoral artery	Embolectomy	Incision into femoral artery and removal of clot
Veins	Esophageal varices due to portal hypertension	Portacaval anastomosis	Joining the portal vein and the inferior vena cava to create a large shunt
Veins	Varicosity	Vein stripping	Ligation of saphenous vein; incision made and stripper introduced into vein; vein extirpated

REFERENCES AND BIBLIOGRAPHY

1. Abel, R. M. *et al.* Survival following free rupture of left ventricular aneurysm. *Annals of Thoracic Surgery,* 21: 175-179, February, 1976.
2. Aker, Umit T. M.D. Personal communications. (Mostly verbatim with permission.)
3. Akhatar, M. *et al.* Clinical uses of His bundle electrocardiography. *American Heart Journal,* 91: 805-809, June, 1976.
4. Akins, C. W. *et al.* Pulmonary valve replacement. *Thoracic and Cardiovascular Surgery,* 71: 721-725, May, 1976.
5. Bahnson, H. T. Occlusive disease of branches of the aorta. In Sabiston, David C. and Spencer, Frank C. *Gibbon's Surgery of the Chest,* 3rd ed. Philadelphia: W. B. Saunders Co., 1976, pp. 954-960.
6. Baily, L. L. *et al.* Improved technique for bedside insertion of the Swan-Ganz pulmonary artery catheter. *Annals of Thoracic Surgery,* 21: 460-461, May, 1976.
7. Barner, H. B., Kaminski, D. L., Codd, J. E., Kaiser, G. and Willman, V. L. Hemodynamics of autogenous femoropopliteal bypass grafts. *Archives of Surgery,* 109: 291-293, August, 1974.

8. Barner, H. B., Kaiser, G. C. and Willman, V. L. Hemodynamics of carotid-subclavian bypass. *Archives of Surgery*, 103: 248-251, August, 1971.

9. Barner, H. B. *et al.* Double internal mammary-coronary bypass. *Archives of Surgery*, 109: 627-630, November, 1974.

10. Barnes, R. W. Evaluating peripheral arterial occlusive disease. *Postgraduate Medicine*, 59: 98-103, February, 1976.

11. Barnett, Ellis and Morley, Patricia. *Abdominal Echography*. London: Butterworths & Co., 1974, pp. 35-38.

12. Barnhorst, D. A. *et al.* Isolated replacement of the mitral valve with the Starr-Edwards prosthesis: An eleven year review. *Thoracic and Cardiovascular Surgery*, 71: 230-237, February, 1976.

13. Barry, W. H. *et al.* Effects of coronary artery bypass grafting on resting and exercise hemodynamics in patients with stable angina pectoris. *American Journal of Cardiology*, 37: 823-830, May, 1976.

14. Behrendt, D. M. *et al.* The Blalock-Hanlon procedure: A new look at an old operation. *Annals of Thoracic Surgery*, 20: 424-432, October, 1975.

15. Benrey, J. *et al.* Permanent pacemaker implantation in infants, children and adolescents. *Circulation*, 53: 245-248, February, 1976.

16. Benzian, S. R. *et al.* Thoracic outlet syndrome. *Radiology*, 111: 275-277, May, 1974.

17. Brodie, B. R. *et al.* Diagnosis of prosthetic mitral valve malfunction with combined echophonocardiography. *Circulation*, 53: 93-100, January, 1976.

18. Carey, J. S. Long-term follow-up of cloth-covered Starr-Edwards prostheses. *Thoracic and Cardiovascular Surgery*, 71: 694-697, May, 1976.

19. Castellanos, Augustin & Myerburg, Robert J. *The Hemiblocks in Myocardial Infarction*. New York: Appleton-Century-Crofts, 1976.

20. Chardack, W. M. Cardiac pacemakers and heart block. In Sabiston, David C. and Spencer, Frank C. *Gibbon's Surgery of the Chest*, 3rd ed. Philadelphia: W. B. Saunders Co., 1976, pp. 1252-1300.

21. Chung, E. K. Artificial cardiac pacing. *Postgraduate Medicine*, 59: 83-90, June, 1976.

22. Cohen, H. C. *et al.* Tachycardias and electrical pacing. *Medical Clinics of North America*, 60: 343-368, March, 1976.

23. Conover, Mary H. and Zalis, Edwin G., *Understanding Electrocardiography*, 2d ed. St. Louis: The C. V. Mosby Co., 1976, pp. 1-198.

24. Cooley, D. A. Technical considerations in cardiovascular surgery for neonates. *Thoracic and Cardiovascular Surgery*, 71: 551-553, April, 1976.

25. Corday, E. (ed.). Symposium on the management of jeopardized ischemic myocardium. *American Journal of Cardiology*, 37: 461-607, March 31, 1976.

26. Curcio, B. M. Ultrasonography and thermography. In Merrill, Vinita. *Atlas of Roentgenographic Positions and Standard Radiologic Procedures*, 4th ed. Vol. III. St. Louis: The C. V. Mosby Co., 1975, pp. 946-950.

27. Denes, P. *et al.* The incidence of typical and atypical A-V Wenckebach periodicity. *American Heart Journal*, 89: 26-31, January, 1975.

28. Dong, E. *et al.* Transplantation of the heart. In Sabiston, David C. and Spencer, Frank C. *Gibbon's Surgery of the Chest*, 3rd ed. Philadelphia: W. B. Saunders Co., 1976, pp. 1507-1521.

29. Durer, D. Medical and surgical treatment of the Wolff-Parkinson-White syndrome. In Creger, William P. (ed.). *Annual Review of Medicine*. Palo Alto, California: Annual Review Inc., 1976. pp. 63-67.

30. Edie, R. N. *et al.* Bypass grafts for recurrent or complex coarctations of the aorta. *Annals of Thoracic Surgery*, 20: 558-566, November, 1975.

31. Eick, R. E. Coronary occlusion. *Medical Clinics of North America*, 60: 49-67, January, 1976.

32. Engel, T. R. *et al.* First-degree sinoatrial heart block: Sinoatrial block in the sick-sinus syndrome. *American Heart Journal*, 91: 303-310, March, 1976.

33. Erskine, J. M. Diseases of the aorta. In Krupp, Marcus A. and Chatton, Milton J. *Current Medical Diagnosis and Treatment*, 15th ed. Los Altos, California: Lange Medical Publications, 1976, pp. 243-247.

34. ————. Arteriosclerotic occlusive disease. *Ibid.*, pp. 247-258.

35. ————. Vasospastic disorders — Vasomotor disorders. *Ibid.*, pp. 259-262.

36. ————. Degenerative and inflammatory venous disease. *Ibid.*, pp. 262-271.

37. Farooki, Z. Q. *et al.* Echocardiographic spectrum of Ebstein's anomaly of the tricuspid valve. *Circulation*, 53: 63-68, January, 1976.

38. Feigenbaum, H. *et al.* Role of echocardiography in patients with coronary artery disease. *American Journal of Cardiology*, 37: 775-786, April, 1976.

39. Fernandez, J. *et al.* Results of mitral replacement with the Beall prosthesis in 209 patients. *Thoracic and Cardiovascular Surgery*, 71: 218-225, February, 1976.

40. Finkstein, N. M. *et al.* Subclavian-subclavian bypass for the subclavian steal syndrome. *Surgery*, 71: 142-145, January, 1972.

41. Fozzard, H. *et al.* Computers for recognition and management of arrhythmias. *Medical Clinics of North America*, 60: 291-298, March, 1976.

42. Freimanis, A. K. Echographic diagnosis of lesions of the abdominal aorta and lymph nodes. *Radiologic Clinics of North America*, 13: 557-572, December, 1975.

43. Friedberg, C. K. *Diseases of the Heart*, 3rd ed. Philadelphia: W. B. Saunders Co., 1966, pp. 12-133.

44. Fruehan, C. T. *et al.* Follow-up catheterization of patients with myocardial infarction during coronary artery bypass surgery. *American Heart Journal*, 91: 186-190, February, 1976.

45. Gallagher, J. J. *et al.* The Wolff-Parkinson-White syndrome and the preexitation dysrhythmias: Medical and surgical management. *Medical Clinics of North America*, 60: 101-123, January, 1976.

46. Geha, A. S. Crossed double internal mammary-to-coronary artery grafts. *Archives of Surgery*, 111: 289-292, March, 1976.

47. Geha, A. S. *et al.* Surgical treatment of unstable angina by saphenous vein and internal mammary

artery bypass grafting. *Thoracic and Cardiovascular Surgery*, 71: 348-354, March, 1976.

48. Gensini, Goffredo G. *Coronary Arteriography*. Mount Kisco, New York: Futura Publishing Co. Inc., 1975, pp. 355-455.

49. Gilette, P. C. Intracardiac electrography in children and young adults. *American Heart Journal*, 89: 36-44, January, 1975.

50. Goldbarg, A. N. Exercise stress testing in the uncovering of dysrhythmias. *Medical Clinics of North America*, 60: 315-324, March, 1976.

51. Grace, W. J. Sudden death and acute myocardial infarction. *American Heart Journal*, 91: 1-2, January, 1976.

52. Green, G. E. Internal mammary coronary artery anastomosis for myocardial ischemia. In Sabiston, David C. and Spencer, Frank C. *Gibbon's Surgery of the Chest*, 3rd ed. Philadelphia: W. B. Saunders Co., 1976, pp. 1378-1383.

53. Green, R. M. *et al.* Arterial embolectomy before and after the Fogarty catheter. *Surgery*, 77: 24-33, January, 1975.

54. Guazzi, M. *et al.* Repetitive myocardial ischemia of Prinzmetal type without angina pectoris. *American Journal of Cardiology*, 37: 923-927, May, 1976.

55. Gutgesell, H. P. *et al.* Transposition of the great arteries. *Circulation*, 51: 32-38, January, 1975.

56. Harrington, O. B. *et al.* Femoral tibial bypass grafts. *Southern Medical Journal*, 69: 393-395, April, 1976.

57. Hauser, R. G. *et al.* Newer developments in pacemakers. *Medical Clinics of North America*, 60: 369-384, March 1976.

58. Herrmann, V., Laks, H., Kaiser, G. C., Barner, H. B., Willmann, V. L. The Blalock-Hanlon procedure: Simple transposition of the great arteries. *Archives of Surgery*, 110: 1387-1390, November, 1975.

59. Higgins, C. B. *et al.* Clinical and arteriographic features of Prinzmetal's variant angina. *American Journal of Cardiology*, 37: 831-839, May, 1976.

60. Humphries, A. W. Technique of bilateral aorto-femoral bypass grafting. *Surgical Clinics of North America*, 55: 1137-1158, October, 1975.

61. Jahnke, E. J. *et al.* Bypass of the right and circumflex coronary arteries with the internal mammary artery. *Thoracic and Cardiovascular Surgery*, 71: 58-63, January, 1976.

62. Kakkar, V. V. Deep vein thrombosis. *Circulation*, 51: 8-19, January, 1975.

63. Kaplan, B. M. The tachycardia-bradycardia syndrome. *Medical Clinics of North America*, 60: 91-100, January, 1976.

64. Kasparian, H. *et al.* Interpreting cardiac catheterization. *Postgraduate Medicine*, 57: 65-72 and 77-83, April, 1975.

65. Kennedy, H. L. *et al.* Practical advantages of two-channel electrocardiographic Holter recordings. *American Heart Journal*, 91: 822-823, June, 1976.

66. Kennedy, H. L. Postmyocardial infarction (Dressler's) syndrome. *American Heart Journal*, 91: 233-239, February, 1976.

67. Killip, T. Arrhythmias in myocardial infarction. *Medical Clinics of North America*, 60: 233-244, March, 1976.

68. Kittredge, R. D. *et al.* Left ventricular aneurysm on lateral chest film. *American Journal of Roentgenology*, 126: 1140-1146, June, 1976.

69. Kones, R. J. *et al.* Reduction in myocardial infarct size. *Southern Medical Journal*, 69: 442-448, April, 1976.

70. Liddicoat, J. E. Intraoperative arteriography during femoral popliteal bypass. *Archives of Surgery*, 110: 839-840, July, 1975.

71. Loop, F. D. Operative technique in myocardial revascularization. *Surgical Clinics of North America*, 55: 1181-1191, October, 1975.

72. Loop, F. D. Internal mammary artery bypass graft in reoperative myocardial revascularization. *American Journal of Cardiology*, 37: 890-895, May, 1976.

73. Loop, F. D. *et al.* Left ventricular aneurysm. In Sabiston, David C. and Spencer, Frank C. *Gibbon's Surgery of the Chest*, 3rd ed. Philadelphia: W. B. Saunders Co., 1976, pp. 1384-1393.

74. Love, J. W. The rechargeable cardiac pacemaker. *Archives of Surgery*, 110: 1186-1191, October, 1975.

75. Ludington, L. G. *et al.* Technique for using soft, flexible catheter stents in aortocoronary vein bypass operations. *Annals of Thoracic Surgery*, 21: 328-332, April, 1976.

76. Marco, J. D., Barner, H. B., Kaiser, G. C., Mudd, G. and Willman, V. Operative flow measurements and coronary bypass graft patency. *Thoracic and Cardiovascular Surgery*, 71: 545-547, April, 1976.

77. Martin, C. E. *et al.* Femoropopliteal bypass for salvage and claudication. *Southern Medical Journal*, 69: 420-423, April, 1976.

78. McConahay, D. R. *et al.* Coronary artery bypass surgery for left main coronary artery disease. *American Journal of Cardiology*, 37: 885-889, May, 1976.

79. McDonald, I. G. Echocardiographic assessment of left ventricular function in aortic valve disease. *Circulation*, 53: 860-864, May, 1976.

80. ———. Echographic assessment of left ventricular function in mitral valve disease. *Circulation*, 53: 865-871, May, 1976.

81. McHenry, P. L. *et al.* Comparative study of exercise-induced ventricular arrhythmias in normal subjects and patients with documented coronary artery disease. *American Journal of Cardiology*, 37: 609-616, March 31, 1976.

82. Meller, J. *et al.* Coronary arterial spasm in Prinzmetal's angina: A proved hypothesis. *American Journal of Cardiology*, 37: 938-940, May, 1976.

83. Meltzer, Lawrence E., Pinneo, R. and Kitchell, J. R. The electrocardiographic basis of arrhythmias. *Intensive Coronary Care*, 2d ed. New York: The Charles Press Publishers Inc., 1970, pp. 109-204.

84. Messmer, K. Hemodilution. *Surgical Clinics of North America*, 55: 659-678, June, 1975.

85. Moran, J. M. *et al.* Surgical treatment of postinfarction ventricular aneurysm. *Annals of Thoracic Surgery*, 21: 107-113, February, 1976.

86. Mudd, Gerard, M.D. Personal communications.
87. Muller, W. H. *et al.* Acquired disease of the aortic valve. In Sabiston, David C. and Spencer, Frank C. *Gibbon's Surgery of the Chest*, 3rd ed. Philadelphia: W. B. Saunders Co., 1976, pp. 1128-1251.
88. Mundth, E. D. Assisted circulation. In Sabiston, David C. and Spencer, Frank C. *Gibbon's Surgery of the Chest*, 3rd ed. Philadelphia: W. B. Saunders Co., 1976, pp. 1394-1415.
89. Oglietti, J. *et al.* Myocardial revascularization: Early and late results after reoperation. *Thoracic and Cardiovascular Surgery*, 71: 736-740, May, 1976.
90. Oglietti, J. *et al.* Supravalvular stenosing ring of the atrium. *Annals of Thoracic Surgery*, 21: 421-424, May, 1976.
91. Pantelis, C. *et al.* Aortic valve closure: Echocardiographic, phonocardiographic and hemodynamic assessment. *American Heart Journal*, 91: 228-232, February, 1976.
92. Payvandi, M. N. Echocardiography in congenital and acquired absence of pericardium. *Circulation*, 53: 86-92, January, 1976.
93. Pease, W. E. *et al.* Familial atrial septal defect. *Circulation*, 53: 759-762, May, 1976.
94. Peter, R. H. Coronary arteriography. In Sabiston, David C. and Spencer, Frank C. *Gibbon's Surgery of the Chest*, 3rd ed. Philadelphia: W. B. Saunders Co., 1976, pp. 1320-1352.
95. Pyle, R. B. *et al.* CPK-MB isoenzyme. *Thoracic and Cardiovascular Surgery*, 71: 884-890, June, 1976.
96. Radford, D. J. *et al.* Echographic assessment of bicuspid aortic valves. *Circulation*, 53: 80-85, January, 1976.
97. Rasten, H. Aortoventriculoplasty. *Thoracic and Cardiovascular Surgery*, 71: 920-927, June, 1976.
98. Ray, J. E. *et al.* Quadruple coronary artery bypass grafting. *Annals of Thoracic Surgery*, 21: 7-11, January, 1976.
99. Resnekov, L. Theory and practice of electroversion of cardiac dysrhythmias. *Medical Clinics of North America*, 60: 325-342, March, 1976.
100. Reul, G. J., Cooley, D. A. *et al.* Long-term survival following coronary artery bypass: Analysis of 4,522 consecutive patients. *Archives of Surgery*, 110: 1419-1424, November, 1975.
101. Robb, G. P. *et al.* Appraisal of the double two-step exercise test — a long-term follow-up study of 3,325 men. *Journal of American Medical Association*, 234: 722-727, November 17, 1975.
102. Robbins, Stanley L. Blood vessels — normal — Congenital anomalies. *Pathologic Basis of Disease*. Philadelphia: W. B. Saunders Co., 1974, pp. 581-586.
103. _____. Arteriosclerosis. *Ibid.*, pp. 586-604.
104. _____. Inflammatory diseases — Other vascular disorders. *Ibid.*, pp. 604-614.
105. _____. Aortic aneurysms — Varicose veins — Others. *Ibid.*, pp. 614-636.
106. _____. Heart — Anatomy — Congestive heart failure. *Ibid.*, pp. 637-643.
107. _____. Major types of heart disease. *Ibid.*, pp. 643-680.

108. _____. Other cardiac diseases classified by anatomic divisions. *Ibid.*, pp. 681-698.
109. Roberts, D. L. *et al.* Long-term survival following aortic valve replacement. *American Heart Journal*, 91: 311-317, March, 1976.
110. Roe, B. B. Ebstein's anomaly. In Sabiston, David C. and Spencer, Frank C. *Gibbon's Surgery of the Chest*, 3rd ed. Philadelphia: W. B. Saunders Co., 1976, pp. 1170-1175.
111. Romero, C. A. Holter monitoring in the diagnosis and management of cardiac rhythm disturbances. *Medical Clinics of North America*, 60: 299-313, March, 1976.
112. Rosch, J. *et al.* Coronary artery stenosis. *Radiology*, 119: 513-520, June, 1976.
113. Roven, R. B. Phenomena of the heart. In Halsted, James A. (ed.). *The Laboratory in Clinical Medicine*. Philadelphia: W. B. Saunders Co., 1976, pp. 239-283.
114. Rushmer, Robert F. Functional anatomy and control of the heart. *Cardiovascular Dynamics*, 4th ed. Philadelphia: W. B. Saunders Co., 1976, pp. 76-131.
115. _____. Systemic arterial hypertension — Postural hypotension. *Ibid.*, pp. 176-245.
116. _____. Atherosclerosis: Occlusive disease of coronary and peripheral arteries. *Ibid.*, pp. 351-381.
117. _____. Congenital malformations of the heart. *Ibid.*, pp. 446-496.
118. _____. Valvular heart disease. *Ibid.*, pp. 497-531.
119. _____. Cardiac compensation, hypertrophy, myopathy and congestive heart failure. *Ibid.*, pp. 532-568.
120. Seybold-Epting, W. *et al.* Repair of ventricular septal defect after pulmonary artery banding. *Thoracic and Cardiovascular Surgery*, 71: 392-397, March, 1976.
121. Simon, J. *et al.* Constrictive pericarditis. *Annals of Thoracic Surgery*, 21: 440-441, May, 1976.
122. Simpson, J. M. *et al.* Prevention of deep-vein thrombosis. *American Heart Journal*, 91: 401-402, March, 1976.
123. Sokolow, M. Congenital heart diseases. In Krupp, Marcus A. and Chatton, Milton J. *Current Medical Diagnosis and Treatment*, 15th ed. Los Altos, California: Lange Medical Publications, 1976, pp. 152-161.
124. _____. Acquired heart diseases. *Ibid.*, pp. 161-186.
125. _____. Atherosclerotic heart disease. *Ibid.*, pp. 187-201.
126. _____. Disturbances of rate and rhythm. *Ibid.*, pp. 201-209.
127. _____. Disturbance of conduction. *Ibid.*, pp. 209-213.
128. _____. Cardiac failure — Diseases of pericardium — Diseases of myocardium. *Ibid.*, pp. 213-242.
129. *Specialized Diagnostic Laboratory Tests*, 11th ed. Van Nuys, California: Bio-Science Laboratories, 1976, pp. 88-97.
130. Spencer, F. C. Bypass grafting for occlusive disease of the coronary arteries. In Sabiston, David C. and Spencer, Frank C. *Gibbon's Surgery of the*

Chest, 3rd ed. Philadelphia: W. B. Saunders Co., 1976, pp. 1364-1374.

131. ————. Unstable (preinfarction) angina. *Ibid.*, pp. 1375-1377.

132. ————. Acquired disease of the mitral valve. *Ibid.*, pp. 1190-1210.

133. Stefanik, G. *et al.* A method for insertion of a stented xenograft valve in the atrioventricular position. *Annals of Thoracic Surgery,* 21: 166-167, February, 1976.

134. Stephen, M. *et al.* Tibial artery bypass. *Archives of Surgery,* 111: 235-238, March, 1976.

135. Taguchi, K. *et al.* Surgical treatment of congenital heart disease with special reference to the application of hypothermia. *Annals of Thoracic Surgery,* 21: 296-303, April, 1976.

136. Taira, A. *et al. Patch* closure of the ductus arteriosus. *Annals of Thoracic Surgery,* 21: 454-455, May, 1976.

137. Thilenius, O. G. Subdivided left atrium: An expanded concept of cor triatriatum sinistrum. *American Journal of Cardiology,* 37: 743-750, April, 1976.

138. Tice, D. A. *et al.* Coronary artery bypass with freeze-preserved saphenous vein allografts. *Thoracic and Cardiovascular Surgery,* 71: 378-382, March, 1976.

139. Truccone, N. J. *et al.* Cardiac output in infants and children after open-heart surgery. *Thoracic and Cardiovascular Surgery,* 71: 410-414, March, 1976.

140. Tyson, K. R. T. Congenital heart disease in children. *Clinical Symposia,* 27: 2-36, November, 1975.

141. Unstable agina pectoris: National Cooperative Study Group to compare medical and surgical therapy. *American Journal of Cardiology,* 37: 896-902, May, 1976.

142. Urschel, H. C. *et al.* Recurrent thoracic outlet syndrome. *Annals of Thoracic Surgery,* 21: 19-25, January, 1976.

143. Vaughan, Victor C. III and McKay, R. James (eds.) Congenital heart disease — Rheumatic diseases. *Nelson Textbook of Pediatrics,* 10th ed. Philadelphia: W. B. Saunders Co., 1975, pp. 522-1074.

144. Walt, A. J. *et al.* The treatment of shock. *Advances in Surgery,* Vol. IX. Chicago: Year Book Medical Publishers, Inc., 1975, pp. 1-39.

145. Weinberg, S. L. Observations on ambulatory electrocardiographic monitoring in clinical practice. *Heart & Lung,* 4: 546-554, July-August, 1975.

146. Weir, Don C., M.D. Personal communications.

147. Whitehouse, Walter M. (ed.). Angiography. *Diagnostic Radiology.* Chicago: Year Book Medical Publishers, 1976, pp. 31-75.

148. Willman, Vallee L. M.D. Personal communications.

149. Willman, V. L. and Barner, H. B. Carotid occlusive disease. In Sabiston, David C. (ed.) *Textbook of Surgery,* 10th ed. Philadelphia: W. B. Saunders Co., 1972, pp. 1683-1692.

150. Zollinger, Robert M. and Zollinger, Robert M., Jr. Vascular procedures. *Atlas of Surgical Operations,* 4th ed. New York: Macmillan Publishing Co. Inc., 1975, pp. 228-274.

Chapter VI
Disorders of the Blood and Blood-Forming Organs

BLOOD

A. Origin of Terms:

1. blast (G) — germ
2. cyto (G) — cell
3. emia (G) — blood
4. erythro (G) — red
5. hemo (G) — blood
6. leuko (G) — white

7. osis (G) — increase, condition
8. penia (G) — decrease, poverty
9. phage (G) — to eat
10. plasma (G) — anything formed
11. polymorph (G) — many forms
12. reticulum (L) — network

B. Hematologic Terms:[3, 53, 83, 88]

1. erythroblasts — immature red blood cells, possess a nucleus and are present in fetal blood.
2. erythrocytes — red blood cells; mature cells have no nucleus.
3. erythropoiesis — the production of red blood cells.
4. hematopoiesis, hemopoiesis — the development of the various cellular elements of the blood — erythrocytes, leukocytes, platelets, others.
5. hemoglobin — a chemical component of erythrocytes containing two substances: globin and hematin, an iron pigment which is responsible for the transport of oxygen to the cells.
6. leukocytes — white blood cells divided according to structure into granulocytes, lymphocytes and monocytes.
7. leukocytes of granulocytic series — the cytoplasm contains granules. This series includes
   a. polymorphonuclear neutrophils — cytoplasmic granules stainable with a neutral dye. Schilling's hemogram or differential leukocyte count distinguishes 4 age groups:
      (1) neutrophilic myelocytes — youngest neutrophils, nucleus round or ovoid-shaped.
      (2) neutrophilic metamyelocytes, junge kernige — immature cells in which the nucleus has become indented.
      (3) neutrophilic band or staff cells — immature non-filamented cells in which the nucleus is T, V or U-shaped without division into segments.
      (4) neutrophilic lobocytes or polymorphonuclear neutrophils — filamented mature cells with distinct segmentation.

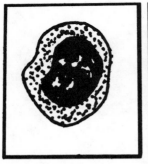 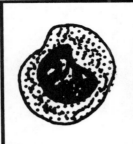 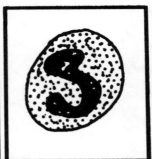 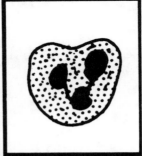

Myelocytes   Metamyelocytes   Bands, nonfilaments 4%   Segments, filaments 66%

Fig. 44 – Developmental phases of neutrophils from immature to mature cells. Eosinophils, basophils, monocytes and lymphocytes make up the remaining 30% of leukocytes.

    b. polymorphonuclear eosinophils — cytoplasmic granules of cells take an acid stain.

    c. polymorphonuclear basophils — cytoplasmic granules of cells take an alkaline stain.

8. lymphocytes — leukocytes derived from lymphoid tissue. The cytoplasm contains no granules or only a few.

9. monocytes — mononuclear leukocytes. The cytoplasm contains no granules or only a few.

10. myelopoiesis — the formation of blood cells and tissue elements from bone marrow.

11. myeloproliferative — referring to an increased production of myelopoietic cells and tissue.

12. normoblasts — nucleated red cells which precede normal erythrocytes in the developmental process.

13. normocytes — normal non-nucleated red blood cells.

14. phagocytes — two classes of white cells.

    a. the macrophages which absorb dead cells and tissues.

    b. the microphages which ingest bacteria.[3, 53]

15. plasma — liquid portion of blood without cellular elements.

16. plasma cells, plasmacytes — leukocytes, normally absent in blood film, occasionally seen in infection but rarely present in circulating blood. Their function is to synthesize immunoglobulins.[3]

17. platelets, thrombocytes — round or oval disks which control clot formation and clot retraction.

18. polymorphonuclear — having nuclei of variable shape.[3, 53, 83]

19. reticulocytes — immature red cells in intermediary stage of development between nucleate and anucleate forms. They contain a fine intracellular network and are normally present in the blood in small numbers.[83, 88]

20. serum — liquid portion of the blood after fibrinogen has been consumed in the process of clotting.[72]

21. sideroblasts — nucleated erythrocytes containing stainable iron granules.[14]

22. siderocytes — circulating red cells containing stainable iron granules.[14]

C. Diagnostic Terms:

1. Conditions primarily affecting the red cells:

    a. anemia — blood disorder characterized by a reduction in erythrocyte count, hemoglobin and hematocrit, although not all 3 findings may be present.
It is usually a manifestation or a complication of a disease, not a diagnosis.[74, 82]
A condensed version of Wintrobe's etiologic classification of anemia is presented:

      (1) anemia of blood loss — disorder develops subsequent to an acute or chronic hemorrhage.

      (2) deficiency factors in red cell production (erythropoiesis)

          (a) iron deficiency anemia — depletion of body's iron storage, which may be followed by an inadequate production of hemoglobin and a reduction of the oxygen carrying capacity of the blood.[3, 18, 74, 84]

          (b) megaloblastic anemias — the common denominator is a disordered synthesis of DNA (deoxyribonucleic acid) due to deficiency of vitamin B_{12} or folic acid.
Normally dietary vitamin B_{12} interacts with a mucoid secretion of the gastric fundus, the intrinsic factor of Castle. In the absence of this factor, B_{12} cannot be absorbed by the ileum and nutritionally utilized by the body.[3, 74, 84]
Folic acid (B_c) deficiency may be caused by malnutrition, malabsorption, increased requirement or loss of folic acid and defective folate metabolism.[74]

          (c) pernicious anemia — prototype of a megaloblastic anemia, usually associated with marked vitamin B_{12} deficiency caused by failure of gastric mucosa to secrete an intrinsic factor. Laboratory findings reveal a very low red count, often below 2,000,000, a hemoglobin relatively less

Table 9

MODIFIED SCHILLING'S HEMOGRAM — DIFFERENTIAL LEUKOCYTE COUNT

| Type of Count | Percentage | | | | | | | | | |
| | Neutrophils | | | | | Total Neutrophils | Eosinophils | Basophils | Lymphocytes | Monocytes |
	Myeloblasts	Myelocytes	Metamyelocytes	Bands, nonfilaments	Segments, filaments					
Normal Range	……	……	……	2 - 6	50 - 70	52 - 76	1 - 4	0 - 1	20 - 40	2 - 8
Shift to left; for example, infections	……	……	4	12	69	85	……	……	12	3
Shift to left; for example, chronic myelocytic leukemia	1	4	10	20	40	75	11	9	3	2
Shift to right; for example, pernicious anemia	……	……	……	2	78	80	……	……	16	4

In most infections the differential leukocyte count reveals a shift to the left. Characteristically, a few metamyelocytes (juveniles or junge kernige) and an abnormally high number of bands are found in the blood smear. The more immature the cells are, the more serious is the condition, as may be gleaned from the shift to the left in myelocytic leukemia. In pernicious anemia there is a shift to the right and the mature neutrophils are polysegmented filaments.

reduced and achylia gastrica (absent or diminished gastric juice). Anorexia, sore tongue, weakness, fatigue, a waxy pallor and neurologic damage are common clinical manifestations.[74, 84]

(d) sideroblastic anemias — hereditary or acquired anemias exhibiting an excess of iron deposits within normoblasts usually in association with hypochromia and microcytosis. The anemia may be present at birth but develops more frequently in young adults. The iron overload tends to initiate cardiac arrhythmias and liver fibrosis. Diabetes is frequently associated with sideroblastic anemia.

(3) failure of bone marrow

(a) aplastic anemia — a marked reduction of red cells, white cells and platelets (pancytopenia) or a selective reduction of red cells or platelets. Fat cells abound in the bone marrow. Clinical features are pallor, lassitude, bleeding and purpura. The disease may be idiopathic or caused by toxic drugs or ionizing irradiation.

(b) Fanconi syndrome, congenital pancytopenia — idiopathic anemia that develops in early infancy, appears to be hereditary and is associated with congenital abnormalities of the bones, heart, kidneys, eyes, microcephaly and an olive brown skin. The dominant hematologic finding is pancytopenia in which there is a profound depression of the cellular elements of the blood.[45, 74, 86]

(4) excessive destruction of erythrocytes

(a) hemolytic anemias — congenital or acquired blood disorders characterized by a shortened life span and an excessive destruction of mature red corpuscles.[12, 74, 85]

(b) hemolytic disease of the newborn (HDN), erythroblastosis fetalis — reduction of the life span of red cells, usually resulting from a hemolytic reaction of the Rh positive infant to the sensitized Rh negative mother. Uncontrolled high bilirubin levels may result in brain damage evidenced by lethargy, characteristic spasms and sharp cries.[3, 26, 39, 74, 85]

(c) hereditary elliptocytosis, elliptocytic anemia — inherited hemolytic disorder noted for the presence of a large proportion of elliptic-shaped erythrocytes in the circulating blood. Occasionally the disorder seems to be associated with leg ulcers, an enlarged spleen and abnormalities of the skeleton. Clinical manifestations are uncommon.[74, 85]

(d) hereditary spherocytosis, spherocytic anemia — familial type of hemolytic anemia characterized by the presence of sphere-shaped red cells, reticulocytosis and increased osmotic fragility. Clinical features may include cholelithiasis, a palpable liver, splenomegaly, nosebleed and a typical skeletal abnormality, the tower skull.[6, 58, 74, 85, 86]

(e) paroxysmal nocturnal hemoglobinuria — hemolytic disorder characterized by a defect of the red cell membrane which causes enzymatic and serologic abnormalities. The hemolysis ranges from mild to severe. Iron deficiency is present due to the loss of hemoglobin in urine at night. Episodes of fever, chills and hemoglobinuria signal acute hemolysis.[25, 63, 74, 85]

(5) enzyme deficiency and increased red cell destruction

(a) glucose-6-phosphate dehydrogenase (G6PD) deficiency — a common erythrocyte metabolic defect or hereditary red-cell enzyme defect. G6PD is necessary for the normal metabolism of erythrocytes. A drug-induced hemolytic anemia develops in G6PD deficiency. Antimalarials, sulfonamides, analgesics and antipyretics are chiefly responsible for the increased red cell destruction.[28, 53, 74, 85]

(b) pyruvate kinase (PK) deficiency — the most common enzymatic deficiency characterized by varying degrees of chronic hemolytic anemia and accelerated symptoms during stress or intercurrent infection.[28, 85]

(6) both, increased destruction and decreased production of erythrocytes

(a) sickle cell anemia — genetic abnormality of red blood cells due to the presence of the gene Hb S* (homozygous genotype). Hemoglobin S produces progressive hemolysis and sickling of cells as the oxygen tension is lowered and deoxygenation increases. The resultant circulatory impairment may lead to vascular occlusions by plugs of sickled red cells causing thrombosis, infarction and leg ulcers. The disease is found among American Negroes.[3, 31, 74, 85]

(b) thalassemias — a group of hereditary, familial anemias of the hypochromic microcytic type due a genetic defect which results in a reduced synthesis of adult hemoglobin (Hb A). They comprise:

(1) thalassemia major, Cooley's anemia — the homozygous genotype (both parents transmit defect) usually causes severe anemia, enlargement of the spleen and liver, jaundice and mongoloid facies.

(2) thalassemia minor — heterogenous genotype (one parent transmits thalassemia trait to offspring) results in mild anemia.

(3) other syndromes of thalassemia.[85]

b. polycythemia — disorder in which the outstanding characteristics are highly increased red cell mass and hemoglobin concentration.[3, 7, 79]

(1) primary polycythemia, polycythemia rubra vera, erythremia — chronic blood condition of unknown cause characterized by hyperplasia of bone marrow, abnormally high red cell count, hemoglobin and hematocrit which may be associated with a high platelet count, leukocytosis and leukemia.

(2) secondary polycythemias — various blood disorders in which tissue hypoxia is a significant feature. The abnormally reduced oxygen supply to the tissues stimulates an excessive production of erythropoietin which in turn increases bone marrow activity and thus red cell formation.

2. Conditions primarily resulting from a defective mechanism of coagulation. The various substances involved in the clotting of the blood are called coagulation factors, designated by Roman numerals I to XIII. According to Wintrobe factor III, tissue thromboplastin, and factor IV, calcium, are rarely used and factor VI does not exist. Effective hemostasis is dependent upon the integrity of the factors below, cellular components of the blood and the walls of the blood vessels. A final step in the complex coagulation process involves the conversion of fibrinogen to fibrin. The coagulation factors are according to International Nomenclature:**

Factor I — fibrinogen

Factor II — prothrombin

Factor V — proaccelerin, labile factor, accelerator globulin, thrombogen (AcG)

Factor VII — proconvertin, stable factor, serum prothrombin conversion accelerator (SPCA)

Factor VIII — antihemophilic factor or antihemophilic globulin, antihemophilic factor A (AHF) or (AHG) or (AHF-A)

Factor IX — plasma thromboplastin component or Christmas factor, antihemophilic factor B (PTC) or (CF) or (AHF–B)

Factor X — Stuart factor or Prower factor

Factor XI — plasma thromboplastin antecedent, antihemophilic factor C (PTA)

---

* Many other abnormal hemoglobins produce sickling without clinical symptoms. Hb S inherited from *one* parent may be asymptomatic.

**Maxwell M. Wintrobe (ed.). *Harrison's Principles of Internal Medicine*, 7th ed. New York: McGraw-Hill Book Co., 1974, p. 302.

Factor XII — Hagemann factor
(HF)

Factor XIII — fibrin stabilizing factor, Laki-Lorand factor, fibrinase.
(LLF)

Bleeding disorders are present in[13, 17, 48, 68, 75, 87]

  a. diffuse intravascular coagulation (DIC), consumption coagulopathy — pathologic clotting which differs from normal coagulation by

    (1) being a diffuse instead of a local process

    (2) damaging the clotting site instead of giving it protection

    (3) consuming some coagulation factors (fibrinogen, Factors V, VIII, XIII) thus predisposing to spontaneous bleeding

    (4) forming fibrin-fibrinogen degradation products (FDP) due to intravascular fibrinogen breakdown which is going on simultaneously with the pathologic clotting. Alternative names of FDP are:

      (a) fibrin-fibrinogen split products

      (b) fibrin-fibrinogen related antigens (FR-antigens).[72]

Diagnostic essentials include platelet reduction, prolonged prothrombin time, marked fibrinolysis, defective clot formation resulting in diffuse bleeding. Intravascular coagulation with massive hemorrhage may follow trauma, surgery, childbirth, gastrointestinal insult and other causes.[13, 17, 20, 75, 87]

  b. Henoch-Schönlein syndrome, anaphylactoid purpura — acquired bleeding abnormality seen primarily in children and characterized by widespread vasculitis affecting many organs. Purpura is the dominant clinical feature. The syndrome may be accompanied by intussusception, abdominal pain, bleeding from digestive and urinary systems, kidney disease and bone pain.[75, 87]

  c. hemophilia-A, Factor VIII deficiency — well known hereditary disease in which a sex-linked trait is transmitted by females while the hemorrhagic disorder develops exclusively in males. In its classic form there is marked deficiency of the antihemophilic factor VIII leading to spontaneous bleeding episodes. Hemarthroses and hematomas are common complications.[10, 75, 87]

  d. hemophilia-B, Factor IX deficiency, Christmas disease — familial disorder of blood coagulation attributed to a deficiency of the thromboplastin component, Factor IX. The clinical picture of the disease hemophilia-B is that of hemophilia-A.[10, 75, 87]

  e. hereditary hemorrhagic telangiectasia, Rendu-Osler-Weber syndrome — a congenital defect in the vascular hemostatic mechanism usually complicated by iron deficiency anemia. Localized dilatations of venules and capillaries are visible on the skin and mucous membranes. Epistaxis is common and bleeding may occur from digestive, urinary and respiratory tracts. The elderly tend to develop spiderlike skin lesions.[87]

  f. purpura — disorder characterized by pinpoint extravasations or petechiae and larger skin lesions, the ecchymoses. Bleeding may occur spontaneously particularly from mucous membranes and internal organs.[32, 75]

  g. thrombocytopenia purpura, idiopathic (cause unknown) — disorder resulting from a marked degree of platelet reduction. Symptoms vary from insignificant purpuric spots to serious bleeding from any body orifice or into any tissue.[1, 3, 23, 32, 68]

  h. von Willebrand's disease, pseudohemophilia, vascular hemophilia — life-long inherited bleeding disorder affecting both sexes, characterized by factor VIII deficiency and prolonged bleeding time. Abnormal bruising and bleeding into the skin and mucosa are usually of the purpuric type.[10, 75, 87]

3. Conditions primarily affecting the white blood cells.

  a. leukemia — a neoplastic disease which primarily involves the bone marrow, lymphatic and reticuloendothelial systems. It is usually characterized by an overproduction of leukocytes. The more common forms are presented.[3, 32, 57, 72, 76]

    (1) acute leukemia, stem cell leukemia — an undifferentiated form of leukemia since the cells are too young to be identified. Immature leukocytes usually

abound in the peripheral blood and bone marrow.   The onset is either abrupt or gradual ushering in fever, pallor, prostration, bleeding, joint and bone pains.[72]   Acute leukemia may occur in differentiated forms such as acute granulocytic, lymphoblastic, myeloblastic, monocytic, basophilic or eosinophilic leukemia and others depending on the dominant cell.   Anemia and thrombocytopenia may coexist.[3, 42, 61, 72]

    (2) chronic lymphocytic leukemia — a great excess of lymphocytes, 50,000-250,000 white cells, enlargement of lymph nodes and spleen, anemia and bleeding episodes.[3, 60]

    (3) chronic myelocytic leukemia — predominance of myelocytes in blood picture, white count ranging between 100,000-500,000 cells per cu mm of blood, anemia, splenomegaly, pallor, weakness, dyspnea, cachexia, pain and hemorrhagic tendencies.[3, 67, 72]

    (4) leukemoid reaction — blood disorder simulating leukemia because of its highly increased white count.

  b. leukopenia, granulocytopenia, agranulocytosis — a low white count of less than 5000 leukocytes per cu mm, caused by certain infections, nutritional deficiencies, hematopoietic disorders, chemical agents and ionizing radiation.

  c. neutropenia — decreased concentration of neutrophils in the blood predisposing to multiple severe infections.   The normal median concentration is 3650 neutrophils per cubic millimeter of blood.[11]

  d. preleukemia — leukemia suspected but no definitive laboratory evidence to justify the diagnosis.   The significant hematologic disorder is the presence of anemia, normochromic or normocytic, hypochromic or microcytic associated with a low or normal reticulocyte count.   Preleukemia occurs in all age groups with some predilection for the elderly.   The majority of children develop later lymphoblastic leukemia, the majority of adults myeloblastic leukemia.[44, 51]

4. Conditions primarily affecting cells produced by myelopoietic tissue of the bone marrow:

  a. chronic granulomatous disease (CGD) — a defect in neutrophil bacteriocidal function, characterized by recurrent infections, enlarged liver, spleen and lymph nodes, eczema and formation of granulomas.   Death usually ensues in the first decade of life.[11, 53]

  b. myeloproliferative disorders — conditions which have their origin in bone marrow and in varying degrees show an overgrowth of bone marrow cells.   Examples are chronic polycythemia vera and granulocytic leukemia.

  c. myelosclerosis, myelofibrosis — the classic form of this myeloprolific disorder reveals a triad of findings: (1) increasing marrow fibrosis, (2) a huge spleen and enlarged liver and (3) progressive anemia.   The patient may experience a dragging sensation and intense pain in the splenic area.[76, 86]

5. Conditions primarily concerned with an unbalanced proliferation of cells, usually plasma cells, and associated with an abnormality of immunoglobulins (gamma globulins).

  a. amyloidosis — the presence of amyloid infiltrates in body tissues.   Amyloid is a complex substance, principally containing protein and carbohydrates.   It is imperfectly understood and undergoing further investigation.

    (1) primary systemic (or local) amyloidosis — a plasma cell dyscrasia and genetic metabolic disorder characterized by cardiac and gastrointestinal involvements, arthropathy, peripheral neuropathy and paresthesias.

    (2) secondary parenchymatous amyloidosis — condition usually associated with infection and chronic tissue breakdown of underlying disease particularly as that seen in multiple myeloma.   Amyloid deposits are found in the spleen, kidney, adrenals, liver, lymph nodes and pancreas.[16]

  b. multiple myeloma, plasma cell myeloma — malignant neoplastic disease characterized by widespread bone destruction, intense bone pain, an excess of atypical plasma cells in the bone marrow, abnormal immunoglobulins, anemia and recurrent pneumonia or other bacterial infections related to defective antibody synthesis.   Renal damage may be associated with elevated calcium levels in blood and urine.[8, 42, 76]

c. **Waldenstrom's macroglobulinemia** — a plasma cell dyscrasia in which the production of gamma M globulin is greatly accelerated.   Bone marrow findings resemble those of chronic lymphocytic leukemia and multiple myeloma.   Anemia and low hemoglobin levels are present in symptomatic disease.   There may be involvement of the heart, nerves, muscles and joints.[32, 76]

D. Terms Related to Transfusions and Marrow Transplantations:

1. **transfusions** — the transfer of blood or its components into the circulating blood of recipients.[2, 3, 5, 15, 46, 71, 75]

    a. **autologous transfusions** — transfusions prepared from recipients' own blood.   They are safe and of particular value to patients who have unusually rare blood types, react severely to homologous blood transfusions or refuse donor blood on religious grounds.   Two forms are used:

    (1) **intraoperative autologous transfusion** — blood salvaged in massive bleeding at surgery and reinfused in patient.

    (2) **predeposit autologous transfusion** — recipient's blood withdrawn weeks prior to an anticipated need and stored in blood bank.   The withdrawal of blood stimulates red cell production.   When erythropoiesis is inadequate, iron supplements aid in maintaining the patient's iron storage.[2]

    b. **homologous transfusions** — donors' blood products obtained prior to an anticipated need of recipient and deposited in blood bank.   Blood preparations are standardized by the *National Institute of Health* (NIH) or *United States Pharmacopeia* (USP) or both.[2, 3, 71, 75]

    (1) whole blood

    (a) **banked whole blood, citrated whole blood, USP** — normal blood collected in acid citrate dextrose solution (ACD) USP to prevent coagulation; primarily used for restoring or maintaining blood volume.

    (b) **heparinized whole blood** — normal blood in heparin solution to prevent coagulation; formerly used for priming heart-lung machine to maintain extracorporeal circulation in open heart surgery.

    (2) blood cells

    (a) **leukocyte transfusion, granulocyte transfusion** — white cell transfusion, of value in neutropenia and granulocytopenia when neutrophils or other granulocytes are needed and in immune deficiency when cellular immune responses should be evoked.   Its therapeutic effect in leukemia and cancer has been established.[2, 5, 15, 43, 72]

    (b) **leukapheresis, leukopheresis** — collection of granulocytes from a normal donor or untreated patient with chronic myelogenous leukemia using a blood cell separator or filtration leukapheresis device.   The granulocytes are transfused into a patient, usually one with cancer, granulocytopenia and sepsis to stimulate bone marrow production of neutrophils.   The leukocyte poor blood is returned to the donor.[43]

    (c) **packed red cells** — concentrated suspension of red blood cells (about 70%) in ACD solution with most of the plasma removed; indicated in anemia and hemorrhage when the oxygen carrying capacity of the blood needs to be increased.[2, 3, 5, 15, 72]

    (d) **platelet concentrate** — platelet rich blood, freshly drawn from single donor; widely used in hematologic disorders with variable results.[2, 5, 15, 43]

    (e) **plateletpheresis** — platelet concentrate obtained from single donor by manual pheresis or mechanical pheresis, a promising but still experimental therapy.[5]

    (f) **red cells deglycerolized** — frozen, thawed red blood cells, using glycerol to prevent cellular damage during freezing and thawing and removing glycerol prior to transfusion. Autologous and rare blood type transfusion products can be preserved in frozen blood centers to meet future needs.[3, 5, 50]

(3) blood proteins and plasma fractions

   (a) antihemophilic human plasma, USP — normal plasma, promptly processed to preserve antihemophilic globulin Factor VIII, a component of fresh plasma. It is indicated in the treatment of hemophilia.[2, 3, 5]

   (b) cryoprecipitate (Cryo) — commercial product prepared by slowly thawing fresh frozen plasma to form cryoprecipitate rich in antihemophilic Factor VIII. Cryo is the treatment of choice in hemophilia and other bleeding disorders.[2, 5, 15]

   (c) fresh frozen plasma (FFP) — plasma separated from whole blood and containing all clotting factors; useful as replacement therapy in depletion of coagulation factors.[5]

   (d) fibrinogen — a plasma protein for controlling bleeding due to fibrinogen deficiency.

   (e) gamma globulin (IgC) — a plasma fraction used for the amelioration of hepatitis and IgC deficiency.[15, 72]

   (f) plasmapheresis — plasma withdrawn from donor according to prescribed size and frequency of donation for the purpose of transfusing patient in need of plasma fraction therapy. The remaining cells are reinfused into the donor.[2, 3]

   (g) plasma protein fraction (PPF) — effective therapeutic agent for hypovolemia. It contains serum albumin (5%) and a number of other plasma proteins.[5]

   (h) serum albumin — a plasma fraction used in the treatment of shock and some protein deficiencies.[20]

   (i) transfusion reaction — untoward response to intravenous infusion of a blood preparation. It may be caused by air embolism, allergy, bacterial contaminants, circulatory overload and hemolysis due to incompatibility of cells. Reactions vary in degree from mild to life-threatening; chills, fever, malaise and headache are common warning signals.[2, 15, 71, 75]

2. bone marrow transplantation — bone marrow grafting in hematologic neoplasia based on the assumption that malignant disorders might be successfully treated by aggressive chemotherapy and life-threatening total body irradiation provided donor marrow would prevent death induced by lethal radiation dosage.[22, 25, 59, 69, 70]

   a. allogenic marrow transplantation — bone marrow obtained from

      (1) donor related to recipient, matched siblings — histocompatibility usually present in members of the same family.[3]

      (2) donor unrelated to recipient — histoincompatibility frequently present. Infused marrow cells are prone to reject the patient's cells and he is likely to develop

         (a) graft-versus-host disease (GVHD) — a major problem in the transplantation of tissues or organs occurring when an immunoincompetent host receives histoincompatible lymphocytes. The chief targets of GVHD are the skin, gut and liver.[70, 88]

         (b) histoincompatibility — tissue incompatibility between a donor and recipient.

         (c) immunoincompetence — deficient response to antigenic stimulus, congenital or acquired disease, or related to therapy and other causes.[72]

   b. autologous marrow transplantation — aspiration of the patient's own bone marrow prior to the initiation of aggressive radiotherapy with or without intensive chemotherapy and its infusion when bone marrow toxicity becomes life-threatening.[69, 70]

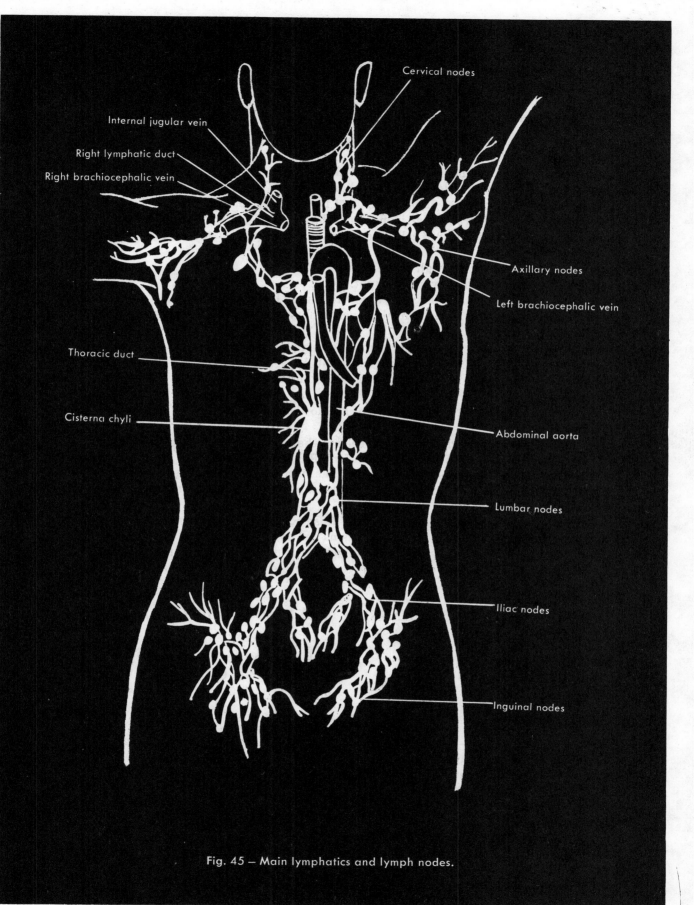

Fig. 45 — Main lymphatics and lymph nodes.

c. isogenic or syngenic marrow transplantation — marrow grafting between identical twins. Since donor and host have the same tissue antigens, no immunologic barrier to transplantation should be present.[69, 70]

E. Symptomatic Terms:

1. anisocytosis — variation in size of red cells, seen in pernicious anemia.
2. blood dyscrasia — morbid blood condition.
3. erythrocytosis — abnormal increase in red blood cells.
4. erythropenia — abnormal decrease in red blood cells.
5. fibrinolysis — dissolution of fibrin; blood clot becomes liquid.
6. hemochromatosis — intracellular iron overload associated with organic damage.[72]
7. hemolysis — destruction of red cells and subsequent escape of hemoglobin into blood plasma.
8. leukocytosis — abnormally high white count.
9. leukopenia — abnormally low white count.
10. macrocytosis — abnormally large erythrocytes in the blood.
11. megaloblastosis — large, usually oval shaped, embryonic red corpuscles found in bone marrow and blood.
12. microcytosis — abnormally small erythrocytes present in the blood.
13. neutropenia — excessively low neutrophil count.[11]
14. neutrophilia — increase in neutrophils including immature forms, seen in pyogenic infections.
15. pancytopenia — an abnormal reduction of all blood cells: erythrocytes, leukocytes and platelets.[86]
16. poikilocytosis — irregularly shaped red cells in the blood seen in pernicious anemia.
17. proliferation — increase in reproduction of similar forms or cells.[72]
18. reticulocytosis — an increase in reticulocytes as seen in active blood regeneration due to stimulation of red bone marrow or in congenital hemolytic anemia and some other anemias.
19. rouleaux formation, pseudoagglutination — false agglutination in which the erythrocytes look like stacks of coins. It is seen in plasma cell dyscrasias such as multiple myeloma.[65]
20. thrombocytopenia — a deficiency of thrombocytes or platelets in the circulating blood.[1, 68]
21. thrombocytosis — an excess of thrombocytes or platelets in the circulating blood.[1, 27]

LYMPHATIC CHANNELS AND LYMPH NODES

A. Origin of Terms:

1. adeno (G) — gland
2. angi, angio (G) — vessel
3. histio, histo (G) — web, tissue
4. lymph (L) — lymph
5. reticulum (L) — little net

B. Anatomic Terms:

1. histiocytes, histocytes — tissue cells or macrophages which belong to the reticuloendothelial system and possess phagocytic properties.
2. lymph — a clear or sometimes milky liquid found in lymphatics.
3. lymphatic duct, right — duct which drains into the right brachiocephalic vein or one of its tributaries.
4. lymphatics — thin-walled vessels widely distributed throughout the body and containing many valves.
5. lymph nodes — encapsulated lymphoid tissue scattered along the lymphatics in chains or clusters.
6. reticuloendothelial system — system includes highly phagocytic cells such as macrophages or histiocytes present in the loose connective tissue of the body, the

sinusoids of the lymph nodes, spleen, liver, as well as in the bone marrow and lungs. It is thought that the function of these cells is

   a. normally the removal of destroyed cells from the circulation and perhaps the storage of iron to be used in the regeneration of erythrocytes
   b. in pathologic disorders the removal of bacteria, dead tissue and foreign bodies.[88]

7. thoracic duct — duct which drains into the left brachiocephalic vein or one of its tributaries.

C. Diagnostic Terms:

1. Burkitt's lymphoma — a malignant tumor of lymphoid tissue which usually involves the facial bones and abdomen of young children. The etiologic agent is the Epstein-Barr virus.[4]

2. histiocytosis X — the term refers to 3 disorders in which there is histiocytic proliferation without the presence of an infective agent or abnormal lipid metabolism.[77]

   a. eosinophilic granuloma of bones — generally a solitary benign osteolytic lesion containing numerous histiocytes and eosinophils. Sites of predilection are the pelvis, vertebrae, head and ribs. The lesion occurs in children and adolescents.[77]

   b. Hand-Schüller-Christian disease — a childhood affliction with diffuse bone involvement due to multiple osteolytic lesions which may be associated with diabetes insipidus, eczema, exophthalmos, otitis media, respiratory disease, enlargement of the liver, spleen and lymph nodes.[77]

   c. Letterer-Siwe disease — histiocytic proliferation present in lymph nodes, spleen, liver, skin, lung and bones. Pantocytopenia occurs frequently since histiocytes are prone to replace the bone marrow. The disorder is primarily seen before the age of 3 and less commonly in older children.[77]

3. Hodgkin's disease — a life-threatening, neoplastic disease producing widespread lymph node involvement, enlargement of the spleen and liver, serious blood disorders, pathologic changes in the bones and other organs, systemic manifestations such as recurrent bouts of fever, night sweats, malaise and weight loss. Exacerbations and remissions are characteristic of the clinical course. In an attempt to gain a better understanding of Hodgkin's disease, four stages have been recognized. Luke and Butler's histologic staging (Table 10) usually reflects the clinical picture of the patient. The purpose of the Ann Arbor staging (Table 11) is to offer a guide to treatment modalities of Hodgkin's disease.[21, 29, 42, 52, 56, 57, 77, 89]

Table 10

HISTOLOGIC CLASSIFICATION OF HODGKIN'S DISEASE

Histologic Classification[a]	Histologic Variants[b]
Lymphocytic predominance	Nodules containing lymphocytes, histiocytes and a few Reed Sternberg (RS) cells
Nodular sclerosis	Bands of collagen in nodes, lacunae of RS cells
Mixed cellularity	Lymph nodes containing lymphocytes, histiocytes, plasma cells, neutrophils, eosinophils and many RS cells
Lymphocytic depletion	Anaplastic variants of RS cells, only a few lymphocytes present

[a]Adapted from R. J. Lukes and J. J. Butler. The pathology and nomenclature of Hodgkin's disease. *Cancer Research*, 26:1063, 1966.

[b]Stanley L. Robbins. Hodgkin's disease. *Pathologic Basis of Disease.* Philadelphia: W. B. Saunders Co., 1974, pp. 760-767.

Table 11

STAGING CLASSIFICATION FOR HODGKIN'S DISEASE[a]

Stage	Pathologic Involvement
I	A single lymph node region or single extralymphatic site or organ
II	Two or more lymph node regions on the same side of the diaphragm or localized disease of an extralymphatic organ or site
III	Lymph node regions on either side of the diaphragm or localized pathology of an extralymphatic site or organ, or spleen, or both
IV	Diffuse disease of one or more extralymphatic organs with or without associated nodal lesions

[a]Adapted from Robert C. Young and Vincent T. DeVita. Hodgkin's disease (The Ann Arbor Classification). In Conn, Howard F. (ed.) *Current Therapy*. Philadelphia: W. B. Saunders Co., 1976, pp. 290-300.

4. lymphadenitis — inflammation of the lymph glands.
5. lymphadenopathy — any diseased condition of the lymph nodes; e.g. enlarged lymph nodes due to an unknown cause.[72]
6. lymphangioma — tumor composed of lymphatics.
7. lymphangitis — inflammation of the lymphatics.
8. lymphedema — congenital or acquired disorder of the lymphatics which prevents the removal of tissue fluids by the lymph channels and the absorption of protein and other substances by lymphatic capillaries resulting in impairment of lymph flow and edema.[64]
9. lymphocytic choriomeningitis (LMC) — acute (rarely fatal) or mild form of aseptic meningitis caused by the LMC virus. Clinical features of the mild form are weakness, malaise, fever, myalgia, back pain and sometimes respiratory symptoms. The cell count of the cerebrospinal fluid (CSF) is highly increased. Lymphocytes predominate.[36]
10. lymphomas — neoplasms which may arise in lymphoid tissue and vary in degree of malignancy. They are distinguished by their histologic components and diffuse or nodular pattern. According to a revised classification malignant non-Hodgkin's lymphomas may be
    a. lymphocytic, well differentiated lymphomas, formerly lymphocytic lymphomas
    b. lymphocytic, poorly differentiated lymphomas, formerly lymphoblastic lymphomas
    c. stem cell lymphomas including Burkitt's lymphomas
    d. histiocytic lymphomas, formerly reticulum cell sarcomas.
    Painful cervical lymph nodes, fever, malaise, sweating and weight loss are early clinical findings, followed later by splenohepatomegaly and the presence of lymphomas in liver, spleen, lungs, other organs as well as thrombocytopenia, hemorrhage and infection.[29, 32, 54, 77]
11. mycosis fungoides, granuloma fungoides — chronic, progressive, lymphomatous tumor of the skin which tends to ulcerate and ultimately cause death.[77]

D. Operative Terms:

1. biopsy of lymph node — removal of small piece of lymphoid tissue for microscopic study.
2. lymphadenectomy — excision of lymph nodes.
3. lymphadenotomy — incision and drainage of lymph gland.
4. multiple lymph node excision — removal of metastatic lymph nodes in a certain region, e.g. the axillary nodal cluster, the periaortic chain or the pelvic and retroperitoneal nodes.

E. Symptomatic Terms:

1. lymphocytosis — abnormal increase of lymphocytes in the blood.
2. lymphocytopenia — deficient number of lymphocytes in the blood.

3. Pel-Ebstein type of fever — seen in Hodgkin's disease.   Fever rises to about 120° for five or six days, then remains normal for five or six days and continues the same cycle.

SPLEEN

A. Origin of Terms:

1. splen (G) — spleen
2. lien (L) — spleen

B. Anatomic Term:

spleen — a lymphoid organ located in the left hypochondriac region   It is active in the destruction of red blood cells and the manufacture of lymphocytes and phagocytes.

C. Diagnostic Terms:

1. accessory spleens — additional spleens, performing the same function as the spleen.   The condition is very common.
2. asplenia — absence of spleen.
3. chronic congestive splenomegaly, hepatolienal fibrosis, Banti's syndrome — condition characterized by longstanding congestion and enlargement of the spleen usually due to liver disease associated with portal or splenic artery hypertension.   Leukopenia, anemia and gastrointestinal bleeding are common manifestations.[55, 81, 88]
4. hypersplenism, hypersplenic syndrome — excessive splenic activity associated with highly increased blood cell destruction leading to anemia, leukopenia and thrombocytopenia.[55, 72]
5. splenic infarcts — relatively common lesions usually caused by embolism, thrombosis or infection.[55, 72]
6. splenitis, lienitis — inflammation of the spleen.
7. splenoptosis — downward displacement of the spleen.
8. splenorrhexis — rupture of spleen due to injury or advanced disease.

D. Operative Terms:

1. splenectomy — removal of the spleen.
2. splenopexy — fixation of a movable spleen.
3. splenorrhaphy — suture of a ruptured spleen.
4. splenotomy — incision into the spleen.

E. Symptomatic Terms:

1. autosplenectomy — small fibrotic spleen in adult with sickle cell anemia.   Multiple splenic infarctions result in shrinkage of the organ.[72]
2. splenomegaly, splenomegalia — enlargement of the spleen.[81]

RADIOLOGY

A. Terms Related to Diagnostic Radiology:

1. lymphadenography — radiographic delineation of lymph nodes after the injection of a contrast medium.
2. lymphangiography (LAG), lymphography — a radiographic study of the lymphatic system following the injection of a radiopaque substance in the lymphatic vessels.[24, 40, 73, 78]
   a. bimanual lymphangiography — delineation of the lymphatic system after the injection of a contrast medium into both hands to visualize the lymphatic and nodal involvement of the upper extremities including the axillary, supraclavicular and periclavicular areas.

    b. bipedal lymphangiography — delineation of the lymphatic system after the injection of radiopaque material into both feet to visualize the lymphatic structures of the lower extremities, groin, pelvis, periaortic region and thoracic duct.

    c. unilateral lymphography — delineation of lymphatics and nodes of one side of the body.

3. ultrasonography of spleen — use of ultrasound or the production of echoes to determine the size of the spleen.[41]

4. xeroradiography of lymph nodes — a radiographic method of obtaining images of soft tissue masses on selenium-coated metal plates, used to delineate normal nodes, inflammatory nodes, metastatic nodes and primary lymph node disease.[38]

B. Terms Related to Therapeutic Radiology:

1. irradiation — subjection of a patient or a substance to the action of light, x-ray or other radiant energy.

    a. external irradiation

        (1) segmental — irradiation confined to local areas.

        (2) total body — irradiation including the entire torso and extremities.[37, 54]

    b. internal irradiation, interstitial — insertion of radon containing capillary tubes or needles into a tissue to shrink a tumor, destroy a cancerous growth or the like.

2. radiation — emission of any form of radiant energy in various directions.

3. radiation therapy, radiotherapy — use of all forms of radiant energy in the treatment of disease. Radiotherapy is an accepted therapeutic modality in leukemia, polycythemia vera, Hodgkin's disease and malignant lymphomas. It is also used as a palliative measure to relieve bone pain in multiple myeloma and other malignant disorders.[47, 54]

    a. megavoltage, megavolt — a unit of electromotive force equal to one million volts.*

    b. megavoltage radiotherapy, supervoltage radiotherapy — the use of rays produced by at least 1,000,000 volts or equivalent such as those of Cobalt-60 Betatron Linear accelerator to treat deep seated tumors including bladder, cervix, uterus and lung neoplasms or lymphomas.[80] Extended field megavoltage radiotherapy to diseased organs and adjacent lymph nodes is the treatment of choice in stages I, II, and III of Hodgkin's disease.[52, 89]

CLINICAL LABORATORY

A. Terms Related to Hematology:

1. bleeding time — duration of bleeding from a standardized wound. It measures the platelet function and the integrity of the vessel wall.

2. capillary fragility tourniquet test — procedure measuring the resistance of the capillaries to pressure and stress. A blood pressure cuff is applied to the upper arm and kept inflated at 80 mm pressure for 5 minutes. If a number of purpuric spots appear below the cuff area a few minutes after the cuff is released, the test is positive.[87]

3. coagulant — substance contributing to clot formation.

4. coagulation time, clotting time — time taken for venous blood to clot.

5. coagulum, blood clot — a lumpy mass formed in static blood in the laboratory and composed of platelets, red and white cells, irregularly scattered in fibrin network.[23]

6. clotlysis — dissolution of a clot.

7. clot retraction — formation of a clot and the exuding of serum: a qualitative platelet function test. Normally the retraction of blood begins within 30 to 60 minutes from the time it was drawn.

8. hemoglobin concentration (Hb) — measurement of the amount of hemoglobin, formerly recorded in grams per 100 milliliters (gm/100 ml), currently in grams per deciliter (g/dl) according to the International System of Units (SI).**

---

*Stedman's Medical Dictionary, 23rd ed., 1976, p. 841. (verbatim)

**The International System of Units (SI) seeks to report the results from scientific investigations of various disciplines in a uniform manner.

9. mean corpuscular hemoglobin (MCH) — weight of hemoglobin in average red blood cells, formerly expressed in micromicrograms ($\mu\mu g$), presently in picograms (pg).[33, 87]

10. mean corpuscular hemoglobin concentration (MCHC) — per cent of hemoglobin concentration in the average red blood cell, currently expressed in grams per deciliter of red cells (g/dl).[33]

11. mean corpuscular volume (MCV) — mean volume of the average red blood cell, formerly recorded in cubic microns ($c\mu$), presently in femoliters (fl).

12. osmotic fragility — measurement of the power of red cells to resist hemolysis in a hypotonic salt solution.

13. volume of packed red cells (VPRC), hematocrit (Hct) — measurement of the volume of packed red blood cells in the venous blood.
    Normal values depend on sex, altitude and method used to measure VPRC. A similar interdependence is observed in other hematologic findings.

14. prothrombin — coagulation factor II present in blood plasma.

15. prothrombin time — time in seconds required for thromboplastin to coagulate plasma.
    Normal findings:
    Quick's method . . . . 11-16 seconds
    Prolonged prothrombin time in vitamin K deficiency, hypoprothrombinemia and obstructive jaundice.

16. thromboplastin — coagulation factor III, thought to initiate clotting by converting prothrombin to thrombin in the presence of calcium ions. Tissue thromboplastin is chiefly found in the brain, thymus, placenta, testes and lungs.[87]

    a. complete thromboplastins — substances causing clot formation as quickly with hemophilic as with normal blood.

    b. partial thromboplastins — substances causing clot formation less quickly with hemophilic than with normal blood.[66]

    c. partial thromboplastin time (PTT) — valuable screening test for abnormalities of blood coagulation measuring coagulation factors involved in the intrinsic pathways.
        Normal findings:
        comparable to normal control.
        Increase in vitamin K deficiency, hepatic disease, von Willibrand's disease, presence of circulating anticoagulants and others.[87]

17. thrombus — structure formed in circulating blood, chiefly composed of a head of agglutinated platelets and white cells and a tail of fibrin and entrapped red cells.[23]

Table 12
CELLULAR CONSTITUENTS OF BLOOD

Constituents	Normal Range Per Cubic Millimeter of Blood[a] (Formerly)	International System of Units (SI)[b] (Currently)	Pathologic Increase	Pathologic Decrease
Erythrocytes — Male Erythrocytes — Female	4,500,000 to 6,000,000 4,000,000 to 5,500,000	4.5 to 6.0 X 10^{12}/L 4.0 to 5.0 G 10^{12}/L	Polycythemia vera	Anemias
Reticulated erythrocytes	Usually 1 per cent or less of total erythrocytes	50 X 10^9/L expressed in absolute numbers	Hemolytic jaundice	Purpura hemorrhagic
Leukocytes	5,000 to 10,000	5.0 X 10^9/L	Infections, leukemias	Agranulocytosis influenza typhoid fever
Platelets or thrombocytes	200,000 to 400,000	200 X 10^9/L	. . . .	Thrombocytopenic purpura acute leukemia

[a] Opal Hepler, *Manual of Clinical Laboratory Methods*, 4th ed. Springfield, Illinois: Charles E. Thomas Publisher, 1955, p. 33.

[b] Maxwell M. Wintrobe. *Clinical Hematology*, 7th ed. Philadelphia: Lea and Febiger, 1974, p. 1897.

Table 13

SOME HEMATOLOGIC FINDINGS IN DISEASE

Test	Normal Values[a, b]	Diagnostic Aid in Disease[a]	Pathologic Response
Bleeding time Duke Ivy	1-6 minutes 2-3 minutes	Thrombocytopenia von Willebrand's disease Coagulation defects	Increase
Clotting time Lee White Silicone	7-12 minutes 2 hours	Hemophilia purpura Hemorrhage of newborn	Increase
Clot retraction time	1-24 hours	Thrombocytopenic purpura	No restriction
Osmotic fragility	0.4-0.2% of Na Cl	Congenital hemolytic jaundice Aplastic anemia	Increase
Capillary fragility (tourniquet test)	0-10 petechiae per unit of area[a]	Thrombocytopenic purpura, Purpura associated with Severe infections, Systemic vascular diseases	Increase
Hemoglobin	15 g/dl........Currently (grams/deciliter) 15 gm/100 ml....Formerly	Polycythemia vera, dehydration Anemias......................	Increase Decrease
Mean corpuscular hemoglobin MCH	28 pg.........Currently (picograms) 28 $\mu\mu$g........Formerly	Hyperchromic anemias........... Hypochromic anemias.............	Increase Decrease
Mean corpuscular volume MCV	87 fl.........Currently (femtoliters) 87 cμ.........Formerly	Macrocytic anemias............. Normocytic hypochromic anemia Microcytic hypochromic anemia	Increase Decrease Decrease
Mean corpuscular hemoglobin concentration MCHC	34 g/dl.........Currently (grams/deciliter of red cells) 34%..........Formerly	Macrocytic hypochromic anemia Microcytic hypochromic anemia	Decrease Decrease

[a] Hepler, op. cit., pp. 40-91.

[b] Normal values given according to (1) SI — International System of Units, (2) formerly used measurements. See Wintrobe, op. cit., p. 1897.

B. Terms Related to Blood Grouping and Immune System[2, 3, 66]

1. ABO system — the international system of Landsteiner in which the 4 main blood groups are designated by the letters A, B, AB and O.   This system is universally used.
2. agglutination — clumping of erythrocytes when mixed with incompatible blood or antisera.
3. agglutinin — a specific antibody in blood serum which causes agglutination.
   a. autoagglutinin — resembles cold agglutinin, reacts at temperature below 37°C with person's own cells and those of other groups.
   b. cold agglutinin — antibody causes clumping of human group O red cells at zero 5°C or below 37°C temperature.[72]
4. agglutinogen — a substance which stimulates the production of agglutinins when introduced into the body.

5. antibody — a molecule belonging to a special group of proteins known as gamma globulins (IgG, IgM, others).

6. antigen — a substance which causes the formation of antibodies.

   a. ABO antigens — genetically determined, specific glycoproteins, primarily located on the surface of red blood cells, but also in other body tissues.[72]

   b. human leukocyte antigens (HLA) — antigens found on the surface of nucleated cells including most body tissues and cellular components of the circulating blood with exception of red cells. Peripheral blood leukocytes are often suitable to assess the HLA antigenic composite of a person.

   It is imperative that HLA typing is done for the detection of HLA antibodies prior to platelet or leukocyte transfusons or transplant procedures of bone marrow, kidney, heart, others.[3, 5, 59, 72]

   c. platelet antigens — antigens specific for platelets and associated with ABO and HLA antigens. Matching for platelet transfusions is complex and problematic.[3, 5, 72]

7. blood factor for hemagglutinogen — serologic factor which occurs on the surface of red blood corpuscles.

8. blood group or blood type — inherited characteristic of human blood which remains unchanged throughout life.

9. blood grouping systems — the classification of blood based on hemagglutinogens in red blood corpuscles. There are different types of blood factors (hemagglutinogens) requiring special methods of typing. The blood group systems refer to these serologic factors: for example:

      ABO system to A, B, AB and O factors

      MN system to M, N, MN factors

      Rh-Hr system to Rh and Hr factors. *

The recent discovery of subgroups (e.g.: A_1, A_2, A_3, A_4 and others for the ABO system) explains why incompatibility of types of blood may occur with the same blood group.

   a. incompatible blood — blood not capable of being mixed without causing hemolysis or clumping of red blood cells.

   b. type-O — universal donor — blood has no agglutinogens, hence no clumping.[2, 66]

10. cross-matching — procedure done to determine the compatibility between the recipient's blood and donor's blood in order to prevent blood transfusion reaction.[2, 66]

11. MN system — classification based on the presence of MN factors in erythrocytes. This system is used in genetic blood group analysis and in medicolegal paternity studies when parental claims are disputed.[2, 66]

12. Rh-Hr system — a system of complex antigenic structure. The Rh factor is an agglutinogen which occurs in the red blood corpuscles of 87% of white people. Originally

Table 14

COMPATIBILITY OF BLOOD FOR TRANSFUSION[a]

Recipient's Blood	Donor's Blood
A	A or O
B	B or O
AB	AB, A, B, or O
O	O only

[a] Rh studies are done routinely on all blood transfusions. In addition, subgroups may be checked to prevent reactions. Universal donor blood is only used for recipients of group A or B or AB in emergency when their respective type is not available.

---

* For information on other blood group systems (Lewis, Kell, P, Duffy, MNS, Kidd, Lutheran, Ii and Vel) consult Israel Davidsohn and John Bernard Henry (eds.). *Clinical Diagnosis by Laboratory Methods*, 15th ed. Philadelphia: W. B. Saunders Co., 1974, pp. 348-413.

only Rh positive and Rh negative agglutinogens were known; at present subgroups of Rh factors are recognized. The Rh determinations are of clinical importance in blood transfusion and obstetrics. There is a reciprocal relationship between Hr and Rh factors.[2, 66]

C. Terms Related to Miscellaneous Blood Tests:

1. blood gas determinations — sensitive indicators of physiologic changes of lung function and tissue perfusion in acute illness. Measurements are obtained from hydrogen, carbon dioxide and oxygen tensions (pressures) of arterial or venous blood. The "p" refers to partial pressure.[19]

   a. P_{CO_2} — pressure or tension of carbon dioxide measured in millimeters of mercury.

   Normal values

   arterial P_{CO_2} ....35-40 mm Hg
   venous P_{CO_2} ... .40-45 mm Hg[19]

   Increase in hypercarbia
   CO_2 retention in respiratory acidosis and metabolic alkalosis.

   Decrease in hypocarbia
   Excessive loss of carbon dioxide in hyperventilation due to respiratory alkalosis or metabolic acidosis.

   b. pH — hydrogen ion concentration or acidity value of blood (or urine)

   Normal values

   arterial pH 7.38-7.44
   venous pH 7.36-7.41

   Increase in acidosis
   Decrease in alkalosis.[19]

   c. P_{O_2} — pressure or tension of oxygen expressed in millimeters of mercury.

   Normal values

   arterial P_{O_2} .... 95-100 mm Hg
   Patients with chronic lung disease normally have an aterial P_{O_2} of 70 mm Hg or less.

   Decreased values

   arterial P_{O_2} in advanced lung or heart disease.
   venous P_{O_2} due to inadequate blood volume, exchange of gases, cardiac output and tissue perfusion.[19]

2. fibrin-fibrinogen degradation products (FDP) — protein fragments resulting from the digestive action of plasmin or related enzymes on fibrin or fibrinogen.[87]

3. fibrinogenolysis — the proteolytic destruction of fibrinogen and other clotting factors in the circulating blood.[87]

4. fibrinolysis — the destruction of fibrin in blood clots or the dissolution of fibrin due to enzymatic action.[87]

5. tests for the detection of FDP

   a. direct latex test (Thrombo-Wellcotest) — a rapid slide test based on a latex reagent, sensitized with anti-FDP antibodies capable of detecting degradation products and fibrin in serum and urine.[75]

   Normal values

   serum FDP in resting adult .... 4.9 ± 2.8 μg/ml
   urine FDP .... 0.25 μg/ml

   Increased values

   serum FDP in thromboembolic disease with peak level of 400 μg/ml and drop to normal in about 24 hours; acute myocardial infarction with serum FDP rising 2-4 days after the attack. If after the peak level subsides, a second rise of serum occurs, this signals extention of myocardial infarction or complications.

   b. red cell haemagglutination-inhibition test (HAI) — immunoassay suitable for quantitative research studies because of its precision and high sensitivity.[75, 87]

6. serum iron and iron binding capacity — valuable diagnostic test used in anemia and related disorders to determine iron excess or iron lack. The calculation of per cent saturation of iron provides additional information for differential diagnosis.[9]

7. transferrin, siderophilin — an iron binding glycoprotein primarily synthesized by functional liver cells and referred to as transport iron due to its iron transferring activity. Transferrin saturated with iron is known as iron-binding capacity (IBC) or total iron-binding capacity (TIBC).[9]

ABBREVIATIONS

A. Related to Hematology:

Ab — antibody
ACD — acid-citrate-dextrose
Ag — antigen
AHF — antihemophilic factor VIII
AHG — antihemophilic globulin factor VIII
bas — basophils
CBC — complete blood count
CF — Christmas factor, factor IX
eos — eosinophils
ESR — erythrocytic sedimentation rate
FDP — fibrin-fibrinogen degradation products
FR — fibrin-fibrinogen related
FSP — fibrin-fibrinogen split products
HAI — haemagglutination-inhibition immunoassay
Hb — hemoglobin

Hb A — adult hemoglobin
Hb F — fetal hemoglobin
Hb S — sickle cell hemoglobin
Hct, Ht — hematocrit
lymph — lymphocytes
MCH — mean corpuscular hemoglobin
MCT — mean circulation time
MCV — mean corpuscular volume
mon — monocytes
PCT — plasmacrit test
PCV — packed cell volume (hematocrit)
PMN — polymorphonuclear neutrophils
PTA — plasma thromboplastin antecedent, factor XI
PTC — plasma thromboplastin component, factor IX
RBC — red blood count
RES — reticuloendothelial system
SI — saturation index
VI — volume index
VPRC — volume packed red cells
WBC — white blood count

B. Related to Radiology:

LAG — lymphangiography
Mev, MeV — megavolt, megavoltage

RAD, rad — radiation absorbed dose
TBI — total body irradiation

C. Related to Hematologic Disorders:

AIHA — autoimmune hemolytic anemia
ALL — acute lymphoblastic leukemia
AML — acute myeloblastic leukemia
CLL — chronic lymphocytic leukemia
CML — chronic myelocytic leukemia
DIC — diffuse intravascular coagulation
G6PD — glucose-6-phosphate dehydrogenase

GvH, GVHD — graft versus host disease
HCD — heavy chain disease
HDN — hemolytic disease of the newborn
HE — hereditary elliptocytosis
HS — hereditary spherocytosis
IMF — idiopathic myelofibrosis
ITP — idiopathic thrombocytopenia purpura
PA — pernicious anemia
PK — pyruvate kinase deficiency
SCA — sickle cell anemia

D. Related to Organizations:

AABB — American Association of Blood Banks

ACS — Association of Clinical Scientists

ASCP — American Association of Clinical Pathologists

ASLM — American Association of Law and Medicine

E. Related to Measurements of the Metric System:

Weights in descending order:

kg	= kilogram	= 1,000 grams	= 10^3gm
gm,g	= gram	= 1,000 milligrams	= 10^3mg
mg	= milligram	= 1,000 micrograms	= 10^{-3}gm
μg	= microgram	= 1,000 nanograms	= 10^{-6}gm
ng	= nanogram	= 1,000 picograms	= 10^{-9}gm
pg	= picogram	= 1,000 femtograms	= 10^{-12}gm
fg	= femtogram	= 1,000 attograms	= 10^{-15}gm

Capacity in descending order:

l, L	= liter	= 1,000 milliliters	= 10 deciliters	(dl)
l, L	= liter	= 1,000 cubic centimeters	= 10 deciliters	(dl)
dl	= deciliter	= 100 milliliters	= 0.10 liter	(l)
cl	= centiliter	= 10 milliliters	= 0.10 deciliter	(dl)
ml	= milliliter	= 1,000 microliters	= 0.10 centiliter	(cl)
μl*	= microliter	= 1,000 nanoliters	= 0.001 milliliter	(ml)
nl	= nanoliter	= 1,000 picoliters	= 0.001 microliter	(μl)
pl	= picoliter	= 1,000 femtoliters	= 0.001 nanoliter	(nl)
fl	= femtoliter	= 1,000 attoliters	= 0.001 picoliter	(pl)

Length in descending order:

m	= meter	= 1,000 millimeters	= 100 centimeters	(cm)
dm	= decimeter	= 100 millimeters	= 10 centimeters	(cm)
cm	= centimeter	= 10 millimeters	= 0.01 meter	(m)
mm	= millimeter	= 1,000 micrometers	= 0.001 meter	(m)
μm	= micrometer	= 1,000 nanometers	= 0.001 millimeter	(mm)
nm	= nanometer	= 1,000 picometers	= 0.001 micrometer	(μm)
pm	= picometer	= 1,000 femtometers	= 0.001 nanometer	(nm)
fm	= femtometer	= 1,000 attometers	= 0.001 picometer	(pm)

Miscellaneous:

mEq — milliequivalent (measure of electrolytes)

mEq/L — milliequivalent per liter

μEq — microequivalent

mμ — millimicron (same as nanogram)

mM — millimol

mOsm — milliosmol (measure of osmolarity)

mIU — milliInternational Unit

μIU — microInternational Unit

μU — microunit

---

*μl — microliter, formerly cu mm — cubic millimeter. For further information see Israel Davidsohn and John B. Henry (eds.). *Clinical Diagnosis by Laboratory Methods*, 15th ed. Philadelphia: W. B. Saunders Co., 1974, pp. 1376-1395.

ORAL READING PRACTICE

Hodgkin's Disease

This peculiar and interesting disease is characterized by a painless enlargement of the lymph nodes which is initially confined to one group, frequently those located in the cervical region. From there the lymph node involvement spreads to the **axillary** and **inguinal** regions and progressively assumes systemic proportions. If **mediastinal spread** and **infiltration** of the lung **parenchyma** and pleura occur, the patient may experience **substernal** pain, cough, **dyspnea** and **stridor.**

Retroperitoneal lymph node involvement may lead to the formation of a mass which presses on the stomach and produces a sense of fullness. This type of involvement tends to exert a deleterious effect resulting in a dislodgment of the kidneys, compression of the **ureters** and **inferior vena cava** and **infiltrations** into the neighboring structures, the spinal nerves and **vertebrae.** **Splenomegaly** and **hepatomegaly** are common signs and may be associated with progressive **anemia, obstructive jaundice** and **ascites.**

Lesions of Hodgkin's disease are sometimes found in the reproductive system. **Osteolytic** and **osteoplastic** changes may occur in the ribs, vertebrae, femur and pelvis and cause bone tenderness or intense pain. As the disease progresses to the terminal phase, the patient manifests high fever and a marked degree of **lassitude, debility, pallor** and **cyanosis.**

The diagnostic feature of Hodgkin's disease is the **Reed-Sternberg** cell, a tumor cell containing irregular shaped **cytoplasm,** a large **nucleus,** heavy clumps of **chromatin** and **distinctive nucleoli,** surrounded by a clear halo.

Pathologic staging of the extent of the disease is of practical significance as a guide to the best **therapeutic** approach. With early diagnosis, improved understanding of Hodgkin's disease and the modality of treatment adapted to the stage of the disease, the **prognosis** formerly fatal, may be favorable.[29, 56, 89]

Dramatic results have been obtained from the judicious use of **megavoltage radiotherapy** or **cobalt** particularly in reducing or controlling cervical and axillary **lymphadenopathy.**[52, 72, 89]

Cyclic combination chemotherapy is the treatment of choice in advanced Hodgkin's disease. **Cancerocidal** agents such as **nitrogen mustard, chlorambucil, cyclophosphamide** with **prednisone** are employed, inducing remissions and a prolongation of life. It is a known fact that the use of antineoplastic drugs requires much caution because of their potential **toxicity.**[56, 89]

The most serious untoward effect of aggressive megavoltage radiotherapy and chemotherapy is **myelosuppression** resulting in a reduction of all cellular elements of the blood (pancytopenia). **Granulocytopenia** with its lowered resistance to infection and **thrombocytopenia** with its hemorrhagic tendencies become life-threatening **sequelae.**

The terminal phase of Hodgkin's disease is signalled by **lymphopenia,** a striking **immunologic** manifestation heralding a **defective response** to previously encountered **antigens.**[21, 29, 42, 52, 56, 57, 77, 89]

Table 15

SOME DISORDERS OF THE BLOOD AND BLOOD FORMING ORGANS AMENABLE TO SURGERY

Cells or Organs Involved	Diagnoses	Operations	Procedures
Red cells Bone marrow	Aplastic anemia	Marrow transplantation[a] Allogenic grafting	Multiple marrow aspirations from iliac bones Intravenous infusion of marrow from histocompatible donor

Cells or Organs Involved	Diagnoses	Operations	Procedures
White cells Bone marrow	Acute lymphoblastic leukemia	Marrow transplantation[a] Allogenic grafting	Same as above
	Acute myelogenous leukemia	Isogenic grafting	Intravenous infusion of marrow from identical twin
	Chronic myelogenous leukemia	Autologous grafting	Aspiration and storage of patient's own marrow Intravenous infusion of autologous marrow when blast crisis develops
Red cells	Hereditary spherocytosis	Splenectomy	Removal of spleen
Platelets	Thrombocytopenia due to increased platelet destruction	Splenectomy	Removal of spleen
Blood cells Spleen	Congestive splenomegaly with cytopenia	Splenectomy	Removal of spleen
Spleen	Traumatic rupture of spleen	Splenectomy	Removal of spleen
Lymph nodes Spleen	Hodgkin's disease Lymphoma	Exploratory laparotomy and splenectomy[b, c]	Surgical opening of abdomen with removal of spleen for the purpose of staging before initiating treatments[b, c]
Lymph nodes	Embryonal cell carcinoma of testis Metastases to lymph nodes	Radical retroperitoneal lymph node dissection (postorchiectomy)	Peritoneal cavity opened peritoneum reflected off the aorta and vena cava Multiple pelvic and periaortic lymph nodes removed

[a] E. D. Thomas. Bone marrow transplantation, Part I. *New England Journal of Medicine*, 292: 832-843, April 17, 1975 (Continuing investigations).

[b] R. R. Schilling. Hereditary spherocytosis: A study of splenectomized patients. *Seminars in Hematology*, 13: 169-176, July, 1976.

[c] H. L. Dameshek, *et al.* Hematologic indications for splenectomy. *Surgical Clinics of North America*, 55: 253-276, April, 1975.

REFERENCES AND BIBLIOGRAPHY

1. Adelson, E. Bleeding disorders secondary to platelet anomalies. In Conn, Howard F. (ed.). *Current Therapy 1976*. Philadelphia: W. B. Saunders Co., 1976, pp. 283-288.
2. American Association of Blood Banks. Plasmapheresis — Blood grouping systems — Transfusions — Adverse reactions — Autologous transfusions. *Technical Methods of Procedures of the American Association of Blood Banks*, 6th ed. Chicago: American Association of Blood Banks, 1974, pp. 20-199 and 310-321.
3. Avoy, Donald R. *Blood: The River of Life*. The American National Red Cross, 1976, pp. 1-76.
4. Banks, P. M. *et al.* American Burkitt's lymphoma. *American Journal of Medicine*, 58: 322-329, March, 1975.
5. Becker, G. A. Therapeutic use of blood components. In Conn, Howard F. (ed.). *Current Therapy 1976*. Philadelphia: W. B. Saunders Co., 1976, pp. 329-333.
6. Bellingham, A. J. Hereditary spherocytosis. *Clinics in Haematology*, 4: 139-144, February, 1975.

7. Bersagel, D. E. Plasma cell myeloma. In Conn, Howard F. (ed.). *Current Therapy 1976*. Philadelphia: W. B. Saunders Co., 1976, pp. 320-322.

8. Berlin, N. I. Diagnosis and classification of the polycythemias. *Seminars in Hematology*, 12: 339-352, October, 1975.

9. *Bio-Science Handbook*, 11th ed. Van Nuys, California: Bio-Science Laboratories, 1976, pp. 117-127.

10. Blatt, P. M. *et al.* Hemophilia and the hemophiloid disorders. In Conn, Howard F. (ed.). *Current Therapy 1976*. Philadelphia: W. B. Saunders Co., 1976, pp. 278-282.

11. Boggs, D. R. Neutropenia. In Conn, Howard F. (ed.). *Current Therapy 1976*. Philadelphia: W. B. Saunders Co., 1976, pp. 270-272.

12. Bowdler, A. J. The spleen and haemolytic disorders. *Clinics of Haematology*, 4: 231-246, February, 1975.

13. Brodsky, I. Coagulation disorders. *Emergency Medicine*, 7: 57-59, April, 1975.

14. Cartwright, G. E. *et al.* Sideroblasts, siderocytes and sideroblastic anemia. *New England Journal of Medicine*, 292: 185-193, January 23, 1975.

15. Cash, J. D. (ed.). Blood transfusions and blood products. *Clinics in Haematology*, 5: 3-222, February, 1976.

16. Cohen, H. J. *et al.* Resolution of primary amyloidosis during chemotherapy. *Annals of Internal Medicine*, 82: 466-473, April, 1975.

17. Coleman, R. W. *et al.* Disseminated intravascular coagulation. *Heart and Lung*, 3: 789-796, September-October, 1974.

18. Conrad, M. E. Anemia due to iron deficiency. In Conn, Howard F. (ed.)., *Current Therapy 1976*. Philadelphia: W. B. Saunders Co., 1976, pp. 254-255.

19. Davidsohn, Israel and Henry, John B. (eds.). Tables of normal values. *Clinical Diagnosis by Laboratory Methods*, 15th ed. Philadelphia: W. B. Saunders Co., 1974, pp. 1376-1392.

20. Davison, A. M. Albumin concentrates. *Clinics in Haematology*, 5: 135-147, February, 1976.

21. Donaldson, S. S. *et al.* Pediatric Hodgkin's disease. *Cancer*, 37: 2436-2447, May, 1976.

22. Dooren, J. J. *et al.* Bone marrow transplantation in children. *Seminars in Hematology*, 11: 369-382, July, 1974.

23. Douglas, A. S. Management of thrombotic diseases. *Seminars in Hematology*, 8: 95, April, 1971.

24. Dunnick, N. R. Repeat lymphography in non-Hodgkin's lymphoma. *Radiology*, 115: 349-354, May, 1975.

25. Fefer, A. *et al.* Paroxysmal nocturnal hemoglobinuria and marrow failure treated by infusion of marrow from an identical twin. *Annals of Internal Medicine*, 84: 692-695, June, 1976.

26. Freda, V. J. Current concepts: Prevention of Rh hemolytic disease. *New England Journal of Medicine*, 292: 1014-1016, May 8, 1975.

27. Ginsburg, A. D. Platelet function in patients with high platelet counts. *Annals of Internal Medicine*, 82: 506-511, April, 1975.

28. Glader, B. E. *et al.* Haemolysis due to pyruvate kinase deficiency and other glycolytic enzymopathies. *Clinics in Haematology*, 4: 123-138, February, 1975.

29. Gladstein, E. *et al.* Staging of Hodgkin's disease and other lymphomas. *Clinics in Haematology*, 3: 77-90, February, 1974.

30. Goldstein, L. M. Aplastic anemia in pregnancy: Recovery after normal spontaneous delivery. *Annals of Internal Medicine*, 82: 537-539, April, 1975.

31. Harkness, D. R. Sickle cell disease. In Conn, Howard F. (ed.). *Current Therapy, 1976*. Philadelphia: W. B. Saunders Co., 1976, pp. 266-270.

32. Heller, Paul (ed.). Blood and blood-forming organs. *Medicine 1976*. Chicago: Year Book Medical Publishers, Inc., 1976, pp. 215-314.

33. Hepler, Opal. *Manual of Clinical Laboratory Methods*, 4th ed. Springfield, Illinois: Charles E. Thomas Publisher, 1955, pp. 40-45.

34. Hyman, C. B. Thalassemia (Cooley's anemia). In Conn, Howard F. (ed.). *Current Therapy 1976*. Philadelphia: W. B. Saunders Co., 1976, pp. 263-265.

35. Jawetz, Ernest, Melnick, Joseph L. and Adelberg, Edward, A. Chlamydiae. *Review of Medical Microbiology*, 12th ed. Los Altos, California: Lange Medical Publications, 1976, pp. 237-244.

36. ————. Lymphocytic choriomeningitis, *Ibid.*, p. 398.

37. Johnson, R. E. Total body irradiation (TBI) as primary irradiation for advanced lymphosarcoma. *Cancer*, 35: 242-246, January, 1975.

38. Kalisher, L. Xeroradiography of axillary lymph node disease. *Radiology*, 115: 67-72, April, 1975.

39. Kandall, S. *et al.* Hemolytic disease of the newborn. In Conn, Howard F. (ed.). *Current Therapy 1976*. Philadelphia: W. B. Saunders Co., 1976, pp. 273-277.

40. Katzen, B. T. Positive lymphoangiography in Gaucher's disease. *Radiology*, 115: 85-86, April, 1975.

41. Koga, T. *et al.* Ultrasonographic determination of the splenic size and its clinical usefulness in various liver diseases. *Radiology*, 115: 157-161, April, 1975.

42. Kyle, R. A. *et al.* Multiple myeloma, acute leukemia and Hodgkin's disease — Occurrence in three of four family members. *Cancer*, 37: 1496-1499, March, 1975.

43. Leavell, Byrd Stuart and Thorup, Oscar Andreas. *Fundamentals of Clinical Hematology*, 4th ed. Philadelphia: W. B. Saunders Co., 1976, pp. 719-740.

44. Linman, J. W. *et al.* The preleukemic syndrome. *Seminars in Hematology*, 11: 93-100, January, 1974.

45. Maldonado, J. E. *et al.* Fanconi syndrome in adults. *American Journal of Medicine*, 58: 354-364, March, 1975.

46. Mc Credie, K. B. *et al.* White blood cell transfusions. *Clinics in Haematology*, 5: 379-394, June, 1976.

47. Mill, W. B. Radiation therapy in multiple myeloma. *Radiology*, 115: 175-178, April, 1975.

48. Morrison, F. S. Hemorrhagic complications in surgery. In Artz, Curtis P. and Hardy, James D. *Management of Surgical Complications*, 3rd ed. Philadelphia: W. B. Saunders Co., 1975, pp. 55-67.

49. Noguchi, S. *et al.* T and B lymphocytes in non-Hodgkin's lymphoma. *Cancer*, 37: 2247-2254, May, 1976.

144

50. Pepper, D. S. Frozen red cells. *Clinics in Haematology*, 5: 53-67, February, 1976.

51. Pierre, R. V. Preleukemia states. *Seminars in Hematology*, 11: 73-92, January, 1974.

52. Piro, A. J. Hodgkin's disease: Radiation therapy. In Conn, Howard F. (ed.). *Current Therapy, 1976*. Philadelphia: W. B. Saunders Co., 1976, pp. 297-300.

53. Quie, P. G. Pathology of bacteriocidal power of neutrophils. *Seminars in Hematology*, 12: 143-160, April, 1975.

54. Rappaport, A. H. *et al.* Erythroleukemia following total body irradiation for advanced lymphocytic lymphoma. *Radiology*, 115: 179-180, April, 1975.

55. Robbins, Stanley L. Blood and bone marrow — Lymph nodes and spleen. *Pathologic Basis of Disease*. Philadelphia: W. B. Saunders Co., 1974, pp. 699-781.

56. Rosenberg, S. A. *et al.* The management of stages I, II and III of Hodgkin's disease with combined radiotherapy and chemotherapy. *Cancer*, 35: 55-63, January, 1975.

57. Rosner, F. Hodgkin's disease and acute leukemia. *American Journal of Medicine*, 58: 339-353, March, 1975.

58. Schilling, R. F. Hereditary spherocytosis: A study of splenectomized patients. *Seminars in Hematology*, 13: 169-176, July, 1976.

59. Shaw, J. F. HLA typing. *Pathology & Laboratory Medicine*, 100: 341-345, July, 1976.

60. Silver, R. T. The chronic leukemias. In Conn, Howard F. (ed.). *Current Therapy 1976*. Philadelphia: W. B. Saunders Co., 1976, pp. 311-316.

61. Simone, J. V. Acute lymphocytic leukemia in childhood. *Seminars in Hematology*, 11: 25-39, January, 1974.

62. Simone, J. V. *et al.* Combined modality therapy of acute lymphocytic leukemia. *Cancer*, 35: 25-35, January, 1975.

63. Sirchia, G. Paroxysmal nocturnal haemoglobinuria. *Clinics in Haematology*, 4: 199-229, February, 1975.

64. Smith, Richard. Factitious lymphedema of the hand. *Journal of Bone and Joint Surgery*, 57-A: 89-94, January, 1975.

65. *Stedman's Medical Dictionary*, 23rd ed. Baltimore: The Williams & Wilkins Co., 1976, p. 1158.

66. Stern, K. *et al.* Blood groups and their applications. In Davidsohn, Israel and Henry, John B. (eds.). *Clinical Diagnosis by Laboratory Methods*, 15th ed. Philadelphia: W. B. Saunders Co., 1974, pp. 348-413.

67. Stryckmans, P. A. Current concepts in chronic myelogenous leukemia. *Seminars in Hematology*, 11: 101-139, April, 1974.

68. Stuart, J. J. Inherited defects of platelet function. *Seminars in Hematology*, 7: 233-253, July, 1975.

69. Thomas, E. D. *et al.* Bone marrow transplantation. Part I. *New England Journal of Medicine*, 292: 832-843, April 17, 1975.

70. _____. Bone marrow transplantation. Part II. *New England Journal of Medicine*, 292: 895-902, April 24, 1975.

71. Trey, C. Treatment by transfusion. *Emergency Medicine*, 7: 96-99, April, 1975.

72. Tucker, Eugene F., M.D. Personal communications.

73. Wallace, Sidney. *et al.* Lymphangiography in tumors of the female genital system. *Radiologic Clinics of North America*, 12: 79-92, April, 1974.

74. Wallerstein, R. O. Anemias — Hemolytic anemias. In Krupp, Marcus A. and Chatton, Milton. *Current Medical Diagnosis and Treatment*, 15th ed. Los Altos, California: Lange Medical Publications, 1976, pp. 273-294.

75. _____. Hemorrhagic disorders — Blood transfusions. *Ibid.*, pp. 307-318.

76. _____. Leukemias — Multiple myeloma — Macroglobulinemia — Myelofibrosis. *Ibid.*, pp. 294-307.

77. _____. Hodgkin's disease — Malignant lymphoma — Mycosis fungoides — Histiocytosis. *Ibid.*, pp. 301-303.

78. Walter, J. F. Lymphangiographic findings in histoplasmosis. *Radiology*, 114: 65-66, January, 1975.

79. Wasserman, L. R. The treatment of polycythemia vera. *Seminars in Hematology*, 13: 57-78, January, 1976.

80. Weir, Don C. M.D. Personal communications.

81. Wintrobe, M. M. and Boggs, D. R. Enlargements of lymph nodes and spleen. In Wintrobe, Maxwell M. (ed.). *Harrison's Principles of Internal Medicine*, 7th ed. New York: McGraw-Hill Book Co., 1974, pp. 309-313.

82. Wintrobe, M. M. and Lee, G. R. Hematologic alterations. In Wintrobe, Maxwell M. (ed.). *Harrison's Principles of Internal Medicine*, 7th ed. New York: McGraw-Hill Book Co., 1974, pp. 288-300.

83. Wintrobe, Maxwell M. *et al.* The normal hematopoietic system. *Clinical Hematology*, 7th ed. Philadelphia: Lea and Febiger, 1974, pp. 41-528.

84. _____. Macrocytic anemias — Anemias characterized by impaired iron metabolism. *Ibid.*, pp. 566-692.

85. _____. Hemolytic anemias — Other red cell disorders. *Ibid.*, pp. 717-1042.

86. _____. Pancytopenias and myelophthistic complications. *Ibid.*, pp. 1741-1790.

87. _____. Disorders of platelets and hemostasis — Coagulation disorders. *Ibid.*, pp. 1043-1252.

88. _____. Leukocytes, spleen and the reticuloendothelial system. *Ibid.*, pp. 221-370.

89. Young, R. C. *et al.* Hodgkin's disease: Chemotherapy. In Conn, Howard F. (ed.). *Current Therapy 1976*. Philadelphia: W. B. Saunders Co., 1976, pp. 290-297.

Chapter VII
Respiratory Disorders

NOSE

A. Origin of Terms:

1. choane (G) — a funnel
2. concha (L) — a shell
3. meatus (L) — a passage

4. osme (G) — sense of smell
5. rhin- (G) — nose
6. septum (L) — partition

B. Anatomic Terms:[10, 28, 53]

1. choana (pl. choanae), posterior aperture — opening of the nasal cavity into the nasopharynx.
2. concha (pl. conchae), turbinate — one of the scroll-like bony projections on the lateral wall of the nasal cavity.
3. naris (pl. nares) — nostril.
4. nasal meatus (pl. meatuses) — space beneath each concha of the nose.
5. nasal septum — partition between the two halves of the nasal cavity.
6. nasopharynx — an open chamber located behind the nasal fossa and below the base of the skull.

C. Diagnostic Terms:

1. atresia of choanae — pathologic closure of posterior nares or congenital absence of the same.[28]
2. coryza — cold in head.
3. deflection of septum — deviation of septum (deviation: departure from normal.)[28]
4. nasal polyp — benign lesion which may cause considerable obstruction of the nasal airway.[16]
5. nasal skin cancer — dermal lesion of the basal cell, squamous cell, epidermoid or melanoma variety, differing in degree of malignancy and metastatic potential.[28]
6. nasopharyngeal cancer — usually an epidermoid carcinoma or lymphosarcoma of the nasopharynx which may spread by direct extension to the meninges, compress cranial nerves and cause cranial nerve paralyses, ptosis of the eyelid and eventually loss of sight. Invasion of lymph nodes occurs frequently. The incidence of nasopharyngeal cancer is high among the Chinese and Maylays and low in Caucasians.[16, 28, 50]
7. nasopharyngitis — inflamed condition of the nasopharynx.
8. rhinitis — inflammation of the nasal mucosa.
   a. allergic rhinitis — hay fever
   b. atrophic — chronic infection with crust formation and nasal obstruction.
   c. hypertrophic — swollen nasal mucosa leading to nasal obstruction.[28, 47]
9. rhinolith — nasal concretion.

D. Operative Terms:

1. rhinoplasty — plastic reconstruction of the nose.
2. septal dermoplasty — excision of septal mucosa in telangiectatic area and its replacement with skin graft or oral mucous membrane to control bleeding.[28]
3. septectomy, submucous resection — excision of the nasal septum or part of it.
4. transantral ligation of maxillary artery — the application of vascular clips on the maxillary artery in uncontrolled recurrent epistaxis.[28]
5. turbinectomy — excision of a turbinate bone.
6. turbinotomy — surgical incision of a turbinate bone.

146

E. **Symptomatic Terms:**

    1. anosmia — absence of sense of smell.

    2. epistaxis — nosebleed.[28]

    3. rhinorrhea — thin, watery discharge from nose.

PARANASAL SINUSES

A. **Origin of Terms:**

    1. antrum (L) — cavity

    2. ethmo (G) — sieve

    3. front (L) — brow

    4. maxilla (L) — jawbone

    5. sinus (L) — hollow

    6. sphen (G) — wedge

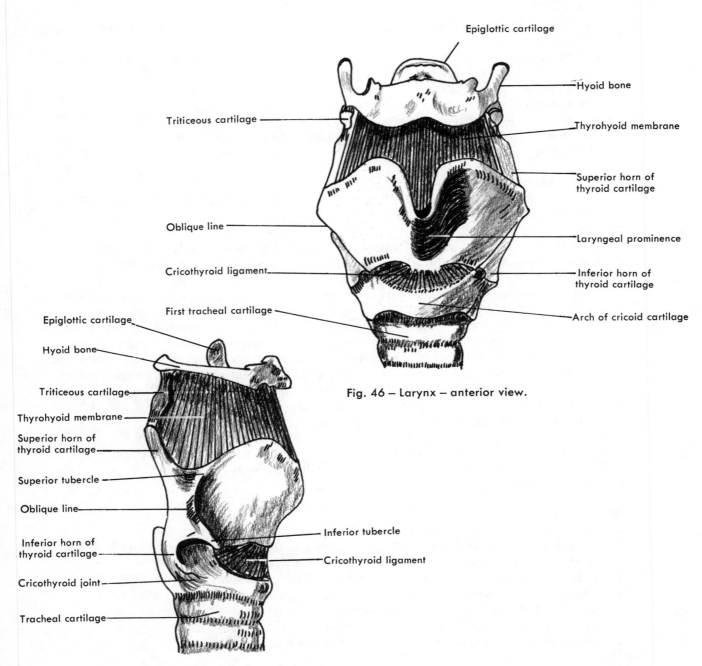

Fig. 46 – Larynx – anterior view.

Fig. 47 – Larnyx – right lateral view.

B. Anatomic Terms:

1. ethmoidal sinus — a collection of small cavities or air cells in the ethmoidal labyrinth between the eye socket (orbit) and nasal cavity.
2. frontal sinus — air space in the frontal bone above each orbit.
3. maxillary sinus, antrum of Highmore — large air sinus of the maxillary bone.
4. sphenoidal sinus — air space, variable in size, in the sphenoid bone. It is divided into right and left halves by a septum.

C. Diagnostic Terms:

1. actinomycosis of sinus — fungus infection in sinus.
2. pansinusitis — inflammation of all the sinuses.
3. sinusitis — inflammation of a sinus or sinuses.[16, 47]

D. Operative Terms:

1. antrotomy — opening of antral wall.
2. Caldwell-Luc operation — radical maxillary antrotomy.
3. ethmoidectomy — excision of ethmoid cells.
4. lavage of sinus — washing out a sinus for removal of purulent material.

LARYNX

A. Origin of Terms:

1. chondros (G) — cartilage, gristle
2. cricoid (G) — ringlike
3. glottis (G) — aperture of larynx
4. larynx (G) — voice box
5. phono- (G) — voice
6. vox (L) — voice

B. Anatomic Terms:[10, 53]

1. cricoid cartilage — ring-shaped cartilage of lowest part of larynx.
2. endolarynx — interior of larynx divided into a supraglottic portion, the glottis and a subglottic portion.
3. epiglottis — thin, leaf-shaped cartilage partially covered with mucous membrane. It closes the entrance of the larynx during swallowing.
4. glottis — two vocal folds with the rima glottidis between them.
5. larynx — tone-producing organ, the voice box, composed of muscle and cartilage. Its interior surface is lined with mucous membrane.
6. rima glottidis — narrowest portion of laryngeal cavity between the vocal folds.
7. vocal folds, vocal cords — mucosal folds each containing a vocal ligament and muscle fibers.

C. Diagnostic Terms:

1. endolaryngeal carcinomas — malignant epithelial tumors of various laryngeal structures such as the glottis, subglottis or supraglottis. Hoarseness is the presenting symptom in cancer of the vocal cord.[4, 5, 16, 25, 50, 56]
2. epiglottitis — inflammation of the epiglottis.
3. hypoplasia of epiglottis — defective development of epiglottis.
4. laryngitis — inflammation of larynx.[16]
5. laryngospasm, laryngismus, laryngeal stridor — adduction of laryngeal muscles and vocal cords resulting in obstruction of airway, marked by sudden onset of inspiratory dyspnea. It is common in children.
6. laryngotracheobronchitis — inflammation of the mucous membrane of larynx, trachea and bronchi.[47]
7. perichondritis — inflammation of the perichondrium, a membrane of fibrous connective tissue which surrounds the cartilage.
8. stenosis of larynx — a narrowing or stricture of the larynx.

D. Operative Terms:

1. dilatation of the larynx — instrumental stretching of the larynx.
2. hemilaryngectomy — removal of half of the larynx.[50]
3. laryngectomy — removal of the larynx for carcinoma.[50]
4. laryngofissure and cordectomy — incision between the cords to open the glottis, inspection of lesion with operating microscope and surgical removal of malignant membranous cord.[14, 56]
5. laryngoplasty — plastic repair of the larynx.
6. laryngoscopy — examination of interior larynx with a laryngoscope.
7. laryngostomy — establishing a permanent opening through the neck into the larynx.
8. laser excision of laryngeal cancer — method of applying a suitable surgical laser to excise malignant vocal cord lesions aided by an operating microscope attached to a laser micromanipulator.[59]

E. Symptomatic Terms:

1. aphonia — loss of voice due to local disease, hysteria or injury to recurrent laryngeal nerve.
2. dysphonia — difficulty in speaking, hoarseness.

TRACHEA

A. Origin of Terms:

1. furca (L) — fork
2. steno- (G) — narrow
3. trachea (G) — windpipe, rough

B. Anatomic Terms:[10, 53]

1. bifurcation — division into two branches.
2. carina — ridge between the trachea at the bifurcation.
3. trachea — windpipe composed of about 18 C-shaped cartilages, held together by elastic tissue and smooth muscle and extending from the larynx to the bronchi.

C. Diagnostic Terms:

1. calcification of tracheal rings — deposit of calcium in trachea.
2. stenosis of trachea — contraction or narrowing of lumen of trachea.
3. tracheoesophageal fistula — communication of esophagus with trachea, a congenital or acquired anomaly.
4. tracheopleural fistula — communication of trachea with the pleura which may be due to postoperative injury or to pressure necrosis of inflated cuff of a tracheostomy tube.

D. Operative Terms:

1. tracheoplasty — plastic operation on trachea.
2. tracheoscopy — inspection of interior of trachea.
3. tracheostomy — formation of a more or less permanent opening into the trachea, usually for insertion of a tube. Tracheostomy (or laryngostomy) is absolutely imperative prior to total laryngectomy, to establish an open airway. It may be necessary after thyroidectomy, brain or lung surgery, to overcome a tracheal obstruction.[16]
4. tracheotomy — incision into the trachea.

BRONCHI

A. Origin of Terms:

1. bronchus (L) — bronchus, windpipe
2. bronchiolus (L) — air passage
3. plasia (G) — to form
4. scope (G) — to examine

B. **Anatomic Terms:**[10, 53]

    1. bronchi, main — the two primary divisions of the trachea resembling it structurally.
        a. right main bronchus is shorter and more vertical than the left and is, therefore, more prone to lodge foreign bodies when aspirated. Its upper and lower parts provide the air passages for the three lobes of the right lung.
        b. left main bronchus gives rise to two lobar bronchi which supply the lobes of the left lung.
    2. bronchioles, bronchioli (sing. bronchiole, bronchiolus) — the smaller subdivisions of the bronchial tubes which do not have cartilage in their walls.

C. **Diagnostic Terms:**

    1. aplasia of bronchus — undeveloped bronchus.
    2. bronchial asthma — distressing affliction, characterized by severe attacks of dyspnea and wheezing triggered by bronchospasm. It may be due to extrinsic factors: pollens, dusts, foods or intrinsic factors: infection, chilling or emotional upset or both.[10, 27, 36, 47]
    3. bronchial carcinoid — slowly growing, highly vascular tumor, potentially malignant, usually found in main stem bronchus as an obstructive endobronchial lesion.[34]
    4. bronchiectasis — dilation of a bronchus or bronchi, secreting large amounts of offensive pus.[27, 36]
    5. bronchiectasic — pertaining to bronchiectasis.
    6. bronchiogenic carcinoma — lung cancer arising in the mainstem bronchus in 75% of patients with this malignant tumor. Metastasis occurs readily because the great vascularity, rich network of pulmonary lymph nodes and constant lung movements facilitate spread to neighboring and remote structures such as the brain, liver and other organs.[2, 22, 36]
    7. bronchitis — inflammation of the bronchial mucous membrane; endobronchial tuberculosis or tuberculous bronchitis due to tubercle bacillus.[6, 60]
    8. bronchopleural fistula — open communication between a bronchus and the pleural cavity. This may be a complication of pulmonary resection.
    9. chronic airway obstruction — disorder of respiratory tract resulting from generalized bronchial narrowing and destruction of functional lung tissue. It is usually characterized by severely impaired expiratory outflow which responds poorly to therapy. Asthma, chronic bronchitis and emphysema are primary respiratory disorders in which chronic airway obstruction is a dominant feature.[27]
    10. status asthmaticus — a prolonged state of severe asthma.[47, 52]

D. **Operative Terms:**

    1. bronchoplasty — plastic operation for closing fistula.
    2. bronchoscopy — examination of the bronchi through a bronchoscope.[36]
    3. bronchotomy — incision into a bronchus.

LUNGS

A. **Origin of Terms:**

    1. alveolus (L) — little tub
    2. apex (L) — tip
    3. phthisis (G) — a wasting
    4. pneumo- (G) — air
    5. pulmo-, pulmon (L) — lung
    6. segment (L) — a portion

B. **Anatomic Terms:**[10, 53]

    1. alveoli (sing. alveolus) — air cells of the lungs in which the exchange of gases takes place.
    2. apex of lung — most superior part of the lung above the clavicle.
    3. base of lung — inferior part of the lung above the diaphragm.

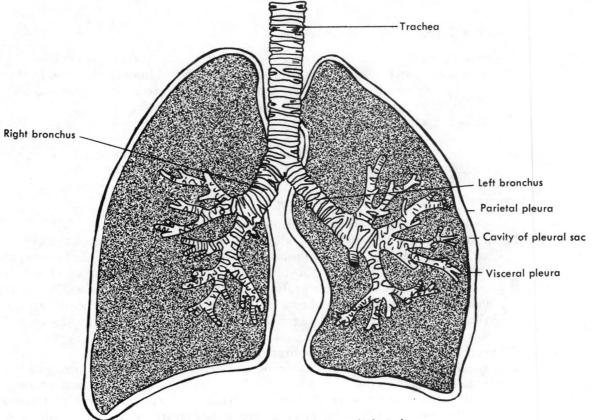

Fig. 48 — Trachea, bronchi, lungs and pleural sacs.

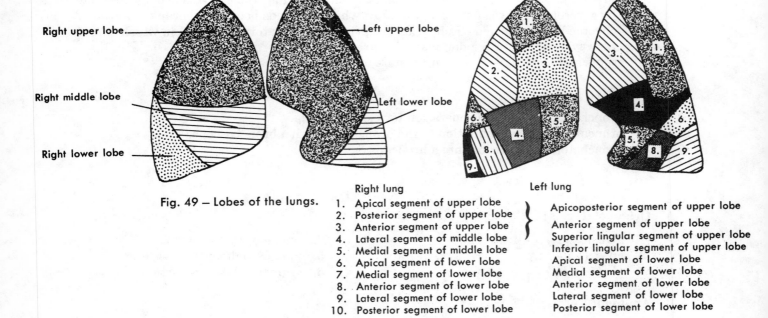

Fig. 49 — Lobes of the lungs.

Right lung

1. Apical segment of upper lobe
2. Posterior segment of upper lobe
3. Anterior segment of upper lobe
4. Lateral segment of middle lobe
5. Medial segment of middle lobe
6. Apical segment of lower lobe
7. Medial segment of lower lobe
8. Anterior segment of lower lobe
9. Lateral segment of lower lobe
10. Posterior segment of lower lobe

Left lung

Apicoposterior segment of upper lobe
Anterior segment of upper lobe
Superior lingular segment of upper lobe
Inferior lingular segment of upper lobe
Apical segment of lower lobe
Medial segment of lower lobe
Anterior segment of lower lobe
Lateral segment of lower lobe
Posterior segment of lower lobe

Fig. 50 — Bronchopulmonary segments of lungs.

4. bronchopulmonary segment — one of the subdivisions of a pulmonary lobe, supplied with a bronchial tube and blood and lymph vessels. The right lung has ten and the left lung nine segments.
5. bronchopulmonary tree — the lung compared to a hollow tree upside down in the thorax. The tree trunk is the trachea kept open and stiffened by C-shaped bars of cartilage. The main bronchi are two large branches which ramify into smaller and smaller ones until they become leaf stems or bronchioles. These, in turn, form tiny airways, the alveolar ducts, which lead to countless clusters of air cells surrounded by capillaries. There the exchange of gases takes place.
6. hilus — triangular depression on the medial surface of the lung which contains the hilar lymph nodes and the entrance or exit of blood and lymph vessels, nerves and bronchi. They form the root of the lung.
7. lobe — a major division of the lung composed of bronchopulmonary segments.
8. parenchyma — the functional tissue of any organ, for example: the respiratory bronchioles, alveolar ducts, sacs and alveoli which participate in respiration.

C. Diagnostic Terms:

1. abscess of lung — a localized area of suppuration in the lung with or without cavitation. It is accompanied by necrosis of tissue.[37, 47]
2. acute respiratory failure — a life-threatening condition characterized by excessively high carbon dioxide tension or abnormally low oxygen tension of the arterial blood. It may be caused by blockage of air passages by tenacious secretions from lung infection, by exposure to atmospheric smog or other irritant inhalants or by brain damage to the respiratory center.[27, 37, 55]
3. anthracosis — a disease of the lungs caused by the prolonged inhalation of fine particles of coal dust.[12, 37]
4. aplasia of lung — incomplete development of the lung.
5. asbestosis — occupational disease due to protracted inhalation of asbestos particles.[12, 37]
6. atelectasis — a functionless, airless lung or portion of a lung.[27]
7. blast injury — internal trauma of lungs, ears, and intestines due to high pressure waves following explosion. It may result in extreme bradycardia, severe cyanosis, dyspnea, hemorrhage and deafness.[12]
8. byssinosis — chronic occupational lung disease due to the inhalation of hemp, flax or cotton.[12, 37]
9. carcinoma of the lung, primary, secondary or metastatic — malignant new growth and the most important of the neoplastic diseases of the lung. Common tumors are:
   a. adenocarcinoma — a tumor containing glandular tissue which may form a mucinous secretion.
   b. oat cell carcinoma, small cell carcinoma — a very malignant tumor, notorious for its early, life-threatening metastases. It is thought to be a variant of bronchial carcinoid.[1]
   c. squamous cell carcinoma — the most common type of lung cancer found almost exclusively in men.
   Metastatic dissemination may occur to any organ, but involves most frequently the liver, brain, adrenals and bones.[1, 20, 21, 22, 45, 47]
10. chronic obstructive lung disease — prolonged airway obstruction causing disabling, progressive, respiratory disease, frequently with irreversible functional deterioration and fatal prognosis.[18, 55]
11. cystic disease of the lungs — condition characterized by the presence of air or fluid containing spaces within the lung:
    a. acquired cystic lesions — secondary to obstructive emphysema, partial bronchial obstruction and tuberculous infection.
    b. congenital cystic lung disease — usually associated with cystic disease of the kidneys, liver and sometimes the pancreas.[47]

12. histoplasmosis — fungus disease caused by *Histoplasma capsulatum;* sometimes associated with calcified pulmonary lesions.
13. pneumoconiosis — a disease of the lungs due to injury by dust from any source.[12]
14. pneumonia — inflammation of the lungs with exudation into lung tissue and consolidation. Predominent etiologic agents are pneumococci and mycoplasmas or pleuropneumonia-like organisms (PPLO) and less frequently staphylococci, streptococci, meningococci, viruses, tubercle bacilli and others. Hospital acquired (nosocomial) infections are usually caused by gram negative organisms.[3, 9, 47, 57]
    Various types are:
    a. bronchopneumonia — inflammation of bronchioli and air vesicles with scattered areas of consolidation.
    b. lobar pneumonia — acute inflammation of one or more lobes of the lung or lungs.
    c. primary atypical pneumonia — infection due to *Mycoplasma pneumoniae* varying from mild to fatal disease.[57]
15. pneumonitis — inflammation of the lung; a virus form of pneumonia.
16. pneumonocele, pneumocele — a pulmonary hernia.
17. pulmonary edema — excess of intra-alveolar and intrabronchial fluid in the lungs inducing cough and dyspnea; common in left heart failure.[37, 41]
18. pulmonary embolism — lodgment of a clot or foreign substance in a pulmonary arterial vessel cutting off the circulation.[12, 40, 41]
19. pulmonary or vesicular emphysema — overdistention of alveoli and smaller bronchial tubes with air.[27, 37, 47]
20. pulmonary hypertension — condition due to increased pressure in the pulmonary artery resulting from obstruction by pulmonary embolism or thrombosis, tuberculosis, emphysema or pulmonary fibrosis.
21. pulmonary infarction — necrosis of functional lung tissue (parenchyma) due to loss of blood supply usually caused by embolism.[12, 40]
22. pulmonary thrombosis — clot formation in any pulmonary blood vessel resulting in circulatory obstruction.[12]
23. pulmonary tuberculosis, phthisis — a specific inflammatory disease of the lungs caused by tubercle bacillus and characterized anatomically by a cellular infiltration which subsequently caseates, softens, and leads to ulceration of lung tissue; manifested clinically by wasting, exhaustion, fever and cough.[15, 40, 42, 47] The classification of the *1974 Diagnostic Standards of Tuberculosis* eliminates previously used terms.[61]
24. shock lung — pulmonary changes due to shock closely resembling severe congestion and edema, both interstitial and intra-alveolar in nature. A shock lung is associated with marked hypoxia, diffuse intravascular coagulation and formation of microthrombi.[48]
25. siderosis — chronic respiratory disorder caused by the inhalation of iron oxide, an industrial hazard of arc welding or steel grinding leading to pulmonary irritation, chronic bronchitis and emphysema.[12, 37]
26. silicosis — occupational disease due to inhalation of silica dust usually over a period of ten years or more.[12, 37]

D. Operative Terms:

1. biopsies:
    a. lung biopsy — small specimen of lung tissue used for pathologic, bacteriologic and spectrographic studies to aid diagnosis.[29, 34, 64]
    b. lymph node biopsy — removal of tissue from scalene or supraclavicular lymph nodes for gross or microscopic examination to aid in the detection of cancer, tuberculosis or other disease.[34]
    c. percutaneous needle biopsy — procedure used when tissue diagnosis is needed to plan radiation therapy and chemotherapy. The area to be biopsied is detected by television fluoroscopy. A biopsy needle is inserted through a small skin incision and cells aspirated are used for cytologic and bacteriologic diagnosis.[21, 64]

2. bronchofiberscopy — endoscopic examination of the tracheobronchial tree using a flexible bronchofiberscope to view the carina and right and left mainstem of bronchus. A 35 mm camera, attached to the bronchofiberscope provides photographic documentation.[51, 64]

3. excisional surgery (extirpative, definitive) — partial or complete removal of the diseased lung.
   a. lobectomy — removal of a pulmonary lobe.
   b. lung resection, pulmonary resection — partial excision of the lung, such as
      (1) segmental resection — removal of a bronchopulmonary segment.
      (2) subsegmental resection — removal of a portion of a **bronchopulmonary segment.**
   c. pneumonectomy — removal of an entire lung.
   d. wedge resection — removal of a triangular portion of the lung, usually a small peripheral lesion, such as a tuberculoma.[34]

4. extrapleural thoracoplasty — multiple rib resection without entering the pleural space.
   a. primary — to effect permanent collapse of the diseased lung and cavity closure.
   b. postlobectomy or postpneumonectomy — to obliterate dead space subject to infection or to reduce empyema space.

5. split rib technique — an approach to lung biopsy which allows wide exposure for exploration. A one centimeter portion of a rib is sectioned posteriorly, then split longitudinally to an anterior point where another rib division is done.[43]

6. surgery for lung embolism:
   a. pulmonary embolectomy — removal of lung embolus in chronic pulmonary obstructive disease.
   b. total cardiopulmonary bypass — operative procedure for massive pulmonary embolism.[19]

E. Symptomatic Terms:

1. anoxemia — deficient oxygen tension in arterial blood.
2. anoxia — oxygen want in tissues and organs.
3. apnea, apnoea — temporary absence of respiration — also seen in Cheyne-Stokes respiration.
4. bronchial or tubular breathing — harsh breathing with a prolonged high pitched expiration which may have a tubular quality.
5. Cheyne-Stokes respiration — irregular breathing beginning with shallow breaths which increase in depth and rapidity to a certain degree; then they gradually decrease and cease altogether. After 10-20 seconds of apnea, the same cycle is repeated.
6. cyanosis — bluish color of skin due to deficient oxygenation.[35]
7. dyspnea, dyspnoea — difficult breathing.[7, 23]
8. expectoration — act of coughing up and spitting out material from the lungs, trachea and mouth.
9. hemoptysis — expectoration of blood.
10. hiccough, hiccup, singultus — spasmodic lowering of the diaphragm followed by spasmodic, periodic closure of the glottis.[27]
11. hypercapnia, hypercarbia — an excess of carbon dioxide in the circulating blood, abnormally high carbon dioxide tension (Pco_2) causing overstimulation of respiratory center.[55]
12. hyperpnea — respirations increased in rate and depth.
13. hyperventilation, hyperaeration — excessive movement of air in and out of the lungs.[27]
14. hyperventilation syndrome — prolonged heavy breathing and long sighing respirations causing marked apprehension, palpitation, dizziness, muscular weakness, paresthesia and tetany. The attack may result from biochemical changes in neuromuscular and neurovascular function or from acute anxiety.
15. hypoxia — oxygen want due to decreased amount of oxygen in organs and tissues.
16. orthopnea, orthopnoea — breathing only possible when person sits or stands.[35]

17. paroxysmal nocturnal dyspnea (PND) — attacks of difficult breathing, usually occurring in heart disease at night.[7]
18. rales — bubbling sounds heard in bronchi at inspiration or expiration.
19. tachypnea — abnormally rapid breathing.

THORAX PLEURA AND MEDIASTINUM

A. Origin of Terms:

1. paries (L) — wall
2. phren (G) — diaphragm, mind
3. pleura (G) — pleura
4. pyon (G) — pus
5. thorax (G) — breast plate, chest
6. viscus, viscer (L) — flesh, vital organ

B. Anatomic Terms:[10, 53]

1. mediastinum — the interpleural space containing the pericardium, heart, major vessels, esophagus and thoracic duct.
2. pleura (pl. pleurae) — a thin sac of serous membrane which is invaginated by the lung and lines the mediastinum and thoracic wall. Each lung has its own pleural sac.
   a. parietal pleura — the costal, mediastinal and diaphragmatic parts of the pleura and the cupola which covers the apex of the lung.
   b. visceral pleura, pulmonary pleura — pleura which invests the lungs and lines the interlobal fissures.
3. pleural cavity — potential space between the parietal and visceral pleurae, lubricated by a thin film of serum.
4. thorax, chest — upper trunk composed of the thoracic vertebrae, sternum, ribs, costal cartilages and muscles. The thoracic cage protects the vital organs of circulation and respiration as well as other mediastinal structures.

C. Diagnostic Terms:

1. abnormal chest:
   a. barrel chest — barrel-like appearance of chest on inspiration in advanced emphysema.
   b. flail chest, flapping chest cage — instability of thoracic cage due to fracture of ribs or sternum or both.[13]
   c. pectus carinatum — keeled chest.
   d. rachitic chest — resembling pigeon breast as in rickets.[7]
2. empyema of pleura, pyothorax — pus in pleural cavity.[38]
3. hemothorax — blood in pleural cavity due to trauma or ruptured blood vessel.[38]
4. hydropneumothorax — watery effusion and air in pleural cavity.
5. mediastinitis — acute or chronic inflammation of the mediastinum.[38]
6. pleural effusion — excessive formation of serous fluid within the pleural cavity.[38, 44]
7. pleurisy, pleuritis — inflammation of the pleura.[38]
8. pyopneumothorax — pus and air in the pleural cavity.
9. spontaneous pneumothorax — entrance of air into the pleural cavity resulting in a collapse of a lung.[38, 58]
10. tension or valvular pneumothorax — entrance of air into pleural cavity on inspiration; air exit blocked by valve-like tissue on expiration; enlargement of pleural cavity and collapse of lung as positive pressure increases resulting in mediastinal shift and depression of diaphragm.[38]

D. Operative Terms:

1. artificial or therapeutic pneumothorax — the introduction of a measured amount of air into the pleural cavity through a needle in order to give the diseased lung temporary rest.
2. biopsies:

    a. mediastinal node biopsy — resection of small piece of tissue from regional lymph node for microscopy and culture.

    b. pleural biopsy — aspiration of cells from parietal pleura with biopsy needle for bacteriologic and histologic studies.

3. cervical mediastinotomy — small incision into the mediastinum in the neck region to obtain biopsy specimen for lymph node for diagnostic evaluation.

4. mediastinoscopy — examination of the mediastinal organs by a mediastinoscope under direct vision to aid in the diagnosis of disease and in assessing the resectability of bronchogenic carcinoma.[34]

5. pleurectomy:

    a. partial — removal of a portion of the pleura.

    b. complete — removal of the entire pleura. This is generally associated with pneumonectomy.[39]

6. pulmonary decortication — removal of fibrinous exudate or pleural peel from the visceral surface of the imprisoned lung to restore its functional adequacy.[34]

7. thoracostomy, open — excision of rib segment for drainage of empyema space.[34, 58]

E. Special Procedures:

1. augmented ventilation — increased capillary circulation and gas exchange in respiration.

    a. intermittent mandatory ventilation (IMV) — the patient breathes on his own, but at intervals mandatory respirations are supplied by a ventilator. This procedure permits a gradual weaning from mechanical ventilation to unaided breathing.[13, 33, 53]

    b. positive end-expiratory pressure (PEEP) — maneuver used to increase the functional residual capacity of the lungs. It affects the airway during expiration preventing intrathoracic pressures from returning to atmospheric pressure.[13, 32, 53]

2. thoracentesis, pleurocentesis — tapping of the pleural cavity to remove pleural effusion for diagnostic or therapeutic purposes.

F. Symptomatic Terms:

1. pleural adhesions — fibrous bands which bind the visceral pleura to the parietal pleura. They may be loose, elastic, avascular or firm, inelastic and vascular.

2. pleural effusion — abnormal accumulation of fluid within the pleural space.[34]

3. pleural exudate — pus or serum accumulating in the pleural cavity. Fibrinous exudate may lead to the formation of adhesions.

4. pleural peel — abnormal layer of fibrous tissue adherent to the visceral pleura and underlying diseased lung. The ever thickening peel may inhibit respiratory function.

5. pleuritic pain, pleurodynia — sharp, intense pain felt in intercostal muscles.

RADIOLOGY

A. General Terms Used in Radiography:

1. aerated — filled with air.
2. calcification — deposit of lime salts in the tissues.
3. consolidation — solidification of the lung as in pneumonia.
4. density — the compactness of structure of a substance.
5. discrete — well defined and clear-cut in appearance.
6. fibrosis — replacement of normal tissue with fibrous tissue.
7. infiltration — the permeation of a tissue with substances that are normally absent.
8. infraclavicular — below the clavicle or collar bone.
9. infrascapular — below the scapula or shoulder plate.
10. inspissated — thickened by absorption of fluid content.
11. peribronchial — pertaining to area around the bronchial tubes.
12. rarefaction — process of decreasing density.
13. rarefied area — area of lessened density.

14. subdiaphragmatic — below the diaphragm.
15. substernal — below the sternum or breast bone.

B. **Terms Related to Diagnostic Radiology:**

1. bronchial brushing, brush biopsy — safe and reliable method of establishing a definite diagnosis in patients with inoperable pulmonary lesion before radiotherapy is instituted.   Under fluoroscopic guidance and topical anesthesia a radiopaque catheter is passed into the bronchial segment where the lesion is located and its proper position is confirmed by spot films.   Minute flexible nylon brushes are then inserted through the catheter to an optimal position.   The lesion is brushed by vigorous, short strokes.   Brush scrapings are used for cytologic and bacteriologic examinations.   A biopsy forceps, passed through the catheter, provides tissue specimens for histologic study of the lesion which is helpful in the identification of benign tumors.   After slightly withdrawing the catheter, selective bronchography is performed.[29, 64]
2. bronchography — radiographic examination of the bronchial tree following the intra-tracheal injection of an opaque solution.[21]
3. laminograms of lung — body section radiograms which delineate sharply a thin layer of lung tissue; thus, the structures lying anteriorly and posteriorly are more or less blurred out.   Laminograms demonstrate the presence of a cavity and many other lung lesions.[21]
4. planigrams, tomograms of lung — same as laminograms.
5. prone chest film — frontal chest radiogram in the prone position for delineating pleural effusion in the posterior lung base.[54]
6. selective segmental bronchography — bronchographic examination of selected parts of the lungs; for example, the apices.   Under local anesthesia a Metras catheter is inserted for the injection of a radiopaque substance.   Aided by fluoroscopic guidance, the contrast medium is allowed to fill the bronchial branches of the pulmonary segments.   Abnormalities are recorded instantly by spot-films.[21]

C. **Terms Related to Special Diagnostic Radiology:**

1. ultrasound in pulmonary disease — lung echograms aiding in the diagnosis of pulmonary embolism or thromboembolism, pleural effusion, pleural thickening and calcification.[31]
2. videodensitometry, densitometry — technique which measures changes in radiographic density during fluoroscopy and provides quantitative measurements of physiologic responses detected by a single static radiogram.   Pulmonary densitometry aids in the diagnosis of lung cancer.[17]
3. xerotomography — xerographic technique applied to tomography, thought to be of considerable value in delineating disorders of the tracheobronchial tree.[24]

D. **Terms Related to Therapeutic Radiology:**

1. interstitial irradiation for unresectable lung cancer (stages I, II, III) — radiotherapy by interstitial implantation of encapsulated sources of radon 222 or iodine 125.   The tumor is considered unresectable in the presence of mediastinal involvement with invasion of the esophagus, trachea or major vessels.[26]
2. radiation therapy for glottic cancer — irradiation of stage I cancer of the glottis, highly curable permitting retention of the larynx; aggressive radiotherapy for advanced glottic cancer about 50 per cent successful.[8, 22]

CLINICAL LABORATORY

A. **Terms Related to Some Essential Bacteriologic Studies:**

1. examination of sputum and gastric washings — tests for demonstrating pathogenic organisms.   Three methods are used:
   a. animal inoculation — injection of prepared material from specimen into a laboratory animal; for example, either a guinea pig or a white mouse.   Smears are made from sacrificed animal after a definite time has elapsed.

    b. culture — material inoculated into an appropriate medium for the purpose of growth and possible identification of the organism.

    c. smear — material spread on a slide for microscopic study of organisms.

2. sensitivity studies — tests for determining the susceptibility of the patient's bacteria to various antimicrobial agents in an effort to evaluate the effectiveness of the therapeutic regime. Results indicate:

    a. drug sensitivity or

    b. drug resistance.

3. skin tests — test for detecting previous exposure and sensitization to tubercle bacilli.

    a. Heaf — intradermal tuberculin test by multiple puncture technique.

    b. Mantoux — intradermal tuberculin test employing purified protein derivative (PPD).[62, 63]

    c. Mono-Vacc — multiple puncture test used in screening programs for tuberculosis.[30]

    d. Tine — intradermal tuberculin test by puncture with four tines dip-dried with old tuberculin.[30, 63]

4. vaccine for tuberculosis, BCG — attenuated vaccine composed of avirulent tubercle bacilli. BCG vaccination produces immunity against tuberculosis, variable in effect and duration.[37]

B. Terms Related to the Evaluation of Lung Function:

1. bronchospirometry — graphic recording of the relative participation of the two lungs in ventilation and oxygen uptake.[34, 49]

2. pulmonary function studies — specific tests for determining the ability of the lungs to perform respiration as compared to the normal for a given age, height and weight. They are primarily concerned with the evaluation of lung volumes, ventilation, the distribution of ventilation and diffusion or oxygen consumption.[34, 35, 49]

ABBREVIATIONS

A. General:

ACD — anterior chest diameter
AFB — acid fast bacillus
A&P — auscultation and percussion
AP — anterior-posterior (projection of x-rays)
ARD — acute respiratory disease
ARF — acute respiratory failure
BCG — bacillus Calmette Guerin (vaccine for tuberculosis)
BS — breath sounds
CMV — controlled mechanical ventilation
COPD — chronic obstructive pulmonary disease
CRF — chronic respiratory failure
FRC — functional residual capacity
IMV — intermittent mandatory ventilation
IPPB — intermittent positive pressure breathing

IS, ICS — intercostal space
LSB — left sternal border
MCL — midcostal line
MSL — midsternal line
OT — old tuberculin
PA — posterior-anterior
PEEP — positive end-expiratory pressure
PND — paroxysmal nocturnal dyspnea
PPD — purified protein derivative
PPLO — pleuropneumonia-like organisms
RD — respiratory disease
RM — respiratory movement
TB — tuberculosis
TF — tactile fremitus
TNM — tumor, nodes and metastases (criteria for staging tumors)
URI — upper respiratory infection
VF — vocal fremitus

B. Organizations:

    ALA — American Lung Association

    ATS — American Thoracic
           Society

    HEW — US Health, Education and
           Welfare Department

ORAL READING PRACTICE

Bronchial Asthma

Bronchial asthma is a condition characterized by **paroxysmal** attacks of dyspnea in which the breathing is wheezy, the expiration is prolonged and the normal **vesicular** murmur is obscured by loud, musical rales.

In some instances nasal **polypi, hypertrophy** of the **conchae; or ethmoiditis** provoke the disease.   An essential factor in many cases is a peculiar susceptibility or **hypersensitivity** to some special protein which is inhaled or ingested.   In some cases of asthma **focal** infection is the essential **etiologic** factor.   Physical overexertion, emotional excitement, seasonal changes and **intercurrent** infections favor the occurrence of attacks.

The paroxysms are excessive at night.   The patient is seized with intense **dyspnea** and a feeling of impending **suffocation** which compel him to sit upright.   The face is anxious, sometimes livid and the skin is covered with cool perspiration.   The respirations are labored and noisy. Cough is usually present and is associated with the **expectoration** of viscid **mucus.**

During the attack the chest is fixed in full inspiratory expansion.   **Percussion** gives **hyperresonance** in chronic **emphysematous** cases.   On **auscultation** there are numerous **rales** especially during inspiration.[11, 27, 36, 47, 62]

Table 16

SOME RESPIRATORY CONDITIONS AMENABLE TO SURGERY

Organs Involved	Diagnoses	Operations	Operative Procedures
Nasal septum	Deflection of nasal septum, congenital or post-traumatic	Septectomy or submucous resection	Removal of nasal septum, partial or complete
Nasal mucosa	Mucous polyp	Excision of lesion	Removal of polyp
Maxillary sinus (antrum of Highmore)	Maxillary sinusitis due to streptococcus	Maxillary sinusotomy, antrum window operation	Opening of the antrum
Larynx	Papilloma or cyst of larynx	Laryngoscopy with excision of lesion	Endoscopic examination with removal of neoplasm
Larynx Epiglottis Vocal cords	Squamous carcinoma of larynx	Total laryngectomy	Removal of entire larynx
Trachea	Carcinoma of larynx	Tracheostomy (preliminary step to laryngectomy)	Fistulization of trachea
Bronchi	Endobronchial tuberculosis	Bronchoscopy with aspiration of bronchial secretions	Endoscopic examination of bronchi

Organs Involved	Diagnoses	Operations	Operative Procedures
Bronchopulmonary segment	Cystic disease of lung, tension air cyst	Segmental resection, lateral segment, middle lobe	Removal of segment including tension air cyst of lung
Bronchopulmonary segment	Moderately advanced tuberculosis with cavitation	Segmental resection, upper lobe	Removal of two segments of upper lobe
Bronchus, Bronchioli Lung	Bronchiectasis, post-infectional	Lobectomy, middle lobe	Removal of middle lobe of lung
Lobe	Tuberculoma	Wedge resection, upper lobe	Excision of triangular shaped tuberculoma
Lung Visceral pleura	Far advanced fibrocaseous tuberculosis Fibrinous pleurisy, lower lobe	Lobectomy, upper lobe Decortication, lower lobe	Removal of upper lobe Excision of thickened fibrotic lesion of visceral pleura
Lung Visceral pleura	Carcinoma of lung or unilateral far advanced tuberculosis	Pneumonectomy, Pleurectomy	Removal of lung including visceral pleura
Lung Thorax	Excessive pleural effusion, empyema	Postpneumonectomy thoracoplasty	Multiple rib resection in two stages

REFERENCES AND BIBLIOGRAPHY

1. Abeloff, M. D. et al. Small cell carcinoma of the lung. *Cancer,* 38: 1394-1401, September, 1976.
2. Baker, R. R. et al. The clinical assessment of selected patients with bronchogenic carcinoma. *Annals of Thoracic Surgery,* 20: 520-528, November, 1975.
3. Barnes, R. V. et al. *Neisseria meningitidis.* A cause of nosocomial pneumonia. *Respiratory Disease,* 111: 229-231, February, 1975.
4. Benisch, B. M. Primary oat cell carcinoma of the larynx: An ultrastructural study. *Cancer,* 36: 145-148, July, 1975.
5. Bocca, E. Supraglottic cancer. *Laryngoscope,* 85: 1318-1326, August, 1975.
6. Burrows, B. Characteristics of chronic bronchitis in a warm, dry region. *Respiratory Disease,* 112: 365-370, September, 1975.
7. Butler, E. K. Dyspnea in the patient with cardiopulmonary disease. *Heart and Lung,* 4: 599-606, July-August, 1975.
8. Constable, W. C. et al. Radiotherapeutic management of cancer of the glottis. *Laryngoscope,* 85: 1491-1503, September, 1975.
9. Crane, L. R. et al. Gram-negative pneumonia in hospitalized patients. *Postgraduate Medicine,* 58: 85-92, September, 1975.
10. Crofton, John and Douglas, Andrew. The structure and function of the respiratory tract. *Respiratory Diseases,* 2d ed. London: Blackwell Scientific Publications, 1975, pp. 1-65.
11. _____. Bronchial asthma. *Ibid.,* pp. 429-460.
12. _____. Pulmonary thromboembolism — Occupational lung disease. *Ibid.,* pp. 488-561.
13. Cullen, P. et al. Treatment of flail chest — Use of intermittent mandatory ventilation and positive end-expiratory pressure. *Archives of Surgery,* 110: 1099-1103, September, 1975.
14. Daly, J. F. et al. Laryngofissure and cordectomy. *Laryngoscope,* 85: 1290-1296, August, 1975.
15. Dandoy, S. et al. Tuberculosis care in general hospitals. *Respiratory Disease,* 112: 757-764, December, 1975.
16. Deatsch, W. W. Ear, nose and throat. In Krupp, Marcus A. and Chatton, Milton. *Current Medical Diagnosis and Treatment,* 15th ed. Los Altos, California: Lange Medical Publications, 1976, pp. 95-105.
17. Densitometry gives a new look at lungs. *Journal of American Medical Association,* 231: 693-696, February 17, 1975.
18. Diener, C. F. et al. Further observations on the course and prognosis of chronic obstructive lung disease. *Respiratory Disease,* 111: 719-724, June, 1975.
19. Ebert, P. A. The role of surgery in the treatment of pulmonary thromboembolism. *Surgical Clinics of North America,* 54: 1107-1113, October, 1974.
20. Feinstein, A. R. Neoplasms of the lung. In Beeson, Paul B. and McDermott, Walsh (eds.). *Textbook of Medicine,* 14th ed. Philadelphia: W. B. Saunders Co., 1975, pp. 867-872.
21. Fennessey, J. J. The radiology of lung cancer. *Medical Clinics of North America,* 59: 95-120, January, 1975.
22. Gelot, R. Primary oat-cell carcinoma of head and neck. *Annals of Otology Rhinology & Laryngology,* 84: 238-244, March-April, 1975.
23. Gracey, D. R. Acute exacerbation of dyspnea in

160

a COPO patient. *Heart & Lung,* 4: 124-127, January-February, 1975.

24. Harle, T. S. *et al.* Xerotomography of the tracheobronchial tree. *American Journal of Roentgenology Radium Therapy and Nuclear Medicine,* 124: 353-357, July, 1975.

25. Hendrickson, F. R. Primary squamous cell carcinoma of the larynx. *Laryngoscope,* 85: 1650-1660, October, 1975.

26. Hilaris, B. S. *et al.* Interstitial irradiation for unresectable carcinoma of the lung. *Annals of Thoracic Surgery,* 20: 491-500, November, 1975.

27. Howell, J. B. L. The diaphragm — Airway obstruction. In Beeson, Paul B. and McDermott, Walsh (eds.). *Textbook of Medicine,* 14th ed. Philadelphia: W. B. Saunders Co., 1975, pp. 816-836.

28. Jaffe, B. F. Diseases and surgery of the nose. *Clinical Symposia,* 26: (1) 2-32, 1974.

29. Janover, M. L. *et al.* Lung biopsy — Bronchial brushing and percutaneous puncture. *Radiologic Clinics of North America,* 9: 73-83, April, 1971.

30. Jenkins, D. W. The tuberculin Tine and Mono-Vacc tests in the patient with active tuberculosis. *Respiratory Disease,* 112: 140-141, July, 1975.

31. Joyner, Claude R. *et al.* The echogram in the study of diseases of the chest. *Ultrasound in the Diagnosis of Cardiovascular-Pulmonary Disease.* Chicago: Year Book Medical Publishers, 1974, pp. 155-168.

32. Kirby, R. R. *et al.* High level positive end expiratory pressure (PEEP) in acute respiratory insufficiency. *Chest,* 67: 156-163, February, 1975.

33. Klein, E. F. Weaning from mechanical breathing with intermittent mandatory ventilation. *Archives of Surgery,* 110: 345-347, March, 1975.

34. Maier, H. C. *et al.* Chest wall, pleura, lung and mediastinum. In Schwartz, Seymour I. (ed.). *Principles of Surgery,* 2d ed. New York: McGraw-Hill Book Co., 1974, pp. 596-675.

35. Manson, R. M. *et al.* Pulmonary function tests — Nonspecific manifestation. In Krupp, Marcus A. and Chatton, Milton. *Current Medical Diagnosis and Treatment,* 15th ed. Los Altos, California: Lange Medical Publications, 1976, pp. 106-107.

36. _____. Disorders of the bronchi. *Ibid.,* pp. 107-111.

37. _____. Disorders of the lungs. *Ibid.,* pp. 111-145.

38. _____. Diseases of the pleura — Diseases of the mediastinum. *Ibid.,* pp. 145-151.

39. Martin, I. N. *et al.* Indications for pleurectomy in malignant effusion. *Cancer,* 35: 734-738, March, 1975.

40. McClement, J. H. Tuberculosis: Chemoprophylaxis and treatment. *Postgraduate Medicine,* 58: 97-101, September, 1975.

41. Meth, R. F. Pulmonary edema and wheezing after pulmonary embolism. *Respiratory Disease,* 111: 693-698, May, 1975.

42. Nakielna, E. M. *et al.* Lifelong followup of inactive tuberculosis. *Respiratory Disease,* 112: 765-772, December, 1975.

43. Narodick, B. G. The split rib technique. *Archives of Surgery,* 110: 442-443, April, 1975.

44. Neef, T. A. *et al.* Tension pleural effusion. *Respiratory Disease,* 111: 543-548, April, 1975.

45. Overholt, R. H. *et al.* Primary cancer of the lung: A 42 year experience. *Annals of Thoracic Surgery,* 20: 511-519, November, 1975.

46. Reed, J. C. *et al.* The air bronchogram in interstitial disease. *Radiology,* 116: 1-10, July, 1975.

47. Robbins, Stanley L. The respiratory system. *Pathologic Basis of Disease.* Philadelphia: W. B. Saunders Co., 1974, pp. 782-851.

48. _____. Fluid and hemodynamic derangements. *Ibid.,* pp. 314-355.

49. Ruppel, Gregg. *Manual of Pulmonary Function Testing.* St. Louis: The C. V. Mosby Co., 1975, pp. 1-116.

50. Rush, B. F. Tumors of the head and neck. In Schwartz, Seymour I. (ed.). *Principles of Surgery,* 2d. ed. New York: McGraw-Hill Book Co., 1974, pp. 555-593.

51. Sackner, M. A. Bronchofiberscopy. *Respiratory Disease,* 111: 62-88, January, 1975.

52. Senior, R. M. *et al.* Status asthmaticus. *Journal of American Medical Association,* 231: 1277-1279, March 24, 1975.

53. Shapiro, Barry A., Harrison, Ronald A. and Trout, Carole A. *Clinical Application of Respiratory Care.* Chicago: Year Book Medical Publishers, Inc., 1975, pp. 1-413.

54. Simonds, B. S. *et al.* The prone chest film. *Radiology,* 116: 11-17, July, 1975.

55. Smith, J. P. Respiratory failure and its management. In Beeson, Paul B. and McDermott, Walsh (eds.). *Textbook of Medicine,* 14th ed. Philadelphia: W. B. Saunders Co., 1975, pp. 836-842.

56. Som, M. L. Cordal cancer with extension to vocal process. *Laryngoscope,* 85: 1298-1307, August, 1975.

57. Stadel, B. V. *et al. Mycoplasma pneumoniae* infection followed by *Haemophilus influenzae* pneumonia and bacteremia. *Respiratory Disease,* 112: 131-134, July, 1975.

58. Stowe, S. M. *et al.* Open thoracotomy for pneumothorax in cystic fibrosis. *Respiratory Disease,* 111: 611-618, May, 1975.

59. Strong, M. S. Laser excision of carcinoma of the larynx. *Laryngoscope,* 85: 1286-1289, August, 1975.

60. Tager, Ira *et al.* Role of infection in chronic bronchitis. *New England Journal of Medicine,* 292: 563-569, March 13, 1975.

61. Weg, J. G. *Diagnostic Standards of Tuberculosis* —Revised. *Journal of American Medical Association,* 235: 1329-1330, March 29, 1976.

62. Werner, William A., M.D. Personal communications.

63. Wijsmuller, G. *et al.* Skin testing: A comparison of the jet injector with the Mantoux method. *Respiratory Disease,* 112: 789-798, December, 1975.

64. Zavala, D. C. Pulmonary biopsy. *Advances in Internal Medicine,* Vol. XXI, 1976, pp. 21-46.

Chapter VIII

Digestive Disorders
MOUTH

A. Origin of Terms:

1. bucca (L) — cheek
2. cheilos (G) — lip
3. dent- (L) — tooth
4. gingiva (L) — gum
5. glossa (G) — tongue
6. labium (L) — lip
7. lingua (L) — tongue
8. odont- (G) — tooth
9. os, pl. ora (L) — mouth
10. staphyle (G) — bunch of grapes
11. stoma (G) — mouth
12. uvula (L) — little grape

B. Anatomic Terms:

1. alveolus — bony tooth socket.
2. hard palate, bony palate — anterior part of roof of mouth.
3. oral cavity — the mouth.
4. soft palate — posterior part of palate partially separating the oral from the nasal part of the pharynx.
5. uvula — small, cone-shaped downward projection from the free lower edge of the soft palate in midline.

C. Diagnostic Terms:

1. aphthous stomatitis — small ulceration of the mucous membrane of the mouth.[25]
2. ankyloglossia — tongue-tie.
3. candidiasis, moniliasis, thrush — curd-like creamy patches in the mouth due to overgrowth of *Candida albicans*. Pain, fever, and lymphadenopathy may be present. The fungal growth is prone to occur when antibiotic therapy or acute illness upsets the balance of the normal flora.[25]
4. cancer of the mouth — malignant lesions of the lips, gums and tongue.[26, 45, 89]
5. cavity of tooth — loss of tooth structure due to decay process, attrition, abrasion, erosion or developmental defect.
6. chilitis, cheilitis — inflammation of the lips.
7. chilosis — morbid condition of the lips due to vitamin deficiency.
8. cleft lip, harelip — congenital anomaly of upper lip consisting of a vertical fissure often associated with cleft palate.
9. cleft palate — a congenital fissure of the roof of the mouth due to nonunion of bones.
10. dental caries — localized progressive decay of tooth structure.[25]
11. epulis, giant cell epulis — a reparative lesion of gingiva which develops in response to trauma or hemorrhage.
12. gingivitis — inflammation of the gums.
13. glossitis — inflammation of the tongue.
14. periapical abscess — abscessed tooth, due to dental decay leading to infection of the pulp.[25]
15. periodontal disease — dental disorders characterized by inflammation of the gums, destruction of alveolar bone, degeneration of periodontal ligament and periodontal pocket formation.[25]
16. stomatitis — inflammation of the mucosa of the mouth and an oral manifestation of systemic disease, allergy or toxic drug effect. Multiple ulcerations and fissures of the corners of the mouth may be present.
17. Vincent's infection, trench mouth — a painful, inflammatory condition of the gums usually associated with fever, ulcerations, bleeding and lymphadenopathy.[25]

D. Operative Terms:

1. cheiloplasty — plastic repair of a lip.
2. cheilostomatoplasty — plastic repair of lip and mouth for cleft lip.
3. clipping of frenum linguae — clipping of membranous fold below tongue to relieve tongue-tie.
4. glossectomy, complete — removal of entire tongue generally done for carcinoma.[33, 45, 89]
5. glossectomy, partial, hemiglossectomy — resection of the tongue.
6. glossorrhaphy — suture of an injured tongue.
7. lip reconstruction — repair of lip which may be done following resection of malignant lesion of lip.[62]
8. oral cavity cancer resection — removal of cancerous tumor usually followed by immediate reconstruction either by direct primary closure of oral cavity defect, local tongue flap or other procedures.[89, 92]
9. palatoplasty — repair of cleft palate.
10. periapical tissue biopsy — microscopic tissue study of the periapex (around the root of a tooth) to determine the benign or malignant character of the pathologic process.[11]
11. radical neck dissection — total removal of all metastatic lesions in the cervical region together with the primary cancer.   This includes lymph nodes, lymphatics, veins, e.g. jugular vein, surrounding muscle, fascia and fat which constitute the repository for metastatic dissemination of the primary cancer.   Neck dissection may be combined with glossectomy, laryngectomy, thyroidectomy, as well as resection of the mandible, palate and maxilla, depending on the extent of the malignant involvement.[10, 33, 45, 89, 92]
12. stomatoplasty — plastic repair of mouth.

E. Symptomatic Terms:

1. glossodynia — a painful tongue due to a chronic inflammatory process of the lingual papillae.[25]
2. leukoplakia of the mouth — white patches on the mucous membrane of the tongue and buccal mucosa.[25]

SALIVARY GLANDS

A. Origin of Terms:

1. mandible (L) — lower jaw
2. parotid (G) — beside the ear
3. ptyalin (G) — saliva, spittle
4. sialon (G) — saliva, spittle
5. sialaden (G) — salivary gland
6. sialangi (G) — salivary duct

B. Anatomic Terms:

1. chief salivary glands — 3 pairs of glands with ducts opening into the oral cavity. They secrete saliva which moistens, dissolves and transports food and produces a starch-splitting enzyme, amylase.
   a. parotid gland and duct (Stensen's duct) located below the ear.
   b. sublingual gland and 10 to 30 ducts situated on the floor of the mouth beneath the tongue; some of the ducts open into the submandibular duct.
   c. submandibular gland and duct (Wharton's duct), situated mainly below the mandible.
2. small salivary glands — numerous glands in tongue, cheeks, lips.

C. Diagnostic Terms:

1. carcinoma of a salivary gland — malignant neoplasm arising from the glandular epithelium of a salivary gland.[25, 45, 89]
2. parotitis — inflammation of parotid gland.
3. ptyalith, sialolith — stone in salivary gland.

4. ptyalocele — cystic tumor of a salivary gland.
5. salivary tumors — adenomas of the mixed type found most frequently on the tongue, palate and lips.   They may undergo malignant transformation.[1, 31, 89]
6. sialadenitis — inflammation of salivary gland.

D. Operative Terms:

1. sialadenectomy — removal of a salivary gland.
2. sialolithotomy — removal of a stone from a salivary gland.
3. subtotal parotidectomy — partial resection of parotid gland with removal of benign tumor.[31]
4. total parotidectomy — wide excision of malignant tumor and gland sometimes including metastatic lesions.[31, 89]

E. Symptomatic Terms:

1. halitosis — offensive odor of breath.[24]
2. ptyalism, salivation — excessive secretion of saliva.

PHARYNX

A. Origin of Terms:

1. fauces (L) — throat
2. palatum (L) — palate
3. pharynx (G) — throat
4. tonsilla (L) — almond, tonsil

B. Anatomic Terms:

1. crypts — follicles or pits in tonsils.
2. palatine tonsil, faucial tonsil — a collection of lymphoid tissue lodged in the tonsillar fossa on either side of the oral part of the pharynx.
3. pharyngeal tonsil — a collection of lymphoid tissue located in the posterior wall of the nasal part of the pharynx.
4. pharynx — fibromuscular tube lined with mucous membrane and divided into oral, nasal and laryngeal parts.   It extends from the nose and mouth to the esophagus and serves as a common pathway for food and air.

C. Diagnostic Terms:

1. adenoids — enlarged pharyngeal tonsils.
2. adenotonsillitis — a bacterial-viral disorder characterized by abnormal oropharyngeal or nasopharyngeal microflora due to streptococci, adenoviruses or other organisms.[111]
3. hypertrophy of tonsils — enlarged palatine tonsils.
4. peritonsillar abscess, quinsy — localized collection of pus around the tonsil.[40, 111]
5. pharyngitis — inflammation of pharynx.
6. tonsillitis — inflammation of the tonsils.

D. Operative Terms:

1. adenotonsillectomy — removal of adenoids and tonsils.[40, 111]
2. pharyngeal flap operation, pharyngeal flap augmentation — a conservative palate repair which permits an essentially normal maxillary and dental arch development thus preventing facial and oral deformities and the hypernasality of cleft palate speech.[15, 38]

E. Symptomatic Terms:

1. aphagia — inability to swallow.
2. deglutition — swallowing.
3. dysphagia — difficulty in swallowing.

ESOPHAGUS

A. Origin of Terms:

1. esophagus (G) — food-carrier, gullet

B. Anatomic Terms:

1. cervical esophagus — portion of esophagus in the neck.
2. thoracic esophagus — portion of esophagus which passes through the thorax.

C. Diagnostic Terms:

1. achalasia, dilation of esophagus — a common disorder due to failure of cardiac sphincter to relax. It is characterized by a dilated and hypertrophied esophagus except for the distal segment which may be atrophied.[3, 8, 87]
2. atresia of esophagus — congenital absence of the esophageal opening or its pathologic closure.[24]
3. carcinoma of esophagus — malignant neoplasm, commonly an epidermoid carcinoma, arising from the epidermis or squamous epithelium; metastatic spread to other organs is a frequent occurrence.[82]
4. diverticula of esophagus (sing. diverticulum) — outpouching of esophageal wall. Two kinds:
   a. pulsion or true diverticula — consist of a bulging of mucosa through weakened parts of the esophageal wall.
   b. traction or false diverticula are due to pull exerted by diseased neighboring structures.
5. esophageal reflux ulceration — ulceration of the esophagus resulting from reflux of acid-peptic secretions into the esophagus due to incompetence of the gastroesophageal sphincter.[65, 86, 87, 88]
6. esophageal trauma — injury to esophagus.
   a. esophageal perforation — a hole in esophageal wall usually due to mechanical injury by ingestion of foreign body, gunshot wound or other causes.
   b. esophageal stricture — narrowing of the esophageal lumen, usually due to chemical injury such as lye ingestion or other caustic agents.[65]
7. esophageal varices — swollen, tortuous esophageal veins which may burst and result in massive hemorrhage. Condition is usually secondary to portal hypertension.[25, 68, 74, 82, 106]
8. esophagitis — inflammation of the esophagus.[88]

D. Operative Terms:

1. bougienage for esophageal stricture — dilation of esophagus with bougies, flexible instruments resembling sounds, used to diagnose and treat strictures of tubular passages.
   A safe procedure is to insert tapered tip Tucker bougies by the retrograde method through a gastrostomy and pull them through the esophagus with a string.[77, 99]
2. esophageal diverticulectomy — excision of diverticulum and closure of the resulting defect.
3. esophagojejunostomy — formation of a communication between the esophagus and jejunum.
4. esophagoplasty — reconstruction or plastic repair of esophageal defect.
5. esophagoplasty with reversed gastric tube — a physiologic method of esophageal replacement using the patient's own stomach to avoid immune reactions caused by rejection of transplants.[56]
6. esophagorrhaphy — suture of injured or ruptured esophagus.
7. fundic patch operation — surgical procedure for repair of ruptured esophagus or acid-peptic stricture and in the treatment of advanced achalasia.[53]
8. fundoplication — operative procedure to relieve gastroesophageal reflux of large amounts of acid-peptic juice to restore gastroesophageal competence.[76, 100]
9. Heller esophagomyotomy — incision into the circular muscle fibers of the distal esophagus to relieve achalasia.[8]

10. radical resection for esophageal cancer — excision of tumor bearing portion of esophagus and regional lymph nodes, followed by restoration of continuity by anastomosis or interposition of loop of colon or jejunum.[20]
11. resection for esophageal stricture — removal of extensive narrow segment followed by colonic bypass. The right colon with terminal ileum and ileocecal valve is tunneled into the neck and anastomosed with the proximal esophagus. The operation is indicated when chronic stricture is unresponsive to bougienage. Sometimes a gastric tube is used as a means of reconstruction.[65, 92, 100]

E. Symptomatic Terms:

1. dysphagia — difficulty in swallowing.
2. odynophagia — painful swallowing.[8]
3. regurgitation — backflow of gastric contents into the mouth.

STOMACH

A. Origin of Terms:

1. fundus (L) — base
2. gaster (G) — stomach, belly
3. omentum (L) — membrane enclosing bowel
4. pyloros (G) — gatekeeper
5. ruga (L) — fold, crease
6. sphincter (G) — binder

B. Anatomic Terms:[82, 107]

1. antrum, gastric — distal nonacid secreting segment of the stomach or pyloric gland region which produces the hormone gastrin.
2. body of stomach — largest portion of the stomach between antrum and fundus.
3. cardia — small area of the stomach near the esophagogastric junction.
4. cardiac orifice — opening at the junction of the esophagus with the stomach.
5. curvatures of stomach:
   a. lesser — right and superior margin of the stomach.
   b. greater — left and inferior margin of the stomach.
6. fundus of stomach — enlarged portion to the left located above the level of the cardiac orifice.
7. omenta (sing. omentum) — peritoneal sheets connecting the stomach with other viscera as the liver, spleen and transverse colon.
8. pyloric part of stomach — distal segment of the stomach including
   a. the antrum or pyloric gland area
   b. the pyloric canal
9. pyloric sphincter — circular muscle around pylorus.
10. pylorus — opening between stomach and duodenum.
11. rugae (sing. ruga) — irregular folds of the mucous membrane of the stomach in which gastric glands are embedded.

C. Diagnostic Terms:

1. gastric neoplasms, benign — new growths of the stomach that rarely interfere with gastric peristalsis.
   a. adenoma — tumor derived from glandular epithelium.
   b. gastrinoma — gastrin-producing adenoma of the stomach, duodenum or pancreas. It may undergo malignant transformation.[97]
   c. papilloma — circumscribed hypertrophy of gastric mucosa.
   d. polyp, polypus — pedunculated outgrowth of mucous membrane.[20, 82]
2. gastric neoplasms, malignant:
   a. carcinoma — usually adenocarcinoma; a malignant new growth of glandular epithelium.

    b. sarcoma — frequently lymphosarcoma, arising from lymphoid tissue.[20, 26, 82]

3. gastric ulcers — localized erosions of gastric mucosa which may result from the digestive action of acid gastric secretion. Secondary involvement of muscle tissue may occur.[26, 82]

    a. acute stress ulcer — acute ulceration of the fragile mucosa of the stomach in response to a stressful situation such as trauma, major surgery, head injury, alcoholic excesses or increased steroid secretion. Erosions occur as single or multiple superficial lesions which may be the source of massive bleeding.[82]

    b. chronic gastric ulcer — chronic peptic ulceration characteristically involving the nonacid secreting antral area and only seldom the acid forming parietal cell region of the stomach.[82]

4. gastritis — acute or chronic inflammation of the gastric mucosa:

    a. atrophic gastritis — a chronic inflammatory process in which atrophic changes of the gastric mucosa are usually irreversible and progressive.[26, 82]

    b. hypertrophic gastritis, Menetrier's disease — a chronic inflammation of the mucous lining of the stomach with greatly enlarged gastric rugae and thickened gastric wall.[3, 82]

5. gastrocele — hernia of stomach; example, diaphragmatic gastric hernia.

6. gastrocolitis — inflammation of stomach and colon.

7. gastroduodenitis — inflammation of stomach and duodenum.

8. gastroenteritis — inflammation of stomach and intestine.

9. gastroptosis, Glenard's disease — downward displacement of stomach.

10. hiatal hernia, hiatus hernia — protrusion of part of the stomach through the esophageal opening of the diaphragm.[3, 26, 76]

11. hypertrophic, pyloric stenosis, congenital — condition seen in the newborn characterized by an overgrowth of muscle fibers which markedly diminishes the lumen of the pyloric canal and gives rise to obstruction.[3, 26, 82]

Table 17

GASTRIC TYPES IN RELATION TO ARCHITECTURAL STRUCTURES OF INDIVIDUALS[a]

Type of Stomach	Description of Type of Stomach	Tonicity of Stomach	Graphic Description
Hypersthenic individual stocky short	Stomach high, wide above, narrow below, transverse position, pylorus to the right	Hypertonic Increased tone	
Sthenic individual well-built	Stomach tubular in shape, as wide above as it is below, pylorus to the right, well above the umbilicus	Orthotonic Normal tone	
Hyposthenic individual more slender	Stomach longer, narrower at the top; a tendency to sag below the greater curvature near the umbilicus; pylorus swinging to the left	Hypotonic Decreased tone	
Asthenic individual still more slender	Stomach sags far down below the umbilicus, being almost collapsed above, expanding into large sac below	Atonic Weak tone	

    [a]L. R. Sante. *Principles of Roentgenological Interpretation*, 10th ed. Ann Arbor, Michigan: Edwards Brothers, Inc., 1956, p. 368.

12. Mallory-Weiss syndrome — longitudinal lacerations of the gastroesophageal mucosa causing upper gastrointestinal bleeding.[101]
13. Zollinger-Ellison syndrome — excessive gastric secretion, rapidly worsening, refractory, or recurrent peptic ulceration and hyperplasia of pancreatic islet cells, which may be due to an ulcerogenic tumor in the pancreas.[43, 82, 92]

D. Operative Terms:

1. anastomosis — surgical formation of a passage or opening between two hollow viscera or vessels; for example, gastrojejunostomy.
2. antrectomy, gastric — removal of the gastrin producing pyloric gland area of the stomach.[101]
3. gastrectomy — partial or subtotal removal of the stomach. Total gastrectomy with jejunal interposition has been advocated for Zollinger-Ellison syndrome.[59, 86, 114]
4. gastric resection — usually the removal of 50-75% of the stomach combined with one of the following procedures:
   a. gastroduodenal anastomosis, Billroth I — joining the resected stomach to the duodenum.
   b. gastrojejunal anastomosis, Billroth II — joining the remaining stomach to the jejunum by either the
      (1) Polya technique — anterior anastomosis, large stoma or
      (2) Hofmeister technique — posterior anastomosis, small stoma.[71, 86, 101]
5. gastrojejunostomy — creation of a communication between the stomach and jejunum.[59, 114]
6. gastrostomy — external fistulization of the stomach. This may be done for the purpose of maintaining nutrition.[114]
7. pyloromyotomy, Fredet-Ramstedt operation — incision of the hypertrophic pyloric muscle down to the mucosa.
8. pyloroplasty — revision of pyloric stoma. Procedures of choice are usually those of Finney and Heinecke-Mikulicz.[34, 71, 101]
9. repair of hiatus hernia — several different methods are used either by the transthoracic or transabdominal approach, for example: freeing the esophagus at the cardia and attaching the region of the esophagogastric junction to the defect in the diaphragm.[76]
10. vagotomy, gastric — the surgical interruption of vagal impulses to the pyloric gland area (antrum) and the gastric parietal cell region.[71, 114]
11. vagotomy, selective gastric — vagal denervation restricted to the parietal cell mass of the stomach.[35, 101]
12. vagotomy and antrectomy — surgical destruction of vagal impulses and excision of the gastric antrum for removing the major stimuli to acid production in gastric and duodenal ulcers.[86, 101]

E. Symptomatic Terms:

1. achlorhydria — absence of hydrochloric acid in the gastric juice.
2. achylia gastrica — absent or reduced gastric secretion due to atrophy of the mucosa of the stomach.
3. anorexia — loss of appetite.
4. bulimia — voracious appetite.
5. cyclic vomiting — periodic vomiting.
6. dumping syndrome — symptoms occurring after meals following gastrectomy. The patient experiences sweating, flushing, warmth, faintness and sometimes diarrhea.[26]
7. dyspepsia — imperfect digestion.
8. epigastric pain — pain over the pit of the stomach.
9. eructation — belching.
10. hematemesis — vomiting blood.[41]
11. hyperchlorhydria — excessive amount of hydrochloric acid in the gastric juice.
12. hypochlorhydria — deficient amount of hydrochloric acid in the stomach.
13. hypergastrinemia — highly increased serum gastrin levels found in Zollinger-Ellison syndrome and pernicious anemia.[94]

14. intrinsic factor, Castle's intrinsic factor — factor normally present in gastric mucosa and gastric juice and required for absorption of vitamin B_{12}. It is absent in pernicious anemia.[23]
15. polyphagia — excessive food intake.
16. pyrosis — heartburn.

SMALL AND LARGE INTESTINES

A. Origin of Terms:

1. appendix (L) — appendage
2. cecum (L) — blind gut
3. colon (G) — large intestine
4. duodenum (L) — twelve, duodenum
5. enteron (G) — intestine
6. ileum (G) — to twist
7. jejunum (L) — empty
8. procto- (G) — anus
9. rectum (L) — straight
10. vermiform (L) — shape of worm

B. Anatomic Terms:[82]

1. small intestine — proximal portion of intestine from pylorus to ileocecal junction.
   a. duodenum — first part of small intestine; extends from pylorus to jejunum.
   b. jejunum — second part of small intestine; extends from duodenum to ileum.
   c. ileum — third part of small intestine; extends from jejunum to cecum.
   d. mesentery — peritoneal fold which carries the blood supply and attaches the jejunum and ileum to the posterior abdominal wall.
2. large intestine — distal portion of intestine including cecum, appendix, colon, rectum and anal canal.
   a. anus — outlet or orifice of anal canal.
   b. appendix vermiformis — an intestinal diverticulum projecting from cecum 3-13 cm and ending blindly.
   c. cecum — blind pouch of large intestine at and below level of ileocecal junction.
   d. colon — large intestine from cecum to rectum including the ascending colon, transverse colon, descending colon and sigmoid or pelvic colon.
   e. flexures of colon
      (1) right colic flexure, formerly hepatic flexure — bend of colon near liver.
      (2) left colic flexure, formerly splenic flexure — bend of colon near spleen.
   f. mesocolon — mesentery attaching the colon to the posterior abdominal wall.

C. Diagnostic Terms:

1. appendicitis — inflammation of the appendix.
2. colitis:
   a. granulomatous colitis — transmural involvement of colon presenting granulomas and fissures.[27]
   b. ischemic colitis — a spontaneous reduction of the arterial blood flow of large intestine associated with abrupt onset of abdominal pain, frequent bloody stools and radiographic changes of colon.[73]
   c. mucous colitis — inflammatory condition marked by large amount of mucus in stool.
   d. ulcerative colitis — inflammation and multiple erosions of the intestinal mucosa leading to hemorrhage and perforations, clinically noted for frequent evacuations of watery, purulent and bloody stools.[27, 60, 82]
3. congenital megacolon, Hirschsprung's disease — excessive enlargement of the colon associated with an absence of ganglion cells in the narrowed bowel wall distally. The aganglionic segment of the colon is the pathologic lesion.[3, 27, 37]
4. diverticulitis — inflammation of a diverticulum or diverticula.[3, 26]
5. diverticulosis — presence of diverticula in the intestinal tract.[3]
6. duodenal ulcer — circumscribed erosion of duodenal wall which may involve full thickness and is usually located near the pylorus.[26, 82]

7. dysentery — inflammation of the intestinal mucosa characterized by frequent small stools, chiefly of blood and mucus. It is due to specific bacillus or ameba.
8. fissure, anal, fissure-in-ano — tear in anal mucosa which may become ulcerated, infected, spastic, scarred and painful.[2]
9. fistula:
    a. anal fistula, fistula in ano — abnormal communication between anal canal or lower rectum and skin near anus.
    b. fecal fistula — abnormal passage from intestine to the body surface or another hollow viscus.
    c. high-output gastrointestinal fistula — a fistula which produces a minimum of 200 ml of gastrointestinal drainage in 24 hours including salivary, gastric, pancreatic and biliary secretions rich in enzymes and electrolytes. Consequently there is a significant loss in energy.[48]
10. enteritis — inflammation of the intestine.
11. hemorrhoids, piles — dilated varicose veins of the anal canal and at anal orifice.
12. ileitis — inflammation of the ileum.
13. intestinal malabsorption syndromes — disorders resulting from a faulty absorption of fat soluble vitamins, proteins, carbohydrates and minerals associated with copious excretion of fatty stools (steatorrhea).[93]
    a. adult celiac disease, gluten enteropathy, celiac sprue — genetic predisposition to gluten (protein of wheat, cereals) intolerance characterized by malnutrition, chronic diarrhea, edema and muscle wasting occurring within the third to sixth decades of life.[93]
    b. childhood celiac disease, gluten enteropathy, celiac sprue — same as adult disease except that it develops in infancy and causes retarded growth.[4]
    c. Crohn's disease of small intestine — nutritional malabsorption due to damaged mucosa, fistulas, strictures and decreased surface for absorption.[60]
    d. short bowel syndrome, short gut syndrome — syndrome characterized by malabsorption of fat soluble vitamins and depletion of fluid and electrolytes.[96]
    e. Whipple's disease — rare disorder characterized by malabsorption of lipids (fat) with resultant steatorrhea, diarrhea, abdominal distress, fever, anemia, lymph node involvement and bouts of arthralgia.[93]
14. intestinal obstruction, ileus — obstruction of small intestine associated with variable symptoms: abdominal distention, colicky pain, nausea, vomiting, obstipation or diarrhea. Interference with the blood flow to the obstructed intestine demands emergency surgery.
    a. adynamic (paralytic) ileus — paralysis of intestinal muscles, absence of bowel sounds. It may be due to electrolyte imbalance or operative handling of intestine.
    b. dynamic (mechanical) ileus — intestinal occlusion from adhesions, strangulated hernia, volvulus, intussusception, emboli or thrombi.[3, 27]
15. intussusception — telescoping of intestine; usually ileum slips into cecum which leads to intestinal obstruction.
16. Meckel's diverticulum — a congenital pouch or sac which usually arises from the ileum and may cause strangulation, intussusception or volvulus.[27]
17. mesenteric artery thrombosis, bowel infarction — vascular syndrome initiated either by a slowly developing or a sudden occlusion of the superior mesentery artery in advanced atherosclerosis or following dissecting aneurysm or the use of oral contraceptives.[73]
18. multiple polyposis — polyps or tumors derived from mucous membrane; scattered throughout intestine and rectum; may undergo malignant degeneration.[12]
19. perforated viscus — a ruptured internal organ due to advanced disease, malignancy, trauma, drugs, gunshot or stab wound. It may be complicated by hemorrhage, shock and peritonitis.
20. proctitis — inflammation of rectum.
21. prolapse of rectum — downward displacement of rectum, seen in infants and old people.
22. rectal cancer — malignant tumor of the rectum or rectosigmoid.[72, 103]

23. rectocele — herniation of rectum into vagina.
24. volvulus — twisting of the bowel upon itself leading to obstruction.

D. Operative Terms:

1. abdominal perineal resection — combined laparotomy and perineal operation for partial or complete removal of colon and rectum.[69, 114]
2. appendectomy — removal of appendix.
3. cecectomy — excision of cecum.
4. cecostomy — external fistulization of the cecum for intestinal obstruction.
5. colectomy — either segmental colon resection or removal of entire colon.[110, 114]
6. colon resection and end-to-end anastomosis — excision of involved colon with or without adjacent lymph glands; joining segments of colon.
7. colostomy — formation of an abdominal anus by bringing a loop of the colon to the surface of the abdomen in an attempt to control fecal discharge.   Another procedure is to bring the proximal segment of the colon to the skin as in abdominoperineal resection.[92, 114]
8. diverticulectomy — removal of diverticulum including resection of involved bowel.
9. hemorrhoidectomy — removal of hemorrhoids.[85]
10. ileostomy — external fistulization of ileum for fecal evacuation often done with total colectomy for ulcerative colitis.[110]
11. jejunoileal bypass — creation of a bypass of a considerable portion of the small intestine by joining the proximal jejunum to the terminal ileum and the distal end of the bypassed segment of the cecum.   The procedure reduces the absorptive capacity of small intestine and induces weight loss.   Various techniques are used to control morbid obesity and hyperlipidemia.[21, 22, 96]
12. operations for aganglionic megacolon (Hirschsprung's disease)
    a. modified Duhamel procedure — side-to-side anastomosis of colon and rectum.
    b. modified Soave procedure — endorectal pull-through of ganglionated bowel to anus.[37]
13. proctocolectomy, total — removal of the entire rectum and resection of the colon which may be done as emergency procedure for colonic perforation from ulcerative colitis.[13]
14. proctoplasty — plastic repair or reconstruction of rectum or anus.
15. reduction of intussusception — normal intestinal continuity restored either by barium enema or if unsuccessful by laparotomy.
16. reduction of volvulus — untwisting of lesion by manipulation.
17. sphincterotomy, lateral internal — effective procedure for the control of an anal fissure using a small circular incision which is closed by suture and avoids fecal soilage.[2]
18. tube cecostomy — surgical decompression of the colon by tube drainage of the cecum.

E. Symptomatic Terms:

1. borborygmus — rumbling or splashing sound of bowels.
2. colic — spasm of any tubular hollow organ associated with pain.
3. diarrhea — frequency of bowel action, soft or liquid stools.[3]
4. fecalith — a fecal concretion.
5. melena — black stool, also black vomit due to blood.
6. obstipation — extreme constipation, often due to obstruction.
7. pruritus ani — itching sensation around the anus.
8. steatorrhea — increased fat content in feces as in malabsorption syndrome or in pancreatitis.[93]

LIVER, BILIARY SYSTEM, PANCREAS, PERITONEUM

A. Origin of Terms:

1. bile (L) — bile, gall
2. celi- (G) — abdomen
3. cholangi (G) — bile duct
4. chole (G) — bile, gall
5. cholecyst (G) — gallbladder
6. choledoch (G) — bile duct
7. cirrho- (G) — yellow, tawny
8. hepato- (G) — liver
9. laparo- (G) — abdominal wall
10. peritoneum (G) — stretching over

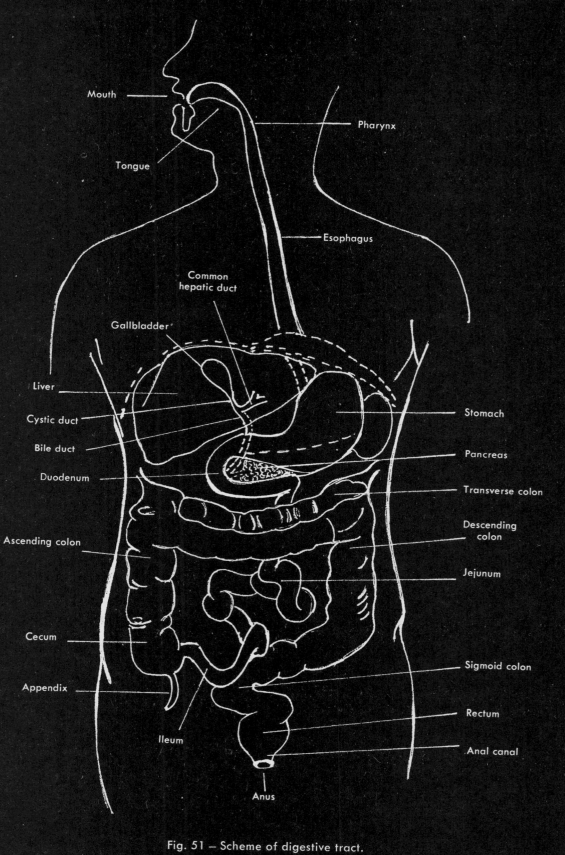

Fig. 51 — Scheme of digestive tract.

172

B. Anatomic Terms:[83]

1. bile duct — duct formed by union of common hepatic duct and cystic duct, carries bile into duodenum.
2. common hepatic duct — duct formed by union of right and left hepatic ducts which receive bile from liver.
3. cystic duct — passageway for bile from gallbladder to bile duct.
4. gallbladder — pear-shaped, sac-like organ which serves as reservoir for bile.
5. pancreas — large endocrine and exocrine gland, its right extremity or head lying within the duodenal curve, its left extremity or tail ending near the spleen.[104]
6. pancreatic duct — main passageway for pancreatic juice containing enzymes; runs from left to right and empties into duodenum.
7. pancreatic islets, islets of Langerhans — clusters of cells producing the hormone insulin.
8. pancreatic juice — clear secretion, 1000-2500 ml of fluid per day, composed of water, electrolytes, proteins and enzymes.[64]
9. peritoneum — a sac of serous membrane composed of a parietal peritoneum which lines the abdominal wall and a visceral peritoneum which invests most viscera and holds them in position.
10. portal circulation — venous blood collected by the portal vein from gastrointestinal canal, spleen, gallbladder and pancreas enters the liver, passes through sinusoids and leaves the liver by the hepatic veins to pour into the inferior vena cava.
11. sphincter of bile duct (of Oddi) — circular muscle fibers around the end of the bile duct.
12. sphincter of hepatopancreatic ampulla — circular muscle fibers around end of ampulla (the union of the bile duct and main pancreatic duct).

C. Diagnostic Terms:

1. liver:
   a. acute yellow atrophy of liver — any severe form of hepatitis marked by shrinkage and necrosis of liver.
   b. Budd-Chiara syndrome — a rare disease characterized by occlusion of hepatic veins usually accompanied by ascites, hepatomegaly and pain in abdomen.[61]
   c. cirrhosis of the liver — organ diffusely nodular and firm.
      (1) portal cirrhosis — Laennec's cirrhosis the most common form, frequently associated with alcoholism and nutritional deficiency.
      (2) biliary cirrhosis — obstructive form is characterized by chronic jaundice and liver failure due to obstruction and inflammation of bile ducts.[61, 66, 83]
   d. fatty liver — abnormal lipid increase in the liver, probably related to reduced oxidation of fatty acids or decreased synthesis and release of lipoproteins causing inadequate lipid clearance from the liver.[61, 83]
   e. hemochromatosis — excess of iron absorption and presence of iron containing deposits (hemosiderin) in liver, pancreas, kidneys, adrenals and heart. It may be associated with hepatic enlargement and insufficiency and esophageal bleeding from varices.[47, 61]
   f. hepatic calculi — stones originating in extrahepatic biliary tract or solely in the liver. They are also found in liver cysts.[83]
   g. hepatic coma, cholemia — peculiar syndrome characterized by slow or rapid onset of bizarre behavior, disorientation, flapping tremors of extended arms, hyperactive reflexes, later lethargy and coma. It seems to be caused by intoxication with ammonia, a product of protein digestion which the diseased liver fails to convert into urea.[83]
   h. hepatic encephalopathy — serious complication of advanced liver disease probably due to cerebral toxins including ammonia, certain amines and fatty acids. It is clinically manifested by personality changes, impaired intellectual ability, awareness and neuromuscular functioning.[61, 67, 90]
   i. hepatic failure, fulminant — clinical syndrome caused by extensive necrosis of the liver

which may be induced by hepatotoxic drugs and may lead to progressive encephalopathy and a fatal prognosis.[6, 71, 90]

j. hepatic injury, drug-induced — liver injury may be
   (1) cholestatic — injury mimicking obstructive jaundice, e.g. due to the use of chlorpromazine, erythromycin, steroids and oral contraceptives.[113]
   (2) cytotoxic — injury leading to severe hepatocellular jaundice, severe liver necrosis and failure, e.g. due to the use of isoniazid, methyldopa, halothane and tetracycline.[14, 61, 113]

k. hepatic necrosis — destruction of functional liver tissue.

l. hepatic trauma — liver injury resulting from blunt trauma or penetrating wounds.[95]

m. hepatitis, viral — acute or chronic inflammation of the liver caused by the hepatitis virus A or B.[61] (See Chapter XV — Systemic Disorders.)

n. hepatoma — a tumor of the liver.

o. hepatorenal syndrome — combined liver and kidney failure usually due to serious injury to the liver associated with hemorrhage, shock and acute renal insufficiency.[61]

p. liver abscess:
   (1) amebic abscess — localized hepatic infection by *Entamoeba histolytica*, a common complication of intestinal amebiasis.
   (2) pyogenic abscess — circumscribed area of suppuration. Infection brought to liver via portal vein, hepatic artery or bile ducts.[83]

q. polycystic liver disease — cystic degeneration of the liver usually associated with congenital polycystic kidneys.[61]

r. portal hypertension — a portal venous pressure above 20 mm Hg associated with splenomegaly, increased collateral circulation, varicosity, bleeding and ascites. Portal hypertension may result from
   (1) intrahepatic block — block within the liver or
   (2) extrahepatic block — block within the portal vein.[83]

s. primary carcinoma of the liver — hepatocellular tumor clinically manifested by an enlarged, tender liver, ascites, jaundice, splenomegaly, edema, fever and hepatic bruit.[30]

t. secondary carcinoma of the liver — metastatic malignant neoplasm, usually from lung, breast or gastrointestinal cancer.

2. biliary system:
   a. biliary stricture — contraction of a biliary duct which is prone to develop after gallbladder surgery and is evidenced by profuse drainage of bile or obstructive jaundice.[105]
   b. carcinoma of gallbladder — scirrhous (hard) type most common; early invasion of adjacent structures.
   c. cholangitis — inflammatory disease of bile ducts.[83]
   d. cholecystitis — inflammatory disease of the gallbladder, frequently associated with the presence of gallstones.[83]
   e. choledocholithiasis — gallstones in the biliary ducts.[50]
   f. cholelithiasis, biliary calculi — the presence of gallstones in the gallbladder.
   g. empyema of gallbladder — pus in the gallbladder.
   h. hydrops of gallbladder — distention of gallbladder with clear fluid.[105]

3. pancreas:
   a. acute hemorrhagic pancreatic necrosis, acute hemorrhagic pancreatitis — major medical emergency apparently caused by the destructive lytic action of pancreatic enzymes, clinically manifested by a sudden onset, acute abdomen, agonizing, constant pain and profound shock.[84]
   b. cystic fibrosis of pancreas, pancreatic fibrosis, mucoviscidosis — a hereditary, familial disease seen in children and adolescents and characterized by a more or less extensive involvement of the exocrine glands, especially those secreting mucus and sweat.[64]
   c. diabetes mellitus — the most significant pancreatic disease in which pathogenic

alterations of the islet cells cause a depletion of the insulin stores.[84]   (See Chapter XII — Metabolic Diseases.)

   d. pancreatic pseudocyst — a fibrous capsule containing pancreatic juice with high levels of pancreatic enzymes, especially amylase.[46, 104]

   e. pancreatic tumors:

   (1) carcinoma of pancreas — a highly fatal malignant tumor, usually derived from glandular epithelium and involving the head of the pancreas (65%).[19, 42, 64]

   (2) islet cell tumors — neoplasms originating from the islets of Langerhans.   They tend to induce hyperinsulinism which in turn produces hypoglycemia. Islet cell lesions may be benign, malignant and metastasizing.[46, 84]

   f. pancreatitis — inflammation of the pancreas, which may be caused by alcoholism or cholelithiasis.   Its pathologic process is due to irritation from enzyme activity which results in pancreatic edema and vascular engorgement.[64]

4. peritoneum:

   a. ascites — collection of fluid within the peritoneal cavity.[73]

   b. hemoperitoneum — blood within the peritoneal cavity.

   c. hernia — rupture or protrusion of a part from its normal location; for example, an intestinal loop through a weakened area in the abdominal wall.

   (1) location:

   (a) femoral — organ passes through femoral ring.

   (b) inguinal — organ protrudes through inguinal canal.

   (c) umbilical — hernia occurs at the navel.

   (2) types:

   (a) incarcerated — hernia causes complete bowel obstruction.

   (b) incisional — hernia complicates surgical intervention.

   (c) strangulated — hernia cuts off circulation so that gangrene develops if emergency operation is not performed.

   d. peritonitis — inflammation of peritoneum.[73]

D. Operative Terms:

1. liver:

   a. biopsy of liver — removal of small piece of tissue for microscopic study.

   b. hepatic lobectomy — removal of lobe of liver.[95]

   c. hepatotomy — incision into liver substance.

   d. shunts for portal hypertension, portal decompression, portosystemic decompression — surgical method of diverting a considerable amount of blood of the hypertensive portal system into the normal systemic venous system in order to prevent or treat variceal hemorrhages.[114]

   (1) mesocaval shunt — surgical communication of the side of the superior mesenteric vein and the upper end of the inferior vena cava for thrombosis of the portal vein.[106]

   (2) portacaval shunt — anastomosis of portal vein to vena cava for intrahepatic block.

   (3) splenorenal shunt — splenectomy followed by an anastomosis between the splenic artery and renal artery for extrahepatic block due to thrombosis of the portal vein.[57, 75, 81, 106]

2. biliary system:

   a. cholecystectomy — removal of the gallbladder.[50]

   b. cholecystojejunostomy — anastomosis between gallbladder and jejunum to bypass the obstruction in the biliary ductal system.[105]

   c. cholecystostomy — surgical creation of a more or less permanent opening into the gallbladder.   This operation is indicated where removal of the gallbladder would be unduly hazardous.[114]

    d. choledochoduodenostomy — surgical joining of the common bile duct to the duodenum.[50, 114]

    e. choledocholithotomy — incision into bile duct for removal of gallstones.[9]

    f. choledochoplasty — plastic repair or reconstruction of bile duct.

    g. Roux-en-Y procedures — jejunal loop or limb surgically used to
        (1) bypass extensive trauma to the bilary ductal system by constructing a choledochojejunostomy
        (2) decompress a choleductal cyst or the biliary tract by performing a cholecystojejunostomy
        (3) anastomose both ends of the completely transected pancreas following pancreatic injury thus accomplishing a pancreaticojejunostomy.[91]

    h. sphincteroplasty (Oddi) — plastic repair of stenotic sphincter of Oddi.[50]

3. pancreas:

    a. pancreatectomy — partial or total removal of pancreas; for example, for islet cell tumor.

    b. pancreatoduodenectomy* — pancreatoduodenal resection indicated in the presence of major injury to the duodenum, pancreas and adjacent viscera which precludes the salvage of these organs.[5, 112]

    c. pancreatojejunostomy — anastomosis of pancreas to jejunum. May be done for carcinoma of the ampulla of Vater.[104]

    d. sphincteroplasty (Vater) — plastic repair of ampulla of Vater for alleviating ampullary obstruction by biliary stones and chronic pancreatitis.[104]

    e. Whipple operation, Whipple pancreaticoduodenostomy* — extensive resection for pancreatic cancer or serious injury including the head, tail and portions of the body of the pancreas, together with the duodenum, part of the bile duct and stomach. The remaining pancreas is anastomosed to the bile duct, jejunum and stomach.[104, 114]

4. peritoneum:

    a. exploratory laparotomy — surgical opening of abdomen for diagnostic purposes.

    b. hernioplasty, herniorrhaphy — repair of hernia.

    c. incision and drainage of abscess — opening and draining peritoneal, retroperitoneal or subphrenic abscess.[73]

E. Terms Related to Special Procedures:

1. balloon tamponade — emergency procedure to control bleeding from esophageal varices using a Boyce or a Linton modification of the Sengstaken-Blakemore tube which permits aspiration of secretions.[68]

2. endoscopy with flexible fiberscope — visualization of a hollow organ using an endoscope with a tip for remote control and a biopsy channel for tissue sampling and histologic study of lesion.

    a. colonoscopy, colonofiberoscopy — a method of examining the colon by using a colonic fiberscope with a 4 way controlled tip to facilitate traversing the flexures of the sigmoid and transverse colon under fluoroscopic guidance. It may permit the removal of polyps up to the ascending colon.[7, 32]

    b. duodenoscopy — the introduction of a flexible duodenoscope into the first part of the duodenum, visualization and cannulation of papilla of Vater. Contrast material is injected into the orifice of the ampulla through a minute cannula to obtain a retrograde cholangiogram or pancreatogram.[16,17, 80]

    c. esophagogastroscopy — visualization of the esophagus, stomach and duodenal bulb using a flexible fiberscope with provision for target biopsy and color photography through the scope. Benign or malignant lesions, bleeding points and hemorrhagic gastritis may be detected by direct vision.[16, 17]

    d. fiberoptic gastroscopy — use of an end-viewing fiberscope as the usual method of

---

*pancreato-, pancreatico — both combining forms are correct.

choice for visualizing the esophagus, stomach, antrum, pylorus, duodenal bulb and an anastomosis after surgery. In addition to the fiberoptic light source the scope contains a channel for biopsies, for suction and air or water instillation and for endoscopic photography.[17]

    e. peritoneoscopy — procedure for visualization of the peritoneal cavity using a peritoneoscope with a fiberoptic light source. It is possible to perform a percutaneous liver biopsy under direct vision, to photograph the lesions, to irrigate the peritoneal cavity, to aspirate ascitic fluid for cytoanalysis and finally arrive at a diagnosis of obscure abdominal disease by peritoneoscopy.[73]

    f. proctosigmoidoscopy — endoscopic procedure for visualization of benign and malignant lesions of the rectosigmoid. It permits excisional biopsy of small lesions, e.g. polyps and segmental biopsy of large ones for diagnosis.[79]

3. exchange transfusion for hepatic coma — exchange of equal volume of blood using a closed transfusion circuit for the purpose of clearing bilirubin, improving the clotting mechanism and reversing coma. Fresh blood is used and electrolytes are added as needed.[90]

4. extracorporeal hemoperfusion — procedure used to remove potential toxins from the patient in hepatic coma including ammonia and various products of deterioration.[90]

5. hyperalimentation — long-term intravenous nutrition with an amino acid-glucose infusate using disposable tubing and infusion pump to maintain a constant infusion rate. A large intravenous catheter is inserted through a central vein and its proper position is radiographically confirmed. Hyperalimentation should be reserved for patients with severe digestive abnormalities.[18, 36, 48]

6. liver perfusion — method of providing extracorporeal support to liver in hepatic coma using regional heparinization and a disposable perfusion circuit primed with 250 to 300 ml of blood. Under aseptic precautions fresh blood is obtained from healthy baboons or from human cadaver, chilled with electrolyte solution and used for liver perfusion until consciousness is restored.[90]

7. pneumatic dilation of the lower esophageal sphincter (LES) — forceful dilation of LES with a bag dilator for reinstituting peristalsis and relaxing the sphincter in early achalasia.[8]

F. Symptomatic Terms:

1. alopecia, pectoral and axillary — absence of hair on chest and axillae (arm pits) in liver damage.

2. arterial spiders, spider nevi — cutaneous vascular lesions occurring on face, neck and shoulders in advanced hepatic disease, also in malnutrition and pregnancy. Each lesion consists of a central arteriole from which small vessels radiate.

3. caput medusae — dilatation of the abdominal veins around the umbilicus seen in severe portal hypertension with liver damage.[61]

4. cholestasis — impaired or obstructed bile flow.[112]

5. fetor hepaticus — a musty, sweet odor to the breath, characteristic of hepatic coma.[61]

6. flapping tremor, liver flap — involuntary movements, elicited in the extended hand by supporting the patient's forearm. It consists of bursts of quick, irregular movements at the wrist similar to waving goodbye. The protruded tongue and dorsiflexed feet may likewise be affected. Flapping tremors occur in severe liver disease and signal impending hepatic coma.[61]

7. hepatic bruit — vascular bruit over liver, a blowing sound or murmur heard on auscultation, probably due to pressure of enlarged liver on aorta.[61]

8. hyperammoniemia — excessive amount of ammonia in the blood as in hepatic coma.[90]

9. icterus, jaundice — yellow discoloration of skin, sclera (white of eyes), membranes and secretions due to excess bilirubin in the blood.[112]

10. palmar erythema, liver palms — a bright or mottled redness of the palms and finger tips seen in liver disease. Palmar erythema also occurs in malnutrition and rheumatoid arthritis.[61]

RADIOLOGY

A. Terms Related to the Diagnostic Radiology of the Digestive Tract:

1. air contrast enema, double contrast enema — examination of the colon using a small amount of barium to coat the walls of the mucosa and air to distend the colon. This procedure may demonstrate intestinal polyps.[44]

2. barium enema examination — fluoroscopic and radiographic examination of the colon after administering a barium sulfate mixture. The colon may be spot-filmed while the enema is effective. Barium enemas are also used in the treatment of intussusception, which is often reduced by the rectal instillation of barium under fluoroscopic guidance.[47]

3. contour — surface configuration or outline of an organ or part; for example, that of the stomach.

4. duodenal cap — freely movable triangular part of the duodenum distal to the pyloroduodenal junction.

5. duodenography, hypotonic — radiologic examination of the duodenum using secretin to inhibit duodenal tonicity and motility thus producing well defined duodenograms.[51, 54]

6. Hampton maneuver — examination of the upper gastrointestinal tract with fluoroscopy and radiography using a barium mixture, but without applying pressure to abdomen. This technique is usually employed in patient with upper gastrointestinal hemorrhage.

7. scout film — a preliminary radiogram of the abdomen before the administration of a radiopaque substance.

8. sialogram — radiographic visualization of the main salivary glands and ducts following the injection of radiopaque material.

9. small intestine series — serial radiograms during the passage of barium through the small intestine.

10. spot film — radiogram of small isolated areas taken during fluoroscopy. Example: sigmoid colon.

B. Terms Related to the Diagnostic Radiology of the Liver and Biliary Tract:

1. barium upper gastrointestinal examination — radiologic demonstration of duodenal, pancreatic or biliary system distortions causing obstructive jaundice.[54, 63]

2. cholangiography — the introduction of radiopaque material into the bile ducts for x-ray examination of the biliary system.
   a. intravenous cholangiography — the intravenous injection of a contrast agent, e.g. methyl glucamine iodipamide (Cholegrafin) to opacify the biliary ductal system.[54]
   b. operative cholangiography — visualization of the ductal system by filling it with a contrast medium and taking radiograms at the time of the operation. This examination seeks to detect the presence of congenital anomalies, neoplasms and elusive gallstones.[70]
   c. percutaneous transhepatic cholangiography — percutaneous needle insertion through functional liver tissue (parenchyma) for injecting a radiopaque substance into a bile duct.[54, 61]
   d. transduodenal endoscopic cholangiography, endoscopic pancreatocholangiography — cannulation of the papilla of Vater with a duodenal fiberscope followed by injection of contrast medium into the pancreatic duct or bile duct or both.[44, 50, 54, 63, 80]

3. cholecystography — x-ray examination of the gallbladder after rendering the bile radiopaque.
   a. intravenous administration of radiopaque material or
   b. oral administration of Telepaque or any other suitable contrast medium.
      Both methods permit adequate gallbladder visualization.[44]

4. cinecholedochography — the routine films combined with cineradiography for visualization of the entire biliary ductal system.
5. cineradiography, cineroentgenography — the making of motion pictures by radiography.
6. portography, portovenography — radiography of the portal vein after injection of radiopaque material.[63]
7. splenoportogram — injection of radiopaque material into the spleen for radiographic study of the splenic and portal veins.

C. Terms Related to Diagnostic Ultrasound of the Abdomen:

1. abdominal echography — the use of noninvasive diagnostic ultrasound for studying the liver, gallbladder and pancreas, spleen, kidney, aorta and retroperitoneal space. It aids in the detection of intra-abdominal abscesses, cysts or tumors.[49]
2. biliary echography — ultrasound imaging of the gallbladder and biliary ducts which may be anechoic or display variable echoes: small, thin or coarse, strong, reflected, few or multiple, depending on the biliary pathology such as dilated bile ducts and gallbladder obstructed by cancer of the ampulla, hydrops of the gallbladder due to obstruction of the cystic duct, fluid-filled gallbladder portrayed by acoustic lucency or gallstones seen by acoustic shadows.[29]
3. hepatic echography — ultrasonic investigation revealing either a normal liver or specific echogenecity as present in hepatic cirrhosis, ascites, liver abscess, fluid-filled cysts, hepatoma, cancer and metastasis.[55]
4. pancreatic echography — noninvasive ultrasound technique producing characteristic echoes which aid in the differential diagnosis of pancreatic cysts and pseudocysts, tumors, cancer and pancreatitis.[46]

D. Terms Related to Therapeutic Radiology:

1. endocavitary irradiation for rectal cancer — conservative method of treating early rectal cancer at 2 or 3 week intervals using an x-ray tube which fits into a special protoscope and is illuminated by a fiberoptic system. If treatment fails, surgery is possible.[108]
2. preoperative supervoltage irradiation for rectal cancer — external high voltage radiotherapy to reduce the size of the malignant tumor and thus facilitate its removal.[108] Preoperative irradiation has also been successfully used in oral carcinoma.[45]

CLINICAL LABORATORY

A. Terms Related to Tests of the Digestive System:

1. amylase (amyl: starch - ase: enzyme) — digestive enzyme acting on starches. It is found in salivary glands, pancreatic juice, liver and adipose tissue.
2. amylolytic — starch-splitting.
3. biliary drainage, medical — a diagnostic and therapeutic measure. Magnesium sulfate, injected through duodenal tube, relaxes the sphincter of Oddi and stimulates bile drainage. Normally, the following distinctions are noted:
    a. the first specimen designated as "A" bile is golden yellow and is collected from the common bile duct.
    b. the second specimen known as "B" bile is green to yellow brown and directly aspirated from the gallbladder.
    c. the third specimen, "C" bile is light yellow and freshly secreted by the liver.
    Bacteriologic studies are done on the second specimen.[23]
4. diastase (syn. amylase) — enzyme digesting starches.
5. duodenal drainage — diagnostic aid in detecting biliary infection. The procedure is the same as that of biliary drainage except that no magnesium sulfate is injected.[23]
6. gastric analysis and related tests:
    a. augmented histalog test — test in which the histalog dose has been calculated

according to body weight to induce maximal gastric acid secretion. If no acid is released, anacidity is present.[23, 98]

    b. augmented histamine test — test in which an optimal histamine dose is used to evoke a maximal gastric acid response thus providing quantitative measurement of the secretory capacity of the stomach.[23, 98]

    c. basal acid output (BAO) — quantitative measurement of gastric acid secretion under basal conditions that is without histamine or histalog stimulation.[23, 98]

    d. gastric analysis (tube) — aspiration of gastric contents for the purpose of determining the secretory ability and motility of the stomach.

      Normal response:
        basal acid output......BAO................0 - 6.0 mEq/hr
        maximal acid output..MAO...............5 - 40 mEq/hr
      (after augmented histamine injection)
      Increase in gastric and duodenal ulcers
      Great increase in Zollinger-Ellison syndrome
      Decrease in gastric cancer and pernicious anemia.[23, 39, 98]

    e. gastric analysis (tubeless) — indirect method without gastric intubation using Diagnex Blue to determine whether the stomach contains acid.[23, 98]

7. gastric exfoliative cytology — valuable method for detecting gastric malignancy by studying cells shed by the mucosa and obtained by aspiration, lavage or abrasive brushes following the liquefaction of the mucosal coating.[102]

8. gastric juice — a composite of water, hydrochloric acid, electrolytes, enzymes, blood group components and the intrinsic factor of Castle.

9. gastrin — hormone formed by cells of the antral mucosa of the stomach and carried by the blood to the gastric fundus stimulating the release of hydrochloric acid and evoking the secretion of pepsin, pancreatic enzymes and the intrinsic factor of Castle.[94]

10. gastrin secretory test — the use of a purified gastrin preparation in gastric secretory studies analogous to those of histamine and histalog.[23]

11. guaiac test — test for occult blood in feces (also in urine).
    Negative reaction — no blood............ no greenish to blue color
    Positive reaction — blood present........ greenish to blue color
    Ulcerated carcinomas of colon or stomach always yield a positive reaction.
    Nonmalignant gastric ulcers intermittently yield a positive reaction.[11]

12. histamine — powerful stimulant to hydrochloric acid secretion, principally acting on the parietal cell mass of the stomach.[23]

13. Hollander insulin hypoglycemia test — use of insulin induced hypoglycemia to evaluate the outcome of vagotomy. Positive results, a few months after surgery, may indicate that vagal nerve fibers are regenerating or the vagotomy was incomplete.[98, 101]

14. intragastric photography — diagnostic procedure accomplished by a minuscule gastrocamera swallowed by the patient to provide color photographs of the interior of the stomach. The procedure is valuable in the detection of ulcers, tumors, polyps and gastritis.

15. intestinal absorption tests — these studies require further development. They are:
    a. D-xylose absorption test (oral)
    b. serum carotene level
    c. vitamin A tolerance test.[11]

16. maximal acid output (MAO) — quantitative measurement of gastric acid secretion after stimulation with augmented dose of histamine or histalog.[23]

17. proteolytic — protein-splitting.

18. secretin — hormone produced by the duodenal mucosa and acting as a potent stimulus to the release of pancreatic secretions.[23]

19. secretin test (Dreiling and Hollander) — the intravenous injection of secretin following the removal of the duodenal contents. The secretin stimulates pancreatic secretions which enter the duodenum and are removed. The study of the duodenal aspirate which includes

volume of output, amylase activity, content of bicarbonate, bile and proteolytic enzymes, aids in the diagnostic evaluation of pancreatic and biliary disorders.[11]

20. serum alpha-fetoprotein (SAFP) — useful test for the detection of hepatic cancer despite its nonspecificity.[30]

21. serum amylase (diastase) determination — test of diagnostic value in pancreatic conditions. Any interference with the outflow of amylase (diastase) causes a rise of the enzyme level.
   Normal values — Method of Somogyi
   serum amylase . . . . 60 - 160 units per dl[11, 39]
   Increase in acute pancreatitis, chronic recurrent pancreatitis and carcinoma of the head of the pancreas and parotitis
   Decrease in carcinoma of liver and pancreatic insufficiency.

22. serum leucine aminopeptidase determination (LAP) — measurement of leucine aminopeptidase, a protein splitting enzyme. Persistent high enzyme levels suggest carcinoma of the pancreas.[39]

23. serum lipase determination — test of usefulness in the early detection of pancreatic cancer.

24. stool examination — macroscopic and microscopic studies, chemical analysis and examinations for parasites and protozoa as diagnostic aids, especially for detecting diseases of the digestive tract.[11]

25. sweat test — diagnostic test in cystic fibrosis of pancreas or mucoviscidosis. Excessively high sweat chloride levels confirm the diagnosis.
   Normal values of sweat chloride range between 4 - 60 mEq/L[39]
   The finger prints or hand print technique of the sweat test is a simplified method for screening children and their relatives. Silver chromate paper moistened with distilled water is used for the test.
   Normal values — imprints of fingers or hand are light and indistinct. In mucoviscidosis imprints of fingers or hand are heavy and distinct. The red silver chromate changes to white silver chloride.

26. transaminase (SGPT) — a valuable diagnostic aid and sensitive index in acute hepatic disease.
   Normal values
   transaminase (SGPT) . . . . 1 - 36 units/ml[39, 94]
   (serum glutamic pyruvic transaminase)
   Increase in acute liver disease . . . . 600 - 700 units/ml
   This rise usually occurs within 25 days after onset of disease. A return to normal is very gradual within 40-80 days.

B. Terms Related to Liver Function:

Liver function tests are of great importance, not only in discovering the severity of hepatic disease, but also in determining the amount of liver damage caused by pathologic conditions of the gallbladder and pancreas. The liver is the largest gland in the body. Useful tests for detecting hepatic impairment are presented.

Table 18
LIVER FUNCTION TESTS

Hepatic Function	Tests	Comments
1. Excretory function chiefly related to bile pigments	a. Bromsulphalein (BSP) Retention of dye indicative of liver damage, metastatic carcinoma of liver and others[a, c]	Most sensitive test of liver function, of value in hepatic blood flow studies[a, c]
	b. Serum Alkaline Phosphatase Elevated in obstructive jaundice, liver abscess and cancer of liver[a, c]	Wide application in the study of hepatic disease[a, c]

Hepatic Function	Tests	Comments
Cont'd.	c. Serum Bilirubin Increased in hepatogenous jaundice, obstructive jaundice, portal cirrhosis, hepatic carcinoma[a, c]	Highly valued hepatic test[a, c]
	d. Bilirubin in Urine Present in hepatitis, hepatogenous and obstructive jaundice	Considerable usefulness
	e. Urobilinogen in Urine Present in hepatogenous jaundice and obstructive jaundice[a, c]	Very helpful
	f. Urobilinogen in Feces Increase in hemolytic jaundice Decrease in obstructive jaundice[a, c]	Helpful
2. Regulation of composition of blood	a. Prothrombin Determination Increased in seconds Decreased in per cent in obstructive jaundice, liver cell damage, vitamin K deficiency[c]	Usefulness established
3. Protein metabolism	a. Total Serum Proteins Serum Albumin Serum Globulin Serum Gamma Globulin Increase of globulin in infectious hepatitis Decrease of total proteins and albumin in liver disease[a, c]	Of value in the detection of hepatic and nonhepatic disorders
	b. Blood Ammonia Levels Increased in hepatic coma[a, c]	Of diagnostic importance
4. Inhibitory action of albumin on gamma globulin and others	a. Cephalin Cholesterol Flocculation Test Grade of flocculation reflecting liver damage b. Thymol Turbidity and Flocculation Test Increased in cirrhosis and infectious hepatitis	Helpful in the detection of hepatic and nonhepatic disorders Diminishing use
	c. Zinc Sulfate Turbidity Altered in prolonged degeneration of liver cells	Diminishing use
5. Carbohydrate metabolism	a. Oral Galactose Test Excretion in a 5 hour period Increased in toxic hepatitis and galactosemia	Decreasing use[a]
	b. Oral Glucose Tolerance Test Excretion of glucose within 30-60 minutes Increased in obstructive jaundice	Rarely of value in hepatic disease
	c. Glucagon Tolerance[a]	Diagnostic aid
	d. Epinephrine Tolerance Decreased in cirrhosis, hepatitis and glycogen storage disease[a, b]	Useful in clinical research[a]

Hepatic Function	Tests	Comments
6. Fat metabolism	a. Determination of Cholesterol	Some definite value Use restricted in liver function study[a, c]
	b. Determination of Cholesterol Esters Both increased in obstructive jaundice Both decreased in liver failure and hepatic necrosis[a]	Limited clinical application[a]
7. Enzyme activity	a. Serum Cholinesterase Decreased in liver disease, slightly low in obstructive jaundice, very low in poisoning from some insecticides	Use uncommon
	b. Serum Glutamic Oxalacetic Transaminase (SGOT) Increased in hepatitis and liver injury	Clinical usefulness
	c. Serum Glutamic Pyruvic Transaminase (SGPT) Highly elevated in acute hepatitis, toxic hepatitis and hepatocellular damage[a, b, c]	Very sensitive test Of greater value than SGOT in liver disease[a, b]
Metals and electrolytes	a. Serum Iron and Iron-binding Capacity Increased in acute hepatitis and hemochromatosis Decreased in cirrhosis[b]	Diagnostic aid Clinical usefulness confirmed
	b. Serum Copper and Ceruloplasmin Decreased in Wilson's disease[b, c] (hepatolenticular degeneration)	Helpful in diagnostic investigation[a]
	c. Urine Copper Increased in Wilson's disease[a, b]	

[a]H. J. Zimmerman. Tests of hepatic function. In Davidsohn, Israel and Henry, John B. *Clinical Diagnosis by Laboratory Study*, 15th ed. Philadelphia: W. B. Saunders Co., 1974, pp. 804-835.

[b]*Bio-Science Handbook*, 11th ed. 1976, pp. 77-185.

[c]Graham H. Jeffries. Diseases of the liver. In Beeson, Paul B. and McDermott, Walsh (eds.). *Textbook of Medicine*, 14th ed. Philadelphia: W. B. Saunders Co., 1975, pp. 1324-1353.

ABBREVIATIONS

A. Related Primarily to Tests:

BA — barium

BAO — basal acid output

BSP — bromsulphalein

CCF — cephalin cholesterol flocculation

CEA — carcinoembryonic antigen

COH — carbohydrate

HAA — hepatitis Australia antigen, hepatitis associated antigen

GI — gastrointestinal

LAP — leucine aminopeptidase

MAO — maximal acid output

PP — postprandial (following a meal)

SAFP — serum alpha-fetoprotein

B. Related to Time-Schedule for Medications:

	Latin	English		Latin	English
ac	ante cibos	before meals	prn	pro re nata	as necessary
bid	bis in die	twice a day	qh	quaqua hora	every hour
hs	hora somni	at bed time	qid	quater in die	4 times a day
pc	post cibos	after meals	stat	statim	immediately
po	per os	by mouth	tid	ter in die	3 times a day

ORAL READING PRACTICE

Malignant Neoplasms of the Oral Cavity

Carcinomas of the mouth include malignant tumors of the lips, tongue and floor of the oral cavity. **Neoplastic** growth may be preceded by gradual development of irregular, white, raised patches known as **leukoplakia.** This condition starts as a chronic, painless inflammation of the **oral mucosa.** It is usually considered a premalignant lesion. Although its **etiology** is unknown, the relationship of tobacco and leukoplakia is a well established fact, since leukoplakia seen in heavy smokers tends to disappear after smoking has been discontinued. The white patches are due to a **keratinization** of the **epithelium.** Fissuring or **ulceration** in a leukoplakic area may be a diagnostic sign that malignant changes are in progress.[26, 45]

Tumors of the upper lip are generally **basal cell carcinomas** which tend to invade adjacent structures, but rarely metastasize. Prompt treatment is imperative.[62]

Carcinoma of the lower lip may show a widespread involvement of the **epidermoid (squamous cell)** type. In its early phase there is a fissure, flat ulcer or chronic leukoplakia which readily forms a **fungating** mass, malignant in character.[62]

Carcinoma of the tongue begins as a fissured ulcer with raised borders. Pain is not present until the cancer may have progressed and metastasized. The areas of **induration** are prone to extend with time. Spontaneous bleeding occurs from ulcerating crevices and is distressing to the patient. With increasing **infiltration** the movement of the tongue becomes restricted. Metastatic **adenopathy** may develop early or late and generally involves the **cervical** and **submaxillary** lymph nodes.[26, 45]

Any ulcer or newgrowth of the lips, tongue or floor of the mouth that does not heal with treatment in a three weeks' period should be **biopsied.** Suspicious lesions must receive prompt attention since progression to inoperability occurs before the patient feels pain.

The treatment of choice in carcinoma of the mouth is surgical removal of the lesion with or without irradiation or, if inoperable, **palliative** radiotherapy alone. For cancer of the lip a V-excision of the malignant lesion may be done to provide relief from discomfort and overcome disfigurement. Some surgeons treat metastatic cancer of the tongue with preoperative **supervoltage** radiotherapy to reduce the size of the tumor and subsequent **hemiglossectomy,** partial **mandibulectomy** and cervical lymph node **dissection.**[33, 89]

Table 19

SOME DIGESTIVE CONDITIONS AMENABLE TO SURGERY

Organ Involved	Diagnoses	Operations	Operative Procedures
Lip	Cleft lip	Cheiloplasty	Plastic repair of lip
Lip (lower)	Squamous cell carcinoma of lower lip	Eslander operation for carcinoma of the lower lip	V-excision of lesion-defect filled by a flap from the upper lip
Lip (upper)	Squamous cell or basal cell carcinoma of upper lip	Eslander operation for carcinoma of the upper lip	V-excision and replacement of operative defect by a triangular flap from the lower lip
Tongue	Epidermoid carcinoma and/or metastatic cervical adenopathy	Partial glossectomy Radical neck dissection or Cautery excision with radon seed implantation in selected cases	Wide excision of malignant lesion including the removal of the jugular vein, muscles of the neck, submaxillary and cervical lymph nodes

Organ Involved	Diagnoses	Operations	Operative Procedures
Parotid gland	Parotid tumor	Resection of parotid gland and tumor under direct vision	Y-shaped incision and dissection for skin flaps Partial removal of parotid gland with tumor keeping facial nerve intact
Parotid gland Facial nerve	Parotid tumor widely infiltrating, facial nerve embedded in tumor	Total parotidectomy Elective excision of facial nerve	Removal of entire gland and tumor including main trunk of facial nerve with plexus
Palate	Cleft palate	Staphylorrhaphy Palatoplasty	Suture of a cleft palate Reconstruction of a cleft palate
Floor of the mouth	Squamous cell carcinoma	Excision of lesion and/or Radiation therapy	Removal of neoplasm and/or irradiation
Tonsils, palatine	Hypertrophy of tonsils Chronic tonsillitis	Tonsillectomy	Removal of tonsils
Tonsils, pharyngeal	Adenoids	Adenoidectomy	Removal of adenoids
Esophagus	Esophageal lesion	Esophagoscopy with biopsy	Direct visualization of the esophagus with removal of bits of tissue
Esophagus	Diverticulum of esophagus	Diverticulectomy	Extirpation of the diverticulum
Esophagus Stomach	Carcinoma of esophagus of the midthoracic portion	Radical resection of the carcinomatous segment of the esophagus Esophagogastric anastomosis or interposition of segment of bowel	Excision of malignant lesion and regional lymph nodes Anastomosis of remaining esophagus and stomach or using a bowel segment as a substitute
Esophagus Stomach	Recurrent hiatus hernia	Repair of hiatus hernia, abdominal or thoracic approach	Direct vision reduction; sac sutured to under surface of diaphragm; inclusion of gastric wall in fixation
Stomach Pyloric muscle	Congenital hypertrophic stenosis of pyloric sphincter	Pyloromyotomy Fredet-Ramstedt operation	Section of hypertrophic pyloric muscle down to mucosa
Stomach	Gastric carcinoma, resectability unknown	Exploratory laparotomy	Opening the abdomen to determine operability of lesion
Stomach Duodenum Jejunum	Early carcinoma of stomach Malignant gastric lesion in upper stomach	Subtotal gastrectomy Gastroduodenostomy or Gastrojejunostomy or Esophagojejunostomy	Partial removal of stomach including lymph glands Joining remaining portion of stomach and duodenum Joining remaining portion of stomach and jejunum Transthoracic approach and esophagojejunal anastomosis

Organ Involved	Diagnoses	Operations	Operative Procedures
Stomach Duodenum Jejunum	Chronic or recurrent gastric ulcer with obstruction or hemorrhage	Gastric resection Billroth I or Billroth II Polya modification or Hofmeister modification	Partial removal of stomach and gastroduodenal anastomosis or gastrojejunal anastomosis using anterior approach or posterior approach
Stomach Duodenum	Duodenal ulcer	Selective vagotomy Mucosal antrectomy[a]	Complete vagal denervation of the stomach Excision of entire gastrin-secreting antral mucosa
Duodenum	Progressive duodenal ulcer with obstruction or hemorrhage	Complete bilateral vagotomy Pyloroplasty	Section of vagus nerve fibers before they enter the stomach Surgical repair of pyloric muscle
Duodenum Jejunum	Large duodenal perforation	Surgical reconstruction of perforated duodenum	Excision of duodenal ulcer Full thickness jejunal pedicle graft for closure of large duodenal defect
Jejunum Ileum	Morbid obesity Hyperlipidemia	Jejunoileal bypass[b]	Division of jejunum a few inches distal to ligament of Treitz, and ileum a few inches proximal to ileocecal valve End-to-end anastomosis to restore continuity Closure of distal jejunum Implantation of proximal ileum into transverse colon or into left colon
Ileum Colon	Regional enteritis	Resection of involved ileum and colon Enteroanastomosis	Radical extirpation of bowel involved in regional enteritis Surgical joining of remaining parts
Colon Ileum	Chronic ulcerative colitis with hemorrhage	Permanent ileostomy with total colectomy	Surgical creation of an ileal stoma for fecal drainage and removal of colon
Colon Cecum	Intestinal obstruction Cancer of left colon	Cecostomy Gibson's technique Transverse colostomy	Creating a communication between cecum and body surface for fecal drainage Diverting fecal content to the body surface
Appendix	Appendicitis	Appendectomy	Removal of appendix
Colon Rectum	Aganglionic megacolon (Hirschsprung's disease)	Modified Duhamel procedure or Modified Soave procedure[c]	Side-to-side colorectal anastomosis Endorectal pull-through of ganglionated bowel to anus

Organ Involved	Diagnoses	Operations	Operative Procedures
Rectosigmoid	Rectal hemorrhage, cause unknown	Rectosigmoidoscopy	Endoscopic examination of the rectosigmoid
Rectosigmoid	Carcinoma of rectum and low sigmoid	Abdomino-perineal resection Miles' operation	Sectioning of bowel above the tumor — creation of permanent colostomy — removal of bowel above and below tumor — excision of anus
Rectum	Hemorrhoids, internal anal or external	Hemorrhoidectomy	Removal of hemorrhoids
Peritoneum	Hernia, inguinal femoral umbilical ventral	Hernioplasty	Surgical repair of hernia
Liver	Hepatic necrosis Hepatic failure Hepatic coma	Exchange transfusion[d] (fresh blood)	Construction of arteriovenous shunt Priming the exchange transfusion circuit Exchange of equal volume of blood
Gallbladder	Cholecystitis Cholelithiasis	Cholecystectomy	Removal of gallbladder
Bile duct	Benign stricture of bile duct	Repair of biliary stricture by end-to-end anastomosis of bile duct	Excision of constricted part and surgical communication of the two ends of the bile duct

[a] R. M. Kirk et al. Vagotomy and mucosal antrectomy in the elective treatment of duodenal ulcers. *American Journal of Surgery*, 123: 323-328, March, 1972.

[b] G. A. Bray *et al.* Intestinal bypass operation as a treatment of obesity. *Annals of Internal Medicine*, 85: 97-109, July, 1976.

[c] J. J. Corkery. Hirschsprung's disease. *Clinics in Gastroenterology*, 4: 531-544, September, 1975.

[d] G. M. Abouna. Improved technique of exchange transfusion for hepatic coma. *Surgery-Gynecology & Obstetrics*, 134: 658-662, April, 1972.

REFERENCES AND BIBLIOGRAPHY

1. Abbey, L. M. Solitary intraductal papilloma of the minor salivary glands. *Oral Surgery — Oral Medicine — Oral Pathology*, 40: 135-141, July, 1975.
2. Abcarian, H. Lateral internal sphincterotomy — A new technique for treatment of chronic fissure-in-ano. *Surgical Clinics of North America*, 55: 143-150, February, 1975.
3. Almy, T. P. Disorders of motility. In Beeson, Paul B. and McDermott, Walsh (eds.) *Textbook of Medicine*, 14th ed. Philadelphia: W. B. Saunders Co., 1975, pp. 1178-1197.
4. Ament, M. E. Intestinal malabsorption. In Vaughan, Victor C. (ed.). *Nelson Textbook of Pediatrics*, 10th ed. Philadelphia: W. B. Saunders Co., 1975, pp. 846-860.
5. Anane-Sefah, J. Operative choice and technique following pancreatic injury. *Archives of Surgery*, 110: 161-166, February, 1975.
6. Andrassy, R. J. *et al.* Liver failure after jejuno-ileal shunt. *Archives of Surgery*, 110: 332-334, March, 1975.
7. Apple, M. F. Colonoscopy: Its principles and applications. *Southern Medical Journal*, 68: 717-718, June, 1975.
8. Arvanitakis, C. Achalasia of the esophagus: A reappraisal of esophagomyomotomy vs forceful pneumatic dilation. *Digestive Diseases*, 20: 841-848, September, 1975.
9. Bartlett, M. K. *et al.* The removal of biliary duct stones. *Surgical Clinics of North America*, 54: 599-611, June, 1974.

10. Bears, O. H. Complications of surgery for cancer of the head and neck. In Artz, Curtis P. and Hardy, James D. *Management of Surgical Complications*, 3rd ed. Philadelphia: W. B. Saunders Co., 1975, pp. 277-290.

11. Beeler, M. F. *et al.* Laboratory evaluation of pancreatic disorders — The examination of feces. In Davidsohn, Israel and Henry, John B. *Clinical Diagnosis by Laboratory Methods*, 15th ed. Philadelphia: W. B. Saunders Co., 1974, pp. 870-920.

12. Behringer, G. E. Polypoid lesions of the colon. *Surgical Clinics of North America*, 54: 699-712, June, 1974.

13. Binder, S. C. *et al.* Emergency and urgent operations for ulcerative colitis. *Archives of Surgery*, 110: 284-292, March, 1975.

14. Black, M. Drug-induced hepatitis. *Emergency Medicine*, 7: 79-82, April, 1975.

15. Blocksma, R. *et al.* A conservative program for managing cleft palate without the use of mucoperiosteal flaps. *Plastic and Reconstructive Surgery*, 55: 160-169, February, 1975.

16. Blumgart, L. H. Endoscopy of the upper gastrointestinal tract. In Longmire, W. P. (ed.). *Advances in Surgery*, Vol. IX. Chicago: Year Book Medical Publishers, 1975, pp. 97-138.

17. Bombeck, C. T. Intraoperative esophagoscopy, gastroscopy, colonoscopy and endoscopy of the small bowel. *Surgical Clinics of North America*, 55: 135-142, February, 1975.

18. Bordos, D. C. Successful long-term intravenous hyperalimentation in the hospital and at home. *Archives of Surgery*, 110: 439-441, April, 1975.

19. Braasch, J. W. Periampullary carcinoma. *Medical Clinics of North America*, 59: 309-314, March, 1975.

20. Brandborg, L. L. Neoplasms of the esophagus — Malignant neoplasms of the stomach — Benign neoplasms of the stomach. In Beeson, Paul B. and McDermott, W. (eds.). *Textbook of Medicine*, 14th ed. Philadelphia: W. B. Saunders Co., 1975, pp. 1290-1297.

21. Bray, G. A. *et al.* Intestinal bypass operation as a treatment of obesity. *Annals of Internal Medicine*, 85: 97-109, July, 1976.

22. Buchwald, H. *et al.* Partial ileal bypass for hyperlipidemia and jejunoileal bypass for obesity. *Current Problems in Surgery.* Chicago: Year Book Medical Publishers Inc., April, 1975, pp. 4-51.

23. Cannon, D. C. Examinations of gastric and duodenal contents. In Davidsohn, Israel and Henry, John Bernard. *Clinical Diagnosis by Laboratory Methods*, 15th ed. Philadelphia: W. B. Saunders Co., 1974, pp. 887-904.

24. Carbone, J. V. *et al.* Nonspecific manifestations. In Krupp, Marcus A. and Chatton, Milton J. *Current Medical Diagnosis & Treatment.* Los Altos: Lange Medical Publications, 1976, pp. 321-328.

25. _____. Diseases of the mouth — Diseases of the esophagus. *Ibid.*, pp. 328-339.

26. _____. Diseases of the stomach — Diseases of the intestines. *Ibid.*, pp. 339-360.

27. _____. Diseases of the colon and rectum — Diseases of the anus. *Ibid.*, pp. 361-370.

28. _____. Diseases of the liver and biliary tract. *Ibid.*, pp. 370-398.

29. Carlsen, E. N. Liver, gallbladder and spleen. *Radiologic Clinics of North America*, 13: 543-556, December, 1975.

30. Chan, C. H. Primary carcinoma of the liver. *Medical Clinics of North America*, 59: 989-994, July, 1975.

31. Chong, G. C. *et al.* Management of parotid gland tumors in infants and children. *Mayo Clinic Proceedings*, 50: 279-283, May, 1975.

32. Christie, J. P. *et al.* Indications for fiberoptic colonoscopy. *Southern Medical Journal*, 68: 881-886, July, 1975.

33. Conley, J. Radical neck dissection. *The Laryngoscope*, 85: 1344-1352, August, 1975.

34. Cooperman, A. M. *et al.* Pyloroplasty. *Surgical Clinics of North America*, 55: 1019-1024, October, 1975.

35. _____. Highly selective vagotomy. *Ibid.*, 55: 1089-1102, October, 1975.

36. Copeland, E. M. *et al.* Intravenous hyperalimentation in patients with head and neck cancer. *Cancer*, 35: 606-611, March, 1975.

37. Corkery, J. J. Hirschsprung's disease. *Clinics in Gastroenterology*, 4: 531-544, September, 1975.

38. Cosman, B. Pharyngeal flap augmentation. *Plastic and Reconstructive Surgery*, 55: 149-155, February, 1975.

39. Davidsohn, Israel and Henry, John B. Table of normal values. *Clinical Diagnosis by Laboratory Methods*, 15th ed. Philadelphia: W. B. Saunders Co., 1974, pp. 1376-1392.

40. Deatsch, W. W. Ear, nose & throat. In Krupp, Marcus A. and Chatton, Milton. *Current Medical Diagnosis and Treatment*, 14th ed. Los Altos, California: Lange Medical Publications, 1976, pp. 100-105.

41. Derezin, M. The upper G.I. bleeder — Looking in from the outside. *Emergency Medicine*, 7: 31-33, April, 1975.

42. Diamond, D. *et al.* Pancreatic cancer. *Surgical Clinics of North America*, 55: 363-376, April, 1975.

43. Dodsworth, J. M. *et al.* Surgical therapy of chronic peptic ulcer. *Surgical Clinics of North America*, 54: 529-547, June, 1974.

44. Donner, M. W. Frontiers in gastrointestinal radiology. In Potchen, E. James. *Current Concepts in Radiology*, Vol. II. St. Louis: C. V. Mosby Co., 1975, pp. 230-257.

45. El-Domeiri, A. A. *et al.* Management of oral and pharyngeal cancer: A multidisciplinary approach. *Surgical Clinics of North America*, 55: 107-116, February, 1975.

46. Elliot, D. W. Pancreatic pseudocysts. *Surgical Clinics of North America*, 55: 339-362, April, 1975.

47. Finch, C. A. Hemochromatosis. In Conn, Howard F. (ed.). *Current Therapy, 1976.* Philadelphia: W. B. Saunders Co., 1976, pp. 289-290.

48. Fischer, J. E. The management of high-output intestinal fistulas. In Longmire, William P. (ed.). *Advances in Surgery*, Vol. IX. Chicago: Year Book Medical Publishers Inc., 1975, pp. 139-176.

49. Friday, R. O. *et al.* Detection and localization of intra-abdominal abscesses by diagnostic ultrasound. *Archives of Surgery,* 110: 335-337, March, 1975.

50. Glenn, F. *et al.* Calculous biliary tract disease. *Current Problems in Surgery.* Chicago: Year Book Medical Publishers Inc., June, 1975, pp. 4-37.

51. Gutierrez, J. G. Use of secretin in hypotonic duodenography. *Radiology,* 113: 563-566, December, 1974.

52. Hartwell, S. W. Surgical treatment of cervical esophagostomy. *Surgical Clinics of North America,* 55: 1103-1105, October, 1975.

53. Hatafuka, T. *et al.* Fundic patch operation in the treatment of advanced achalasia of the esophagus. *Surgery Gynecology & Obstetrics,* 134: 617-624, April, 1972.

54. Hawkins, I. F. *et al.* Radiologic approach to obstructive jaundice and pancreatic disease. *Medical Clinics of North America,* 59: 121-143, January, 1975.

55. Hebert, G. *et al.* Hepatic echography. *American Journal of Roentgenology-Radium Therapy and Nuclear Medicine,* 125: 51-59, September, 1975.

56. Heimlich, H. J. Esophagoplasty with reversed gastric tube. Review of fifty-three cases. *American Journal of Surgery,* 123: 80-92, January, 1972.

57. Herman, R. E. Shunt operations for portal hypertension. *Surgical Clinics of North America,* 55: 1073-1088, October, 1975.

58. Hightower, N. C. Applied anatomy and physiology of esophagus. In Bockus, Henry (ed.). *Gastroenterology,* 3rd ed. Philadelphia: W. B. Saunders Co., 1974, pp. 127-142.

59. Inberg, M. V. *et al.* Surgical treatment of gastric carcinoma. *Archives of Surgery,* 110: 703-707, June, 1975.

60. Janowitz, H. D. Inflammatory diseases of the intestine. In Beeson, Paul B. and McDermott, Walsh (eds.). *Textbook of Medicine,* 14th ed. Philadelphia: W. B. Saunders Co., 1975, pp. 1256-1274.

61. Jeffries, G. H. Diseases of the liver. In Beeson, Paul B. and McDermott, Walsh (eds.). *Textbook of Medicine,* 14th ed. Philadelphia: W. B. Saunders Co., 1975, pp. 1324-1353.

62. Kelly, D. E. Lip reconstruction following resection of an unusual basal-cell carcinoma. *Oral Surgery — Oral Medicine — Oral Pathology,* 40: 19-26, July, 1975.

63. Klaude, J. V. Hepatomegaly — Radiology in Internal Medicine. *Medical Clinics of North America,* 59: 145-167, January, 1975.

64. Knowlessar, O. D. Diseases of the pancreas. In Beeson, Paul B. and McDermott, Walsh (eds.). *Textbook of Medicine,* 14th ed. Philadelphia: W. B. Saunders Co., 1975, pp. 1243-1255.

65. Larrain, A. *et al.* Surgical correction of reflux — An effective therapy for esophageal stricture. *Gastroenterology,* 69: 578-583, September, 1975.

66. Leey, C. H. *et al.* Liver disease of the alcoholic. *Medical Clinics of North America,* 59: 909-918, July, 1975.

67. Maddrey, W. C. *et al.* Chronic hepatic encephalopathy. *Medical Clinics of North America,* 59: 937-944, July, 1975.

68. Malt, R. A. Emergency and elective operations for bleeding esophageal varices. *Surgical Clinics of North America,* 54: 561-571, June, 1974.

69. ————. Rectal carcinoma: Abdominoperineal and anterior resections. *Ibid.,* pp. 741-750.

70. McCormick, J. S. C. *et al.* The operative cholangiogram. *Annals of Surgery,* 180: 902-906, December, 1974.

71. Menguy, R. Stomach. In Schwartz, Seymour I. (ed.). *Principles of Surgery,* 2d ed. New York: McGraw-Hill Book Co., 1974, pp. 1049-1088.

72. O'Brien, T. F. Neoplasms of the small intestine — Neoplasms of the large intestine. In Beeson, Paul B. and McDermott, Walsh. *Textbook of Medicine,* 14th ed. Philadelphia: W. B. Saunders Co., 1975, pp. 1297-1302.

73. Ockner, R. K. Vascular diseases of the intestine — Diseases of the peritoneum, mesentery and omentum. In Beeson, Paul B. and McDermott, Walsh (eds.). *Textbook of Medicine,* 14th ed. Philadelphia: W. B. Saunders Co., 1975, pp. 1281-1290.

74. Orloff, M. J. Emergency treatment for bleeding esophageal varices. *Hospital Physician,* 4: 28-37, April, 1975.

75. ————. The liver — The biliary system. In Sabiston, David C. (ed.). *Davis — Christopher Textbook of Surgery,* 10th ed. Philadelphia: W. B. Saunders Co., 1972, pp. 1003-1091.

76. Ottinger, L. W. Clinical management of hiatus hernias and gastroesophageal reflux. *Surgical Clinics of North America,* 54: 475-488, June, 1974.

77. Payne, W. S. *et al.* Complications of esophageal and diaphragmatic surgery. In Artz, Curtis P. and Hardy, James D. *Management of Surgical Complications,* 3rd ed. Philadelphia: W. B. Saunders Co., 1975, pp. 326-357.

78. Pilla, Lawrence A., M.D. Personal communications.

79. Powers, J. H. Proctosigmoidoscopy in private practice. *Journal of American Medical Association,* 231: 750-751, February 17, 1975.

80. Raskin, J. B. Recent developments in gastrointestinal endoscopy. *Postgraduate Medicine,* 57: 85-91, January, 1975.

81. Resnick, R. H. Portal hypertension. *Medical Clinics of North America,* 59: 945-954, July, 1975.

82. Robbins, Stanley L. The gastrointestinal tract. *Pathologic Basis of Disease.* Philadelphia: W. B. Saunders Co., 1974, pp. 901-984.

83. ————. The liver and biliary tract. *Ibid.,* pp. 985-1055.

84. ————. The pancreas. *Ibid.,* pp. 1056-1077.

85. Rodkey, G. V. Colonic diverticular disease with surgical treatment. *Surgical Clinics of North America,* 54: 655-674, June, 1974.

86. Roth, J. L. Indications for operation and selection of operative procedure for peptic ulcer. In Bockus, Henry (ed.). *Gastroenterology,* 3rd ed. Philadelphia: W. B. Saunders Co., 1974, pp. 871-887.

87. ————. Achalasia and other motor disorders of the esophagus. *Ibid.,* pp. 191-246.

88. _____. Reflux esophagitis and esophageal ulcer. *Ibid.*, pp. 247-288.

89. Rush, B. F. Tumors of the head and neck. In Schwartz, Seymour I. (ed.). *Principles of Surgery*, 2d ed. New York: McGraw-Hill Book Co., 1974, pp. 555-593.

90. Scharschmidt, B. F. Approaches to the management of fulminant hepatic failure. *Medical Clinics of North America*, 59: 927-935, July, 1975.

91. Schwartz, Seymour I. Gallbladder and extrahepatic biliary system. In *Principles of Surgery*, 2d ed. New York: McGraw-Hill Book Co., 1974, pp. 1221-1254.

92. Sherwin, Charles S., M.D. Personal communications.

93. Sleisenger, M. H. Diseases of malabsorption. In Beeson, Paul B. and McDermott, W. (eds.). *Textbook of Medicine*, 14th ed. Philadelphia: W. B. Saunders Co., 1975, pp. 1217-1243.

94. *Specialized Diagnostic Laboratory Tests*, 11th ed. Van Nuys, California: Bio-Science Laboratories, 1976, pp. 77-185.

95. Steichen, F. M. Hepatic trauma in adults. *Surgical Clinics of North America*, 55: 387-407, April, 1975.

96. Storer, E. H. Small intestine. In Schwartz, Seymour I. (ed.). *Principles of Surgery*, 2d ed. New York: McGraw-Hill Book Co., 1974, pp. 1090-1107.

97. Stremple, J. F. Gastrinomas: Gastrin-producing tumors. *Surgical Clinics of North America*, 55: 303-324, April, 1975.

98. Sun, D. C. *et al.* Tests employed in analysis of the stomach contents and their clinical application. In Bockus, Henry I. (ed.). *Gastroenterology*, 3rd ed. Philadelphia: W. B. Saunders Co., 1974, pp. 419-453.

99. Talbert, J. L. Corrosive strictures of the esophagus. In Sabiston, David C. (ed.). *Davis — Christopher Textbook of Surgery*, 10th ed. Philadelphia: W. B. Saunders Co., 1972, pp. 755-760.

100. Thomas, T. V. Restoration of cardioesophageal competence. *Postgraduate Medicine*, 51: 171-175, March, 1972.

101. Thompson, J. C. The stomach and duodenum. In Sabiston, David C. (ed.). *Davis — Christopher Textbook of Surgery*, 10th ed. Philadelphia: W. B. Saunders Co., 1972, pp. 817-859.

102. Vilardell, F. Exfoliative cytology in gastric disorders. In Bockus, Henry L. (ed.). *Gastroenterology*, 3rd ed. Philadelphia: W. B. Saunders Co., 1974, pp. 475-486.

103. Wallack, M. K. *et al.* Cancer of the colon and rectum. *Postgraduate Medicine*, 57: 99-105, April, 1975.

104. Warren, W. D. *et al.* The pancreas. In Sabiston, David C. (ed.). *Davis — Christopher Textbook of Surgery*. Philadelphia: W. B. Saunders Co., 1972, pp. 1092-1121.

105. Way, L. W. Diseases of the gallbladder and bile ducts. In Beeson, Paul B. and McDermott, Walsh. *Textbook of Medicine*, 14th ed. Philadelphia: W. B. Saunders Co., 1975, pp. 1308-1324.

106. Webster, M. W. Current management of esophageal varices. *Surgical Clinics of North America*, 55: 461-472, April, 1975.

107. Weinshelbaum, E. I. Applied anatomy of the stomach. In Bockus, Henry L. (ed.). *Gastroenterology*, 3rd ed. Philadelphia: W. B. Saunders Co., 1974, pp. 389-404.

108. Weir, Don C., M.D. Personal communications.

109. Weisman, M. I. The importance of biopsy in endodontics. *Oral Surgery — Oral Medicine — Oral Pathology*, 40: 153-155, July, 1975.

110. Wheelock, F. C. Surgical management of regional ileitis, ulcerative colitis and granulomatous colitis. *Surgical Clinics of North America*, 54: 675-688, June, 1974.

111. Workshop on Tonsillectomy and Adenoidectomy. *Annals of Otology-Rhinology & Laryngology*, Supplement 19, 84: 7-79, March-April, 1975.

112. Yellin, A. E. *et al.* Pancreatoduodenectomy for combined pancreatoduodenal injuries. *Archives of Surgery*, 110: 1177-1183, October, 1975.

113. Zimmerman, H. J. Liver disease caused by medicinal agents. *Medical Clinics of North America*, 59: 897-907, July, 1975.

114. Zollinger, Robert M. and Zollinger, Robert M., Jr. Gastrointestinal procedures. *Atlas of Surgical Operations*, 4th ed. New York: Macmillan Publishing Co., Inc., 1975, pp. 22-217.

Chapter IX
Urogenital Disorders

KIDNEYS

A. Origin of Terms:

1. calyx (G) — cup
2. cortex (L) — rind, outer
      portion
3. glomerulus (L) — little skein
4. medulla (L) — marrow, inner
      portion
5. nephron (G) — kidney
6. ren (L) — kidney

B. Anatomic Terms:[51, 66]

1. kidneys — paired, bean-shaped organs situated behind the peritoneum on either side of the lumbar spine.   Their function is to preserve the ionic balance of the blood and extract its waste products.
2. nephron, renal tubule — the functional unit of the kidney which is composed of a
   a. glomerular capsule, Bowman's capsule — a double-layered envelope of epithelium which encloses a capillary tuft.   It filters water and solutes out of the blood into the tubule.
   b. glomerulus (pl. glomeruli) — capillary cluster or tuft which is concerned with the initial phase of urine formation.
   c. renal corpuscle — both glomerular capsule and glomerulus.
   d. secretory tubule — tubule which completes urine formation and is functionally divided into a proximal tubule, a thin segment and a distal tubule or thick segment.
   e. collecting tubule — tubule which conveys urine to the renal pelvis.
3. renal cortex — outer portion of the kidney.
4. renal medulla — inner portion of the kidney containing the renal pyramids which include collecting tubules and parts of the secretory tubules.
5. renal papillae — apices of the pyramids which indent the calices.
6. renal pelvis — funnel-shaped enlargement of the ureter as it leaves the kidney.   It contains
   a. calices, formerly calyces (sing. calyx) — cuplike indentations in the kidney pelvis. The collecting tubules open into the calices.
   b. hilus — a notch on the medial surface of the kidney through which the ureter and blood vessels enter or leave the kidney.

C. Diagnostic Terms:

1. acute tubular necrosis of kidney, acute reversible renal failure — a cellular necrosis affecting the renal tubules following shock, trauma, nephrotoxic damage, transfusion reaction, septicemia and other causes.[38, 41, 51]
2. arteriolar nephrosclerosis — renal disorder characterized by an intimal thickening of the afferent glomerular arterioles resulting in a narrowing of the arteriolar lumen and reduced blood supply to nephrons.
   a. benign type — common nephropathy with benign hypertension.
   b. malignant type — uncommon nephropathy with malignant hypertension.[33, 51]
3. congenital anomalies of kidneys:
   a. agenesis — absence of one kidney.
   b. dysplasia — multicystic kidney forming an irregular mass.
   c. ectopy — displaced kidney, usually low in position.[41]
   d. vascular abnormalities — aberrant arteries or veins sometimes compressing the ureter thus causing hydronephrosis.

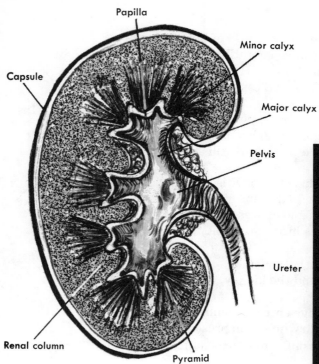

Fig. 52 – Longitudinal section of kidney.

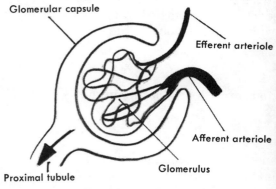

Fig. 53 – Structure of renal corpuscle.

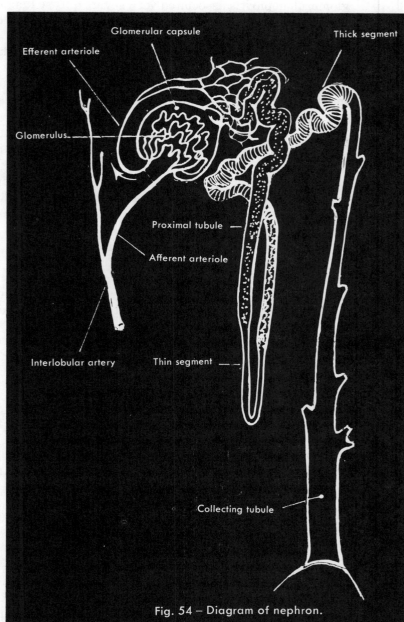

Fig. 54 – Diagram of nephron.

4. glomerulonephritis — form of nephritis involving the renal glomeruli of both kidneys. There is evidence that the glomeruli may be injured by antigen-antibody complexes which develop from the immune responses to streptococcal infection. Hypertension, headache, malaise, puffiness around the eyes, oliguria; blood, protein and casts in the urine are common clinical findings.[33, 34, 85]

5. Goodpasture's syndrome, antiglomerular basement membrane nephritis — acute glomerulonephritis associated with severe diffuse lung disease, hemorrhagic and inflammatory, involving the basement membranes of the glomeruli and lungs. Recovery is rare.[34]

6. hereditary nephritis, Alport's syndrome — familial glomerulonephritis associated with defective hearing and sight. Renal failure may be the final event in males.[15, 62, 85]

7. hydronephrosis — accumulation of fluid chiefly in pelvis and calices, resulting in enlargement of kidney and pressure atrophy. If fluid becomes infected, pyonephrosis develops.[71, 72]

8. infections of the kidney:
   a. abscess of kidney — usually a focal suppuration of the cortex.
   b. perinephric abscess, perinephritis — infection around the kidney.
   c. pyelonephritis — bacterial kidney infection.
      (1) acute form, commonly caused by gram-negative enteric bacilli.
      (2) chronic form, generally no symptoms of urinary infection present.[18, 33, 35, 49, 55, 82]

9. injuries to the kidney — uncommon pathologic lesions usually due to athletic, occupational and traffic accidents. They comprise:
   a. avulsion — separation of kidney from blood supply.
   b. contusions — simple bruising of functional tissue of kidney.
   c. ecchymoses — black and blue spots of kidney substance due to escape of blood.
   d. fissures — slits in renal capsule or pelvis, may cause hematuria.
   e. hematoma — a local mass of clotted blood which may develop especially after injury to renal pelvis.
   f. lacerations — tears may involve renal pelvis and renal capsule and result in severe hematuria.
   g. rupture — an extensive tear of the kidney may be the cause of massive bleeding and death.[13, 64, 65, 69]

10. interstitial nephritis — renal disease in which the interstitial connective tissue is involved. Its acute form appears to be a reaction to systemic infection or drug sensitivity; its chronic form exhibits a diffuse interstitial fibrosis and widespread atrophy of the renal tubules.[34, 47]

11. neoplasms of the kidney
    a. benign tumors:
       (1) cortical adenoma — small nodule or papillomatous growth originating in the renal tubule and embedded in the renal cortex.
       (2) fibroma, lipoma and others
    b. malignant tumors:
       (1) embryoma, nephroblastoma, Wilms' tumor — neoplasm common in children, infrequent in adults; may form huge abdominal mass which exerts pressure on functional renal tissue and metastasizes to the lungs, liver, bones and brain.
       (2) renal cell carcinoma, hypernephroid carcinoma, Grawitz tumor — tumor clinically manifested by a palpable mass, hematuria and pain in the costovertebral region. Widespread metastases are common.[27, 37, 51, 58, 73]

12. nephrolithiasis, renal calculi — stones in the kidney, generally in the pelvis and calices. They may be caused by renal tubular syndromes, enzyme disorders, hypercalcemia, increased uric acid and other factors.[51, 69, 83]

13. nephropathy — any disease of the kidney such as the nephropathy of
    a. acute hyperuricemia — disorder resulting from a sudden high increase of serum uric acid level prone to occur in patients receiving massive antineoplastic therapy for lymphoma or leukemia.[59]

    b. hypercalcemia — abnormal increase in serum calcium associated with hypercalciuria, renal calculi and pyelonephritis. In its early phase polyuria and tubular injury are present, in its late phase there is progressive renal insufficiency.[59]

    c. hypercalcemia crisis — serum calcium 15 - 20 mg/dl (formerly mg/100 ml) or more; may lead to renal failure.[59]

    d. potassium depletion — inability of kidneys to concentrate urine due to potassium deficiency.

14. nephroptosis — a movable, floating kidney which is displaced downward.

15. nephrotic syndrome — clinical state characterized by massive edema, excessive loss of protein in urine and low albumin blood levels. It may develop during the course of glomerulonephritis, a collagen disease, toxic drug reaction or specific allergy.[34, 51, 85]

16. obstructive uropathy — obstruction occurring anywhere along the urinary tract from the renal pelvis to the external urethral meatus, causing changes in renal function, volume of urine and amount of protein and sediment in urine. Obstructive lesions include renal, ureteral, vesical and urethral calculi, strictures, prostatic lesions all of which may lead to hydronephrosis and renal failure.[46, 71]

17. renal artery occlusion — acute blockage of renal artery due to embolus, thrombus or other cause. The kidney is deprived of its blood supply when the occlusion is complete. Renal infarction and renal failure are rare complications.[13, 20]

18. renal calcinosis, nephrocalcinosis — scattered foci of calcification within functional renal tissue.

19. renal cystic diseases — hereditary kidney diseases presenting various cystic lesions of the medulla or cortex. They may be solitary cysts, simple, multilocular and of the dermoid type or polycysts replacing and compressing normal renal tissue and associated with cystic disease of the liver and pancreas[34, 41, 56, 67]

20. renal failure and related disorders:

    a. azotemia — a biochemical abnormality characterized by impaired renal function, an increase of blood urea nitrogen, and creatinine associated with retention of nitrogenous wastes in the blood. When in addition to the biochemical abnormality clinical manifestations are present, uremia is the proper term to be used.[51]

    b. renal failure, acute — clinical state marked by a sudden decrease in glomerular filtration rate and cessation of renal function subsequent to severe kidney damage due to toxins, disease or trauma. Renal tubular necrosis is a dominant characteristic. The lumen of the renal tubules is occluded by debris usually containing protein, epithelial cells and hemoglobin. If the initial oliguric phase is followed by a diuretic phase the patient recovers. Residual damage is common.[1, 4, 51]

    c. renal failure, chronic — clinical state resulting from irreversible slowly progressive renal disorder such as chronic glomerulonephritis or pyelonephritis, drug toxicity, systemic disease or urinary tract obstruction. Marked glomerular damage, as evidenced by electrolyte imbalance and retention of nitrogenous wastes, signals a fatal prognosis.[2, 31, 39, 51]

    d. uremia — syndrome resulting from greatly reduced excretory function in progressive bilateral kidney disease. Clinical symptoms vary widely from lassitude and depression in the early phase to anuria, uremic frost and peripheral neuropathy in the terminal phase.[51]

21. renal hypertension, renovascular hypertension — high blood pressure of kidney resulting from marked thickening of arteriolar walls or stenosis of renal artery by atheromatous plaques and thrombi. It is not known why the ischemic kidney elevates the blood pressure.[70]

22. renal medullary necrosis, renal papillary necrosis — tissue death of renal papillae and medulla, usually a complication of pyelonephritis.[34]

23. renal tuberculosis — degeneration of kidney substance due to infection with tubercle bacilli.[51]

24. renal vein thrombosis — occlusion of the renal vein by a thrombus which may result in an

elevation of the renal pressure, excessive proteinuria and other manifestations of the nephrotic syndrome.   A complete occlusion of the renal vein may be complicated by a hemorrhagic infarction of the kidney.[67, 86]

D. Operative Terms:

1. nephrectomy — excision of kidney primarily for advanced calculous pyonephrosis, hydronephrosis or malignant tumor.
2. nephrolithotomy — incision into kidney for removal of stones.
3. nephrolysis — surgical destruction of renal adhesions.
4. nephropexy — surgical fixation of a displaced kidney.
5. nephrorrhaphy — suture of an injured kidney.
6. nephrostomy — surgical creation of a renal fistula for drainage.
7. nephrotomy — incision into kidney.
8. nephroureterectomy — removal of ureter and kidney for tumor of the renal pelvis or for malignant tumor of the ureter.[2]
9. pyelolithotomy — incision into renal pelvis for removal of calculi.
10. pyeloplasty — plastic repair of renal pelvis.
11. pyelotomy — incision into renal pelvis.
12. renal biopsy, kidney biopsy, percutaneous renal biopsy — removal of renal tissue by a pronged biopsy needle.   The procedure, usually performed under fluoroscopic control, aids in the diagnosis and prognosis of renal disease and serves as guide in its therapeutic management.[34]
13. renal transplantation, kidney transplantation — a form of replacement surgery in which a healthy donor kidney is implanted in a patient after his irreversibly diseased kidneys have been removed.   The renal homograft may be obtained from a living donor or from a cadaver of a person who met with a fatal accident.   Bilateral nephrectomies are imperative in the presence of renal infection or severe hematuria since invariably the donor transplant will develop the disease of the collateral recipient's kidney if only one kidney has been removed.   After the donated homograft is placed extraperitoneally, vascular anastomoses to the iliac vessels and hypogastric artery are performed and an opening is surgically created between a ureter and the bladder (ureteroneo-cystostomy).[2, 11, 32, 36, 54]
14. surgery for renovascular hypertension — operative procedures for the restoration of normal blood flow to the kidney:
    a. bypass grafting for unilateral or bilateral renal artery stenosis.
    b. excision of occluded lesion of renal artery followed by end-to-end anastomosis.
    c. renal endarterectomy or surgical removal of intimal plaques from renal artery with or without patch grafting.[70]

E. Symptomatic Terms:

1. anuria — total suppression of urine due to renal failure or blockage of urinary tract.
2. Dietl's crisis — recurrent attacks of lumbar and abdominal pain, nausea and vomiting, caused by ureteral kinking or by vascular tension in cases of hypermobile kidney.
3. renal insufficiency, renal shut-down, lower nephron nephrosis — severe disturbance of excretory kidney function in renal disease or following surgery or trauma.   Anuria may develop from blood transfusions, overhydration and electrolyte imbalance.[64]
4. renal pain — various degrees from dull, aching to severe, stabbing or throbbing pain in lumbar region.
5. uremic frost — powdery deposit of urea on the skin due to the excretion of urea through perspiration.

URETERS

A. Origin of Terms:

1. junction (L) — joining
2. pyelo- (G) — pelvis, tub
3. pyo- (G) — pus
4. ureterovesical junction — meeting point

B. Anatomic Terms: [51, 66]

    1. ureter — muscular, distensible tube lined with mucous membrane. It carries urine from each kidney to the bladder.

    2. ureteric orifice — opening of the ureter at the outer, upper angle of the trigone (base) of the urinary bladder.

    3. ureteropelvic junction — meeting point between ureter and renal pelvis.

    4. ureterovesical junction — meeting point between ureter and urinary bladder.

C. Diagnostic Terms:

    1. calculus in ureter — ureteral stone causing obstruction.

    2. congenital malformations of the ureter:
        a. duplication of ureters — the most common ureteral abnormality.
           There are two kinds:
           (1) complete duplication — both ureters enter bladder on the same side.
           (2) incomplete duplication — ureters join supravesically.[41]
        b. ectopic ureteral orifice — displaced opening, a developmental defect seen more frequently in women than men. It may result in incontinence.[5, 72]
        c. incomplete ureter — embryonic development ceased before ureter reached kidney. Kidney may be absent or multicystic.
        d. stricture of ureter — abnormal narrowing of the duct, usually at the
           (1) uteropelvic junction or
           (2) ureterovesical orifice.
           It may be complicated by ureteral dilatation and hydronephrosis. The condition may be acquired.[5, 72]
        e. ureterocele — cystic protrusion or ballooning of lower end of ureter into bladder. It may be asymptomatic or obstructive, complicated by ureteral dilatation and hydronephrosis.[72]

    3. hydroureter — ureter overdistended with urine due to obstruction.[52]

    4. injuries to ureter — uncommon pathologic states which may be due to external trauma, be associated with pelvic fractures or occur inadvertently during surgery. A penetrating wound from a bullet may perforate a ureter and result in leakage of urine into the peritoneal cavity.[69]

    5. obstruction of ureter — blocking of ureter, usually resulting from pressure. It interferes with passage of urine.

    6. occlusion of ureter — complete or partial closure of ureter.

    7. pyoureter — infection in the ureter, generally secondary to infection of the bladder or kidney.

    8. ureteritis — inflammation of the ureter.

D. Operative Terms:

    1. ureteral resection — local excision of benign ureteral lesion.

    2. ureterectomy — partial or complete removal of ureter.

    3. ureterocystostomy, ureteroneocystostomy — reimplantation of ureter into bladder.[69]

    4. ureterolithotomy — incision into ureter for removal of calculi.[69]

    5. ureterolysis — freeing the ureter from adhesions to relieve secondary obstruction.

    6. ureteropelvioplasty — plastic operation at the ureteropelvic junction.

    7. ureteropyelostomy — anastomosis of ureter and renal pelvis.

    8. ureterostomy, cutaneous — transplantation of ureter to skin.[68]

    9. ureterovesicoplasty — corrective surgery for persistent reflux by repair of the ureterovesical junction.[71]

E. Symptomatic Terms:

    1. ureteral colic — excruciating, stabbing pain usually caused by the passage of a stone or

large clot into the ureter.   It may be accompanied by prostration, diaphoresis, shock and collapse.[74]

2. ureteral spasm — contraction of ureter, frequently resulting from painful overdistention of ureter by stone.

BLADDER AND URETHRA

A. Origin of Terms:

1. cysto- (G) — bladder
2. trigone (G) — triangle
3. urethra (G) — urethra
4. vesica (L) — bladder

B. Anatomic Terms:[52, 66]

1. bladder, urinary — a hollow, muscular, distensible organ.   It serves as a temporary reservoir for urine.
2. detrusor urinae muscle — a muscular network with bundles of muscle fibers running in various directions, intermingling and decussating.   Their contraction effects the expulsion of urine from the bladder.[66]
3. neck of bladder — lowest angle of bladder.
4. vesical sphincter — thickened detrusor muscle fibers which surround the bladder neck.
5. trigone — triangular internal surface of the posterior wall of the bladder.
6. urethra — fibromuscular channel of communication between the urinary bladder and external urethral orifice.
   a. female urethra — passageway for urine.
   b. male urethra — passageway for urine and seminal fluid.   It is composed of a
      (1) prostatic portion — passes through prostate.
      (2) membranous portion — passes through the pelvic and urogenital diaphragms.
      (3) spongy portion — passes through the penis.[52, 66]

C. Diagnostic Terms:

1. atony of bladder — enormous distention of bladder associated with reduced expulsive force. It occurs in some diseases of the central nervous system.
2. bladder neck obstruction — blockage of the lumen of the bladder outlet resulting in overdistention of the urinary bladder, frequency, dysuria, persistent pyuria, retention with overflow and urinary back flow, dilatation of the ureters, hydronephrosis, renal pain, stone formation and chronic pyonephrosis.   The obstruction may be due to
   a. contracture of vesical outlet, congenital or acquired — a form of urethral stricture. The bladder neck may be narrowed by hypertrophic muscle, fibrous tissue or chronic inflammatory disease or
   b. obstructive lesions of vesical outlet — blood clots, calculi, diverticula, tumors, especially prostatic enlargement.[69, 73, 75]
3. calculus (pl. calculi) of bladder — bladder stone.[69]
4. cord bladder — bladder dysfunction due to injury or lesion of spinal cord.   Residual urine, incontinence and vesicoureteral reflux are usually present.[52]
5. cystitis, acute or chronic — inflammation of bladder due to infection.
6. exstrophy of bladder — a congenital absence of the lower abdominal and anterior vesical walls with eversion of the bladder; absence of closure or formation of the anterior one half of the bladder.[52, 75]   It is often associated with epispadias.[41]
7. injuries to
   a. urinary bladder — direct trauma to the distended bladder may cause vesical compression or rupture; a bony spicule of a fractured bone may pierce the bladder; blood and urine may spill into the peritoneal cavity; a hematoma may form. Accidental perforation of the bladder may occur during surgery.
   b. urethra — injury to the posterior urethra may be more serious than to the bladder including contusions, lacerations and rupture associated with extravasation of urine

and blood and formation of hematoma. Shearing injuries are likely to be complicated by urethral stricture.[69]

8. interstitial cystitis, submucous fibrosis of bladder, Hunner's ulcer — a bladder disorder predominantly seen in middle-aged women. Fibrosis of the vesical wall reduces the bladder capacity which is clinically manifested by frequency, nocturia, distention of the bladder and suprapubic tenderness or pain.[52, 75]

9. megalocystis, megabladder — enormous dilatation of urinary bladder.

10. neoplasms:
    a. benign: papilloma, polyp, others.
    b. malignant: transitional cell carcinoma, epidermoid carcinoma, others.[12, 52, 60, 73]

11. neurogenic bladder — there are 2 main types:
    a. flaccid atonic type — condition caused by lower motor neuron lesion due to trauma, ruptured intervertebral disk, meningomyelocele or other disorders and resulting in vesical dysfunction. The bladder has a large capacity, low intravesical pressure and a mild degree of trabeculation (hypertrophy) of the bladder wall.
    b. spastic automatic type — condition caused by upper motor neuron lesion due to injury, multiple sclerosis or other factors. The bladder capacity is reduced, the intravesical pressure is high, there is marked hypertrophy of the bladder wall and spasticity of the urinary sphincter.[78]

12. prolapse of bladder — a downward displacement of the bladder.

13. stress incontinence — inability to retain urine under any tension and when sneezing, coughing or laughing.[41]

14. stricture of urethra — narrowing of lumen of urethra, due to infection or trauma.[75]

15. stricture of vesicourethral orifice — narrowing of the opening between the bladder and urethra.

16. syphilis of bladder and urethra — venereal infection due to *Treponema pallidum*.

17. Trichomonas infection — a parasitic infection which may occur in bladder and male urethra.

18. trigonitis — inflammation of the trigone, the triangular base of the bladder.

19. urethritis, acute or chronic — inflammation of urethra which may be due to gonococcic infection.[52]

20. vesical fistulas — pathologic openings of bladder leading to adjacent organs:
    a. vesicoenteric fistula — sinus tract between bladder and intestine.
    b. vesicorectal fistula — fistulous connection between bladder and rectum.
    c. vesicovaginal — pathologic opening between bladder and vagina.[75]

D. Operative Terms:

1. cold punch transurethral resection of the vesical neck — endoscopic procedure for relief of bladder neck obstruction using a cold punch resectoscope for transurethral resection of tumor tissue, calcareous deposit or cicatrix. The new Kaplan resectoscope permits:
   a. fiberoptic illumination
   b. magnification and sharp visualization of surgical area
   c. the free flow of irrigation fluid and
   d. controlled movement of the knife.[30]

2. cystectomy — excision of bladder.
   a. partial — resection of bladder.
   b. complete — removal of entire viscus.[16]

3. cystolithotomy — incision into bladder for removal of stones.

4. cystoplasty — surgical repair of the bladder.

5. cystorrhaphy — suture of a ruptured or lacerated bladder.

6. cystoscopy — endoscopic examination of the bladder.[43]

7. cystostomy — surgical creation of a cutaneous bladder fistula for urinary drainage.[69, 71]

8. meatotomy — incision of urinary meatus to increase its caliber.

9. suprapubic vesicourethral suspension, Marshall-Marchetti repair — elevation and

immobilization of the bladder neck and urethra by suturing them to the pubis and rectus muscles for the establishment of urinary control.[75]

10. transurethral resection of the bladder neck — endoscopic resection of the bladder neck for removal of inelastic tissue using the transurethral approach.[45]

11. urethroscopy, panendoscopy — endoscopic examination of the male urethra or distal female urethra using a special panendoscope.[43]

12. urinary diversion operations for incapacitated bladder

    a. ileal conduit, ureteroileostomy — transplantation of both ureters to an isolated segment of the ileum. The urine drains through an external ileal stoma into a bag glued to the skin. Candidates for an elective ileal conduit may be children with bladder exstrophy and incontinence or adults with neurogenic bladders due to injury or neurologic disease or victims of a vesical carcinoma. In malignancy and persistent bladder infection a cystectomy is done with ileal conduit.[22, 68]

    b. sigmoid bladder, neobladder, colocystoplasty — replacement of bladder by creating a substitute bladder. A sigmoid segment is isolated and the ureters and urethra are implanted in the segment. The cecum may also be used for urinary diversion.[41, 61, 81]

E. Symptomatic Terms:

1. albuminuria, proteinuria — albumin or protein in urine.
2. dysuria — difficult or painful urination.
3. enuresis — incontinence or involuntary discharge of urine when asleep at night.
4. frequency of urination — voiding at close intervals, more often than every two hours. This is normal in infancy.[33]
5. glycosuria — sugar in urine.
6. hematuria — blood in urine.[26]
7. hesitancy — dysuria due to nervous inhibition or to obstruction of vesical outlet.
8. micturition — urination.
9. nocturia — frequent voiding during the night, may be due to renal inability to concentrate urine.
10. obstruction in bladder or urethra — blockage causing backflow of urine and renal damage.[71]
11. oliguria — scanty urinary output due to acute tubular necrosis, advanced fluid and electrolyte imbalance, organic kidney lesions, obstructive uropathy and other causes.[26, 38]
12. orthostatic proteinuria, benign postural proteinuria — protein in urine when in upright position, no proteinuria during recumbency.[86]
13. overflow incontinence — involuntary urination caused by overdistention of bladder.
14. polyuria — excessive urinary output.[26]
15. pyuria — pus in the urine.
16. residual urine — inability to empty bladder at micturition resulting in urinary retention and vesical overdistention.[78]
17. spinal shock — sequela of transverse injury to cord. It may cause autonomous bladder paralysis and later automatic voiding.[78]
18. suprapubic discomfort — uncomfortable sensation which may be due to interstitial cystitis, ulceration of the vesical mucosa or other disorders. It is usually present when the bladder fills and disappears when the bladder empties.
19. tenesmus of vesical sphincter — painful spasm at the end of micturition.
20. trabeculation, vesical — hypertrophy involving all muscle layers of the bladder. It may occur in benign prostatic hypertrophy.[41]
21. ureteral pain — usually acute, colicky pain radiating from renal pelvis to groin; may be due to stone pressing against the ureteral wall.[33]
22. urethral discharge — clear, thin, mucoid or purulent, scanty or profuse excretion from the urethra.
23. urgency — intense need to urinate at once.
24. urinary retention — inability to expel urine. This may be acute or chronic, complete or

incomplete. It is frequently caused by obstruction of urinary outflow due to stone, stricture, tumor and the like.

25. vesicoureteral reflux — backflow of urine into kidney, usually due to bladder neck obstruction. It may cause severe renal damage.

F. Terms Related to Special Procedures:

1. cystometrogram — a graphic record of pressure reactions while the patient's bladder is being filled with water. Bladder capacity, residual urine and sensory responses are checked. In cord bladders sensations are absent.[78]

2. cystometry — measurement of intravesical pressure during filling of the urinary bladder with fluid.[78]

3. dialysis — the passage of solutes back and forth across a semipermeable membrane placed between two solutions. Each solute moves toward the fluid in which its concentration is lower. Dialysis is used in acute renal failure to remove urea from the body and terminate electrolyte imbalance. Hemodialysis and peritoneal irrigation are the methods of choice.[24, 32]

4. intermittent hemodialysis — circulation established outside the body with the renal dialyzer one to three times a week depending on the patient's residual kidney function. An arteriovenous fistula is surgically created or an artery and vein are cannulated permitting the repetitive use of hemodialysis. The blood of the patient who is connected to the renal dialyzer passes into a coil of semipermeable membrane immersed in a bath of rinsing fluid. This membrane substitutes for the glomerular membrane. The concentration of solutes in the blood differs from that in the bath to promote a solute transfer through the semipermeable membrane which restores the electrolyte balance. After the solute exchange is completed the blood re-enters the patient's vein. Hemodialysis is a life-sustaining procedure in irreversible renal failure since it removes excess water and the end-products of protein metabolism and corrects acidosis as well as electrolyte imbalance.[2, 24]

5. peritoneal dialysis, peritoneal lavage, intermittent method — perfusion of the peritoneum using commercially prepared electrolyte solutions, special catheters and a closed system of infusion and drainage in the treatment of renal failure. The peritoneum functions basically as an inert semipermeable membrane permitting the exchange of solutes in both directions.[24]

6. prophylactic dialysis — the use of peritoneal dialysis to prevent renal failure.

MALE GENITAL ORGANS

A. Origin of Terms:

1. balano- (G) — glans
2. deferens (L) — carrying away
3. didymos (G) — testis, twin
4. orchido- (G) — testis
5. semen (L) — seed
6. vas (L) — vessel, duct

B. Anatomic Terms:[53, 66]

1. penis — a highly vascular organ containing three erectile tissue components. The distal end is the glans penis over which is folded the prepuce or foreskin.

2. prostate — organ composed of smooth muscle, fibrous and glandular tissue and divided into two lateral lobes and one median lobe. The prostate is structurally an extension of the urinary bladder. It is pierced by the prostatic urethra and ejaculatory ducts. Its secretion is part of the seminal fluid.

3. scrotum — sac of loose redundant skin which encloses the testes and epididymides.

4. testes (sing. testis) — paired male reproductive glands lying in the scrotum and divided into lobules by septa which are inward extensions of the outer covering. The lobules contain threadlike coils, the seminiferous tubules. The testes produce spermatozoa, a

minute part of the seminal fluid and androgen, the male hormone responsible for the secondary sex characteristics.   Three ducts share in the transport of spermatozoa on each side:

    a. epididymis (pl. epididymides) — structure lying on top and at the side of the testis and composed of head, body and tail.   It stores spermatozoa before they are emitted. The greatly coiled duct of the epididymis, about six meters in length, merges into the ductus deferens.

    b. ductus deferens, vas deferens — duct conveying spermatozoa from the epididymis to the ejaculatory duct.

    c. ejaculatory duct — duct formed by union of ductus deferens with duct of seminal vesicle.   Its fluid is carried into the urethra.

5. tunica vaginalis testis — double-layered serous sheath partially covering the testis and epididymis.   An abnormal collection of serum between the layers is known as hydrocele.

C. Diagnostic Terms:

1. actinomycosis — a fungus disease which may affect the genital organs.

2. adenocarcinoma — malignant tumor of glandular epithelium.   It most commonly involves the prostate, less commonly the other genital organs.   Metastases to bone occur frequently.[53, 73]

3. anorchism — absence of testes.

4. balanitis — inflammation of the glans penis.

5. cryptorchism — inproperly descended testis, descent arrested.[40, 53, 75]

6. ectopy of testicle — testicle outside the path of normal descent.[75]

7. epididymitis — inflammation of the epididymis.[53]

8. hydrocele

    a. tunica vaginalis — a collection of fluid within the tunica of the testis.

    b. spermatic cord — a collection of fluid along the spermatic cord usually within the inguinal canal.[53, 75]

9. hypertrophy of prostate, benign — a diffuse enlargement of the prostate, frequently seen in elderly men.   The gland interferes with micturition and eventually results in hydronephrosis and dilatation of ureters.

10. orchitis — inflammation of the testes.[53]

11. paraphimosis — foreskin retracted behind the glans with subsequent edema preventing restoration to normal position.[5]

12. phimosis — stenosis of the orifice of the prepuce or foreskin.   It may be congenitial or due to infection.   The opening may be pinpoint or absent.[53]

13. polyorchism, polyorchidism — more than 2 testes present.[75]

14. prostatitis — inflammation of the prostate gland.

15. syphilis — venereal disease due to *Treponema pallidum*.   Involvement of genital organs is common.

16. testicular tumors — usually malignant neoplasms seen in young adults, 18-35 years of age, less frequently in children and rarely in other age groups.   They include:

    a. choriocarcinoma — malignant tumor secreting chorionic gonadotropin.

    b. embryonal carcinoma — aggressive, lethal, testicular neoplasm which is highly invasive and readily spreads to lymph nodes and internal organs.[53]

    c. seminoma — common testicular germ cell tumor.[29, 53]

    d. teratoma, differentiated — benign cystic dermoid containing multiple tissues including hair and teeth.

    e. teratocarcinoma — malignant testicular tumor composed of various poorly differentiated tissues.

17. tuberculosis — systemic, contagious disease caused by tubercle bacilli.   Involvement of genital organs is infrequent.

18. varicocele — swelling and distention of veins of spermatic cord.[73]

D. Operative Terms:

1. circumcision — removal of an adequate amount of prepuce to permit exposure of the glans.
2. epididymectomy — excision of the epididymis.
3. excision of hydrocele — evacuation of serous fluid or removal of serous tumor from tunica vaginalis.
4. orchiectomy, orchectomy, orchidectomy — removal of testis.
5. orchiopexy — suturing an undescended testis in the scrotum.[75]
6. orchioplasty — plastic repair of a testis.
7. prostatectomies:[73]
    a. perineal prostatectomy — removal of prostate through an incision in the perineum.
    b. retropubic prostatectomy — a form of extravesical removal of prostate with partial or complete resection of gland.
    c. suprapubic prostatectomy — removal of gland through an opening into the bladder from above.
    d. transperineal urethral resection of the prostate — endoscopic resection of prostate combined with perineal urethrotomy to avoid the formation of a postoperative urethral stricture.
    e. transurethral cryogenic prostatectomy — use of special endoscope and freezing technique for destruction of prostatic tumor.
    f. transurethral prostatectomy — removal of obstructing glandular tissue using a special endoscope and electrocautery.[73]
8. vasectomy — removal of a short segment of the vas deferens and ligation of the severed ends.[5]
9. vasoligation — tying the vas deferens with ligature to produce sterility or to prevent epididymitis.[5]
10. vasovasostomy, epididymovasostomy — anastomosis of the vas deferens to epididymis to produce fertility by circumventing the obstructive lesion in the vas.

E. Symptomatic Terms:

1. azoospermia — semen without living spermatozoa causing infertility in the male.
2. dragging inguinal pain — pain may be due to enlargement of the testes.
3. edematous swelling — enlargement of an organ or part resulting from its infiltration with an excessive amount of tissue fluid.
4. lumbosacral pain — pain felt in the small of the back.
5. mucopurulent discharge — drainage of mucus and pus.
6. oligospermia — scanty production and expulsion of spermatozoa.
7. prodromal pain — initial pain signalling that a more severe attack is approaching.
8. prostatism — urinary difficulty resulting from obstruction at the bladder neck by hypertrophy of prostate gland or other causes.
9. strangury — painful urination, drop by drop, due to spasmodic muscular contraction of bladder and urethra.

RADIOLOGY

A. Terms Related to Diagnostic Urography:

1. plain film of abdomen (KUB) — radiogram made without injection of air or radiopaque solution to serve as contrast media. The procedure is a preliminary step when urologic diagnosis is anticipated. It presents renal shadows, the ureters and bladder, bones and intestines.[33, 73, 76]
2. urogram — any radiogram either of the entire urinary tract or of a particular organ. A radiopaque solution is used for the visualization of the organs.

a. cystogram — urogram of bladder

        (1) lateral cystogram — retrograde diagnostic procedure for the detection of true stress incontinence.[75]

        (2) retrograde cystogram — radiopaque substance injected suprapubically into bladder to reveal ureterovesical reflux, urinary extravasation or other abnormalities.[76]

    b. nephrogram — comparative study of urograms of both kidneys in order to detect urinary obstruction, if present.

    c. pyelogram — urogram of kidney pelvis.

    d. ureterogram — urogram of ureter.

    e. urethrogram — urogram of urethra and prostate.

    f. voiding cystogram, voiding cystourethrogram — urogram made while patient voids the contrast medium.

3. urographic medium (pl. media) — a radiopaque solution used for the visualization of the various organs of the urinary tract. The following contrast media of low toxicity are used:

iothalamate (Conray) — diatrizoate (Hypaque or Renografin)

These media may also be employed in the x-ray examination of other organs.[76]

4. urography — radiography concerned with the detection of urologic conditions.[15] Some special procedures are:

    a. cineradiography of urinary tract (cinecystogram) — urographic motion pictures to demonstrate transient or persistent vesicoureteral reflux after having gradually filled the bladder with radiopaque medium.[76]

    b. computed tomography — noninvasive diagnostic technique using an EME scanner to differentiate between normal renal tissue, renal tumors and cysts.[50]

    c. cystourethrography — cystography combined with urethrography to visualize abnormalities of the bladder and urethra.[76]

    d. drip infusion pyelography — intravenous infusion of a large volume of dilute contrast medium in conjunction with nephrotomograms to provide detailed visualization of renal pelves and ureters. The procedure is of special value in the detection of renal cysts.[84]

    e. excretory urography — urograms demonstrating renal excretory function. They are obtained by intravenous injection of a contrast medium or less frequently by retrograde filling of renal calices and pelves with radiopaque solution. Excretory urograms visualize tumors, cysts, hydronephrosis, pyelonephritis, calculi and other obstructive lesions of the urinary tract as well as vesicoureteral reflux.[48, 73, 76]

    f. nephrotomography — body section radiography of the kidney.[73, 76]

    g. pneumocystography — radiographic examination of the urinary bladder after it has been filled with air. This method aids in the detection of vesical tumors.

    h. retrograde pyelography — x-ray examination of the urinary tract after the injection of opaque solution which is introduced through ureteral catheters during cystoscopy. The calices, pelves and ureters are usually well demonstrated.

    i. retroperitoneal pneumography — delineation of retroperitoneal organs by presacral insufflation using carbon dioxide as contrast medium.[76]

B. Term Related to Urologic Angiography:

1. angionephrotomography — rapid intravenous infusion of a radiopaque solution to obtain a series of angiograms of the renal blood vessels. The presence or absence of vascular opacification is of diagnostic significance.[73, 76]

2. angiography — radiographic visualization of blood or lymph vessels following the injection of a contrast medium into an artery or lymphatic.

    a. lymphangiography — opacification of the lymphatic systems, pelvic, inguinal, periaortic, retroperitoneal and subclavicular in order to demonstrate metastatic involvement of the lymph nodes.[6, 9, 76]

    b. renal angiography — under fluoroscopic guidance a catheter, inserted percutaneously in the femoral or axillary or brachial artery, is advanced to the level of the renal arteries and a contrast medium is rapidly injected into the aorta. One to three series of film exposures taken within seconds demonstrate the renal circulation.[73, 76]

    c. renal arteriography — infusion of radiopaque medium into the renal artery to demonstrate the state of the renal cortex and parenchyma which cannot be seen in retrograde pyelography.[19]

    d. selective renal angiography — a catheter is directly passed into a renal artery, radiopaque solution is injected and about 16 exposures are made within seconds. This method offers a great deal of vascular detail and aids in differential diagnosis.[76]

    e. selective renal venography — a special technique for visualizing thrombosis of the renal vein.[76]

    f. venacavography — a radiographic procedure demonstrating enlarged metastatic lymph nodes located behind the peritoneum.[76]

    g. vesical angiography — a method for revealing the size and depth of a bladder tumor, its invasive characteristic if present, thus providing evidence for staging of vesical tumors.[76]

C. Terms Related to Diagnostic Ultrasound:

1. nephrosonography — the delineation of deep renal structures by measuring the transmission of ultrasonic vibrations. Renal sonography is an important method for investigating a renal mass. The calyceal echoes are usually displaced in the presence of a renal cyst or tumor and the lesion is surrounded by an anechoic area. If the tumor enlarges, the echoes multiply within the mass.[7, 28]

2. renal sonogram, nephrosonogram — a record of ultrasonic waves passing through the renal tissue for the purpose of determining the size and location of the kidney. Sonograms may detect congenital anomalies: horseshoe kidney, agenesis, renal ectopy, aid in differentiating between hydronephrosis, unilateral multicystic kidney and polycystic kidney and demonstrate cyst-tumor deformity.[7, 28]

3. ultrasonic scanning of renal transplant — serial volume measurements of kidney transplant by ultrasound to detect changes in size such as
    a. an increase in renal size with or without scattered echoes from collecting tubules in acute rejection of transplant.
    b. a decrease in size, usually present in chronic rejection of transplant.[3]

4. ultrasonic vesical scanning — echographic imaging of intravesical calculi, clots, diverticula, papillomas, primary or metastatic bladder tumors, prostatic hypertrophy, chronic granulomatous cystitis and other disorders.[3]

5. urologic ultrasonography — the diagnostic use of sound beam echoes in the detection of renal tumors or cysts, perirenal abscess, retroperitoneal mass or hemorrhage, polycystic kidneys, testicular torsion and prostatic disorder.[7, 73, 79]

D. Terms Related to Therapeutic Radiology:

1. radiation therapy for tumors of the urinary tract:
    a. carcinoma of the urinary bladder — favorable response to external radiation reported when tumors were located near the ureteral orifice and trigone.
    In general the more undifferentiated the vesical tumor, the more radiosensitive, the more differentiated, the more radioresistant is the tumor.[73] Megavoltage radiation therapy has been used with a measure of success in bladder cancer.[23]
    b. adenocarcinoma of kidney — beneficial results may be obtained from courses of therapy after the surgical removal of the tumor.
    c. Wilms' tumor — temporary relief from symptoms following deep x-ray therapy may result.

2. radiation therapy of prostate gland — treatment gaining wide acceptance.
    a. in early stages (A and B) of prostatic cancer its value is doubtful.

b. in stage C it is curative in many cases.

c. in metastatic carcinoma the relief from pain is remarkable.[73]

3. radiation therapy of testicular tumors — a common treatment modality together with chemotherapy and surgery.[23, 73]

CLINICAL LABORATORY

A. Terms Concerned with Urine Findings:

1. urinalysis — examination of physical and chemical properties of urine. Physical properties comprise quantity, color, specific gravity, odor and others. Chemical properties are concerned with quantitative or qualitative tests dealing with protein, glucose, bile pigments, ketone bodies, blood, calculi and the like. In conditions of the urinary system albumin and casts are frequently present and the pH concentration is altered.

a. albumin, protein — abnormal constituent of urine in renal and febrile diseases and toxemias of pregnancy. It is due to increased permeability of the glomerular filter.

b. casts — cells abnormally formed in the renal tubules and shed in the urine as hyaline, granular, epithelial, blood and pus casts.

c. hydrogen ion concentration (chemical symbol pH) — the reaction of the urine.
(1) pH concentration ...... 7 .... normal neutrality
(2) pH concentration below 7 .... acid in reaction
(3) pH concentration above 7 .... alkaline in reaction
In acidosis the urine is strongly acid; in chronic cystitis and in urinary retention the urine is usually alkaline in reaction.[77]

d. porphyrins (coproporphyrin, uroporphyrin, porphobilinogen) are pigments resembling bilirubin and apparently derived from the hemoglobin of the blood. Minute amounts of porphyrins are normally present in the urine. An increase is abnormal.
(1) coproporphyrin urinary excretion — a valuable test in the detection of lead poisoning, acute porphyria, pellagra and liver damage.
(2) uroporphyrin urinary excretion — diagnostic aid in acute porphyria and acute intermittent porphyria.[83]

2. urinary calculi — stones found in the pelvis of the kidney, ureter and bladder in the form of

a. cystine stones — white or pale yellow granules.

b. oxalate stones (calcium oxalate) — crystalline structure.

c. phosphate and carbonate stones — compact balls.

d. uric acid stones — smooth, round pebbles.[69]

B. Terms Related to Proprietary Urine Tests:

1. Clinistix, Clinitest — reagent strip or tablet for testing glucose in urine.

2. Combistix — 3 separate reagent areas: pH, protein and glucose in urine providing information on acid-base balance, renal function and carbohydrate metabolism.

3. Keto-Diastix — reagent strip for detecting glucose and ketones in urine.

4. Ketostix — reagent strip for checking ketones in urine, serum and plasma.

C. Terms Related to Renal Function Studies:

1. blood urea nitrogen (BUN) — a renal function test which measures the concentration of urea in the blood. In health the blood levels are low since urea, an end-product of protein metabolism, is freely excreted in the urine. In renal impairment and failure urea nitrogen accumulates in the blood and the patient may lapse into coma.
Normal values 8-18 mg of urea nitrogen per 100 ml of blood
Increase in nephritis, urinary obstruction, uremia
Decrease in amyloidosis, nephrosis, pregnancy.[10]

2. concentration and dilution test — this test measures the functional capacity of the kidney to concentrate and dilute urine.

Failure to concentrate urine indicates kidney damage. It may be partially caused by a faulty mechanism of the antidiuretic hormone (ADH) released from the pituitary gland.[8]

3. creatinine determination — a renal function test comparable to blood urea nitrogen. Creatinine is derived from catabolism (breakdown) of creatine phosphate from muscle tissue. It is eliminated by glomerular filtration and excreted in the urine. In a healthy individual the amount of creatinine remains almost constant from day to day.

4. endogenous creatinine clearance — renal function test which measures the removal of creatinine from plasma as it is reflected by the glomerular filtration rate (GFR).[63, 77]

5. Howard test, excretion of water, salt and creatinine — renal function study to detect ischemia of the kidney due to stenosis of the renal artery or its branch or to chronic pyelonephritis with arteriolar involvement. A low urine volume, low sodium and high creatinine concentrations are positive findings and indicate that the patient may benefit by renovascular surgery.[70]

6. phenolsulfonphthalein (PSP) — a dye test for the detection of kidney impairment. About 90% of the PSP is eliminated through the renal tubules and only 10% through glomerular filtration.

Normal values — PSP . . . . . first hour 40 - 60% ; second hour 20 - 25%

A low urinary excretion of the dye of 40% or less in 2 hours is usually associated with nitrogen retention in the blood. Elimination of the dye is delayed in hypertrophy of prostate gland complicated by hydronephrosis, in malignant hypertension, and cystitis with urinary retention.[8, 10, 63, 77]

7. plasma renin activity (PRA) — bioassay method of Gunnels measuring the enzyme activity of renin to screen patients for renovascular hypertension or malignant hypertension.[70, 80]

8. renin — enzyme originating in the glomerulus. Renin levels rise with lowered perfusion pressure and lowered delivery of water and sodium to the glomerulus. High levels of renin formed by the diseased kidney may lead to renal hypertension and primary aldosteronism.[80]

9. Stamey test — sodium chloride-urea-ADH-PAH test designed to demonstrate abnormal reabsorption of water by the ischemic kidney by revealing its reduced urine volume and elevated PAH concentration in comparison with its urate.[70]

10. urea clearance — test measures the glomerular function of the kidneys to remove urea from the blood. It is calculated as plasma cleared of urea in one minute.[8]

D. Terms: Related to Special Studies:

1. follicle stimulating hormone (FSH) — measurement of FSH type of pituitary gonadotropin excretion.

Normal male urine . . . . detectable amount of FSH
Increase of FSH . . . . adult seminiferous tubule failure, Klinefelter's syndrome, others
Decrease of FSH . . . . androgen or estrogen secreting tumors of the adrenal, ovary or testis, others.[80*]

2. luteinizing hormone (LH) — a specific protein hormone, synthesized in the pituitary and acting on both male and female gonadal tissue. Its primary function in the male is testosterone production. FSH and LH combined stimulate the maturation of spermatozoa in the tubules aided by high serum testosterone levels.[80*]

3. semen culture — a study of the seminal flora useful in confirming a diagnosis of bacterial prostatitis.[41]

4. serum acid phosphatase — test measures acid phosphatase, an enzyme freely present in the normal prostate gland which produces it and releases a small amount into the blood serum.

---

*See comment p. 206.

Normal value — Method of Gutman and King-Armstrong
Serum acid phosphatase is............. 1.0 to 4.0 U/ml[10, 73]
Increase is seen in metastatic carcinoma of the prostate gland. The test aids in the detection of obscure bone lesions.

5. serum alkaline phosphatase — test measures the activity of alkaline phosphatase, a prostatic enzyme which is found in small quantity in the blood serum.
   Normal value — Method of Bodansky
   Serum alkaline phosphatase is .... 1.5 to 4.5 U/dl[10, 73]
   Increase may occur in metastases of prostatic carcinoma to bone, in bone growth and repair, bone injury, Paget's disease, biliary tract blockage and liver disease.

6. testicular biopsy for meiotic study — tissue cells of testis appraised in the cytogenetic laboratory as to the progression of spermatogenesis or meiosis predicting a favorable response to hormone therapy in male infertility. A marked degree of arrest or total absence of spermatogenesis suggest probable ineffectiveness of treatment in the sterile male.[40]

7. testosterone — a steroid hormone and very potent androgen.
   Decrease in males .... in hypogonadism, hypopituitarism, Klinefelter's syndrome and after orchidectomy.[80]*

ABBREVIATIONS

ADH — antidiuretic hormone
AG — albumin/globulin (ratio)
BNO — bladder neck obstruction
BNR — bladder neck resection
BPH — benign prostatic hypertrophy
BUN — blood urea nitrogen
CBI — continuous bladder irrigation
CC — chief complaint
CUG — cystourethrogram
Cysto — cystoscopic examination
DL — danger list
ERPF — effective renal plasma flow
GBM — glomerular basement membrane
GFR — glomerular filtration rate
GU — genitourinary
ICU — intensive care unit

IVP — intravenous pyelogram
KUB — kidney, ureter, bladder
NPO — nothing by mouth
PAH — p-aminohippuric acid
pH — hydrogen ion concentration
PRA — plasma renin activity
PSP — phenolsulfonphthalein
PU — prostatic urethra
RER — renal excretion rate
RPF — renal plasma flow
RTA — renal tubular acidosis
TPUR — transperineal urethral resection
TRBF — total renal blood flow
TUR — transurethral resection
UP — urine/plasma (ratio)
VCUG — voiding cystourethrogram

ORAL READING PRACTICE

Hydronephrosis

This condition is a byproduct of mechanical obstruction of the urinary tract. When the interference with the outflow of urine is below the bladder, as in **urethral stricture** or **hypertrophy** of the prostate gland, **bilateral hydronephrosis** develops. When above the bladder, as in **unilateral, ureteral stricture, calculus** or **neoplasm,** the condition affects only one kidney. In addition, pressure from tumors, adhesions, or the **pregnant uterus** outside the urinary tract may interfere with the flow of urine and lead to **hydronephrosis. Congenital anomalies** of the **ureter** or **urethra** may also be responsible for this condition.

There are various degrees of **dilatation** of the **renal pelvis** and ureter. In the initial phase of the disease the pathologic changes are slight. As the condition progresses, the amount of

---

*Hormone studies are increasingly done by radioimmunoassay methods which combine exquisite sensitivity with a high degree of reliability and specificity.

fluid increases, the **papillae** assume a flattened appearance, the **renal cortex** becomes thinned and the pyramids of the medulla undergo atrophic changes. The kidney resembles a hollow shell filled with fluid. In extreme cases several liters of fluid may accumulate in the renal pelvis leading to a complete loss of physiologic capacity. If the **hydronephrosis** is unilateral, the healthy kidney undergoes compensatory hypertrophic changes to adapt itself to the increased functional work load. In this case renal insufficiency does not develop. However, in the presence of advanced bilateral hydronephrosis, the downhill clinical course is steady and terminates in fatal uremia.

The fluid in the kidney differs from normal urine in its reduced content of urea. Since it is locked up in the renal shell and unable to escape to its proper destination, it becomes easily a breeding place for invading bacterial organisms. Another deleterious **sequela** of fluid retention in the kidney is the formation of **renal calculi** which adds insult to injury and completes the physiologic destruction of the organ.

In the early phase of hydronephrosis symptoms may be absent or so mild that they escape notice. As the condition progresses, the kidney becomes palpable, tender and painful. With unrelieved obstruction continued over weeks, the only symptom may be a dull pain. If intermittent obstruction occurs, attacks of pain develop periodically and are accompanied by oliguria which is promptly reversed to **polyuria** when the obstruction is abolished. Should the damaged kidney become infected, **leukocytosis**, fever and **pyuria** signal the onset of **pyonephrosis**.

The treatment of hydronephrosis consists in removing the cause of obstruction such as the ureteral stricture or compressing **prostatic** or vesicular tumor. If done early, the kidney may be saved. In advanced cases the presence of irreparable damage demands the excision of the diseased organ since it serves no useful function and is a constant threat of focal infection.[69, 71, 72, 73, 78]

Table 20
SOME UROGENITAL CONDITIONS AMENABLE TO SURGERY

Organs Involved	Diagnoses	Operations	Operative Procedures
Kidneys	Chronic glomerulo-nephritis, preterminal Irreversible renal failure	Renal homotransplantation including a. bilateral nephrectomy b. revascularization of homograft c. ureterocystostomy	Removal of both kidneys Extraperitoneal donor homografting with vascular anastomoses to iliac and hypogastric vessels Creation of an opening between a ureter and bladder
Kidney	Nephroptosis	Nephropexy	Fixation or suspension of movable or displaced kidney
Kidney	Posttraumatic fistula of kidney	Nephrorrhaphy	Suture of kidney
Kidney	Bilateral nephrolithiasis Unilateral calculous pyonephrosis and infection of ureter	Nephrolithotomy Nephrectomy Ureterectomy	Removal of stones from better kidney first Removal of kidney and ureter
Kidney Ureter	Calculous anuria due to acute ureteral obstruction	Nephrostomy Pyelostomy	Creation of communication between the kidney and the skin for drainage

Organs Involved	Diagnoses	Operations	Operative Procedures
Kidney Ureter	Adenocarcinoma of kidney Papillary carcinoma of kidney pelvis Carcinoma of ureter	Total nephrectomy Nephroureterectomy Partial cystectomy	Removal of kidney Removal of kidney, ureter and bladder cuff
Kidney Ureter	Hydronephrosis due to obstruction from impacted ureteral calculus Dilatation of infected ureter	Total nephrectomy Ureterectomy	Excision of severely damaged kidney and ureter
Renal pelvis	Calculus in renal pelvis, small	Pyelolithotomy	Removal of calculus from renal pelvis
Ureter	Calculus in ureter associated with renal obstruction	Ureterolithotomy	Incision into ureter with removal of calculus
Ureter	Postinfectional stricture of ureter	Ureteroplasty	Plastic repair of ureter
Bladder	Diverticulum of bladder	Diverticulectomy of urinary bladder	Local excision of diverticulum
Bladder	Cystocele	Cystoplasty	Plastic repair of cystocele
Bladder	Hemorrhage from urinary bladder	Cystoscopy with evacuation of blood clots	Endoscopic examination of the bladder
Bladder	Early carcinoma of urinary bladder, no metastasis	Partial cystectomy with wide local excision of tumor	Removal of bladder wall including the carcinoma and a surrounding cuff of normal bladder wall
Bladder	Papilloma encroaching on ureteral orifice	Suprapubic cystostomy with excision of tumor Ureterocystostomy	Surgical opening of the bladder above the symphysis pubis and removal of tumor Anastomosis of ureter to bladder and reimplantation of ureter into bladder
Bladder	Rupture of bladder due to injury	Cystorrhaphy	Suture of bladder
Bladder Ureters	Bladder neck obstruction, vesicoureteral reflux	Bladder neck reconstruction (Y-V plasty) Ureteroneocystostomy	Surgical bladder neck revision and reimplantation of ureters into bladder to correct vesicoureteral reflux
Bladder Ureters	Neurogenic bladder associated with vesical calculi and recurrent pyelonephritis Carcinoma of bladder Exstrophy of bladder	Ureteroileostomy (Ileal conduit) Cystectomy	Transplantation of both ureters to an isolated segment of the ileum for conveying urine to an external stoma Removal of bladder in vesical malignancy and uncontrolled infection

Organs Involved	Diagnoses	Operations	Operative Procedures
Bladder Ureters Urethra	Carcinoma of bladder	Cystectomy Colocystoplasty (Neobladder or Sigmoid bladder)	Excision of urinary bladder Creation of a new bladder by isolating a sigmoid segment and implanting the ureters and urethra in the segment
Prostate	Hypertrophy of prostate	Transurethral resection of prostate cryosurgery of prostate	Partial removal of prostate using a special endoscope and the electrocautery or localized freezing of prostate
Prostate Seminal vesicles Vasa deferentia	Carcinoma of prostate	Retropubic prosta- tectomy Radical perineal prostatectomy	Radical extravesical removal of the prostate Removal of prostate, seminal vesicles and vasa deferentia through perineal incision
Testis Spermatic cord	Torsion of spermatic cord complicated by testicular gangrene	Orchiectomy Orchiopexy	Removal of testis Scrotal fixation of the opposite testis
Testes	Advanced carcinoma of the prostate gland with bone metastases	Orchiectomy, bilateral (castration for andro- gen control)	Removal of both testes
Testis	Undescended testis, unilateral	Orchioplasty Orchiopexy	Surgical transfer of testis to scrotum

REFERENCES AND BIBLIOGRAPHY

1. Abbott, W. M. *et al.* Renal failure after ruptured aneurysm. *Archives of Surgery,* 110: 1110-1112, September, 1975.
2. Amend, W. J. *et al.* Chronic renal failure, dialysis and renal transplantation. In Smith, Donald R. *General Urology,* 8th ed. Los Altos, California: Lange Medical Publications, 1975, pp. 375-381.
3. Barnett, Ellis and Morley, Patricia. *Abdominal Echography.* London: Butterworths & Co., 1974, pp. 53-80.
4. Bricker, N. S. Acute renal failure. In Beeson, Paul B. and McDermott, Walsh (eds.). *Textbook of Medicine,* 14th ed. Philadelphia: W. B. Saunders Co., 1975, pp. 1107-1113.
5. Byrne, John E., M.D. Personal communications.
6. Cerny, J. C. *et al.* An evaluation of lymphangiography in staging carcinoma of the prostate. *Journal of Urology,* 113: 367-370, March, 1975.
7. Coggs, C. G. Ultrasonic examination of the urinary tract. In Smith, Donald R. *General Urology,* 8th ed. Los Altos: Lange Medical Publications, 1975, pp. 75-84.
8. Conn, R. B. Normal laboratory values of clinical importance. In Beeson, Paul B. and McDermott, Walsh. *Textbook of Medicine,* 14th ed. Philadelphia: W. B. Saunders Co., 1975, pp. 1884-1892.
9. Cosgrove, M. D. *et al.* Lymphangiography in genitourinary cancer. *Journal of Urology,* 113: 93-95, January, 1975.
10. Davidsohn, Israel and Henry, John Bernard. Tables of normal values. *Clinical Diagnosis by Laboratory Methods,* 15th ed. Philadelphia: W. B. Saunders Co., 1974, pp. 1376-1392.
11. Delmonico, F. L. *et al.* Renal transplantation in the older age group. *Archives of Surgery,* 110: 1107-1109, September, 1975.
12. DeMeester, L. J. *et al.* Inverted papillomas of the urinary bladder. *Cancer,* 36: 505-513, August, 1975.
13. Depner, T. A. *et al.* Posttraumatic renal artery stenosis. *Archives of Surgery,* 110: 1150-1151, September, 1975.
14. Doornbos, J. F. *et al.* Radiotherapy for pure seminoma of the testis. *Radiology,* 116: 401-404, August, 1975.
15. Elkin, M. Radiology of urinary tract: Some physiological considerations. *Radiology,* 116: 256-270, August, 1975.
16. Evans, R. A. *et al.* Partial cystectomy in treatment of bladder cancer. *Journal of Urology,* 114: 391-393, September, 1975.
17. Finlayson, B. What is new in surgery: Urology. *Surgery Gynecology & Obstetrics,* 140: 224-227, February, 1975.
18. Finley, R. A. Salmonella urinary tract infection. *Southern Medical Journal,* 68: 895-922, July, 1975.

19. Foley, W. D. *et al.* Arteriography of renal transplants. *Radiology*, 116: 271-277, August, 1975.

20. Foster, J. H. Renovascular occlusive disease. *Journal of American Medical Association*, 231: 1043-1048, March 10, 1975.

21. Frazier, W. J. Manipulation of torsion of testicle. *Journal of Urology*, 114: 410-411, September, 1975.

22. Frenay, Sr. Agnes Clare. A dynamic approach to the ileal conduit patient. *American Journal of Nursing*, 64: 80-84, January, 1964.

23. Goffinet, D. R. Bladder cancer: Results of radiation therapy in 384 patients. *Radiology*, 117: 149-154, October, 1975.

24. Hampers, C. L. Dialysis. In Beeson, Paul B. and McDermott, Walsh (eds.). *Textbook of Medicine*, 14th ed. Philadelphia: W. B. Saunders Co., 1975, pp. 1119-1127.

25. Hepler, Opal E. *Manual of Clinical Laboratory Method*, 4th ed. Springfield, Ill.: Charles C. Thomas, Publisher, 1955, pp. 13-28 and pp. 312-315.

26. Hoffmann La Roche Inc. *Handbook of Differential Diagnosis — The Pelvic Region*, 3rd ed. Vol. 3. Nutley, New Jersey: Rocom Press, 1975, pp. 9-151.

27. Holland, J. M. Natural history and staging of renal cell carcinoma. *Ca — A Cancer Journal for Clinicians*, 25: 121-133, May-June, 1975.

28. Holmes, J. H. Urologic ultrasonography. In King, Donald L. (ed.). *Diagnostic Ultrasound*. St. Louis: The C. V. Mosby Co., 1974, pp. 242-259.

29. Johnson, D. E. *et al.* Anaplastic seminoma. *Journal of Urology*, 114: 80-82, July, 1975.

30. Kaplan, J. H. A new cold punch resectoscope. *Journal of Urology*, 107: 1054-1055, June, 1972.

31. Kerr, D. N. S. Chronic renal failure. In Beeson, Paul B. and McDermott, Walsh (eds.). *Textbook of Medicine*, 14th ed. Philadelphia: W. B. Saunders Co., 1975, pp. 1093-1107.

32. Kincaid-Smith, Priscilla. Treatment of irreversible renal failure by transplantation and dialysis. In Beeson, Paul B. and McDermott, Walsh (eds.). *Textbook of Medicine*, 14th ed. Philadelphia: W. B. Saunders Co., 1975, pp. 1114-1119.

33. Krupp, M. A. Genitourinary tract. In Krupp, Marcus A. and Chatton, Milton. *Current Medical Diagnosis and Treatment*, 15th ed. Los Altos, California: Lange Medical Publications, 1976, pp. 521-552.

34. _____. Diagnosis of medical renal diseases. In Smith, Donald R. *General Urology*, 8th ed. Los Altos, California: Lange Medical Publications, 1975, pp. 357-368.

35. Kunin, C. M. Urinary tract infections and pyelonephritis. In Beeson, Paul B. and McDermott, Walsh (eds.). *Textbook of Medicine*, 14th ed. Philadelphia: W. B. Saunders Co., 1975, pp. 1144-1148.

36. Leary, F. J. *et al.* Urologic problems in renal transplantation. *Archives of Surgery*, 110: 1124-1128, September, 1975.

37. Lokish, J. J. Renal cell carcinoma: Natural history and chemotherapeutic experience. *Journal of Urology*, 114: 371-374, September, 1975.

38. Lyon, R. P. Oliguria. In Smith, Donald R. *General Urology*, 8th ed. Los Altos, California: Lange Medical Publications, 1975, pp. 369-374.

39. Major, Georges and Zingg, Ernst J. *Urologic Surgery*. New York: John Wiley & Sons, Inc., 1976.

40. Mehan, D. J., Chehval, M. J. and Sister Leo Rita Volk. A study of meiotic preparation of human spermatocytes and their relationship to infertility. *Journal of Urology*, 115: 284-287, March, 1976.

41. Mehan, Donald J., M.D. Personal communications.

42. Morales A. *et al.* Intracavitary bacillus Calmette Guérin in the treatment of superficial bladder tumors. *Journal of Urology*, 116: 180-183, August, 1976.

43. Morel, Alice and Wise, Gilbert Jane. Cystoscopy — panendoscopy. *Urologic Endoscopic Procedures*. St. Louis: The C. V. Mosby Co., 1974, pp. 50-63.

44. _____. Bladder biopsy, fulguration and ureteral instrumentation. *Ibid.*, pp. 64-78.

45. _____. Transurethral resection — Other urologic procedures. *Ibid.*, pp. 79-129.

46. Muldowney, F. P. Obstructive nephropathy. In Beeson, Paul B. and McDermott, Walsh (eds.). *Textbook of Medicine*, 14th ed. Philadelphia: W, B. Saunders Co., 1975, pp. 1156-1158.

47. Murray, T. *et al.* Chronic interstitial nephritis: Etiologic factors. *Annals of Internal Medicine*, 82: 453-459, April, 1975.

48. Naber, K. G. Continuous infusion urography in unilateral hydronephrosis. *Journal of Urology*, 114: 337-342, September, 1975.

49. Papper, S. Chronic pyelonephritis. In Beeson, Paul B. and McDermott, Walsh (eds.). *Textbook of Medicine*, 14th ed. Philadelphia: W. B. Saunders Co., 1975, pp. 1148-1150.

50. Pickering, R. S. *et al.* Computed tomography of the excised kidney. *Radiology*, 113: 643-648, December, 1974.

51. Robbins, Stanley L. The kidney — Renal failure. *Pathologic Basis of Disease*. Philadelphia: W. B. Saunders Co., 1974, pp. 1078-1147.

52. _____. The lower urinary tract. *Ibid.*, pp. 1148-1170.

53. _____. Male genital system. *Ibid.*, pp. 1171-1200.

54. Salvatierra, O. *et al.* Pediatric cadaver kidneys: Their use in renal transplantation. *Archives of Surgery*, 110: 181-183, February, 1975.

55. Sanford, J. P. Urinary tract infection. *Postgraduate Medicine*, 58: 167-173, September, 1975.

56. Schreiner, G. E. Cysts of the kidney. In Beeson, Paul B. and McDermott, Walsh (eds.). *Textbook of Medicine*, 14th ed. Philadelphia: W. B. Saunders Co., 1975, pp. 1168-1172.

57. _____. Toxic nephropathy. *Ibid.*, pp. 1159-1164.

58. _____. Tumors of the kidneys — Miscellaneous renal disorders. *Ibid.*, pp. 1172-1176.

59. Schwartz, W. B. Other special renal diseases. In Beeson, Paul B. and McDermott, Walsh (eds.). *Textbook of Medicine*, 14th ed. Philadelphia: W. B. Saunders Co., 1975, pp. 1150-1156.

60. Seemayer, T. A. Further observations on carcinoma in situ of the urinary bladder: Silent but

extensive intraprostatic involvement. *Cancer*, 36: 514-520, August, 1975.

61. Segura, J. W. *et al.* Long-term results of ureterosigmoidostomy in children with bladder exstrophy. *Journal of Urology*, 114: 138-140, July, 1975.

62. Seward, C. W. *et al.* Hereditary nephritis (Alport's syndrome) in a new kindred. *Southern Medical Journal*, 68: 871-875, July, 1975.

63. Shaw, S. T. *et al.* Renal function and its evaluation. In Davidsohn, Israel and Henry, John Bernard. *Clinical Diagnosis by Laboratory Methods*, 15th ed. Philadelphia: W. B. Saunders Co., 1974, pp. 84-99.

64. Shires, G. T. Acute renal insufficiency complicating surgery and trauma. In Artz, Curtis P. and Hardy, James D. *Management of Surgical Complications*, 3rd ed. Philadelphia: W. B. Saunders Co., 1975, pp. 83-92.

65. Silber, S. Renal trauma. *Archives of Surgery*, 110: 206-207, February, 1975.

66. Smith, Donald R. Anatomy of the genitourinary tract. In *General Urology*, 8th ed. Los Altos, California: Lange Medical Publications, 1975, pp. 1-12.

67. ———. Disorders of the kidney. *Ibid.*, pp. 336-368.

68. ———. Nonspecific infections of the urinary tract — Specific infections of the urinary tract. *Ibid.*, pp. 136-192.

69. ———. Urinary stones — Injuries to genitourinary tract. *Ibid.*, pp. 200-238.

70. ———. Renovascular hypertension. *Ibid.*, pp. 449-455.

71. ———. Urinary obstruction and stasis — Vesicoureteral reflux. *Ibid.*, pp. 112-135.

72. ———. Disorders of the ureters. *Ibid.*, pp. 382-392.

73. ———. Tumors of the genitourinary tract. *Ibid.*, 247-299.

74. ———. Symptoms of disorders of the genitourinary tract. *Ibid.*, pp. 25-33.

75. ———. Disorders of the bladder, prostate & seminal vesicles — Disorders of the testis, scrotum and spermatic cord. *Ibid.*, pp. 393-430.

76. ———. Roentgenographic examination of the urinary tract. *Ibid.*, pp. 50-74.

77. ———. Urologic laboratory examination. *Ibid.*, pp. 41-50.

78. ———. The neurogenic bladder. *Ibid.*, pp. 300-319.

79. Smith, E. H. Ultrasonic evaluation of pararenal masses. *Journal of American Medical Association*, 231: 51-55, January 6, 1975.

80. *Specialized Diagnostic Laboratory Tests*, 11th ed. Van Nuys, California: Bio-Science Laboratories, 1976, pp. 55-76.

81. Spence, H. M. *et al.* Exstrophy of the bladder: Long-term results in a series of 37 cases treated by ureterosigmoidostomy. *Journal of Urology*, 114: 133-137, July, 1975.

82. Straffon, R. A. Urinary tract infections. *Medical Clinics of North America*, 58: 545-554, May, 1974.

83. Thomas, W. C. Renal calculi. In Beeson, Paul B. and McDermott, Walsh (eds.). *Textbook of Medicine*, 14th ed. Philadelphia: W. B. Saunders Co., 1975, pp. 1164-1168.

84. Weir, Don C., M.D. Personal communications.

85. Wrong, O. M. Glomerular disease. In Beeson, Paul B. and McDermott, Walsh (eds.). *Textbook of Medicine*, 14th ed. Philadelphia: W. B. Saunders Co., 1975, pp. 1124-1142.

Chapter X
Gynecologic Disorders

VULVA AND VAGINA

A. Origin of Terms:

1. colpo- (G) — vagina
2. fistula (L) — pipe, tube
3. hymen (G) — membrane
4. krauros (G) — dry
5. labia (L) — lips
6. vagina (L) — sheath
7. vestibule (L) — antechamber
8. vulva (L) — covering

B. Anatomic Terms:[22, 33]

1. perineum — space between vulva and anus.
2. Skene's glands — urethral glands in female.
3. vagina — musculomembranous tube which connects the uterus with the vulva.   It is the lower part of the birth canal.
4. vulva, pudendum — external female genital organ.   Some of the vulvar structures of gynecologic importance are the following:
   a. clitoris — small body of erectile tissue which enlarges with vascular congestion.
   b. hymen — membranous fold which partially covers the vaginal opening in a virgin.
   c. labia majora (sing. labium majus) — two raised folds of adipose and erectile tissue covered on their outer surface with skin.[15]
   d. labia minora (sing. labium minus) — two small folds covered with moist skin lying between labia majora.
   e. vestibular glands (greater), Bartholin's glands — two small ovoid or round glands which secrete mucus.   They lie deep under the posterior ends of the labia majora.
   f. vestibule of vagina — space between the labia minora which contains the vaginal and urethral orifices and openings of greater vestibular glands.

C. Diagnostic Terms:

1. atresia of:
   a. vagina — congenital absence of vagina.
   b. vulva — congenital absence of vulva.
2. Bartholin's adenitis — inflammation of Bartholin's glands, generally due to gonococcus.[3]
3. Bartholin's retention cysts — tumors retaining glandular secretions.   They tend to undergo suppuration and form abscesses.[3]
4. carcinoma of vagina — usually
   a. clear-cell type — cancer characterized by glands and tubules lined by clear cells (hobnail cells) clustering in solid nests and containing glycogen.   It occurs in adolescents and young women.
   b. epidermoid type — cancer arising from epidermal cells.   It occurs in women over 50 years of age.   Cells are devoid of glycogen.[24, 33]
   Other forms of vaginal cancer are rare.
5. carcinoma of vulva — usually a squamous cell cancer which begins with a small nodule, later undergoes ulceration and may become invasive.   It is the third most common of cancers of the female organs.[23, 32, 33]
6. condylomas — warty growths scattered over vulva.[33]
7. fistula:
   a. rectovaginal — opening between rectum and vagina.
   b. vesicovaginal — opening between bladder and vagina.[3, 26]

8. kraurosis of vulva — excessive shrinkage and atrophy of vulva, commonly seen during postmenopause.[23]
9. leukoplakia of vulva — whitish plaques on vulva which tend to form cracks and fissures. Condition results in leukoplakic vulvitis.[23]
10. vaginitis — inflammation of vagina.
    a. gonorrheal — due to gonococcal infection.
    b. mycotic, monilial — due to fungus infection.
    c. senile — due to atrophic changes; occurs in elderly women.
    d. Trichomonas — due to infection with *Trichomonas vaginalis*.[24, 31]
11. vulvar dystrophies — disorder of epithelial growth and nutrition resulting in changes of the superficial cell layers of the vulva.   The **International Society for the Study of Vulvar Disease** recommends that
    a. the terms atrophic dystrophy, kraurosis, leukoplakia, leukoplakic vulvitis, hyperplastic vulvitis and neurodermatitis be deleted and
    b. histiopathologic definitions be adopted as follows:
       (1) hyperplastic dystrophy of vulva
           (a) with atypia — atypical hyperplasia or dystrophy, mild, moderate or severe, depending on the vulvar alterations
           (b) without atypia — the presence of epithelial hyperplasia[12]
       (2) lichen sclerosus — thinning of the vulvar epithelium with the dermis being characteristically acellular.[23, 32]
12. vulvar Paget's disease — a form of vulvar cancer in situ, recurrent, noninvasive, spreading slowly and presenting a discrete eruption which is initially velvety, soft and red and later eczemoid and weepy with white plaques scattered about in the well localized lesion. Pruritus and burning are distressing symptoms.   The presence of Paget's cells in the lesion clinches the diagnosis.[23, 32, 33]
13. vulvovaginitis — inflammation of the vulva and vagina.

D. Operative Terms:[30]
1. colpectomy — removal of vagina.
2. colpocleisis — closure of vagina, one indication being prolapse of vagina following total hysterectomy.[15, 42]
3. colpomicroscopy — use of the colpomicroscope which affords higher magnification than a colposcope in studying the superficial cervical epithelium for cytologic diagnosis.[25]
4. colpoperineoplasty — repair of rectocele.
5. colpoperineorrhaphy — suture of vagina and perineum.
6. colporrhaphy — suture of vagina.
    a. anterior — repair of cystocele.
    b. posterior — repair to rectocele.[3, 6, 26, 42]
7. colposcopy — examination of the vagina and cervix uteri usually with a binocular microscope that allows the study of tissues under direct vision by magnifying the cells, makes possible colpophotography and the colposcopic selection of target biopsy sites.[15]
8. colpotomy — incision into the vagina to induce drainage.
9. episioplasty — plastic repair of the vulva.
10. excision of Bartholin's gland — removal of the gland.
11. marsupialization of Bartholin's gland cyst — incision and drainage of the cyst and partial excision of the cyst wall followed by suture of the cyst lining to the surrounding surface epithelium.   Lubrication is preserved since the gland is not removed.[15]
12. vulvectomy:
    a. simple vulvectomy — removal of vulvae which may be done for vulvar carcinoma in situ.
    b. radical vulvectomy — total removal of the vulvae with or without dissection of the regional lymph nodes.[7, 23, 39]
13. vulvovaginoplasty — various surgical techniques for creating a neovagina in the presence of vaginal agenesis, the absence of the vaginal canal.[5, 30]

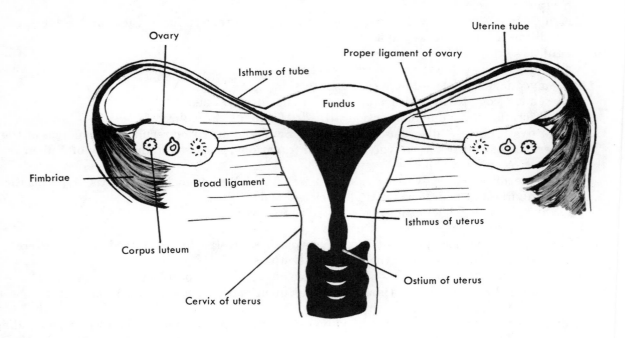

Fig. 55 — Uterus, uterine tubes and ovaries (schematic).

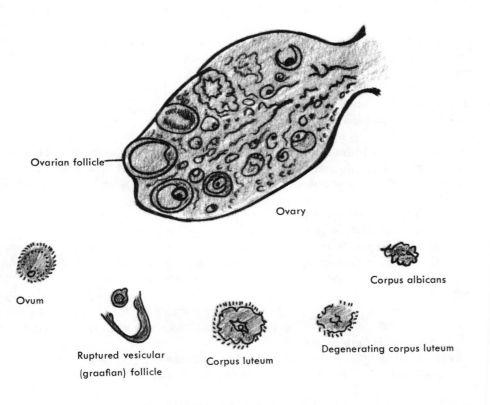

Fig. 56 — Normal ovulatory cycle.

E. Symptomatic Terms:

1. leukorrhea — abnormal cervical or vaginal discharge of white or yellowish mucus.[3, 24]
2. pruritus vulvae — severe itching of vulva.[23]

UTERUS AND SUPPORTING STRUCTURES

A. Origin of Terms:

1. cervix (L) — neck
2. fundus (L) — base
3. hyster (G) — womb
4. isthmus (G) — narrow passage
5. ostium (L) — small opening
6. metra (G) — womb
7. trachelo- (G) — neck
8. uterus (L) — womb

B. Anatomic Terms:[22, 33]

1. cul-de-sac, rectouterine pouch, Douglas' pouch — a pocket between the rectum and posterior uterus, formed by an extension of the peritoneum.
2. ligaments of uterus.
   a. broad ligaments — double-layered peritoneal sheets which extend from the side of the uterus to the lateral pelvic wall.
   b. round ligaments — two fibromuscular bands, one on each side arising anteriorly from the fundus, passing through the inguinal canal and inserting into the labia majora.[15]
3. myometrium — muscular wall of uterus.
4. uterus (nonpregnant) — a pear-shaped, thick-walled, muscular organ, situated in the pelvis between the urinary bladder and the rectum. It is about three inches ($7\frac{1}{2}$ cm) long and two inches (5 cm) wide in its upper segment. It is divided into
   a. body of uterus — main part extending from fundus to isthmus of uterus.
      (1) body cavity, uterine cavity — triangular space within the body.
      (2) endometrium — mucous membrane lining the body cavity.
   b. cervix of uterus — lower part of uterus extending from isthmus to vagina.
      (1) cervical canal — passageway between uterine cavity and vagina.
      (2) ostium of uterus, external os — opening of cervix into vagina.
   c. fundus of uterus — superior dome-shaped portion of uterus above the openings of the uterine tubes into the body cavity of uterus.
   d. isthmus of uterus — constriction of uterus between body and cervix.[33]

C. Diagnostic Terms:

1. diseases of the cervix uteri:
   a. carcinoma of the cervix — malignant cervical lesion which may present as an ulceration or tumor associated with excessive and irregular uterine bleeding and a leukorrheic vaginal discharge.[3, 25]
      (1) adenocarcinoma — highly malignant cancer assuming a glandular pattern.
      (2) squamous cell or epidermoid carcinoma — most frequent form arising from squamous epithelium.[3, 25]
      Terms adopted by the **International Federation of Gynecology and Obstetrics**:
      (1) invasive carcinoma — cancer of cervix including the 4 stages presented in Fig. 57.
      (2) microinvasive carcinoma — Stage 1A preclinical cancer characterized by early stromal invasion. Diagnosis is based on microscopic examination from biopsy specimen.
      (3) preinvasive carcinoma — Stage O intraepithelial carcinoma, carcinoma in situ.[3, 25, 34]
   b. cervicitis — inflammation of the cervix uteri.
      (1) acute — typically due to acute gonorrheal infection.
      (2) chronic — a common condition due to low grade infection.[3, 25]

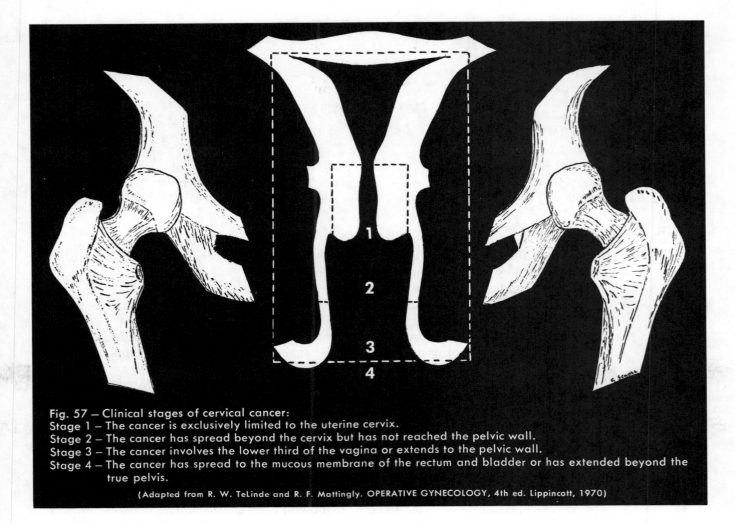

Fig. 57 — Clinical stages of cervical cancer:
Stage 1 — The cancer is exclusively limited to the uterine cervix.
Stage 2 — The cancer has spread beyond the cervix but has not reached the pelvic wall.
Stage 3 — The cancer involves the lower third of the vagina or extends to the pelvic wall.
Stage 4 — The cancer has spread to the mucous membrane of the rectum and bladder or has extended beyond the true pelvis.

(Adapted from R. W. TeLinde and R. F. Mattingly. OPERATIVE GYNECOLOGY, 4th ed. Lippincott, 1970)

    c. endocervicitis — inflammation of the mucous membrane of the cervix uteri.

    d. erosion of cervix — a red area produced by the replacement of squamous epithelium by columnar epithelium.

    e. eversion of cervix, ectropion — a rolling outward of swollen mucous membrane resulting from chronic cervicitis.   It may be associated with lacerations, cysts and erosions.

    f. polyps of cervix — soft, movable, pedunculated tabs that bleed readily.[3, 25]

2. diseases and malfunctions of the corpus uteri:

    a. adenomyosis — endometrial invasion of the myometrium which may be associated with dysmenorrhea and excessive uterine bleeding.[3, 34]

    b. dysfunctional uterine bleeding — functional bleeding not due to any local disease.[15] It may result from an irregular production of estrogen and/or progesterone by the ovary and may occur during puberty, the reproductive period of life or during menopause.[29]

    c. endometriosis — aberrant endometrial tissue found in various pelvic and abdominal organs.[3, 27]

    d. endometritis — inflammation of the mucous membrane lining the corpus uteri.

    e. parametritis — cellulitis of the tissue adjacent to the uterus.

    f. perimetritis — pelvic peritonitis.

3. displacements of the uterus:

    a. anteflexion — uterus, abnormally bent forward.

    b. prolapse, procidentia, descensus uteri — downward displacement of the uterus which may protrude from the vagina.

    c. retroflexion — corpus uteri, abnormally bent backward.

    d. retroversion — corpus uteri, abnormally turned backward with cervix directed toward symphysis pubis.

4. neoplasms of the uterus:

    a. benign tumors including

        (1) endometrial polyps — small projecting lesions which may be sessile, multiple and resemble cystic hyperplasia.

        (2) leiomyomas, myomas — benign smooth muscle tumors, erroneously referred to as fibroids, forming single or multiple, large or small, firm, encapsulated masses which may be

            (a) intraligamentous — myoma protrudes into broad ligament

            (b) intramural — myoma is embedded in myometrium

            (c) submucous — sessile or pedunculated, myoma is located beneath the endometrium, may bleed profusely and rarely undergoes sarcomatous transformation.[3, 27]

    b. malignant tumors including

        (1) adenocarcinoma of the corpus uteri — endometrial cancer characteristically affecting the postmenopausal woman in 2 ways:

            (a) as a circumscribed lesion — small portion of endometrium is diseased although myometrial invasion may be extensive

            (b) as a diffuse type — the entire endometrium is involved; ulcerations and necrotic areas are present.

        Endometrial cancer may result from prolonged estrogen stimulation with inadequate progesterone or without progesterone and from other causes.[15, 17, 27, 41]

        (2) leiomyosarcoma — neoplasm usually arises from the uterine wall, recurs readily after removal and metastasizes to bone, brain and lung.[27, 34]

D. Operative Terms:

1. cold conization, cold knife cone biopsy of uterine cervix — cold knife removal of lining of cervical canal for locating the site of abnormal exfoliative cells in the absence of a visible lesion. The procedure is valuable in the detection of preinvasive lesions, cancer in situ and occult cancer.[25]

2. culdocentesis — surgical puncture of the cul-de-sac used as diagnostic procedure whenever intraperitoneal bleeding is suspected, as for example in ectopic pregnancy.

3. culdoscopy — endoscopic examination of the rectouterine pouch (cul-de-sac) and pelvic viscera to detect whether or not endometriosis, adnexal adhesions, tumors or ectopic pregnancy are present or to determine the cause of pelvic pain, sterility or other disorders.[29]

4. dilatation and curettage — instrumental expansion of the cervix and scraping of the uterine cavity to remove

    a. endocervical tissue and endometrial tissue for diagnosis.

    b. placental tissue to control bleeding as in an incomplete abortion.

    c. small submucous myoma, polyp or other lesion in the management of uterine bleeding.[4, 25, 42]

5. electrocautery of endocervix — removing the mucous lining of the cervical canal by a high frequency current to control chronic cervicitis.[15] The procedure is also used to repair an incompetent cervix so that successful pregnancy may be achieved.

6. hysterectomy — removal of the uterus.

    a. partial or subtotal excision; for example, supracervical removal.

    b. total hysterectomy — excision of entire uterus and cervix.

    c. radical, Wertheim's operation — removal of entire uterus and dissection of regional lymph nodes.[4, 18, 27]

    d. vaginal hysterectomy — removal of the uterus by the vaginal approach.[4, 18, 27, 42]

7. hysteroscopy, fiberoptic — endoscopic examination for intrauterine diagnosis or therapy by
    a. endometrial biopsy
    b. identification of uterotubal junction, submucous myomas, polyps and septa
    c. detection and lysis of intrauterine adhesions
    d. female sterilization.
    Special features are the use of carbon dioxide or hyperviscosity dextran and the
    Storz hysteroscope (4 mm) which permits microphotography of the endometrium.[1, 13]

8. laparoscopy — endoscopic visualization of abdominal organs, especially the pelvic viscera:
    the uterus, tubes and ovaries. The procedure is of diagnostic value in primary and
    secondary amenorrhea, polycystic ovarian syndrome, unruptured ectopic pregnancy, pelvic
    inflammatory disease and other disorders.[3, 27]

9. myomectomy:
    a. abdominal approach — removal of intramural myoma or myomas from the uterus.
    b. vaginal approach — removal of cervical myoma from uterine cervix.[27, 42]

10. panhysterectomy, total hysterectomy — removal of entire uterus including the cervix.[3, 18, 42]

11. suspension of uterus — correction of retrodisplacement of the uterus:
    a. Baldy-Webster procedure — creation of a surgical opening for the passage of the round
        ligaments which are then sutured to the back of the uterus.[26]
    b. modified Gilliam procedure — surgical shortening of the round ligaments through the
        internal inguinal ring. This allows the stronger portion of the round ligament to
        bring the uterus forward.[26]

12. trachelectomy, cervicectomy — removal of uterine cervix.

13. tracheloplasty, Sturmdorf procedure — cone or core excision of endocervix; cervical
    canal covered with mucosal flap.

E. Symptomatic Terms:

1. amenorrhea — absence of menstruation for 3 months or more
    a. primary amenorrhea — no menstrual cycle initiated by the age of 18 or older.
    b. secondary amenorrhea — menstrual cycle ceased after initial menarche.[10, 29]

2. cryptomenorrhea — menses occur, but there is no external manifestation, due to
    obstructive lesion of lower genital canal.[29]

3. dysmenorrhea — painful menses. There are 2 types:
    a. primary dysmenorrhea — menstrual distress is a functional disturbance, precipitated by
        emotional tension. It is prevalent in adolescence, but may occur later in life.
    b. secondary dysmenorrhea — menstrual pain has an organic basis and its onset is
        usually postadolescence.[3, 29]

4. hypermenorrhea, menorrhagia — abnormal premenopausal bleeding due to irregular
    endometrial shedding, endometrial polyposis, uterine myoma or hypertrophy or
    bleeding disorder.[3]

5. hypomenorrhea — diminished bleeding and number of days of menstrual period.[29]

6. metrorrhagia — irregular bleeding from uterus not due to menses, but to hormone
    imbalance; sometimes induced by estrogen administration or hypothyroid state or caused
    by myoma, cervical or endometrial cancer, polyposis or other disorders.[3]

7. oligomenorrhea — infrequent menstrual bleeding; interval of cycles is over 38 days but
    less than 3 months.[29]

8. polymenorrhea — recurrent uterine bleeding within a 24 days period related to an
    exceptionally short cycle or the interruption of the cycle by psychic or physical trauma.[3]

9. premenstrual tension — syndrome recurring monthly prior to menstruation characterized
    by fluid retention, weight gain, depression or agitation. It is thought to be an
    exaggerated response to the impending period.[3, 29]

OVARIES AND UTERINE TUBES

A. Origin of Terms:

1. albus (L) — white
2. ampulla (L) — little jar
3. dehiscere (L) — to gape
4. fimbria (L) — fringe
5. folliculus (L) — little bag
6. infundibulum (L) — funnel
7. luteum (L) — yellow
8. ovarium (L) — egg holder
9. ovum, ova (L) — egg, eggs
10. salpingo (G) — tube, trumpet

B. Anatomic Terms:

1. ova (sing. ovum) — female reproductive cells.
2. ovaries (sing. ovary) — two female reproductive glands producing ova after puberty.
    a. ovarian follicle — small excretory structure of the ovary. The primary ovarian follicle is immature consisting of a single layer of follicular cells. The vesicular ovarian or graafian follicle develops, ruptures and discharges the ovum. It also secretes the follicular hormone, estrogen.
    b. corpus luteum — small yellow body formed in ruptured ovarian follicle. It secretes the corpus luteum hormone, progesterone.
    c. corpus albicans — white body which develops from corpus luteum. It leaves a pitlike scar on ovary.
3. uterine tubes, fallopian tubes, oviducts — two muscular canals about four inches (10 cm) long which provide a passageway for the ovum to the uterus and a meeting place for the ovum and spermatozoon in fertilization. An ovum entering the tube through the abdominal opening of the fimbriated infundibulum passes through the
    a. ampulla — wider, thinner-walled longest part of the tube.
    b. isthmic portion — interstitial portion of the tube, narrower and thicker-walled than the ampulla.[15]
    c. uterine part — tube within the myometrium.
    d. uterine opening — entrance into the uterine cavity.[35]

C. Diagnostic Terms:

1. abscess, tuboovarian — localized suppuration of the uterine tube and ovary.
2. Brenner tumor — peculiar, usually benign ovarian tumor containing epithelial cell nests within a matrix of fibrous tissue. It may undergo mucinous transformation or increased epithelial proliferation as seen in malignancy.[3, 28, 35]
3. cyst of ovary — a fluid containing tumor of the ovary.
    a. graafian follicle cyst — retention cyst appearing on the ovary as a fluid filled bleb due to the inability of the partially formed follicle to reabsorb.
    b. corpus luteum cyst — functional ovarian enlargement resulting from the fluid increase by the corpus luteum following ovulation.
    c. endometrial ovarian cyst — cyst formed by ectopic endometrial tissue and filled with decomposed blood due to bleeding into the cystic cavity. This cyst may be attached to other pelvic structures.[3]
    d. theca lutein cyst — cyst, prone to occur in both ovaries, is filled with straw colored or serosanguineous fluid and may rupture. It develops in the presence of hydatidiform mole, choriocarcinoma and excessive therapy with chorionic gonadotropin.[3, 14, 28, 35]
4. cystadenoma of ovary — silent tumor, nonproductive of hormone constituting 70% of ovarian neoplasms.
    a. pseudomucinous cystadenoma — usually a multilocular, encapsulated, slowly growing, glandular cyst containing brownish fluid and sometimes enlarging enormously.
    b. serous cystadenoma — encapsulated multilocular glandular cyst filled with yellowish thin fluid, growing in size, but not to great excess.[3, 14, 28, 35]

5. dysgerminoma — germ cell tumor occurring in small girls or in first decades of life, exhibiting variability in size and malignancy. The tumor may be associated with streak ovaries, rudimentary gonads seen in chromosome aberration.[3, 28]

6. dehiscence of wound, burst abdomen, evisceration, wound disruption — a bursting open of a sutured wound, followed by protrusion of intestine through the incision, a serious surgical complication; also dehiscence of a graafian follicle.

7. hydrosalpinx — uterine tube distended by clear fluid.

8. infertility, female — temporary or permanent inability to conceive or become pregnant depending on multiple etiologic factors such as
   a. anovulation
   b. defects of the luteal phase
   c. the condition of the cervix
   d. the status of the uterine tubes
   e. immunologic responses and
   f. male factors.[3]

9. Meigs syndrome — solid, fibromatous, unilateral tumor of the ovary associated with hydrothorax and ascites. Other pelvic tumors may also form pleural and peritoneal effusions which promptly disappear with surgical removal of the tumor.[3, 28, 35]

10. oophoritis, acute and chronic — inflammation of the ovary or ovaries.

11. pelvic inflammatory disease — broad terms including pelvic inflammations due to gonococcal, streptococcal postabortal infections as well as intestinal parasites in juveniles; multiple infectious organisms may coexist.[9]

12. polycystic ovarian syndrome, Stein-Leventhal syndrome — a symptom complex characterized by bilateral enlarged ovaries containing multiple follicular microcysts. Amenorrhea, infertility, obesity, hypertension and hirsutism (hairiness) are common symptoms.[3, 28, 35, 38, 41]

13. pyosalpinx — pus in the uterine tube.

14. ruptured tuboovarian abscess — a breaking open of the abscess and escape of purulent drainage into peritoneal cavity.[16]

15. salpingitis, acute and chronic — inflammation of the uterine tube or tubes.

16. torsion of ovarian pedicle — twisting of the pedicle of an ovarian cyst resulting in circulatory disturbance and sharp persistent pain.

17. tumors of the ovary:
    The **International Federation of Gynecology and Obstetrics** classifies ovarian tumors as follows (condensed classification):
    a. benign tumors:
       (1) cystic, non-neoplastic — follicular, luteal, others.
       (2) cystic, neoplastic — epithelial, dermoid, others.
       (3) solid — fibroma, Brenner tumor, others.
    b. malignant tumors:
       (1) cystic — cystadenocarcinoma, carcinoma.
       (2) solid — carcinoma, endometrioid, mesonephroma.
       (3) other malignant tumors — teratoma, etc.
       (4) tumors with endocrine potential — feminizing or virilizing tumors.
       (5) metastatic or by direct extension.[2, 11, 21, 28]

18. tumors of the uterine tubes:
    a. benign tumors — adenomyoma, others.
    b. malignant tumors — carcinoma, sarcoma.
    c. metastatic tumors.[35]

D. Operative Terms:

1. adnexectomy — removal of uterine adnexa, the tubes and ovaries[18]
2. complete ovarian ablation — surgical removal of the entire ovary.
3. oophorectomy, ovariectomy

   a. partial removal of an ovary.

   b. complete removal of one ovary.

   c. castration, bilateral, complete removal of ovaries.[12, 42]

4. oophoropexy — fixation of a displaced ovary.

5. oophoroplasty — plastic repair of an ovary.

6. ovarian wedge resection — removal of a triangular wedge of the ovary for the purpose of stimulating ovarian activity in anovulation and infertility.[38]

7. panhysterectomy and bilateral salpingo-oophorectomy — removal of complete uterus, both tubes and ovaries.[18, 42]

8. salpingectomy — partial or complete removal of the uterine tubes.

9. salpingolysis — the breaking up of peritubal adhesions which damage the fimbriated end of the tube. This procedure is considered an effective means of correcting infertility.

10. salpingo-oophorectomy — removal of tubes and ovaries.[18, 42]

11. tubal implantation — correction of the cornual block and implantation of the unobstructed tubes into the uterine cavtiy, to restore tubal patency following sterilization surgery.[29]

12. tubal insufflation, uterotubal insufflation, Rubin test — procedure used for diagnostic and therapeutic purposes:

   a. to detect whether the tubes are blocked or patent.

   b. to relieve tubal obstruction by dislodging mucous plugs and breaking up adhesions at the fimbriated ends of the tubes. Successful pregnancy may follow.[3, 29]

13. tubal ligation — tying the tubes to prevent pregnancy; sterilization surgery.

14. tuboplasty, salpingoplasty — reconstructive tubal surgery for the correction of infertility. The constricted or occluded end of the uterine tube is excised and the distal portion of the tube is reimplanted into the uterus. Recently the use of cone-shaped, spiral stents has been advocated as an effective method of maintaining tubal patency.[18, 29, 33]

E. Symptomatic Terms:

1. anovulation — absence of ovulation due to cessation or suspension of menses.

2. menopause — cessation of menses and reproductive period of life.

3. ovulation — expulsion of an ovum from the ruptured graafian follicle.

4. septic shock — sudden hypotension, renal dysfunction, peripheral blood pooling and metabolic acidosis caused by gram-negative bacteremia due to septic abortion, puerperal sepsis or pelvic infection.[12]

RADIOLOGY

A. Terms Related to Diagnostic Ultrasound:

gynecologic ultrasonography — the diagnostic use of ultrasound in detecting ovarian masses, pelvic inflammations, abnormalities of uterus, ectopic pregnancy and tuboovarian abscesses.

B. Terms Related to Therapeutic Radiology:

1. radiotherapy — use of ionizing radiation (x-rays) in the treatment of diseases. Depending on the disease it is used either as the primary and only method of treatment or in conjunction with surgery or chemotherapy. Over 95% of the diseases treated are malignancies.[30]

2. radiotherapy, preoperative — effective treatment in the management of radiosensitive tumors prior to surgery. Irradiation devitalizes cancer cells and shrinks the tumor. Carcinomas of the cervix and endometrium generally respond well to radiotherapy.[27, 30]

3. radiotherapy, postoperative — following surgery irradiation used as a palliative and therapeutic measure, if the tumor has been incompletely removed or the patients are poor risk, elderly and obese. In incurable patients with uterine and ovarian cancer radiotherapy prolongs the patient's useful life.[28, 30]

Table 21

ULTRASONIC DIAGNOSIS OF OVARIAN LESIONS

Ovarian Cysts and Tumors		*Ultrasonic Identification*[a, b]
Small lesions	Intrapelvic cysts	High percentage undetectable
	Solid dermoids	Detectability questionable
Large lesions	Dermoid cysts	Cystic and solid components and sometimes septa detectable
	Unilocular cysts	Classic characterization usually identified
	Multilocular cysts	Linear echoes reflected from septa
	Malignant cysts	Cyst echoes from solid tissue projections into the lumen usually present
	Ovarian fibromas	Less transonic than uterine fibromas
	Ovarian carcinomas or sarcomas	Ultrasonic characteristics similar to any abdominal malignancy; differential diagnosis difficult

[a]Ellis Barnett and Patricia Morley. *Abdominal Echography.* London: Butterworths & Co., 1974, pp. 112-126.
[b]W. J. Cochrane. Ultrasound in gynecology. *Radiologic Clinics of North America,* 13: 457-466, December, 1975.

C. Terms Related to Radiation Injury:

1. overirradiation — excessive radiation therapy. It may cause a syndrome characterized by nausea, vomiting, diarrhea, anorexia and malaise within hours after overexposure followed by blood dyscrasia, within weeks or months.
2. radiation anemia — usually aplastic anemia; no red blood cells are formed due to suppression of bone marrow activity. It occurs following excessive whole body radiation.
3. radiodermatitis — inflammation of skin resulting from exposure to radiation.
4. radioepithelitis — disintegration of epithelial tissue due to radiation, notably to that of the mucous membrane.
5. radionecrosis — disintegration or death of tissue caused by radiation.
6. radionephritis — acute condition due to overexposure of kidney to radiation. It is manifested by hypertension, edema, casts and protein in urine.
7. radioneuritis — nerve involvement resulting from overexposure to radioactivity.
8. radiation sickness — untoward effects of radiotherapy, usually manifested by nausea, vomiting and diarrhea, resulting from the breakdown of body tissue.

CLINICAL LABORATORY

A. Cytologic Studies for Gynecologic Conditions:

1. cytopathologic studies — they include cytogenetic, cytologic and hormonal evaluation of gynecologic disorders with specimens for study usually obtained by microbiopsy.[12]
2. cytogenetic studies — they deal with the chromosomal makeup for clarifying issues of hermaphroditism, intersexuality and antenatal sex determination.[12]
3. cytologic studies — the detection of tumors of the cervix and endometrium in the preinvasive state when proper treatment can be instituted. Several methods have been devised to obtain smears for cytologic diagnosis.

a. Ayre's surface cell biopsy method — the smear is obtained from cervical scrapings by means of a wooden spatula.[12]

b. Gravlee jet washer — a vacuum suction technique of intrauterine washing for collecting cytology specimens from the endometrium for an early detection of cancer.[3, 20]

c. Papanicolaou's method — a curved glass pipette with rubber bulb for aspirating vaginal fluid with its cellular components.

The smear technic is based on the fact that vaginal and uterine epithelia, like all epithelial tissue, undergo continual exfoliation or shedding of cells. Similarly, tumors which reach the lining surface may exfoliate cells which fall into the vagina and become mixed with the vaginal secretion. Experts in exfoliative cytology recognize incompletely developed malignant cells which gradually and progressively change from a benign, preinvasive, preclinical stage to an early invasive and late malignant stage.[3, 12, 37]

4. hormonal studies — cytopathologic evaluation for detecting abnormal cytohormonal patterns which may suggest the presence of functional ovarian neoplasms, endocrine or breast tumors and endometrial or tubal lesions.[12]

5. microbiopsy — the cellular specimen obtained for tissue examination by the pathologist.

B. Other Tests:

1. culture for *Neisseria gonorrhoeae* — use of Thayer-Martin (TM) medium in cultures for the detection of the gonococcus.[19]

2. dark-field examination — most specific means of direct demonstration of *Treponema pallidum* obtained from moist lesions of primary, secondary or relapsing syphilis.[3, 36]

3. Schiller test — test helpful in the detection of superficial cancer particularly that of the cervix. Normal epithelium is rich in glycogen and stained deeply by iodine solution. Cancerous epithelium has almost no glycogen and takes no stain. The test has its limitations.

ABBREVIATIONS

A. General Terms:

CIS — carcinoma in situ
D&C — dilatation and curettage
FSH — follicle stimulating hormone
GC — gonorrhea
Gyn — gynecology
IUD — intrauterine device
HPO — hypothalamic-pituitary-ovarian
LH — luteinizing hormone

LTH — luteotropic hormone
LMP — last menstrual period
MH — marital history
PID — pelvic inflammatory disease
PMP — previous menstrual period
TM — Thayer-Martin (culture medium for gonococcus)
WF — white female

B. Organizations:

ACOG — American College of Obstetricians and Gynecologists
ACS — American College of Surgeons

FIGO — International Federation of Gynecology and Obstetrics
ISSVD — International Society for the Study of Vulvar Disease

ORAL READING PRACTICE

Ovarian Neoplasms

Ovarian neoplasms may occur at any age; however, the majority develop during the reproductive period. Of these the proportion of **benign** to **malignant** neoplasms is about three to four.

The new growths tend to be larger than 6 cm in diameter. The ovaries and related **embryonic** rests are frequent sources of cyst formation. Smaller or plum-sized **cysts** occasionally are **non-neoplastic** growths. **Follicular** cysts are derived from the **graafian follicles** and vary in size from 2 to 20 mm, though sometimes are larger. They are usually **bilateral** and **multiple** and lined with flattened epithelium which is lost in some areas. Characteristically, their contents appear watery to serous, straw-colored or blood-tinged.

Simple cystadenomata of the ovary are prone to reach an enormous size, containing several gallons of fluid. They are usually globular, **lobulated** and **multilocular** with a smooth surface and a pedicle attachment through which nutrient blood vessels pass.

The lining epithelium of cystadenomas may proliferate markedly forming an irregular wide-spread ingrowth which contains **papillary projections** extending into the cyst cavity. The neo-plasm thus formed is usually quite **vascular** and the epithelial covering of its tree-like branches is **hyperplastic** and often **anaplastic**. It may exhibit a marked tendency to **invade** adjacent struc-tures and reach the **peritoneal** surface from which point widespread peritoneal invasion and meta-stasis take place. The outcome is a gelatinous **carcinomatosis** of the **peritoneum**. The same fatal complication may develop if rupture of a **papillary cystadenoma** results in freeing neoplastic cells and bits of tissue in the peritoneal cavity.

Ovarian cysts may be entirely asymptomatic. When manifestations do result, they fall into the following categories: (1) those involving functional disturbances, such as **menorrhagia** and **metrorrhagia**, (2) those resulting from mechanical factors incident to the size of the cyst, (3) those characterized by obvious enlargement of the abdomen often without associated manifestations and, finally, (4) those resulting from **torsion** of the **pedicle** of the cyst.[2, 3, 11, 14, 21, 28, 35]

Table 22
SOME GYNECOLOGIC CONDITIONS AMENABLE TO SURGERY

Organs Involved	Diagnoses	Operations	Operative Procedures
Hymen	Atresia of hymen	Hymenotomy Hymenectomy	Incision of hymen Excision of hymen
Clitoris	Congenital hypertrophy of clitoris due to adrenal cortical hyperplasia	Reconstruction of external genitals Clitorectomy	External genitals reconstructed along normal female lines and clitoris removed
Bartholin's gland	Abscess of Bartholin's gland	Incision and drainage of Bartholin's gland	Surgical opening and evacua-tion of abscess
Bartholin's gland	Chronic bartholinitis and cysts of Bartholin's gland	Marsupialization of Bartholin's gland cyst	Partial excision of cyst wall Suture of cyst lining to the surrounding surface epithelium
Vulva	Leukoplakia of vulvae	Vulvectomy	Removal of vulvae
Vulva	Vulvar carcinoma, epidermoid type	Basset operation: Vulvectomy Lymphadenectomy	Excision of vulva, superficial inguinal lymph nodes and wide dissection of deep fe-moral and inguinal glands
Vulva Perineum	Burn of vulva and perineum	Episioperineoplasty	Plastic repair of vulva and perineum
Vagina Bladder	Vesicovaginal fistula	Closure of vesicovaginal fistula	Suture of fistula

Organs Involved	Diagnoses	Operations	Operative Procedures
Vagina Bladder	Urinary stress incontinence	Suprapubic vesicourethral suspension Marshall-Marchetti operation	Surgical elevation and fixation of the bladder neck and urethra by suturing them to the pubis and rectus muscles
Vagina Bladder	Urinary stress incontinence associated with cystocele	Kelly operation modified technique	Construction of a firm shelf of periurethral tissue to sup- port bladder and urethra
Vagina Bladder	Cystocele	Colpoplasty	Plastic repair of vagina; repair of cystocele
Vagina Perineum	Rectocele	Colpoperineoplasty	Plastic repair of vagina and perineum; repair of rectocele
Cervix uteri	Chronic endocervicitis	Conization Sturmdorf procedure Plastic repair of cervix uteri	Removal of mucous lining of cervical canal by high fre- quency current Conized area covered with mucosal flap
Cervix uteri	Eversion of cervix (ectropion)	Striping by cautery Cryosurgery	Hot cautery Freezing technique
Cervix uteri	Squamous cell carcinoma of cervix uteri, early phase, radioresistant lesion	Radical hysterectomy Pelvic lymphadenectomy	Excision of entire uterus Removal of pelvic lymph glands
Corpus uteri	Submucous myoma	Myomectomy	Complete enucleation of myoma
Corpus uteri Tubes Ovaries	Adenocarcinoma of corpus uteri Metastasis to adnexa uteri	Panhysterectomy Salpingectomy Oophorectomy	Removal of corpus and cervix uteri, tubes and ovaries
Uterus	Prolapse of uterus	Manchester-Fothergill operation	Amputation of cervix and fixation of ligament to anterior uterus
Uterus	Severe retroversion of uterus Slight descensus uteri	Suspension of uterus Modified Gilliam procedure	Surgical shortening of the round ligaments through the internal inguinal ring
Uterine tube	Tuboövarian abscess	Incision and drainage of abscess	Surgical opening and evacua- tion of abscess
Ovary	Torsion of ovarian pedicle	Oophorectomy	Excision of ovary
Ovary	Cystadenocarcinoma, serous type	Panhysterectomy Bilateral salpingo- oophorectomy	Removal of entire uterus, both tubes and ovaries, including regional lymph nodes

REFERENCES AND BIBLIOGRAPHY

1. Averette, H. E. Gynecology and Obstetrics. *Surgery Gynecology & Obstetrics*, 142: 201-205, February, 1976.

2. Barber, H. R. K. Ovarian cancer in children. *Ca — A Cancer Journal for Clinicians*, 25: 334-337, November-December, 1975.

3. Benson, R. C. Gynecology. In Krupp, Marcus A., Chatton, Milton J. *Current Medical Diagnosis & Treatment*, 15th ed. Los Altos, California: Lange Medical Publications, 1976, pp. 415-448.

4. _____. Common surgical procedures in Obstetrics and Gynecology. *Ibid.*, pp. 448-450.

5. Carparo, V. J. *et al.* Vaginal agenesis. *American Journal of Obstetrics and Gynecology*, 124: 98-107, January, 1976.

6. Clark, D. H. Repair of vesico-vaginal fistulas: Simultaneous transvaginal-transvesical approach. *Southern Medical Journal*, 68: 1410-1416, November, 1975.

7. Cruz-Jimenez, P. R. Cutaneous basal cell carcinoma of vulva. *Cancer*, 36: 1860-1868, November, 1975.

8. Danforth, David N. (ed.). *Textbook of Obstetrics and Gynecology*, 3rd ed. New York: Harper & Row, Publishers, 1977.

9. Eschenbach, D. A. *et al.* Acute pelvic inflammatory disease. *Clinical Obstetrics and Gynecology*, 18: 35-56, March, 1975.

10. Farber, M. *et al.* Amenorrhea: A review of 40 cases. *Obstetrics and Gynecology*, 47: 115-118, January, 1976.

11. Fraumeni, J. F. *et al.* Six families prone to ovarian cancer. *Cancer*, 36: 364-369, August, 1975.

12. Frost, J. K. Gynecologic and obstetric cytopathology. In Novak, Edmund R. and Woodruff, J. Donald. *Gynecologic and Obstetric Pathology*, 7th ed. Philadelphia: W. B. Saunders Co., 1974, pp. 634-728.

13. Greenhill, J. P. (ed.). *Obstetrics and Gynecology*, 1975. Chicago: Year Book Medical Publishers, Inc., 1975, pp. 253-300.

14. Greenwald, E. F. Ovarian tumors. *Clinical Obstetrics and Gynecology*, 18: 61-86, December, 1975.

15. Hamilton, Eugene G., M.D. Personal communications.

16. Heaton, F. C. *et al.* Postmenopausal tuboovarian abscess. *Obstetrics and Gynecology*, 47: 90-94, January, 1976.

17. Henriksen, E. The lymphatic dissemination of endometrial carcinoma. *American Journal of Obstetrics and Gynecology*, 123: 570-576, November 15, 1975.

18. Herbst, A. L. *et al.* Gynecology. In Schwartz, Seymour I. *Principles of Surgery*, 2d ed. New York: McGraw-Hill Book Co., 1974, pp. 1589-1630.

19. Kellogg, D. S. New developments in the laboratory diagnosis of gonorrhea. *Clinical Obstetrics and Gynecology*, 18: 153-160, March, 1975.

20. Lukeman, J. M. An evaluation of the negative pressure "Jet Washing" of the endometrium in menopausal and postmenopausal patients. *Obstetrical and Gynecological Survey*, 30: 400-401, June, 1975.

21. Mikuta, J. J. A rational approach to carcinoma of the ovary. *Southern Medical Journal*, 68: 1401-1406, November, 1975.

22. Novak, Edmund R., Jones, Georgeanna Seegar, Jones, Howard W. Anatomy. *Novak's Textbook of Gynecology*, 9th ed. Baltimore: Williams & Wilkins Co., 1975, pp. 1-17.

23. _____. Diseases of the vulva. *Ibid.*, pp. 182-212.

24. _____. Diseases of the vagina. *Ibid.*, pp. 212-231.

25. _____. Cervicitis and cervical polyp — Carcinoma of the cervix. *Ibid.*, pp. 232-291.

26. _____. Relaxations, incontinence, fistulas and malpositions. *Ibid.*, pp. 292-317.

27. _____. Adenocarcinoma of the corpus uteri — Myoma of the uterus — Adenomyosis of the uterus — Sarcoma of the uterus. *Ibid.*, pp. 332-394.

28. _____. Benign tumors of the ovary — Malignant tumors of the ovary — Functioning tumors of the ovary. *Ibid.*, pp. 444-541.

29. _____. Infertility and abortion — Amenorrhea — Dysmenorrhea, premenstrual tension and related disorders. *Ibid.*, pp. 625-730.

30. Pilla, Lawrence A., M.D. Personal communications.

31. Rein, M. F. *et al.* Trichomoniasis, candidiasis and the minor venereal diseases. *Clinical Obstetrics and Gynecology*, 18: 73-88, March, 1975.

32. Report of the Committee on Terminology. New nomenclature for vulvar disease. *Obstetrics and Gynecology*, 47: 122-124, January, 1976.

33. Robbins, Stanley L. Female genital tract. *Pathologic Basis of Disease*. Philadelphia: W. B. Saunders Co., 1974, pp. 1201-1214.

34. _____. Cervix — Body of the uterus and endomentrium. *Ibid.*, pp. 1214-1238.

35. _____. Fallopian tubes — Ovaries. *Ibid.*, pp. 1238-1255.

36. Rudolph, A. H. *et al.* Syphilis — Diagnosis and treatment. *Clinical Obstetrics and Gynecology*, 18: 163-182, March, 1975.

37. Shulman, J. J. The Pap smear: Take two. *Obstetrical and Gynecological Survey*, 30: 710-711, October, 1975.

38. Toaff, R. *et al.* Infertility following wedge resection of the ovaries. *American Journal of Obstetrics and Gynecology*, 124: 92-96, January 1, 1976.

39. Twombly, G. H. Radical vulvectomy and bilateral superficial and deep groin and pelvic lymphadenectomy. *Clinical Obstetrics and Gynecology*, 18: 2-32, March, 1975.

40. Van Nagell, J. R. *et al.* Diagnostic and therapeutic efficacy of cervical conization. *American Journal of Obstetrics and Gynecology*, 124: 134-139, January 15, 1976.

41. Wood, G. P. *et al.* Endometrial adenocarcinoma and the polycystic ovary syndrome. *American Journal of Obstetrics and Gynecology*, 124: 140-142, January 15, 1976.

42. Zollinger, Robert M. and Zollinger, Robert M., Jr. Gynecologic procedures. *Atlas of Surgical Operations*, 4th ed. New York: Macmillan Publishing Co., Inc., 1975, pp. 275-305.

Chapter XI
Maternal, Antenatal and Neonatal Conditions

A. Origin of Terms:

1. gravida (L) — pregnancy
2. multi (L) — many
3. nulli (L) — none
4. pario (L) — to bear
5. pelvis (L) — basin
6. placenta (L) — cake
7. primi (L) — first
8. puer (L) — boy, child

B. General Terms:

1. basal body temperature — body temperature taken under basal conditions before arising in the morning. Relatively lower levels are present in the preovulatory phase than in the postovulatory phase.[9]
2. biphasic curve — curve referring to the two basic general temperature levels in the menstrual cycle:
   a. the lower temperature level, known as the estrogenic phase, extends from the onset of menstruation to a short period after ovulation. The woman's basal temperature is usually below 97.9°F (36.6°C) orally. The early part of this estrogenic phase is nonfertile. The time and extent of this period of infertility can be approximated (see rhythm).
   b. the higher temperature level follows ovulation. The woman's basal temperature is usually above 97.9°F (36.6°C). Since the life of an ovum is limited, the period which follows the first 3 days of the rise is nonfertile.[20]
3. blighted ovum — an impregnated ovum which has ceased to grow within the first trimester.
4. contraception — voluntary prevention of pregnancy.[9]
5. gestation — intrauterine development of infant.
   a. embryonic period — approximately the first trimester.
   b. fetal period — approximately the second and third trimesters.[47, 74]
6. gravida — a pregnant woman.
7. high risk gravida — there are multiple reasons for considering a pregnant woman a high risk patient. She may be too young or too old, underweight or overweight, have diabetes, hypertension, urinary infection, rubella, hepatitis, Rh incompatibility, alcoholic or narcotic addiction and many other health hazards. By identifying the problem during early gestation appropriate treatment may be instituted to protect the mother and growing fetus.[6, 47, 48, 72]
8. high risk neonate — newborn in need of resuscitation due to abnormally brief or prolonged gestation, too low or too high birth weight, defective Apgar score, fetal diseases, congenital anomalies, chromosomal aberrations and a host of maternal factors.[7, 72]
9. multipara — a woman who has given birth to two or more children.
10. natural childbirth — childbirth in a normal physiologic manner without anesthetic or instruments. The woman participates actively and consciously in her delivery.
    a. Read's method, childbirth without fear — antenatal program for the mother-to-be including education, psychologic conditioning, exercises and relaxation techniques preparatory to the 3 stages of labor. The relaxation is active and may induce sleep and amnesia. A minimum of pain is experienced during delivery.
    b. psychoprophylactic method as practiced by Lamaze, childbirth without pain — verbal analgesia based on antenatal training of the expectant mother. Words are used as therapeutic agents to create in the woman's mind a chain of conditioned reflexes

applicable to childbirth (Pavlov's second system). The mother-to-be learns to give birth: to breathe, push and relax effectively and to bring forth the child in a mentally alert state. The couple's united efforts make childbirth without pain a victory for both, since the husband plays an active part in the entire program.

11. natural family planning — a method based on the recognition of the fertile period of the menstrual cycle.[10, 20, 46, 39, 53]
    a. calendar rhythm — a method of determining the approximate time of ovulation related to the length of a series of a woman's menstrual cycles. It is assumed that
       (1) ovulation takes place within a range of 12-16 days before menstruation
       (2) the maximal survival of the ovum is about 48 hours
       (3) the maximal survival of the sperm is about 72 hours.
       Rhythm refers, in obstetrics, to the alternating periods of sterility and fertility. Since fertility depends on the availability of the ovum, pregnancy may be avoided by practicing continence a few days before and after ovulation.[20, 53]
    b. ovulation method, Billings method — a study of the mucus pattern of fertility in order to predict the fertile period of the menstrual cycle. After menstruation a a mucous discharge of sticky, cloudy secretion appears and lasts about 6 days. It is followed by a peak symptom of lubricative, clear, slippery mucus resembling egg white which is present for one or two days. Typically ovulation takes place within this phase. After the peak symptom another kind of mucus forms. It is so thick, viscoid and tenacious that the sperm cannot penetrate it. Conception may be avoided by practicing abstinence from the onset of the mucous discharge until 4 days after the appearance of the peak symptom.[10, 46, 53]
    c. temperature method — the recognition of body temperature changes during the normal menstrual cycle with a rise of temperature occurring following ovulation. The infertile period includes a preovulatory and postovulatory phase. Exact temperature recording during the postovulation phase may pinpoint the fertile period. After a temperature elevation for 3 consecutive days, the fertilization of the ovum is no longer possible.[10, 46, 53]
12. parturient — woman in labor.
13. perinatology — the study of the infant before, during and after birth.
14. primipara — a woman who has delivered her first child after the period of viability.
15. teratogens — noxious agents: actinic, infectious, chemical, mechanical or nutritional, capable of disrupting normal gestation with subsequent antenatal death or the birth of a misshapen, deformed neonate.[74]
16. teratology — the study of disfiguring malformations due to arrested embryonic growth and fetal development of organs or structures.[74]

C. Anatomic Terms:

1. pelvis (pl. pelves) — bony ring adapted to childbearing in female. It is composed of sacrum, coccyx and hip bones.
   a. false pelvis — bounded posteriorly by lumbar vertebrae; serves to support pregnant uterus.
   b. true pelvis — bounded posteriorly by sacrum, of practical significance in child bearing.
   c. pelvic brim, pelvic inlet — upper opening into true pelvic cavity.
   d. pelvic outlet — the lower opening of the pelvis.
   e. promontory of the sacrum — the upper projecting part of the sacrum.
2. placenta — vascular structure which provides nutrition for the fetus.
3. secundines, afterbirth — fetal membranes and placenta; their expulsion occurs in third stage of labor.

D. Diagnostic Terms:

1. abortion — expulsion of the product of conception before the fetus has attained viability.[62]
   a. habitual abortion — 3 or more consecutive, spontaneous abortions.[35]

    b. imminent, threatened abortion — vaginal bleeding with or without pain, and cervical dilatation, usually terminating in expulsion of fetus.

    c. incomplete abortion — fetal expulsion with retention of total or partial placenta and subsequent bleeding.

    d. induced abortion — voluntary expulsion of fetus, brought about by mechanical means or drugs.[16, 50, 61, 71]

    e. inevitable abortion — rupture of membranes associated with cervical dilatation and followed by fetal expulsion.

    f. missed abortion — fetus dead, but retained in utero for days or weeks.

    g. septic abortion — abortion with fever without any other known cause for temperature elevation, usually referred to as septic.   Patients who have had interference, even if afebrile, may have a septic abortion.   A foul smelling vaginal discharge is a dominant feature.[35]

2. ectopic pregnancy — fertilized ovum implanted outside of uterine cavity: in tube, ovary or free in abdomen attached to a viscus.[9, 62]

3. hyperemesis gravidarum — severe nausea and vomiting during the first months of pregnancy which may cause dehydration and serious metabolic disturbances in mother and fetus.[9]

4. hypertensive disorders of pregnancy — high blood pressure of 140/90 and above, preceding pregnancy or developing during gestation or in early puerperium.   Proteinuria, edema, convulsions and coma may be present.

    a. eclampsia — major disorder of pregnancy and puerperium manifested by high blood pressure, convulsions, renal dysfunction, headache, edema and severe cases of coma.

    b. preeclampsia — usually a disorder of a first pregnancy but may also occur in multiparas who are severely hypertensive or diabetic.   Characteristically there is an upward trend in high blood pressure, sudden and excessive weight gain related to fluid retention and kidney dysfunction, proteinuria or albuminuria.[28, 62]

5. involution of uterus — postpartum return of uterus to its former shape and size.

6. oligohydramnios — deficient amount of amniotic fluid.

7. phlegmasia alba dolens — phlebitis of femoral vein; may occur postpartum.

8. placenta ablatio, placenta abruptio — premature detachment of the placenta generally causing severe hemorrhage.

9. placenta accreta — adherent placenta; remains attached to uterus after delivery.[9]

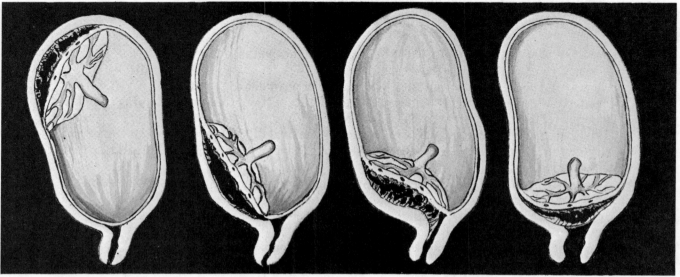

Fig. 58 — Normal placenta.   Fig. 59 — Marginal placenta previa.   Fig. 60 — Partial placenta previa.   Fig. 61 — Complete placenta previa.

(Adapted from J. W. Huffman, M.D. *Gynecology and Obstetrics*. Philadelphia: W. B. Saunders Co. 1962 — with permission).

10. placenta previa — a displaced placenta, implanted in lower segment of uterine wall.
    a. marginal insertion — placenta comes up to the ostium uteri, but does not cover it.
    b. partial placenta previa — placenta covers the ostium uteri incompletely.
    c. complete or central placenta — placenta entirely obstructs the ostium uteri.
11. polyhydramnios, hydramnios — excessive amount of amniotic fluid.
12. puerperal hematoma — escape of blood into the mucosa or subcutaneous tissues of the external genitalia forming painful vaginal or vulvar hematomas (blood tumors). They may also form in broad ligaments.[35]
13. puerperal infection, puerperal fever, childbed fever, puerperal septicemia, puerperal sepsis — infection of the genital tract occurring within the postpartum period. Fever is the dominant characteristic of puerperal infection; however, the puerpera may have fever from other causes, e.g. kidney or lung infections.
14. rupture of uterus, hysterorrhexis, metrorrhexis — laceration of uterus, a torn uterus.
15. subinvolution — failure of the uterus to reduce to its normal size after delivery.
16. trophoblast — a layer of ectoderm which attaches the conceptus to the uterine wall, nourishes the embryo and has invasive propensities, thus malignant potentials.
17. trophoblastic disease (TRD) — disease originating in trophoblast.
    a. chorioadenoma destruens — malignant nonmetastasizing, invasive tumor which may penetrate the muscular coat and even the serosa of the uterus and neighboring structures rendering its removal difficult. Trophoblastic proliferation tends to be excessive.[35, 55, 62]
    b. choriocarcinoma — highly malignant, invasive tumor derived from fetal trophoblast. Neoplastic cells infiltrate the myometrium and readily metastasize to the liver, lungs, brain and pelvic organs. Choriocarcinoma may be a complication of a hydatidiform mole.
    c. hydatidiform mole — developmental abnormality of the placenta characterized by the conversion of chorionic villi into a mass of vesicles that resemble hanging grapes. Embryonic growth is usually terminated but if it continues to full term, the neonate will probably be stillborn.[19, 55, 62]
18. uteroplacental apoplexy, Couvelaire uterus — sudden, severe retroplacental bleeding into the myometrium.[9]
19. various conditions associated with pregnancy or puerperium — disorders or states affecting the nonpregnant women may also affect the gravida and puerpera. Chlamydial, cytomegaloviral, herpetic, mycoplasmal and venereal infections of the mother are readily transmitted to the fetus and may cause congenital defects.[3, 48, 49, 69, 77]

E. Operative Terms:

1. Cesarean section — removal of the fetus through an incision into the uterus.
   a. classic — incision into corpus uteri.
   b. lower uterine segment — incision into the lower segment of the uterus.
   c. Cesarean hysterectomy — delivery of the child by section, followed by supravaginal or supracervical hysterectomy.[60]
   d. vaginal hysterectomy, colpohysterectomy — removal of the uterus through the vagina.[9]
2. breech extraction — method of delivery when the presenting parts are the buttocks or feet. The fetus is pulled out.
3. episiotomy — incision of perineum to facilitate delivery and prevent perineal laceration.
   a. median episiotomy — midline incision of perineum.
   b. mediolateral episiotomy — the incision is directed toward one side of the midline.[35]
4. forceps operations — instrumental delivery of child.
   a. low forceps — application of forceps when head is on perineum.
   b. high forceps — application of forceps before head has passed through the pelvic inlet.
   c. mid-forceps — application of forceps when head is at level of ischial spines.[35]
5. saline abortion — intra-amniotic injection of hypertonic salt solution after 14 weeks of gestation to induce abortion.[50, 61]

6. vacuum extraction — instrumental delivery of infant with a vacuum extractor, indicated in
   a. fetal distress, malpresentation, prolapse of arm
   b. maternal inertia, prolonged labor, heart-lung disease, shock, toxemia.[56]
7. version — the process of turning the fetus in the uterus.
   a. cephalic version — the head is made the presenting part.
   b. podalic version — the breech is made the presenting part.

F. Symptomatic Terms:

1. attitude, obstetric — the intrauterine position of the fetus.
2. ballottement — method of detecting pregnancy or testing for engagement of fetal head. The examiner sharply taps against the lower uterine segment with his forefinger in the vagina and tosses the embryo upward.
3. Bandl's ring — a groove seen on the abdomen between pubis and umbilicus after hard labor.
4. Braxton-Hicks sign — painless contractions of the uterus throughout gestation. They occur periodically and last to term.[35]
5. bruit of placenta — blowing sound heard on auscultation. It is due to maternal circulation.[35]
6. Chadwick's sign — violet discoloration of the vaginal mucosa, presumptive evidence of pregnancy.[9]
7. colostrum — yellowish fluid secreted by the mammary gland during pregnancy and for the first 2 or 3 days postdelivery.[9]
8. dilatation of cervix — gradual opening of the cervix to permit passage of fetus.
9. dystocia — difficult birth.[21, 58]
10. effacement — obliteration of cervix; the process of thinning and shortening of the uterine cervix.
11. engagement — descent of the fetal head through the pelvic inlet.
12. engorgement — excessive venous and lymph stasis of lactating breasts, usually referred to as caked breasts.[9]
13. gestation — pregnancy.
14. Goodell's sign — softening of the uterine cervix, indicative of pregnancy.[9]
15. Hegar's sign — softening of lower uterus; occurs in pregnancy.
16. hemorrhage — excessive blood loss.
    a. antepartum — before birth.
    b. intrapartum — during delivery.
    c. postpartum — after delivery.
17. labor — normal uterine contractions which result in the delivery of the fetus.
    a. missed labor — a few contractions at full-term, then cessation of labor and fetal retention, usually due to death of fetus in utero or extrauterine pregnancy.
    b. precipitate labor — hasty labor.
    c. premature labor — before full-term.
    d. protracted labor — unduly prolonged.[21]
18. labor — 3 stages:
    a. cervical dilatation — first stage begins with uterine contractions terminates with complete cervical dilatation.
    b. expulsion — second stage, from complete dilatation of the cervix to the birth of the baby.
    c. placental separation and expulsion — third stage, from delivery of neonate to expulsion of the placenta.[21]
19. lochia — discharge from the birth canal following delivery.
20. pica — peculiar cravings of the pregnant woman for strange food or nonedibles.
21. presentation or lie — the relation which the long axis of the fetus bears to that of the mother. Accordingly, distinction is made between longitudinal and transverse presentations. Longitudinal presentations occurs in 99.5% of cases and includes the following varieties:

   a. breech presentation — presentation of the fetal buttock.
       (1) complete breech — thighs flexed on abdomen and legs flexed upon thighs.
       (2) footling — the foot presents.
       (3) frank breech — legs extended over ventral body surface.
       (4) knee — the knee presents.
   b. face presentation — presentation of the fetal head.
       (1) brow — the forehead presents.
       (2) sinciput — the large fontanel presents.
       (3) vertex — the upper and back part of the head presents.   This is the most
           common variety.[29]
    Transverse presentation occurs in 0.5% of cases.

22. quickening — the pregnant woman's first perception of fetal life.[9]
23. sterility — infertility, reproductive failure.[9]

THE ANTENATAL PERIOD

A. Origin of Terms:

1. amnion (G) — membrane around fetus
2. antigen (G/L) — against begetting
3. chorion (G) — membrane around fetus
4. fetus (L) — offspring
5. teras (G) — monster
6. toxico (G) — poison

B. Anatomic Terms:

1. amnion — the innermost fetal membrane which forms the bag of waters and encloses the fetus.
2. amniotic fluid — fluid contained in the amniotic sac.
3. chorion — outer envelope of the fetus.
4. embryo — the product of conception, especially during the first three months of life.
5. fetus — the unborn child after the first three months of development.

C. Diagnostic Terms:

1. abortus (pl. abortuses) — a fetus which weighs about 500 grams (17 ounces) when expelled from the uterus, thus is unable to survive.
2. fetal anomaly, preventable — malformed fetus due to mother taking teratogenic drugs during pregnancy, e.g.:
   a. anticarcinogens as aminopterin, cytoxin, methotrexate, others
   b. ovarian or testicular steroids as androgen, estrogen, progesterone
   c. thalidomide, others.[9, 31, 35, 52]
3. fetal anoxia, intrauterine asphyxia — oxygen want of the fetus which may result from prolapse of the cord, placenta abruptio, compression of the umbilical vein or other causes. Death is inevitable if fetus is not delivered promptly.[6, 8, 22]
4. fetal distress — a life threatening condition due to fetal anoxia, hemolytic disease or other causes.[6]
5. fetal hemolytic disease — blood disorder caused by antibody antigen reaction in ABO, Rh or other blood group incompatibility. Maternal antibodies cross the placenta, agglutinate fetal blood cells and destroy them. Fetal anemia develops.[2, 12, 26, 35, 70]
6. fetotoxicity — toxic effects of maternal medication on fetus and neonate. Some high risk agents are:

	Drugs	Toxicity
a. analgesics	acetylsalicylic acid	Bleeding of neonate
	(Aspirin — excessive	Convulsions
	use)	Encephalopathy
	other salicylates	
b. antianxiety	diazepam	Bleeding of neonate
drugs	(Valium)	
(ataractics-	meprobamate	Retarded growth
tranquilizers)	(Equanil)	

c. anticoagulants (coumarin)	coumadin dicumarol warfarin	Bleeding of neonate Hypoprothrombinemia Fetal death
d. hypnotics sedatives	barbiturates phenobarbital pentobarbital thiopental	Abstinence syndrome Retarded growth Bleeding of neonate Hyperbilirubinemia
e. narcotics	heroin meperidine (Demerol) methadone (Dolophine) morphine	Abstinence syndrome Convulsions Nerve damage Retarded growth Neonatal death

Among the many other hazards of fetotoxicity are maternal immunization (Sabin) for poliomyelitis, smallpox vaccination and compulsive nicotine smoking.[6, 9, 30, 31, 38, 40, 54]

7. prolapse of cord — premature descent of the umbilical cord, a cause of fetal death.

D. Terms Related to Special Procedures:

1. amniocentesis — puncture of the amniotic cavity:[6, 25, 65]
    a. to aspirate fluid for amniotic fluid analysis.[78, 81]
    b. to inject radiopaque substance for amniography.[65]
    c. to administer intrauterine transfusions to the fetus with severe hemolytic disease.[42, 72, 79]
    d. to determine pressure changes of amniotic fluid which permit the continuous monitoring of uterine contractibility.
    e. to monitor the fetal heart rate.[41]
    f. to detect possible genetic disorder antenatally.[73]

2. anti-D antibody injection — preparation for passive immunization of Rh negative mothers of D-positive babies administered intramuscularly or intravenously within 72 hours after delivery. Its purpose is to prevent Rh isoimmunization and fetal hemolytic disease in future pregnancies. The individual sterile vaccine vials are prepared from plasma obtained from severely sensitized Rh-negative women who had still-born hydropic fetuses or from gamma globulin from naturally or artificially sensitized donors.[35, 36, 37]

3. fetal electrocardiography — a method of detecting and recording electric impulses of the fetal heart. In contradistinction to the larger, slower deflections of the maternal heart, the normal fetal heart beat yields smaller and more rapid deflections. Fetal distress may be evidenced by a delay in the conduction time.[35]

4. fetal monitoring — continuous recording of fetal heart rate (FHR) patterns from a direct fetal electrocardiogram (FECG) electrode and uterine contractions using a transcervical catheter. Indications are clinical signs of fetal distress, FHR changes, suspected cephalopelvic disproportions and high risk pregnancies.[41]

5. fetal phonocardiography — the detection of fetal heart sounds by means of a phonocardiograph.

6. fetal telemetry — a wireless radio transmission which provides remote recordings of the fetal electrocardiography or other data.

7. intrauterine transfusion — the injection of red cell concentrate prepared from Rh-negative whole blood (packed erythrocytes) into the peritoneal cavity of the fetus to combat fetal hemolytic anemia and prevent fetal death.[2, 42, 72, 79]

THE NEONATAL PERIOD

A. Origin of Terms:

1. natus (L) — birth
2. neo (G) — new, recent
3. neonate (L) — newborn
4. umbilicus (L) — naval

B. Anatomic Terms:

1. fontanel, fontanelle — the junction point of cranial sutures which remains widely open in the newborn.
2. umbilical cord — cord connecting placenta with fetal umbilicus. At birth chiefly composed of one umbilical vein and two umbilical arteries surrounded by gelatinous substance.

C. Diagnostic Terms:

1. asphyxia neonatorum — lack of oxygen in the blood of the newborn.
2. atelectasis neonatorum — failure of the lungs to expand at birth.[59]
3. caput succedaneum — tumor-like edema of presenting part of child's head.[8]
4. cerebral hemorrhage — brain hemorrhage due to birth injury or coagulation defects resulting in anoxia, cyanosis and convulsions.[8, 21]
5. congenital stridors — breathing disorders associated with a crowing or stridulous noise from birth or first week of life due to malformation, abnormal position or functioning of glottis, trachea or vocal cords.
6. cord hemorrhage — bleeding from umbilical cord.
7. Down's syndrome, mongolism, trisomy G_{21} — a chromosome aberration characterized by mental retardation and many physical features such as slanting eyes, flat facial profile, thick, fissured tongue protruding from open mouth, pudgy, broad neck, hypotonia and absence of the Moro reflex in the newborn.[74]
8. drug addiction in neonate — withdrawal symptoms in the newborn appearing soon after birth. The infant is restless, has a shrill cry, tremors, twitchings and convulsions. Its manifestations may closely parallel those of adult withdrawal, such as yawning, sneezing, anorexia and diarrhea.[8, 54]
9. erythroblastosis fetalis — hemolytic disease of the newborn.
   a. anemic type — damage to bone marrow, liver and spleen, excessive hemolysis.
   b. hydropic type — extremely edematous, stillborn or neonatal death.
   c. icteric type — marked jaundice, may be followed by kernicterus.[2, 8, 12, 78]
10. hydrocephalus — abnormal fluid collection in the ventricles of the brain resulting in an enlargement of the head.[8]
11. hyperbilirubinemia, neonatal — abnormally high bilirubin content of the circulating blood predisposing the newborn to kernicterus due to unconjugated bilirubin concentration within brain tissue.[8, 78]
12. idiopathic respiratory distress syndrome, hyaline membrane disease — serious breathing difficulty due to hyaline material, a sticky exudate, filling the alveolar ducts and alveoli, thus obstructing the airway and preventing oxygenation. The condition, which occurs primarily in premature infants, may be fatal.[24, 59, 63]
13. imperforate anus, atresia of anus — rectum ending in a blind pouch.
14. infections of the newborn:
    a. congenital rubella syndrome — neonate born with a rubella virus infection due to transplacental transmission which is particularly serious when it occurs during the first trimester. The contagion lasts from 12 to 18 months after birth. The newborn may have cataracts, cardiovascular anomalies, microcephaly, mental retardation, deafness and other defects.[11, 25, 51, 66]
    b. epidemic diarrhea — loose, yellow green stools, dehydration and acidosis.
    c. impetigo contagiosa — skin disease, appearance of vesicles which change to pustules and later to crusts. It is caused by staphylococci.

  d. neonatal chlamydial, cytomegaloviral, herpetic and other infections.[3, 49]

  e. ophthalmia neonatorum — purulent conjunctivitis.

  f. thrush — fungus infection of oral mucous membrane forming white patches or aphthae.[8]

15. kernicterus, nuclear jaundice, biliary encephalopathy — irreparable brain damage complicating severe erythroblastosis. Excess serum bilirubin, liberated by destroyed erythrocytes and not converted into an excretable form, stains the brain nuclei and results in mental retardation, cerebral palsy or deafness. The most severe cases die within a few days. Kernicterus can be prevented by exchange transfusions.[8, 78]

16. meningocele — meninges protruding through a defect in the spine or skull.[8]

17. phocomelia — congenital deformities such as absence or stunting of extremities. Infants, born of mothers, who took thalidomide during the first trimester of pregnancy, developed these malformations.[9]

18. prematurity — infant born before his development is complete. A birth weight below 2500 Gm marks prematurity according to the World Health Organization.[7, 70]

19. retrolental fibroplasia — disorder seen in premature infants who receive continuous oxygen therapy. The retina becomes edematous and detached. Partial or total blindness develops.[7]

20. tongue-tie, ankyloglossia — short frenulum linguae preventing neonate from taking feeding.

21. umbilical hernia, omphalocele — rupture of the umbilicus associated with protrusion of intestine. It occurs in the first weeks of life.[8]

D. Operative Terms:

1. exchange transfusion — replacing the blood of a neonate who has a severe antibody-antigen reaction due to hemolytic disease with blood devoid of the offending antigen.[2, 35]

2. clipping of frenulum linguae — minor operation to relieve tongue-tie.

3. repair of imperforate anus — surgical creation of an opening.

E. Symptomatic Terms:

1. Apgar score — assessing a neonate's physical condition by evaluating his heart rate, respiratory effort, reflex irritability and skin color according to a scoring system.[14, 33]

2. Chvostek's sign — facial irritability in tetany evoked by a slight tap over the facial nerve. The spasm is unilateral.

3. congenital — born with a certain condition.

4. eructation — belching.

5. meconium — black stools of the newborn.

6. Moro reflex, startle reflex — reflex indicating an awareness of balance in the neonate. The reflex is stimulated by a sudden jarring of the crib or jerking of a blanket. The infant draws up his legs and throws his arms symmetrically forward.[7]

7. premature — before the proper time, in obstetrics before full term.

8. pylorospasm — spasm of circular muscle of lower end of stomach.[35]

9. vernix caseosa — fatty substance which covers the newborn.

RADIOLOGY

A. Terms Related to Diagnostic Radiology:

1. amniography — radiography of the pregnant uterus after injecting a radiopaque substance into the amniotic fluid. The procedure permits an evaluation of the fetus, placenta and amniotic sac.

2. fetography — radiographic study of the fetus in utero using a contrast medium with lipid affinity which coats the vernix and thus outlines the fetus.[59]

3. hysterosalpingography, uterotubal radiography, uterosalpingography — introduction of a

contrast medium into the uterus and uterine tubes.   This procedure is done under radiographic control to determine the patency of the tubes in reproductive failure.[9]

4. neonatal radiography — radiologic investigation of the newborn to diagnose a major health problem such as congenital heart disease, increased size of head and cerebral ventricles, esophageal atresia, tracheobronchial fistula, urinary tract or large bowel disorder.[59]

5. pelvimetry — radiographic measurement of various obstetric diameters of the bony pelvis.

6. pelvimetry and cephalometry — radiographic measurement of the relationship of the size of the fetal head to the size of the pelvic diameters.

7. placentography — radiography of the placenta after the injection of a contrast medium or without opaque substance using a compensating filter to even up the x-ray exposure of the pregnant uterus.[58]

B. Terms Related to Diagnostic Ultrasound:*

1. B-mode scan of fetus and placenta — ultrasound technique which aids in detecting
   a. fetal growth rate, maturity or death in utero and twin or multiple pregnancy
   b. location of the placenta, various degrees of placenta previa and twin placentas.[5, 18]

2. B-mode time motion (TM) scan — complex ultrasonic technique for the determination of the fetal heart rate.[5]

3. obstetric echocardiography — cardiac evaluation of maternity patient with pericardial effusion, mitral valve disease or cardiomyopathy by using ultrasound to assess the cardiac status and estimate the volume overload of the heart.[1]

4. obstetric ultrasonography — ultrasound technique for detecting fetal abnormalities, e.g. fetal hydrops or anencephaly and maternal disorders: hydramnios, extrauterine pregnancy, hydatidiform mole, fibroids or cysts associated with pregnancy and other conditions.[5, 17, 44, 64]

5. ultrasonic cephalometry — A-mode and B-mode ultrasonic techniques combined for determining the biparietal diameter (BPD) as a means of estimating the size, weight and probable gestational age of the fetus.[5, 18, 35]

6. ultrasonic placentography — this technique shows the precise location of the placenta for selecting the best puncture site prior to amniocentesis and the degree of displacement in placenta previa.[5, 18, 44]

7. ultrasonography in abortion — ultrasonic detection of complete or incomplete abortion. No echoes in the uterus may indicate a complete abortion and preclude the need for curettage.   Retained products of conception are echoic, but since other intrauterine disorders are likewise echogenic, a differential diagnosis is imperative.[64]

8. ultrasound monitoring of fetus — continuous recording by a Doppler ultrasound instrument with the transducer placed in a location where the fetal heart sounds are sharpest, thus best picked up as audible signals.[35]

CLINICAL LABORATORY

A. Terms Related to Pregnancy Tests:

1. immunologic pregnancy tests, immunoassays for pregnancy — sensitive tests for human chorionic gonadotropin (HCG) in serum and urine.   Excess chorionic gonadotropin is present in pregnancy.   Techniques are simple and results are read in 2 hours or less (actually in 5 minutes).   The tests are designed for office use.
   However, immunologic tests also yield positive results in choriocarcinoma and hydatidiform mole.   In menopause elevated pituitary gondotropin may produce a false positive test.[68]   The following commercial immunologic pregnancy tests are in current use:
   a. hemagglutination-inhibition tests:[68]
      (1) Pregnosticon tube test

---

*See Chapter IV — Neurologic and Psychiatric Disorders for Basic Terms of Diagnostic Ultrasound.

(2) Pregnosticon Accuspheres (a free-dried reagent).
  b. latex agglutination-inhibition tests:
    (1) Gravindex — use of latex particles with adsorbed HCG.[9, 68]
    (2) Placentex — tube test
        Positive for pregnancy — no flocculation within 90 minutes since HCG in urine inhibits flocculation
        Negative for pregnancy — flocculation within 90 minutes since lack of HCG in urine permits flocculation of latex particles.[68]
  2. Other hormone tests:
    a. alpha fetoprotein (AFP) serum determination — maternal α-fetoprotein serum measurement is usually adequate for the antenatal diagnosis of fetal abnormality.[15, 73]
    b. alpha fetoprotein in amniotic fluid — α-fetoprotein level may serve as a nonspecific but reliable index of neural tube defects e.g. anencephaly, spina bifida and others.[73, 76]
    c. human placental lactogen (HPL) determination — serum assay shows that HPL levels rise progressively during pregnancy, are very high in diabetes and low in placental insufficiency.
    d. oxytocin challenge test (OCT) — test seeks to induce the stresses of labor in order to observe their effect on the fetal heart rate. It is indicated when fetal life is endangered by high risk pregnancy.[23]
    e. urinary estriol determination — measurement of estriol which is excreted more plentifully than the other 2 estrogens, estrone and estradiol. Normally urinary estriol excretion rises progressively during pregnancy and reaches it peak level at full term. A marked decline in placental estriol during the second or third trimester signals placental insufficiency.[45, 68]

B. Terms Related to Fertility Studies:

  1. biopsy:
    a. endometrial biopsy and histologic study — method of determining evidence of ovulation. If absent, the ovarian factor is thought to be the cause of sterility. However the biopsy does not indicate whether the ovary is primarily or secondarily involved.[35]
    b. ovarian biopsies, bilateral — removal of ovarian tissue for the detection of the cause of infertility, evaluation and resumption of ovarian function. Large ovarian biopsies with use of Palmer biopsy forceps may be done under laparoscopic control.
  2. laparoscopy — endoscopic examination of pelvic and reproductive organs for diagnostic appraisal and/or therapeutic control.
  3. testicular biopsy — cytologic examination of tissue section from testis in oligospermia and azoospermia to detect the underlying pathology of infertility in the male.[9]
  4. tubal insufflation (Rubin test) — tubal patency test in reproductive failure. Blocked tubes are a cause of sterility.[9]

C. Terms Related to Parental, Antenatal and Neonatal Tests and Procedures:

  1. ABO incompatibility — incompatibility in the A,B,AB, and O blood types. Usually the mother is type O and the baby type A or B. This incompatibility occurs in a considerable number of pregnancies, but erythroblastosis develops in a relatively small percentage of them.
  2. amniotic fluid analyses — spectrophotometric tracings or other determinations on amniotic fluid in the antepartum management of Rh incompatibility, diabetes, etc. Fetal involvement exists if there is an abnormal increase in the pigments that absorb light at wave lengths between 450 and 460mμ.* Repeated amniotic fluid analyses are valuable guides for timing intrauterine transfusion or induction of labor.[78]
  3. antiglobulin reaction, Coombs test — a test for antibodies.

*1 mμ = 1 millimicron = 0.001 of a micron = 1 nm = 1 nanometer.

    a. direct Coombs test — a test for antibody coating of erythrocytes.

        Negative reaction — direct Coombs, no antibody coating on newborn's red cells

        Positive reaction — direct Coombs, antibody coating on newborn's red cells indicative of hemolytic disease.[78]

    b. indirect Coombs test — test determines presence of antibodies in serum.[35]

4. bilirubin — a pigment in bile derived from degenerated hemoglobin of destroyed blood cells. In newborns and particularly in premature and erythroblastotic babies the liver is unable to cope with the large amount of bilirubin liberated by destroyed erythrocytes. This results in an excess of bilirubin in the blood.

5. bilirubin determinations using cord blood of neonate.

    Normal values of serum bilirubin

      full-term newborn .... 1.0 - 3.0 mg per dl

    Increase in serum bilirubin

      physiologic jaundice .... 5.0 mg per dl and over

      hyperbilirubinemia ....18.0 - 20.0 mg per dl

      kernicterus ....25.0 mg per dl and over or below.[8, 78]

    The more immature the neonate, the more marked is his susceptibility to kernicterus.[8]

6. blood group analysis of prospective parents — a study of the parental blood groups in order to detect maternal and paternal grouping differences, predictive of mother-child incompatibilities. Routine procedures include ABO grouping, Rh typing and screening for irregular antibodies.[2, 79]

7. blood group analyses for exclusion studies — tests used in medicolegal practice on the basis that parental blood groups are inherited by the child.

    The American Medical Association accepts only the findings of the ABO, MN and Rh-Hr analyses for legal purposes except when experts use other systems.

    Determinations are made to exclude allegation or denial of paternity. To clarify the issue an example of the MN system of blood typing should be of interest.

          Disputed Father   **Mother**

            Type M   **Type N**

                    Child

            Type N — Genotype NN

    Since the child does not have the gene M, the person in question is not his father.[2, 79]

8. glucuronyl transferase — enzyme absent from the liver of premature infants at birth and incompletely developed in full-term newborns. This enzyme lack seems to account for the liver's inability to handle the load imposed by the increased destruction of red cells in the first days of life.[8]

9. phenylalanine — essential amino acid present in protein foods. A blocking of its conversion into tyrosine causes phenylalanine blood levels to rise and phenylketone bodies to be excreted in the urine. As a result brain development ceases. Mental retardation is preventable by early treatment with a low phenylalanine diet.[4]

10. phenylketonuria detection — diagnostic tests for detecting PKU, an inborn error of protein metabolism.

    a. ferric chloride tests (5 or 10%) on urine:

        (1) diaper test

        (2) tube test

        (3) Phenistix reagent strip test.

      Negative reaction — no color change

      Positive reaction — blue green or gray color of urine

      Phenylpyruvic acid is one of the metabolites excreted in phenylketonuria.

    b. Guthrie test — a simple screening test requiring several drops of blood from the heel of the newborn before the baby is taken home from the hospital.

      Negative test — phenylketonuria unlikely to develop

      Positive test — diagnosis to be confirmed by other tests.

      In states where mandatory testing of the neonate for phenylketonuria is done, the Guthrie test is considered legally acceptable. Thus the detection of this hereditary disorder is becoming a legal as well as a professional obligation in medicine.

c. serum phenylalanine test — procedure measures phenylalanine levels in blood serum.
Normal level — serum phenylalanine .... 0.5 - 2.0 mg/dl
Increase in phenylketonuria .... 60 mg/dl and above.[4]

11. phototherapy for neonate — effective method of lowering unconjugated bilirubin levels by exposing the newborn to fluorescent or other light according to need:
   a. infants with physiologic jaundice due to mildly elevated serum bilirubin benefit by the fluorescent lighting system of the nursery.
   b. infants with hyperbilirubinemia threatening encephalopathy are exposed to intense fluorescent light therapy in special incubators to reduce their excessive serum bilirubin.[8]

12. Rh isoimmunization — sensitization that occurs when red cells containing Rh antigens, not present in the cells of the recipient, enter the circulation. This develops most commonly in Rh negative women carrying Rh positive babies or receiving transfusion with Rh positive blood. It usually occurs during the second Rh positive pregnancy or subsequent pregnancies.[35, 36, 37]

13. rubella, German measles, in early pregnancy — a relatively mild disease with fever, rash and lymph node involvement which causes serious deformities in the growing fetus when it occurs during the first trimester. Preventive measures are presented:
   a. active immunization against rubella — live virus vaccine prepared in tissue cell culture derived from various sources and given as a single subcutaneous injection to nonpregnant, nonimmune women.
   b. hemagglutination (HI) test for rubella — routine test to be performed within 10 days of exposure to rubella. An antibody titer of 1:10 or above is usually indicative of patient being immune and will not develop rubella. An antibody titer below 1:10 suggests that the patient may develop rubella.
   c. immune serum globulin (ISG) — prophylactic agent thought to prevent maternal and congenital rubella and rubella-induced congenital malformations. This passive immunization against rubella should be given to pregnant, nonimmune women within 7 or 8 days after exposure.
   d. postpartum rubella immunization — procedure perfomed on nonimmune women during the puerperium to prevent rubella infection in future pregnancies.[11, 25, 51, 66]

14. sickle cell disease screening tests — screening procedures for sickle cell hemoglobin (HbS) during the first months of life, preferably at the infant's first checkup. Tests primarily indicated include the tube solubility or a microscopic test for HbS and a blood smear to detect sickled cells.[78]

15. spectrophotometry — instrumental measurement of the intensity of various wave lengths of light transmitted under standardized conditions by a substance under study.[78]

ABBREVIATIONS

A. **General:**

AFP — alpha (α) fetoprotein
BBT — basal body temperature
BPD — biparietal diameter
CDC — calculated day of confinement
CS — Cesarean section
CWP — childbirth without pain
EDC — estimated day of confinement
FECG — fetal electrocardiogram
FHR — fetal heart rate
FHT — fetal heart tone
FTND — full term normal delivery

HCG — human chorionic gonadotropin
HDN — hemolytic disease of newborn
HPL — human placental lactogen
HSG — hysterosalpingography
IUP — intrauterine pressure
LBW — low birth weight
LMP — last menstrual period
NB — newborn
OB — obstetrics
OGN — obstetric-gynecologic-neonatal

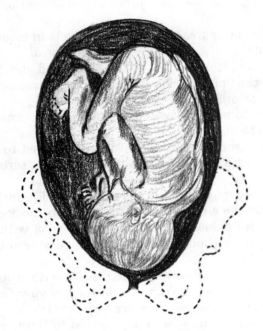

Fig. 62 – Right occiput anterior (ROA) position.

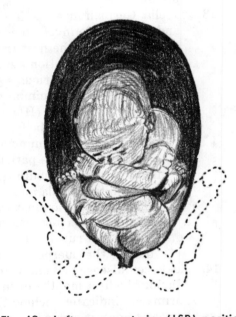

Fig. 63 – Left sacro-posterior (LSP) position.

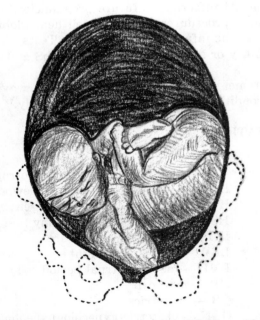

Fig. 64 – Right scapulo-posterior (RScP) position.

PPA pos. — phenylpyruvic acid positive
(phenylketonuria present)
PU — pregnancy urine
RML — right mediolateral (episiotomy)

Rh neg. — rhesus factor negative
Rh pos. — rhesus factor positive
UC — uterine contractions

B. Vertex Presentation:

LOA — left occipitoanterior
LOP — left occipitoposterior
LOT — left occipitotransverse

ROA — right occipitoanterior
ROP — right occipitoposterior
ROT — right occipitotransverse

C. Face Presentations:

LMA — left mentoanterior
LMP — left mentoposterior
LMT — left mentotransverse

RMA — right mentoanterior
RMP — right mentoposterior
RMT — right mentotransverse

D. Breech Presentations:

LSA — left sacroanterior
LSP — left sacroposterior

RSA — right sacroanterior
RSP — right sacroposterior

E. Tranverse Presentations:

LScA — left scapuloanterior
LScP — left scapuloposterior

RScA — right sacroanterior
RScP — right sacroposterior

F. Organizations:

AAMIH — American Association for
Maternal and Infant Health
ACNMW — American College of Nurse
Midwifery
ACOG — American College of Obstetricians
and Gynecologists
FACOG — Fellow of American College
of Obstetricians and
Gynecologists

FSAA — Family Service Association of
America
ICM — International Confederation
of Midwives
NAACOG — Nurses Association of the
American College of Obstetricians and Gynecologists
USCB — United States Children's Bureau

ORAL READING PRACTICE

Clinical Signs of Fetal Hydrops

There are three clinical types of fetal **erythroblastosis, hydrops fetalis, neonatal icterus gravis** and hemolytic anemia of the newborn. Of these types hydrops fetalis is the most serious condition since its mortality rate is one hundred per cent.

The clinical signs of fetal hydrops are manifold and are sequels of the massive destruction of blood. They include

1. anemia due to hemolysis
2. **hyperplasia** of the marrow which is thought to be a compensatory reaction of the marrow to the hemolytic process
3. foci of **extramedullary** production of red cells (erythropoiesis) in the spleen, liver, kidneys and other tissues, resulting in **splenomegaly, hepatomegaly** and other tissue reactions
4. a marked increase of immature erythrocytes (**erythroblasts**) in the circulation
5. anemic anoxia associated with tissue damage, particularly of the endothelial cells, cerebral nuclei and liver

6. hemolytic jaundice due to the excessive increase in blood destruction
7. obstructive jaundice caused by the occlusion of biliary capillaries
8. **hepatocellular jaundice** resulting from oxygen want of liver cells
9. edema due to **hepatic hypoproteinemia** and damage to **endothelial** tissues.[8, 34, 44]

Table 23

SOME OBSTETRIC AND NEONATAL CONDITIONS AMENABLE TO SURGERY

Organs Involved	Diagnoses	Operations	Operative Procedures
Cervix uteri Endometrium	Early incomplete abortion	Dilatation and curettage	Instrumental expansion of cervix and scraping of endometrium to remove blood clots and tissue
Cervix uteri	Dystocia Cervical stenosis Carcinoma of cervix in pregnancy, viable fetus	Cesarean section	Removal of fetus through incision into uterus
Uterine tube	Ruptured ectopic pregnancy with massive hemorrhage	Salpingectomy, unilateral	Removal of one fallopian tube
Perineum	Second stage of labor, tense perineum	Episiotomy, mediolateral or midline	Incision into perineum
Perineum	Obstetric laceration of the perineum	Perineorrhaphy	Suture of the torn perineum
Pelvis	Inlet contraction of pelvis	Cesarean section	Abdominal delivery of fetus
Pelvis	Prolonged labor, dystocia	Elective forceps delivery	Fetus delivered by horizontal traction
Uterus	Total placenta previa antepartum or intrapartum hemorrhage	Cesarean section	Incision into corpus uteri and delivery of fetus through abdomen
Uterus	Rupture of uterus, fatal hemorrhage, maternal death	Postmortem Cesarean section	Delivery of fetus by incision through abdominal wall and uterus after death of mother
Cervix uteri	Obstetric laceration of cervix	Trachelorrhaphy	Suture of torn cervix uteri
Blood of fetus	Fetal hemolytic disease, severe	Amniocentesis Intrauterine transfusion	Surgical puncture of amniotic cavity Injection of Rh negative packed red cells into the fetal peritoneal cavity
Blood of newborn	Erythroblastosis fetalis, Rh positive Hyperbilirubinemia	Exchange transfusions within 24 hours after birth	Replacing the infant's red cells by transfusing him with Rh negative erythrocytes which will remain unharmed by maternal antibodies
Intestine of newborn	Meconium ileus with intestinal obstruction due to mucoviscidosis	Intestinal resection	Surgical intervention to relieve intestinal obstruction

REFERENCES AND BIBLIOGRAPHY

1. Allen, J. W. Noninvasive cardiology in the pregnant and postpartum patient. *Clinical Obstetrics and Gynecology*, 18: 133-143, September, 1975.

2. American Association of Blood Banks. Hemolytic disease of the newborn. *Methods and Procedures of the American Association of Blood Banks*, 6th ed. Chicago: American Association of Blood Banks, 1974, pp. 144-158.

3. Amstey, M. S. Genital herpesvirus infection. *Clinical Obstetrics and Gynecology*, 18: 89-100, March, 1975.

4. Auerbach, V. H. *et al.* Defects in metabolism of amino acids. In Vaughan, Victor C., McKay, R. James *Nelson's Textbook of Pediatrics*. Philadelphia: W. B. Saunders Co., 10th ed. 1975, pp. 407-463.

5. Barnett, Ellis and Morley, Patricia. *Abdominal Echography*. London: Butterworths & Co., 1974, pp. 2-132.

6. Behrman, R. E. The fetus — High risk pregnancies — The newborn infant. In Vaughan, Victor C., McKay, R. James, Nelson, Waldo E. *Textbook of Pediatrics*, 10th ed. Philadelphia: W. B. Saunders Co., 1975, pp. 322-337.

7. _____. The high risk infant — Prematurity and low birth weight. *Ibid.*, pp. 337-350.

8. _____. Diseases of the newborn infant: Premature and full term. *Ibid.*, pp. 351-406.

9. Benson, Ralph C. Gynecology & Obstetrics. In Krupp, Marcus A. and Chatton, Milton. *Current Medical Diagnosis and Treatment*, 15th ed. Los Altos, California: Lange Medical Publications, 1976, pp. 412-473.

10. Billings, John and Billings, Lyn. The ovulation method of family planning. Conference. St. Louis University School of Medicine, Department of Gynecology and Obstetrics, December 13, 1974.

11. Blattner, R. J. German measles. In Vaughan, Victor C. and McKay, R. James (eds.). *Nelson Textbook of Pediatrics*, 10th ed. Philadelphia: W. B. Saunders Co., 1975, pp. 653-662.

12. Bowman, J. M. Rh erythroblastosis fetalis 1975. *Seminars in Hematology*, 12: 189-207, April, 1975.

13. Bowman, H. S. Effectiveness of prophylactic immunosuppression. *American Journal of Obstetrics and Gynecology*, 124: 80-87, January 1, 1976.

14. Chick, L. *et al.* Prediction of the one-minute Apgar score from fetal heart rate data. *Obstetrics and Gynecology*, 48: 452-455, October, 1976.

15. Cowchock, F. S. *et al.* Diagnostic use of maternal serum alpha-fetoprotein levels. *Obstetrics and Gynecology*, 47: 63-68, January, 1976.

16. Craig, J. M. The pathology of birth control. *Obstetrical and Gynecological Survey*, 30: 750-752, November, 1975.

17. Cunningham, M. E. *et al.* Ultrasound in the evaluation of anencephaly. *Radiology*, 118: 165-168, January, 1976.

18. Curcio, B. M. Ultrasonography and thermography. In Merril, Vinita. *Atlas of Roentgenographic Positions and Standard Radiologic Procedures*, 4th ed., Vol. III. St. Louis: The C. V. Mosby Co., 1975, pp. 946-959.

19. Curry, S. L. *et al.* Hydatidiform mole — Long-term follow-up of 347 patients. *Obstetrical and Gynecological Survey*, 30: 471-473, July, 1975.

20. Dahm, C. H. Natural methods of family planning. Unpublished material, December, 1974.

21. Deonna, T. *et al.* Neonatal intracranial hemorrhage in premature infants. *Obstetrical and Gynecological Survey*, 31: 790-792, November, 1976.

22. Dimmick, J. *et al.* Antenatal infection: Adequate protection against hyaline membrane disease? *Obstetrics and Gynecology*, 47: 56-62, January, 1976.

23. Farahani, G. *et al.* Oxytocin challenge test in high risk pregnancy. *Obstetrics and Gynecology*, 47: 159-168, February, 1976.

24. Farrell, P. M. *et al.* Hyaline membrane disease. *Respiratory Disease*, 111: 657-688, May, 1975.

25. Fleet, W. F. *et al.* Gestational exposure to rubella vaccines. A population surveillance study. *Obstetrical & Gynecological Survey*, 30: 732-734, November, 1975.

26. Freda, V. J. *et al.* Current concepts: Prevention of Rh hemolytic disease. *New England Journal of Medicine*, 292: 1014-1016, May 8, 1975.

27. Freeman, R. K. An evaluation of the significance of a positive oxytocin challenge test. *Obstetrics and Gynecology*, 47: 8-13, January, 1976.

28. Friedman, E. A. Hypertensive states of pregnancy. In Conn, Howard F. (ed.). *Current Therapy 1976*. Philadelphia: W. B. Saunders Co., 1976, pp. 763-766.

29. Friedman, E. A. *et al.* Station of the fetal presenting part. *Obstetrics and Gynecology*, 47: 129-136, February, 1976.

30. Gennser, G. *et al.* Maternal smoking and fetal breathing movements. *American Journal of Obstetrics and Gynecology*, 123: 861-867, December 15, 1975.

31. Goodman, Louis S. and Gilman, Alfred. *The Pharmacological Basis of Therapeutics*, 5th ed. New York: Macmillan Publishing Co., Inc., 1975.

32. Greenhill, J. P. (ed.). Placenta lactogen. *Obstetrics and Gynecology*. Chicago: Year Book Medical Publishers Inc., 1975, p. 69.

33. _____. Fetal and neonatal biochemistry of Apgar scores. *Ibid.*, p. 197.

34. Greenhill, J. P. and Friedman, E. A. *Biological Principles and Modern Practice of Obstetrics*. Philadelphia: W. B. Saunders Co., 1974, pp. 550-553.

35. Hamilton, Eugene G., M.D. Personal communications.

36. Hamilton, E. G. Ten years experience with high-titer anti-D plasma for the prevention of Rh immunization. *Obstetrics and Gynecology*, 40: 692-696, November, 1972.

37. _____. High-titer anti-D plasma for the prevention of Rh isoimmunization. *Obstetrics and Gynecology*, 36: 331-340, September, 1970.

38. Hathaway, W. E. The bleeding newborn. *Clinics in Perinatology*, 2: 83-98, March, 1975.

39. Hilgers, T. W. Why natural family planning. Unpublished material, December, 1974.

40. Holden, K. R. Neonatal seizures and their treat-

244

ment. *Clinics in Perinatology,* 2: 3-14, March, 1975.

41. Hon, E. H. Clinical value of fetal heart rate monitoring. *Clinical Obstetrics and Gynecology,* 18: 1-23, December, 1975.

42. Jewett, J. F. Amniotic fluid infusion. *New England Journal of Medicine,* 292: 973-974, May 1, 1975.

43. Kaplan, N. M. Clinical complications of oral contraceptives. *Advances in Internal Medicine,* Vol. XX. Chicago: Yearbook Medical Publishers, Inc., 1975, pp. 197-214.

44. Kassner, E. G. Sonographic diagnosis of fetal hydrops. *Radiology,* 116: 399-400, August, 1975.

45. Katagiri, H. *et al.* Estriol in pregnancy. *American Journal of Obstetrics and Gynecology,* 124: 272-280, February 1, 1976.

46. Klaus, H. The ovulation method. *St. Louis University Magazine,* 47: 12-14, Spring, 1974.

47. Lesinski, J. High risk pregnancy: Unresolved problems of screening, management and diagnosis. *Obstetrics and Gynecology,* 46: 599-603, November, 1975.

48. Manning, P. R. (ed.). Cardiac disease in pregnancy. *Clinical Obstetrics and Gynecology,* 18: 27-179, September, 1975.

49. McCormack, W. M. Management of sexually transmissible infections during pregnancy. *Clinical Obstetrics and Gynecology,* 18: 57-71, March, 1975.

50. McDonald, T. W. *et al.* Medical complications of induced abortions. *Obstetrical and Gynecological Survey,* 30: 30-33, January, 1975.

51. Menser, M. A. *et al.* The pathology of congenital rubella. *Obstetrical and Gynecological Survey,* 30: 256-258, April, 1975.

52. Monif, G. R., Rennert, O. M. (eds.). Clinical teratology. *Clinical Obstetrics and Gynecology,* 18: 139-263, December, 1975.

53. Moore, W. M. O. Family planning by periodic abstinence. *Obstetrical and Gynecological Survey,* 30: 670-672, October, 1975.

54. Neuman, L. L. *et al.* The neonatal narcotic withdrawal syndrome: A therapeutic challenge. *Clinics in Perinatology,* 2: 99-110, March, 1975.

55. Novak, Edmund R., Jones, Georgianna S., Jones, Howard W. Trophoblastic disease. *Novak's Textbook of Gynecology,* 9th ed. Baltimore: Williams and Wilkins Co., 1975, pp. 587-620.

56. Ott, W. J. Vacuum extraction. *Obstetrical and Gynecological Survey,* 30: 643-649, October, 1975.

57. Pilla, Lawrence A., M.D. Personal communications.

58. Pritchard, Jack A. and Macdonald, Paul C. *Williams Obstetrics,* 15th ed. New York: Appleton-Century-Crofts, 1976.

59. Reilly, B. J. (ed.). Symposium on neonatal radiology. *Radiologic Clinics of North America,* 13: 167-368, August, 1975.

60. Reis, R. A. *et al.* Cesarean hysterectomy. *Obstetrics and Gynecology,* 46: 687-691, December, 1975.

61. Risk, A. *et al.* Second trimester abortions. *Obstetrical and Gynecological Survey,* 31: 139-141, February, 1976.

62. Robbins, Stanley L. Placental diseases. *Pathologic Basis of Disease.* Philadelphia: W. B. Saunders Co., 1974, pp. 1255-1264.

63. Roberton, N. R. *et al.* Prognosis for infants with idiopathic respiratory distress syndrome. *Obstetrical and Gynecological Survey,* 31: 133-134, February, 1976.

64. Sanders, R. C. *et al.* Sonography in obstetrics. *Radiologic Clinics of North America,* 13: 435-456, December, 1975.

65. Schwarz, R. H. Amniocentesis. *Clinical Obstetrics and Gynecology,* 18: 1-22, June, 1975.

66. Siegel, M. Unresolved issues in the first 5 years of the rubella immunization program. *American Journal of Obstetrics and Gynecology,* 124: 327-332, February, 1976.

67. Sitarz, A. L. *et al.* Management of isoimmune neonatal thrombocytopenia. *American Journal of Obstetrics and Gynecology,* 124: 39-42, January 1, 1976.

68. *Specialized Diagnostic Laboratory Tests,* 11th ed. Van Nuys, California: Bio-Science Laboratories, 1976, pp. 33-167.

69. Stagno, S. *et al.* Cervical cytomegalovirus excretion in pregnant and nonpregnant women. *Obstetrical and Gynecological Survey,* 31: 118-119, February, 1976.

70. Stockman, J. A. Anemia of prematurity. *Seminars in Hematology,* 12: 163-173, April, 1975.

71. Tatum, H. J. *et al.* The Dalkon shield controversy — structural and bacteriological studies of IUD tails. *Journal of American Medical Association,* 231: 711-717, February 17, 1975.

72. Turner, J. H. Fetal and maternal risks associated with intrauterine transfusion procedures. *American Journal of Obstetrics and Gynecology,* 123: 251-256, October 1, 1975.

73. Walker, J. Prognostic value of antenatal screening. *American Journal of Obstetrics and Gynecology,* 124: 30-38, January 1, 1976.

74. Warkany, J. *et al.* Prenatal disturbances. In Vaughan, Victor C., McKay, R. James (eds.). *Nelson Textbook of Pediatrics,* 10th ed. Philadelphia: W. B. Saunders Co., 1975, pp. 289-320.

75. Weir, Don C., M.D. Personal communications.

76. Weis, R. R. *et al.* Amniotic fluid α-fetoprotein as a marker in prenatal diagnosis of neural tube defects. *Obstetrics and Gynecology,* 47: 148-151, February, 1976.

77. Williamson, A. P. Varicella-Zoster virus in the etiology of severe congenital defects. *Obstetrical and Gynecological Survey,* 31: 28-30, January, 1976.

78. Wintrobe, Maxwell M. Hemoglobinopathies — Hemolytic disease of the newborn (HDN). *Clinical Hematology,* 7th ed. Philadelphia: Lea and Febiger, 1974, pp. 822-910.

79. ———. Blood groups and blood transfusions. *Ibid.,* pp. 451-497.

80. ———. Diffuse intravascular coagulation — DIC in neonates and infants. *Ibid.,* pp. 1211-1226.

81. Wood, G. P. The evaluation of the fetal lung maturity by amniotic fluid analysis. *Southern Medical Journal,* 68: 538-542, May, 1975.

Chapter XII
Endocrine and Metabolic Disorders

ENDOCRINE GLANDS

A. Origin of Terms:

1. acro (G) — extremity
2. crine (G) — to secrete
3. edema (G) — swelling
4. goiter (L) — throat
5. hormone (G) — to excite
6. physis (G) — growth
7. pituita (L) — phlegm
8. thyro (G) — shield
9. tropho (G) — nourishment

B. Anatomic Terms:

1. endocrine glands — ductless glands producing internal secretions which are absorbed directly into the blood stream and influence various body functions.
2. hormone — active principle of an internal secretion.
3. hypophysis, pituitary gland — small ovoid body situated in the hypophysial fossa of the sphenoid bone. It is composed of the adenohypophysis and neurohypophysis, each performing distinct functions. The adenohypophysis or anterior pituitary is known as the master endocrine gland because of its physiologic effect upon the suprarenals, gonads, pancreas and thyroid. Some important hormones of the adenohypophysis are
   a. adrenocorticotropic hormone (ACTH) affecting the adrenal cortex and combating inflammatory processes. (ACTH is essential to maintain life.)
   b. follicle stimulating and luteinizing hormones regulating the reproductive cycle.
   c. growth hormone promoting normal bone development.
   d. prolactin stimulating the secretion of milk.
   e. thyrotropic hormone evoking increased uptake of iodine by the thyroid.[12, 17, 39, 60]
   The neurohypophysis is thought to be not a true endocrine but a depot for neurosecretions known as the antidiuretic hormone (ADH) containing vasopressin and oxytocin.[39, 45, 60]
4. parathyroids — two to four small glands, usually a pair attached to each thyroid lobe. They secrete a hormone which regulates the metabolism of calcium and phosphorus[40, 59, 71]
5. suprarenals, adrenals — two glands, one on top of each kidney. They are composed of an inner medullary substance and an outer cortex. The medulla produces adrenalin and noradrenalin. The adrenal cortex forms the adrenocortical steroids known as the corticosteroids or corticoids. They include the glucocorticoids and mineralocorticoids. C-19 derivatives yield androgens and C-18 derivatives estrogens.[41, 58]
   Adrenocortical steroids help to regulate sodium, potassium and chloride metabolism, the water balance and carbohydrate, protein and fat metabolism.
6. thymus — endocrine gland secreting thymin, a hormone which inhibits neuromuscular transmission.[60]
7. thyroid — the gland consists of two large lateral lobes and a central isthmus. It produces the hormones, thyroxine and triiodothyronine, with different physiologic properties.[59, 71]

C. Diagnostic Terms:

1. acromegaly — disease characterized by enlarged features, particularly of the face and hands. This is the result of oversecretion of the pituitary growth hormone.[17, 39, 68]
2. Addison's disease — primary adrenal cortical insufficiency, a chronic syndrome. Pigmentation is a dominant trait.[41, 48]
3. adrenal apoplexy — adrenal infarction associated with hemorrhage. It is usually a complication of anticoagulation therapy or septicemia. Hypotension is present.[48]
4. adrenal crisis, Addisonian crisis — acute adrenocortical insufficiency and a life-threatening

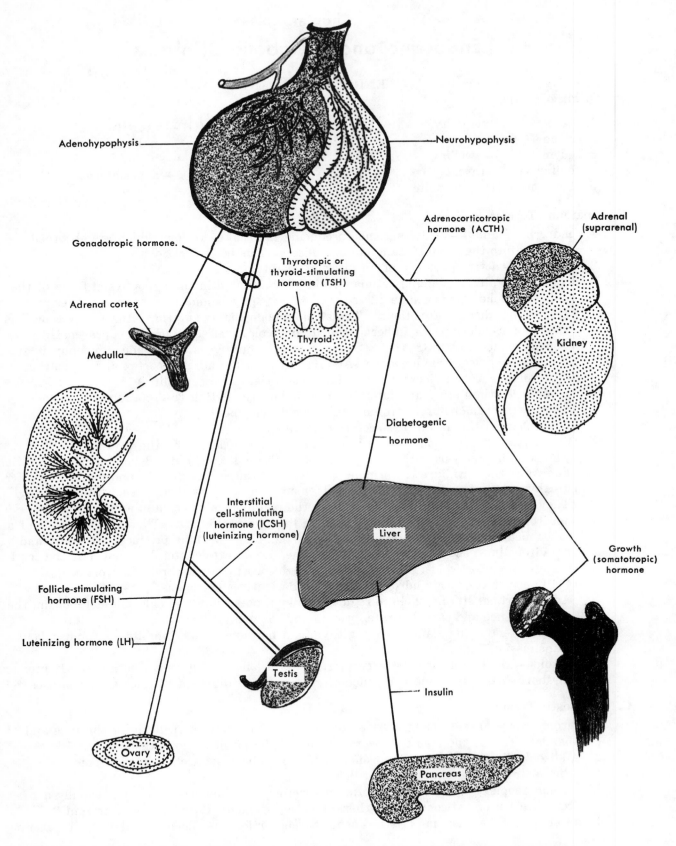

Fig. 65 — Hormones of the adenohypophysis; direct and indirect effect on target organs.

event resulting from a lack of glucocorticoids, hyperkalemia and depletion of extracellular fluid during acute stress. Clinical manifestations are lassitude, headache, mental confusion, gastric upset, circulatory collapse, coma and death.[41]

5. adrenal neoplasms:
   a. adenomas and adenocarcinomas — benign or malignant glandular tumors arising from the adrenal cortex. Oversecretion of androgen by the tumor may cause virilization in women and children; excess estrogen production by tumor may result in feminization in men. [26, 29, 48]
   b. neuroblastomas — tumors arising from the adrenal medulla. They are generally associated with metastases to bones.[26, 48]
   c. pheochromocytomas — tumors usually arising from adrenal medulla and characterized by paroxysmal hypertension.

6. Conn's syndrome, primary aldosteronism — excessive secretion of aldosterone associated with pathology of adrenal cortex resulting in potassium depletion, sodium retention, extreme exhaustion, paresthesias, cardiac enlargement and increased CO_2 combining power.[26, 48]

7. craniopharyngioma — pituitary tumor of the intrasellar or suprasellar area which may compress the optic chiasm causing blindness, raise intracranial pressure followed by severe headaches, and contain calcifications, cystic components and cholesterol.[12, 52]

8. Cushing's disease — syndrome attributed to the hyperproduction of cortisone and hydrocortisone by the adrenal cortex. Obesity, weakness and hypertension are typical manifestations.[17, 26, 41, 48]

9. dwarfism, pituitary — congenital underdevelopment due to hyposecretion of the growth hormone.[38, 39]

10. eunuchism — total gonadal underdevelopment.[38]

11. eunuchoidism — partial gonadal underdevelopment.[38]

12. Froehlich's syndrome, adiposogenital dystrophy — panhypopituitarism resulting primarily from deficient secretion of the gonadotropic hormone. Its features are marked obesity, eunuchoidism with or without nonpituitary brain lesions which may increase the intracranial pressure.[60]

13. giantism — abnormal growth, particularly of long bones before the closure of the epiphyseal lines. It is due to overproduction of the growth hormone of the anterior pituitary.[17, 39]

14. goiter — an enlargement of the thyroid gland. It may be classified as:
   a. nontoxic diffuse goiter
   b. toxic diffuse goiter
   c. nontoxic nodular goiter
   d. toxic nodular goiter.[20, 40]

15. hypercalcemic syndrome — abnormally high calcium levels of the blood seen in bone malignancies, endocrine and metabolic disorders such as multiple myeloma, acute adrenal insufficiency, hyperthyroidism, vitamin D intoxication, sarcoidosis and milk-alkali syndrome. It may be due to prolonged bed rest in osteoporosis, Paget's disease and other disorders.[2]

16. hyperinsulinism due to islet cell tumor — condition marked by hypoglycemic episodes with a blood sugar below 30 or 40 mg/dl (deciliter) convulsions increasing in frequency and severity and eventually coma.[25]

17. hyperparathyroidism, primary — overproduction and overactivity of the parathyroid hormone present in hypercalcemia, osteitis fibrosa and tissue calcification.[2, 73]

18. hyperthyroidism, thyrotoxicosis, exophthalmic goiter, Graves disease — thyrotoxic state currently considered an immunologic disorder. The antigen, probably of thyroid origin, is still unknown. Excessive hormone secretion increases oxygen consumption and thus accounts for the high metabolic rate. Clinical characteristics are goiter, protrusion of the eyeballs, tachycardia, tremors, emotional instability, sweating and weight loss.

19. hypoparathyroidism — abnormally decreased production of the parathyroid hormone causing hypocalcemia. It may be associated with reduced serum calcium and elevated serum phosphate levels.

20. hypothyroidism — condition resulting from insufficiency of thyroid hormones in the blood.[20, 40]
21. multiple endocrine adenomatoses (MEA) — endocrinopathies of tumors, genetically distinct and of autosomal dominant inheritance.
    a. MEA, type I, Wermer's syndrome — a familial disorder of pituitary, pancreatic and parathyroid gland tumors exhibiting great variability in endocrine involvement and clinical manifestations.
    b. MEA, type II, Sipple's syndrome — an inherited disorder, usually comprising medullary thyroid carcinoma associated with bilateral pheochromocytomas of the adrenal medulla.[62, 65]
22. myxedema — hypothyroidism causing lethargy, nonpitting edema, weakness and slow speech.[20, 40]
23. reactive hypoglycemia — a common hormonal disturbance initiated by an anxiety state which stimulates both increased consumption of carbohydrates and gastric emptying. This is followed by a high blood sugar which in turn accelerates insulin production and causes reactive hypoglycemia. It is also known as postprandial reactive hypoglycemia.[24, 36]
24. Simmond's disease, pituitary cachexia — primary chronic pituitary insufficiency causing extreme weight loss and general debility.[39, 60]
25. tetany — hypofunction of the parathyroids, resulting in intermittent, tonic spasms due to calcium deficiency.[2]
26. thymitis, autoimmune — autoimmune reaction in thymus, probably the basic thymus lesion in myasthenia gravis.[6]
27. thymoma — tumor of thymus which may be invasive and associated with myasthenia gravis or other syndromes. It tends to recur after removal.[64]
28. thymotoxicosis — excessive secretion of thymin causing toxic effects.
29. thyroid dysfunction — malfunction of the thyroid hormones resulting in several thyrotoxic myopathies associated with muscular atrophy and weakness, depletion of energy and other manifestations.[54]
30. thyroiditis — inflammation of the thyroid gland.
    a. acute thyroiditis — sudden onset of inflammatory process with local tenderness of thyroid.
    b. Hashimoto's thyroiditis, struma lymphomatosa — lymphoid goiter or lymphocytic thyroiditis, thought to be an autoimmune, hereditary disease and not as the name suggests an infectious or inflammatory disorder. It occurs almost exclusively in women. A medium sized, rubbery, firm goiter, low metabolism and hypothyroidism are common clinical findings.[20, 59]
    c. Riedel's struma — a rare chronic type of the old age group characterized by fibrotic changes and a wooden sensation in neck.[59]
    d. subacute thyroiditis — inflammation usually subsequent to viral infection in the respiratory tract indicative of an immunologic response to the virus.
31. thyroid neoplasms:
    a. adenomas — benign glandular tumors.
    b. carcinomas — malignant tumors, with subsequent metastases to cervical lymph nodes, the long bones and lungs.[1, 11, 19]

D. Operative Terms:

1. adrenalectomy — removal of adrenal gland or glands.[8, 16, 32]
2. cryohypophysectomy — one of several procedures which uses the stereotaxic transsphenoidal approach, achieves pituitary ablation (removal of hypophysis) by the application of a cryoprobe.[10, 32]
3. microneurosurgery of pituitary gland — microdissection of tumor under magnification and with intense illumination using a binocular surgical microscope.
    Techniques are:
    a. Hardy's oronasal-transphenoidal approach — entering the sphenoid sinus via nasal septum for removal of intrasellar tumor.

b. Rand's transfrontal-transphenoidal approach — opening the sphenoid sinus through a frontal craniotomy for removal of tumor attached to optic chiasm.[21, 32, 74]

4. parathyroidectomy — removal of parathyroid tissue to control hyperparathyroidism.
5. thymectomy — removal of thymus gland.[64]
6. thyroid surgery:
    a. lobectomy of thyroid — usually the removal of the isthmus and involved lobe for solitary thyroid nodule.
    b. partial thyroidectomy — method of choice for removal of fibrous nodular thyroid.
    c. subtotal thyroidectomy — the removal of most of the thyroid to relieve hyperthyroidism.[71]

E. Symptomatic Terms:

1. exophthalmos — abnormal protrusion of the eyeballs.
2. hirsutism — excessive growth of hair.
3. hyperkinesia, hyperkinesis — hypermotility, abnormally increased motility.
4. malignant exophthalmos — excessive protrusion of the eyeballs which fails to respond to treatment and leads to loss of sight.
5. paroxysmal hypertension — sudden recurrence of high blood pressure after a remission. It may be caused by conditions of the adrenal gland.
6. postural hypertension — high blood pressure associated with changes in posture.
7. pressor effect — stimulating effect.
8. proptosis — forward displacement of the globes in the orbit, same as exophthalmos.
9. virilism — masculinization in women.
10. vitiligo — white patches on the skin of the hands and feet. They may be seen in hyperthyroidism.

METABOLIC DISEASES

A. Origin of Terms:

1. keton (G) — ketone
2. melano- (G) — black
3. meli, melit (G) — honey
4. metabole (G) — change
5. porphyr- (G) — purple
6. tophus (L) — porous stone

B. Diagnostic Terms:

1. acid-base imbalance — disturbance in acid-base balance of the blood concerned with carbon dioxide (carbonic acid) as the acid component and bicarbonate as the base component of the equation. As a result abnormal changes develop in the carbon dioxide tension (Pco_2) and hydrogen ion concentration (pH). Lungs and kidneys play major roles in:
    a. metabolic acidosis — primary alkali deficit characterized by a low pH and Pco_2. It occurs in Addison's disease, starvation, diarrhea, renal and liver diseases, overtreatment with acids, etc.[2, 17]
    b. metabolic alkalosis — primary alkali excess marked by increased pH and Pco_2. It is caused by excessive loss of acid, gastric suction, potassium deficit, Cushing's syndrome, overtreatment with alkaline salts, etc.
    c. respiratory acidosis — primary CO_2 excess, low pH and high Pco_2 indicative of impaired gaseous exchange and hypoventilation resulting in carbon dioxide retention. It may develop in overdepression of respiratory center, lung disease and heart failure.
    d. respiratory alkalosis — primary CO_2 deficit, high pH and low Pco_2 present in hyperventilation. It is seen in overstimulation of respiratory center, high altitudes, fever, hysteria and anxiety.[33]
2. alkalosis — abnormal increase of alkalinity in the blood.
3. carcinoid syndrome, carcinoidosis — peculiar metabolic disorder characterized by flushing, diarrhea, dyspnea and valvular heart disease. The symptoms are related to an overproduction of serotonin by the malignant carcinoid tumor of the gastrointestinal tract, usually the terminal ileum. Metastases to the liver and adjacent lymph nodes may occur.[23, 28]

4. diabetes insipidus — metabolic disorder due to hyposecretion of the antidiuretic hormone of the pituitary gland.   Its clinical manifestation are polydipsia and polyuria.[33]

5. diabetes mellitus — a chronic metabolic disease genetically determined and in its advanced stage clinically manifested in a nonstressed patient by fasting hyperglycemia, ketoacidosis, atherosclerotic and microvascular pathologic changes, protein breakdown and neuropathies.[10, 36, 61]

6. diabetes mellitus in situ, occult diabetes — a prediabetic state in which the glucose tolerance curve is normal and the correlated insulin tolerance abnormal.   In the earliest detectable phase dietary carbohydrate control may correct the condition.[42]

7. galactosemia — inborn error of carbohydrate metabolism resulting in an incapacity for metabolizing galactose.   Consequently galactose blood levels increase abnormally and galactose may be present in the urine.   The neonate is normal.   Gastrointestinal disorders, ascites, cirrhosis, proteinuria, mental retardation and cataracts develop in infancy if galactose is not eliminated from the diet.[4]

8. Gaucher's disease — a hereditary metabolic defect resulting in faulty lipid storage. Abnormal reticuloendothelial (Gaucher) cells proliferate and cause progressive splenomegaly, pigmentation of the skin, anemia, and frequently bone involvement.

9. glycogenoses — glycogen storage diseases caused by enzymic defect in building up and breaking down glycogen.[61]

10. gout, gouty arthritis — disorder of purine metabolism and recurrent form of arthritis manifested by an abnormal increase of uric acid in the blood, tophi, joint involvement and in severe cases, uric acid nephrolithiasis or renal failure.

11. hyperglucagonemia — excess of glucagon in the circulating blood.   It does not cause glucose intolerance in normal subjects or bring about deterioration of diabetic control. Glucagon in the insulin deprived patient can worsen the condition.[25, 56, 67]

12. lipidosis, pl. lipidoses — any disorder in which abnormal lipid concentrations are found in extracellular fluid and body tissues.[5,7, 27, 31, 37, 46]   According to Fredrickson abnormally high plasma lipids and lipoproteins occurring in various metabolic disorders present problems of classification and treatment.[27]
   These disorders comprise
   a.   abnormal plasma lipoproteins including
       (1)   hyperlipoproteinemia, 6 types
       (2)   dyslipoproteinemia
       (3)   hypolipoproteinemia
   b.   lipid storage diseases caused by functional deficiency of a certain enzyme.   Gaucher's disease and Wolman's disease belong in this category as well as many other disorders.
   c.   granulomatous diseases with lipid storage, e.g. histiocytosis
   d.   other xanthomatoses
   e.   adipose tissue disorders
       (1)   lipoatrophy, partial (lipodystrophy)
       (2)   lipoatrophy, complete
   f.   other lipidoses.
   The complexity of the subject matter precludes the definition of terms.   For Fredrickson's classic exposition of disorders of lipid metabolism see *Harrison's Principles of Internal Medicine*, 7th ed., 1974, pp. 634-644.[27]

13. metabolic stone disease — nephrolithiasis classified according to etiology.   Kidney stones may form in hypercalcemia states, renal tubular syndromes, hyperuricemia, defective enzyme metabolism and other disorders.

14. obesity — excess of adipose tissue which presents a potential risk to good health.   The metabolic factor causing obesity may be the steroid excess of glucocorticoids in Cushing's syndrome.   Since obese persons usually have hypertriglyceridemia and hypercholesterolemia they are more prone to develop atherosclerosis, hypertension and diabetes mellitus than nonobese persons.[5]

15. phenylketonuria — hereditary metabolic disorder causing mental retardation.   Phenyl-

ketone bodies are found in serum and urine.   The disease is due to an inborn error of amino acid metabolism.

16. porphyria — inborn faulty porphyrin metabolism resulting in porphyrinuria.
    a. congenital, erythropoietic type — porphyria characterized by skin lesions due to photosensitivity from porphyrin in subcutaneous tissue.
    b. hepatic intermittent acute type — porphyria noted for liver damage, brownish pigmentation of the skin and neurologic symptoms.[66]

17. Wolman's disease — rare familial xanthomatosis characterized by punctuate calcium deposits throughout the enlarged adrenal glands, hepatosplenomegaly and visceral foam cells filled with triglyceride and cholesterol.   The disease is lethal.[27, 61]

18. xanthomatosis — a widespread eruption of xanthomas on the skin and tendons.   The xanthomas are yellow, lipid-containing plaques which are usually associated with hyperlipoproteinemia.[5, 27]

C. Symptomatic Terms:

1. exacerbation — aggravation of symptoms.
2. glycosuria — the presence of sugar in the urine.
3. hyperchloremia — excessive chloride concentration in the circulating blood.
4. hypercholesterolemia — excessive cholesterol concentration in the circulating blood.[5, 7]
5. hyperchylomicronemia — excessive chylomicron concentration in the circulating blood.[37]
6. hyperglycemia — excessive sugar concentration in the circulating blood.[25, 62]
7. hyperkalemia — excessive potassium concentration in the circulating blood.
8. hypernatremia — excessive sodium concentration in the circulating blood.
9. hypertriglyceridemia — excessive triglyceride concentration in the circulating blood.
10. hyperuricemia — excessive uric acid concentration in the circulating blood.
11. hyponatremia — abnormally low serum sodium level due to a disturbed ratio of water to sodium.
12. ketosis — excess ketone bodies in the body fluids and tissues due to incomplete combustion of fatty acids which may result from a faulty or absent utilization of carbohydrates. Ketosis may produce severe acidosis.   It develops in uncontrolled diabetes mellitus and starvation.[10, 13, 36]
13. Kussmaul breathing — classic manifestations in diabetic acidosis marked by unusually deep respirations associated with dyspnea.   This type of breathing is due to an abnormally increased acid content of the blood resulting in continuous overstimulation of the respiratory center.
14. melanosis — black pigments deposited in body tissues.
15. polydipsia — excessive thirst.
16. polyphagia — overeating.
17. remission — symptoms decreased in severity.
18. steatorrhea — excess fecal fat due to malabsorption of lipids, enzyme deficiency of pancreas, or intestinal disease.
19. tophi (sing. tophus) — sodium biurate deposits near a joint.   Condition is peculiar to gout.

HORMONAL DISORDERS AND CYTOGENETICS

A. Origins of Terms:

1. acro- (G) — extremity
2. centre (G) — center
3. chroma (G) — color
4. cyto- (G) — cell
5. gamete (G) — spouse
6. gen (G) — to produce
7. idio- (G) — distinct
8. karyo- (G) — nucleus
9. mitos (G) — thread
10. mono- (G) — single
11. mutant (G) — to change
12. ovum (G) — egg
13. soma (G) — body
14. sperm (G) — seed
15. spermato (G) — to sow seed
16. syndrome (G) — running together

B. Cytogenetic Terms:[51, 76]

1. acrocentric — centromere located at one end.
2. autosomal aberration — abnormality of chromosomes.
   a. acquired — developed after birth as in chronic myeloid leukemia.
   b. congenital — present at birth as in mongolism.
3. autosomal dominant inheritance — one abnormal dominant gene of a pair is passed on to 50% of the sons and daughters although the affected parent has a normal mate.
   As the rule autosomal dominant inheritance delineates the following pattern:
   a. equal distribution of the abnormal trait among males and females.
   b. direct transmission of the trait over 2 generations or more.
   c. abnormal trait affecting close to 50% of the members of the pedigree.[75]
4. autosomal recessive inheritance — abnormality is produced by paired defective genes since both parents contribute one recessive abnormal gene. Criteria for establishing recessive inheritance are:
   a. consanguinity increases the chance that the affected gene is passed on by the two related parents.
   b. the same genetic disorder occurs in collateral family branches.
   c. the disease is present in 25% of the siblings.[75]
5. autosome, autosomal chromosome — nonsex chromosome.
6. banding — banded or striped appearance of chromosomes when special staining is done to chromosomes at metaphase using the Giemsa Band method for karyotyping.[22, 70]
7. centromere — constriction in center of chromosome.
8. chromosomal aberration — abnormality of chromosomes.
   a. acquired — developed after birth as in chronic granulocytic leukemia in which the Philadelphia (Ph[1]) chromosome is present.
   b. congenital — present at birth as in mongolism.[51]
9. chromatin — deoxyribonucleic acid, known as DNA, found in chromosomes and stainable by basic dyes.
10. chromosome — threadlike body of chromatin in cell nucleus. Chromosomes are bearers of hereditary substances, called genes. Normally the number of chromosomes for each species remains constant. At present chromosomes have become the prime target of genetic investigation.
11. chromosome analysis — karyotyping.
12. chromosome defects — two types occur:
    a. aneuploidy — abnormal chromosome number:
       (1) aneuploid mosaics — modal numbers differing in 2 or more distinct cell populations.
       (2) heterosomal aneuploidy — all cells possessing uniform aneuploidy including
          (a) complex aneuploidy — 2 or more individual chromosomes in the same person show defects in numbers.
          (b) monosomy — one member of a chromosome pair is absent.
          (c) polysomy — the same chromosome is present 4 times or more.
          (d) triploidy — each chromosome occurs in triplicate.[69]
          (e) trisomy — one chromosome occurs in triplicate.[22, 43, 47, 70]
    b. structural defects of chromosomes:
       (1) deletion — partial loss of a chromosome which is prone to occur during cell division and may be a long arm or short arm deletion. Usually there are 2 breaks in a chromosome and the segment between fractures is lost.[22]
       (2) duplication — a condition in which a portion of a chromosome is represented more than once.[76]
       (3) isochromosome — transverse division of the centromere during meiosis which causes a chromosomal aberration.[22]
       (4) translocation — a chromosome segment which shifts to a different position. It is balanced if there is a full complement of genetic material even if the

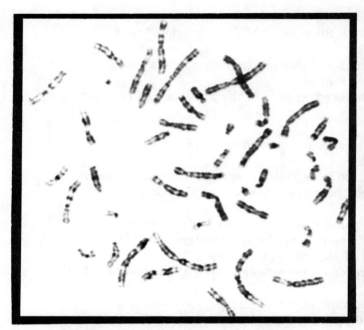

Fig. 66 – Chromosomes from a normal human male cell, grown in tissue culture and arrested at the metaphase.

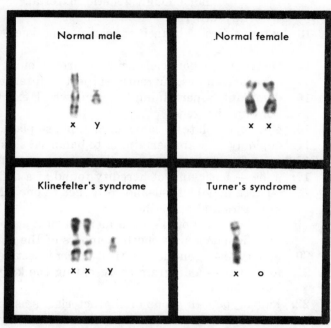

Fig. 67 – Human sex chromosomes, normal pattern and chromosomal aberrations.

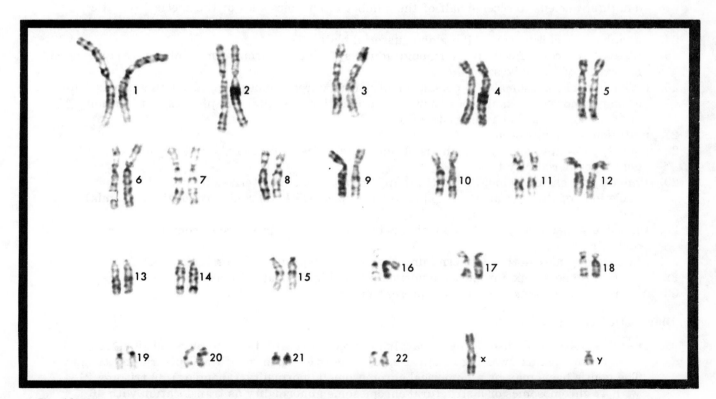

Fig. 68 – Karyotype or idiogram of a normal human male, constructed from fig. 66. Note banding of chromosomes.

(Sister Leo Rita Volk, SSM. Cytogenetic Research Laboratory
St. Mary's Health Center, St. Louis, Missouri)

arrangement happens to be unusual.   It is unbalanced if there is too much or not enough genetic material.[22, 49, 70]

    (5) others.

13. cytogenetics — branch of science concerned with the origin and development of cells in heredity.

14. DNA-deoxyribonucleic acid — chromosomal material thought to transmit hereditary characteristics, currently subject to intense research.

15. dominant — pertaining to a gene which exerts its effect even in the presence of a contrasting or opposite gene.

16. equatorial plate — same as metaphase plate.

17. euploidy — state pertaining to balanced sets of chromosomes in every number.

18. gamete — mature germ cell, sperm or ovum.

19. gene — basic unit of heredity found at a definite locus (place) on a particular chromosome. There may be thousands of genes to one DNA molecule.   Genes, like chromosomes, come in pairs and are either

    a. heterozygous — each member of a gene pair carries a different instruction or

    b. homozygous — both members of the gene pair carry the same instruction.[72, 75]

20. genotype — genetic constitution irrespective of external appearance.

21. idiogram — a diagram representing the karyotype (chromosome pattern) of the cells of an individual.

22. karyotype — a group of characteristics as form, number and size used to identify an individual's chromosomal pattern.   A karyotype of a normal person has 46 chromosomes including 22 autosomal pairs and 2 sex chromosomes.   They are arranged and numbered according to the 1961 International Classification System of Denver, Colorado.   This is known as karyotyping.

23. meiosis — special cell division which occurs in maturation of sex cells and causes each daughter nucleus to receive half of the number of chromosomes of the species' somatic cells.

24. metaphase — chromosomes lying on equatorial plate.

25. mitosis — process of cell division; longitudinal splitting of chromosomes into halves and migration of the halves.

26. mosaicism, chromosomal — a population of normal chromosomes together with a population of one or more abnormal types varying in proportion.   Mental and physical retardation are common clinical characteristics.[70]

27. mutation — change occurring in genes.

28. phenotype — apparent type with visible characteristics which may be independent of genotype (hereditary type).

29. Philadelphia chromosome, Ph[1] — G group chromosome characterized by partial loss (deletion) of the long arm.   It is present in typical CML (chronic myelocytic leukemia) and absent in atypical CML.[22, 49, 70]

30. recessive — pertaining to a gene which is ineffective in the presence of contrasting or opposite genes.

31. sex chromosomes — those determining the sex of offspring; XX for female, XY for male.

32. X-chromosome — sex chromosome normally found in male and female.

33. Y-chromosome — sex chromosome present in male.

C. Diagnostic Terms:

1. Down's syndrome — disorder with varying degrees of retardation and physical signs of mongolism such as dwarfing of stature, slanting eyes, open mouth and protruding tongue. The gentic basis may be a numerical chromosome abnormality (aneuploy) as trisomy 21 with 47 chromosomes or a structural chromosome abnormality as translocation with 46 chromosomes.[49, 70, 72]

2. D-trisomy, trisomy 13-15 — a common chromosome abnormality with 47 chromosomes clinically characterized by hemangiomas, polydactylia and microphthalmia.   Less evident

are cardiovascular and neurologic anomalies which are detectable by chromosome analysis.[22, 49, 51, 70]

3. Klinefelter's syndrome, seminiferous tubule dysgenesis — disorder in which chromosomal aberration results in sterility due to defective embryonic development of the seminiferous tubules. The symptom complex comprises various degrees of
   a. aspermia or oligospermia — lack or scanty secretion of semen.
   b. eunuchoidism — sparsity of hair on face and body.
   c. gynecomastia — overdevelopment of the mammary glands in the male.
   d. hypoplasia of testes, hypogonadism — small, firm testes.
   Mental retardation and psychiatric disorders are common.[49, 51]

4. Noonan's syndrome, Turner's male phenotype — a condition characterized by cryptorchism, insufficient spermatogenesis, webbed neck, short stature, cardiovascular defects and other anomalies. It is not a chromosomal abnormality.[51, 76]

5. Turner's syndrome, gonadal dysgenesis, ovarian dysgenesis — a complex inherited disorder caused by chromosomal aberration. Constant clinical signs are rudimentary ovaries composed of a fibrotic streak in each broad ligament and infertility. The classic syndrome includes different degrees of
   a. estrogen deficiency — inadequate secretion of female hormones.
   b. hypomastia — abnormally small breasts.
   c. malformations — structural defects such as dwarfism, shieldlike chest, webbed neck, coarctation of the aorta and others.
   d. true primary amenorrhea — absence of menses.[49]

Table 24
CYTOGENETIC STUDIES*

Chromosomal Findings	Normal Male	Normal Female	Klinefelter's Syndrome	Turner's Syndrome
Chromosome count	46	46	47	45
Chromosomal pattern	XY	XX	XXY	XO
Chromatin nuclear sex	Chromatin negative	Chromatin positive	Chromatin positive — genetic female	Chromatin negative — genetic male
Major clinical signs	Proper size and function	Proper size and function	Testicular hypoplasia Sterility	Ovarian hypoplasia Infertility

* Cf. Sir Eric Riches (ed.) *Modern Trends in Urology.* London: Butterworths, 1960, pp. 255-261. Other chromosomal patterns and chromatin nuclear sex have been reported, less frequently.

RADIOLOGY

A. Terms Related to Diagnostic Radiology:

1. computer tomography (CT) of the brain — the patient's head is placed in the center of the scanning ring and the x-ray beam is directed to scan the brain from 180 different angles. CT scanning, when concerned with endocrine disorders, tends to detect
   a. pinealomas including solid and cystic teratomas, pineal blastomas, cytomas and gliomas.
   b. cystic changes within the pituitary gland or a craniopharyngioma, an avascular mass in the suprasellar area with calcifications and cystic components.[52]

2. radiogram of adrenals — method of obtaining radiologic evidence of adrenal calcifications of tumors.   Abdominal x-ray pictures, urography and tomography may be used.[55]

3. radiogram of the soft tissues of the neck — method of demonstrating compression of the trachea and calcification with a thyroid neoplasm.

4. ultrasonography of the thyroid gland — diagnostic ultrasound, a simple noninvasive method for ascertaining the size of the thyroid gland and nodule and differentiating solid from cystic lesions.   B mode ultrasonography offers information about hypofunctioning thyroid nodules and aids in establishing patterns for cystadenoma, multinodular goiter and thyroiditis.   It is a safe procedure in the assessment of pediatric and pregnant patients with thyroid lesions.[50, 63]

B. Terms Related to Therapeutic Radiology:

1. neuroblastomas of adrenal medulla — these tumors are considered radiosensitive and radiocurable.

2. thyroid tumors — there is convincing evidence that irradiation causes thyroid cancer.[35]

CLINICAL LABORATORY

A. Terms Primarily Related to Endocrine Function Studies:

1. adrenal gland:
   a. adrenal cortex — outer portion of adrenal gland.   The cortex produces many steroid hormones including 3 major groups:
      (1) steroids controlling the salt and water metabolism.
          Example — aldosterone.
      (2) steroids regulating the glucose metabolism and promoting gluconeogenesis.
          Example — hydrocortisone.
      (3) steroids affecting androgenic activity.
          Example — androsterone.[34]
   b. adrenal medulla — inner portion of adrenal gland which secretes adrenalin (epinephrin) and noradrenalin (norepinephrin).
   c. aldosterone — potent salt-retaining hormone of adrenal cortex which affects electrolyte balance.
   d. aldosterone in urine — quantitative measurement of aldosterone excreted in urine.
      Normal values
      urinary aldosterone level .... 2-26 µg (micrograms) in 24 hours
      Increase in primary and secondary aldosteronism, nephrosis with edema, congestive heart failure with edema, hepatic cirrhosis with ascites and in the second and third trimesters of normal pregnancy.[18, 34, 69]
   e. catecholamines in urine — determination of the excretion of adrenalin and noradrenalin and their metabolites, vanillylmandelic acid and metanephrines.
      Normal values:
      adrenalin-noradrenalin .... below 18 µg/dl (deciliters) in random urine
      adrenalin-noradrenalin .... below 135 µg/dl (deciliters) in 24 hour urine
      metanephrines .... 0.3-0.9 mg (milligrams) in 24 hour urine
      vanillylmandelic acid (VMA) .. 0.7-6.8 mg (milligrams) in 24 hour urine
      Increase in pheochromocytoma and vigorous exercise.[15, 69]
      Related to vanillylmandelic acid (VMA) is homovanillic acid (HVA) which is elevated in the presence of neuroblastomas.[15, 69]
   f. corticosteroids — steroid hormones secreted by the adrenal cortex.[3]
   g. 17-hydrocorticosteroids
      Normal values — Method of Porter-Silber
      17-OH corticosteroids in men .... urine .... 5-15 mg in 24 hours
      17-OH corticosteroids in women .... urine .... 5-13 mg in 24 hours

Increase usually in Cushing's syndrome, in marked stress, acute pancreatitis and in eclampsia

Decrease in hypopituitarism and Addison's disease.[31]

h. 17-ketosteroids in urine — in men measurement of the metabolites of the adrenocortical steroids, adrenal and gonadal androgens; in women and children primarily measurement of adrenal gland secretion. The levels of the 17-KS in urine aid in the detection of endocrine disorders.

Normal values — Method of Vestergaard

17-KS excretion in men ....urine.......8.0-15.0 mg in 24 hours

17-KS excretion in women ......urine.......6.0-11.5 mg in 24 hours

Increase in adrenocortical tumor especially if malignant, interstitial neoplasm of testes, adrenogenital syndrome and occasionally in Cushing's disease

Decrease in Addison's disease and myxedema.[18, 31]

2. thyroid gland — See Chapter XX for tests.

B. Terms Primarily Related to Metabolic Studies:

1. basal metabolic rate — measurement of number of calories needed for the support of basic metabolic functions such as respiration, circulation, body temperature in a resting individual. The normal range is from -10 to $+10$ per cent.

2. blood sugar level — concentration of glucose in the blood.

3. calcitonin — calcium reducing hormone derived from thyroid, parathyroids and sometimes thymus. It effects calcium metabolism, regulates plasma calcium levels and bone remodeling Calcitonin secretion is excessive in medullary carcinoma of the thyroid.[2, 41, 57]

4. carbohydrate tolerance tests:

a. glucose tolerance tests — the intravenous or oral administration of a measured glucose load to discover disorders of carbohydrate metabolism.[10, 24, 31]

Normal values — the true blood sugar method — oral test

fasting blood sugar ....below 100 mg/dl

peak level ....below 160 mg/dl

two hour value ....below 120 mg/dl

Diabetes mellitus

peak level ....above 160 mg/dl

two hour value ....above 120 mg/dl.[14]

b. postprandial blood sugar determination — a screening procedure for the detection of diabetes mellitus. Blood to determine sugar content is drawn 2 hours after the patient started to eat a meal containing 50-100 gm of carbohydrates.

Normal value — the true blood sugar method

blood sugar ....below 100 mg/dl

Increase in hyperglycemia

blood sugar ....above 100 mg/dl

Decrease in hypoglycemia

blood sugar ....below 60 mg/dl.[31]

c. tolbutamide (orinase) tolerance tests — the intravenous or oral administration of tolbutamide sodium to determine the presence or absence of diabetes mellitus when the standard glucose tolerance test fails to provide relevant results. Other indications are (1) hepatic disease, as a means of distinguishing hepatogenic from insulin deficient carbohydrate abnormalities, (2) pancreatic disease and (3) insulin-secreting pancreatic islet cell tumors or insulomas.[24]

5. carbon dioxide combining power — a test for determining the acid-base balance in the blood. In health and with normal activity the acid waste products of metabolism exceed the basic. (See Table 25 for specific information.)

6. 5-HIAA — simple test measuring the urinary excretion of 5-hydroxyindole acetic acid, a metabolic product of serotonin. A marked increase is diagnostic of metastatic carcinoid. Further confirmatory evidence is provided by elevated serotonin blood levels.

Table 25

SOME ESSENTIAL TESTS IN METABOLIC DISORDERS

Test	Normal Values[a]	Increased Values	Decreased Values
Blood Sugar—fasting Adults—Folin-Wu Adults—True Newborns—True	80-120 mg/dl 60-100 mg/dl 30- 50 mg/dl	Diabetes mellitus Hypoinsulinism Hyperpituitarism Hyperthyroidism	Insulin effect Hyperinsulinism Hypopituitarism Addison's disease Hypothyroidism
CO_2 capacity Adults Infants	53-70 vol. % or 24-32 mEq/L 40-55 vol. % or 18-25 mEq/L	Alkalosis Hypercortico-adrenalism Excessive alkali therapy Respiratory conditions	Acidosis Diabetes Nephritis Eclampsia Severe diarrhea

a Cf. Opal E. Hepler. *Manual of Clinical Laboratory Methods*, 4th ed. Springfield, Illinois: Charles C. Thomas, 1955, p. 296.

Normal values — Method of Sjoerdsma
5-HIAA . . . . less than 16 mg urinary excretion in 24 hours
In metastatic carcinoidosis . . . . 50 - 600 mg urinary excretion in 24 hours.
Normal values
serotonin blood levels . . . . 0.1 - 0.3 µg (micrograms) per ml
In metastatic carcinoidosis . . . . 0.5 - 3.0 µg (micrograms) per ml.[14, 23]

7. glucagon — polypeptide hormone secreted by the alpha cells of the pancreatic islets.[10, 24, 56, 67]

8. glucose tolerance — according to Allen: the more sugar a healthy person takes, the more he utilizes. The reverse is true of the diabetic.

9. insulin resistance — tolerance to high daily dosage (200 units) due to obesity or to the development of antibodies which bind insulin.

10. insulin tolerance test — the intravenous administration of regular or crystalline insulin to detect the presence of insulin resistance in patients with a tentative diagnosis of acromegaly or Cushing's syndrome.
    Normal value — return to pre-injection level within 90 to 120 minutes
    Increase — prolonged fall, sometimes associated with hypoglycemic symptoms, indicative of abnormal sensitivity to insulin
    Decrease — lesser fall suggestive of insulin resistance.[24]

11. ketone bodies — acetone bodies, products of faulty metabolism in diabetic acidosis. Since sugar is not utilized normally in diabetes mellitus, excessive fat is mobilized and employed in energy production.   Other clinical states characterized by faulty fat metabolism which result in ketoacidosis are starvation, prolonged diarrhea and vomiting, von Gierke's disease, etc.
    In ketoacidosis ketone bodies accumulate in the blood (ketonemia) and are excreted in the urine (ketonuria).[13, 36]
    Ketone body determination:
    Normal value
        no ketone bodies in blood and urine
    Ketoacidosis
        serum ketone test (serum acetone test) . . . . above 2.0 mg/dl
        urine ketone test (Acetest or Ketostix) . . . . purple color reaction with diacetic acid 5 - 10 mg/dl.[18]

12. lactic acidosis — excess lactic acid in the blood due to its inadequate removal in circulatory, respiratory, renal and hepatic failure, septic shock and terminal cancer.

Its clinical manifestations are hyperventilation, mental confusion followed by coma and collapse.

Table 26

LABORATORY FINDINGS IN DIABETIC COMA[a]

	Ketoacidosis	Lactic Acidosis
Plasma		
acetone	4 plus	0 or 1 plus
bicarbonate	low	low
glucose	high	normal or high or low
Urine		
acetone	4 plus	0 or 1 plus
sugar	4 plus	0 or 1 plus

[a] Adapted from J. H. Karam. Diabetes mellitus. In Krupp, Marcus A and Chatton, Milton. *Current Medical Diagnosis and Treatment*, 15th ed., Los Altos, California: Lange Medical Publications, 1976, p. 740.

13. lipids — a group of organic substances, mostly composed of carbon, hydrogen and some oxygen. Lipids may also contain nitrogen and phosphorus. They are soluble in hydrocarbon and ether and insoluble in water.

Normal values — serum lipids

total lipids	400 - 800 mg/dl
cholesterol	150- -250 mg/dl
triglycerides	10 - 190 mg/dl
phospholipids	150 - 380 mg/dl
fatty acids	9 - 15 mM/l
neutral fat	0 - 200 mg/dl
phospholipid-P	8 - 11 mg/dl.[18]

14. lipoproteins — lipids and proteins combined. Lipids alone cannot enter the circulation, but lipoproteins can be transported by the blood stream. They comprise:

a. alpha lipoproteins — tiny particles containing much protein. They do not predispose to atherosclerosis.

b. beta lipoproteins — particles very small, cholesterol content high predisposing to atherosclerosis.

c. pre-beta lipoproteins — particles are relatively large and appear to be active in the transport of triglycerides.

d. chylomicrons — large particles present in serum during digestion of fat-containing foods. They disappear from serum 12 hours after the meal.[5, 27, 46, 69]

15. metabolite — any product of metabolism, for example, the mineral metabolites: sodium, potassium and chloride which are profoundly influenced by the activity of the adrenal cortex.

a. chloride salts are chiefly bound to sodium. In the gastric juice chlorides are present in the form of hydrochloride.

Normal values — Method of Schales

serum chloride .... 100 - 106 mEq/L[14]

Increase in many conditions resulting from decreased excretion or increased intake.

b. potassium salts, as potassium chloride, phosphates and bicarbonates, are found within tissue cells, especially in muscle cells and blood plasma.

Normal values — Method: Flame photometer

serum potassium .... 3.5 - 5 mEq/L

Increase in Addison's disease

Decrease in Cushing's syndrome.[14, 69]

c. sodium salts, in the form of sodium chloride and sodium bicarbonate, are present in the blood plasma and extracellular fluids.

Normal values — Method: Flame photometer
serum sodium .... 136 - 145 mEq/L
Increase in Cushing's syndrome
Decrease in Addison's disease.[14]

16. osmolality — solute concentration per unit of water, usually expressed in milliosomols per liter of a solution (mOsm/L).

Normal values — serum osmolality .... 285 - 295 mOsm/L.[14, 18]

17. phenotype — the external expression of the genetic constitution of an organism.
18. transferrin — a glycoprotein which transports iron in plasma.
19. triglycerides — simple or neutral fats composed of 3 molecules of fatty acid that are esterified to glycerin.[31]

C. Terms Related to Cytogenetic Tests for Chromosomal Sex Determination:

1. biopsy of human skin — this is a microscopic examination of a small piece of epithelium to detect characteristic chromatin masses alongside the nuclear membrane in somatic cells.   They are usually only found in females.[76]

2. buccal or oral smear test, sex chromatin test, Barr test of nuclear sex — a stained smear of epithelial cells, scraped from the mucosa of the cheek, is studied under the microscope for chromatin bodies.   Normally males are chromatin negative and females chromatin positive.[22, 76]

3. leukocyte cell smear from peripheral blood — a cytologic test for chromosomal sex differentiation.   A small number of circulating neutrophils possess a characteristic drumstick chromatin attachment distinguishable from the remaining nucleus.   This drumstick formation on the cell nucleus has not been found in males.[22, 70, 76]

4. tissue culture of human cells — new method of culturing permits growth without chromosomal disorganization.   Tissue is cultured in vitro to obtain sufficient mitoses.   The culture is treated with colchicine to arrest mitosis in metaphase and with hypotonic saline to attain spreading of the chromosomes.   Preparations are then squashed, stained and photographed under a microscope.   The photomicrograph is enlarged and the chromosomes cut out and paired to make a karyotype.[70]

ABBREVIATIONS

ACTH — adrenocorticotropic hormone
ADH — antidiuretic hormone
ATP — adenosine triphosphate
BMR — basal metabolic rate
CO_2 — carbon dioxide
CRF — corticotropic releasing factor
CZI — crystalline zinc insulin
DOC — desoxycorticosterone
ECF — extracellular fluid
EFA — essential fatty acids
FBS — fasting blood sugar
FFA — free fatty acids
FSH — follicle stimulating hormone
FTI — free thyroxine index
GTT — glucose tolerance test
ICF — intracellular fluid

ICSH — interstitial cell stimulating hormone
IF — interstitial fluid
K — potassium
LATS — long-acting thyroid stimulator
LH — luteinizing hormone
MSH — melanocyte-stimulating hormone
NaCl — sodium chloride
NPH — neutral protein Hagedorn (insulin)
P — phosphorus
PGH — pituitary growth hormone
PP — postprandial
PZI — protamine zinc insulin
17-KS — 17 ketosteroids
17-OH — 17 hydroxycorticoids
TSH — thyroid stimulating hormone
TTH — thyrotropic hormone

ORAL READING PRACTICE

Hypothyroidism

Hypothyroidism is a functional disorder caused by insufficiency of the circulating thyroid hormones.   Any biologic, chemical or physical factors which reduce the hormone supply may result in thyroid failure.

In primary hypothyroid states the condition may be congenital as in **cretinism,** or acquired as in juvenile **myxedema** or adult **myxedema.** Surgical excision, atrophy or disease of the thyroid gland stop or lower hormone production and a lack of iodine in food seriously hampers hormone synthesis.

In secondary hypothyroid states the pituitary gland elaborates an inadequate amount of the thyroid stimulating hormone (TSH) which drastically reduces thyroid function. This deficit of thyrotropin (TSH) occurs in **pituitary necrosis** or Sheehan's disease and primary chronic hypopituitarism or Simmond's syndrome. A total absence of TSH is seen in **hypophysectomized** patients.

The judicious use of replacement therapy with **thyroxine** or **triiodothyronine** in thyroid failure and a thyrotropin preparation in pituitary failure is imperative to maintain relatively normal metabolic processes and overcome hypothyroidism.[20, 39, 60]

Table 27

SOME ENDOCRINE CONDITIONS AMENABLE TO SURGERY

Organs Involved	Diagnoses	Operations	Operative procedures
Adrenal gland	Adenoma of the adrenal cortex, unilateral, anterior to kidney	Unilateral adrenalectomy with excision of neoplasm	Abdominal approach with preliminary exploration of ovaries in the female followed by removal of neoplasm
Adrenal gland	Cushing's syndrome associated with (1) psychosis (2) multiple bone fracture (3) severe diabetes	Subtotal adrenalectomy Bilateral adrenalectomy	Removal of one adrenal gland Removal of adrenals by the subdiaphragmatic route, transthoracic or transabdominal approach
Adrenal glands	Metastatic cancer of the breast	Bilateral adrenalectomy	Excision of both adrenals
Parathyroid	Parathyroid adenoma Hyperparathyroidism	Excision of adenoma of parathyroid gland	Removal of neoplasm to prevent recurrent renal calculi
Thyroid gland	Solitary thyroid nodule of unknown nature	Surgical exploration	Tissue from thyroid nodule removed — frozen section made
Thyroid gland	Hyperthyroidism-exophthalmic goiter	Partial or subtotal thyroidectomy	Removal of part of thyroid gland
Thyroid gland	Papillary carcinoma with metastases to adjacent lymph nodes	Complete or total thyroidectomy with neck dissection	Excision of entire thyroid gland with dissection of the upper portion of neck
Thyroid gland	Postthyroidectomy hemorrhage	Thyroidotomy	Reopening of thyroid wound for removal of hematoma and control of hemorrhage
Thymus gland	Myasthenia gravis nonthymomatous	Thymectomy transcervical[a]	Incision across the suprasternal notch Removal of thymus

[a] D. S. Girnar. Anesthesia for transcervical thymectomy in myasthenia gravis. *Anesthesia and Analgesia . . . Current Researches,* 55: 13-17, January-February, 1976.

REFERENCES AND BIBLIOGRAPHY

1. Alderson, P. O. The single palpable thyroid nodule. *Cancer*, 37: 258-265, January, 1976.

2. Aurbach, G. D. Parathyroid. In Beeson, Paul B. and McDermott, Walsh (eds.). *Textbook of Medicine*, 14th ed. Philadelphia: W. B. Saunders Co., 1975, pp. 1802-1818.

3. Bauman, G. *et al.* Prolonged corticotropic action of synthetic human ACTH in man. *Clinical Endocrinology and Metabolism*, 42: 160-162, January, 1976.

4. Beutler, E. Galactosemia. In Beeson, Paul B. and McDermott, Walsh (eds.). *Textbook of Medicine*, 14th ed. Philadelphia: W. B. Saunders Co., 1975, pp. 1624-1625.

5. Bierman, E. L. *et al.* Disorders of lipid metabolism. In Williams, Robert H. (ed.). *Textbook of Endocrinology*, 5th ed. Philadelphia: W. B. Saunders Co., 1974, pp. 890-937.

6. Blackstock, R. *et al.* The role of thymus and bone marrow cells in immunologic competence. *Southern Medical Journal*, 69: 209-216, February, 1976.

7. Brown, M. S. Familial hypercholesterolemia. *Advances in Internal Medicine*, Vol. II. Chicago: Yearbook Medical Publishers, Inc., 1975, pp. 273-296.

8. Brown, P. W. *et al.* Bilateral adrenalectomy for metastatic breast carcinoma. *Archives of Surgery*, 110: 77-81, January, 1975.

9. Brunzell, J. D. *et al.* Relationships between fasting plasma glucose levels and insulin secretion during intravenous glucose tolerance tests. *Clinical Endocrinology and Metabolism*, 42: 222-229, February, 1976.

10. Cahill, G. F. Diabetes mellitus. In Beeson, Paul B. and McDermott, Walsh (eds.). *Textbook of Medicine*, 14th ed. Philadelphia: W. B. Saunders Co., 1975, pp. 1599-1619.

11. Chong, G. C. Medullary carcinoma of the thyroid gland. *Cancer*, 35: 695-704, March, 1975.

12. Christy, N. P. The anterior pituitary. In Beeson, Paul B. and McDermott, Walsh (eds.). *Textbook of Medicine*, 14th ed. Philadelphia: W. B. Saunders Co., 1975, pp. 1677-1699.

13. Clements, R. S. *et al.* Ketoacidosis. *Southern Medical Journal*, 69: 217-221, February, 1976.

14. Conn, R. B. Normal laboratory values of clinical importance. In Beeson, Paul B. and McDermott, Walsh (eds.). *Textbook of Medicine*, 14th ed. Philadelphia: W. B. Saunders Co., 1975, pp. 1884-1892.

15. Coulombe, P. *et al.* Catecholamines metabolism in thyroid diseases. *Clinical Endocrinology and Metabolism*, 42: 125-131, January, 1976.

16. Dao, T. L. Adrenalectomy with radical mastectomy in the treatment of high-risk breast cancer. *Cancer*, 35: 478-482, February, 1975.

17. Daughaday, W. H. The adenohypophysis. In Williams, Robert H. (ed.). *Textbook of Endocrinology*, 5th ed. Philadelphia: W. B. Saunders Co., 1974, pp. 31-79.

18. Davidsohn, Israel and Henry, John B. Tables of normal values. *Clinical Diagnosis by Laboratory Methods*, 15th ed. Philadelphia: W. B. Saunders Co., 1974, pp. 1376-1392.

19. DeCosse, J. J. *et al.* Carcinoma of the thyroid. *Archives of Surgery*, 110: 783-789, June, 1975.

20. DeGroot, Leslie J. and Stanbury, John B. *The Thyroid and Its Diseases*. 4th ed. New York: John Wiley & Sons, 1975, pp. 314-748.

21. DeJong, Russel and Sugar, Oscar. Tumors. *Neurology and Neurosurgery 1976*. Chicago: Year Book Medical Publishers, Inc., 1976, pp. 435-450.

22. Eggen, R. R. Cytogenetics. In Davidsohn, Israel and Henry, Bernard J. *Clinical Diagnosis by Laboratory Methods*, 15th ed. Philadelphia: W. B. Saunders Co., 1974, pp. 1307-1339.

23. Engelman, K. The carcinoid syndrome. In Beeson, Paul B. and McDermott, Walsh. *Textbook of Medicine*, 14th ed. Philadelphia: W. B. Saunders Co., 1975, pp. 1795-1802.

24. Ensinck, J. W. *et al.* Disorders causing hypoglycemia. In Williams, Robert H. (ed.). *Textbook of Endocrinology*, 5th ed. Philadelphia: W. B. Saunders Co., 1974, pp. 80-94.

25. Fajans, S. S. Hyperinsulinism, hypoglycemia and glucagon secretion. In Wintrobe, Maxwell M. (ed.). *Principles of Internal Medicine*, 7th ed. New York: McGraw-Hill Book Co., 1974, pp. 554-560.

26. Forsham, P. H. Disorders of the adrenal glands. In Smith, Donald R. *General Urology*, 8th ed. Los Altos, California: Lange Medical Publications, 1975, pp. 320-325.

27. Fredrickson, D. S. Disorders of lipid metabolism and xanthomatosis. In Wintrobe, Maxwell M. (ed.). *Principles of Internal Medicine*, 7th ed. New York: McGraw-Hill Book Co., 1974, pp. 634-644.

28. Godwin, J. D. Carcinoid tumors — An analysis of 2837 cases. *Cancer*, 36: 560-569, August, 1975.

29. Hajjar, R. A. Adrenal cortical carcinoma — A study of 32 patients. *Cancer*, 35: 549-554, February, 1975.

30. Hamburger, J. I. Recurrent hyperthyroidism after thyroidectomy. *Archives of Surgery*, 111: 91-92, January, 1976.

31. Henry, J. B. Clinical chemistry — Endocrine measurements. In Davidsohn, Israel and Henry, John B. *Clinical Diagnosis by Laboratory Methods*. Philadelphia: W. B. Saunders Co., 1974, pp. 516-771.

32. Hume, D. M. *et al.* Pituitary and adrenal. In Schwartz, Seymour. *Principles of Surgery*, 2d ed. New York: McGraw-Hill Book Co., 1974, pp. 1363-1427.

33. ————. Endocrine and metabolic responses to injury. *Ibid.*, pp. 1-64.

34. Huq, M. S. *et al.* Concurrence of aldosterone, androgen and cortisol secretion in adrenal venous effluents. *Clinical Endocrinology and Metabolism*, 42: 230-238, February, 1976.

35. Kaplan, E. L. *et al.* Recent developments in radiation-induced carcinoma of the thyroid. *Surgical Clinics of North America*, 56: 199-206, February, 1976.

36. Karam, J. H. Diabetes mellitus — Hypoglycemia. In Krupp, Marcus A. and Chatton, Milton. *Current Medical Diagnosis & Treatment*, 15th ed. Los Altos, California: Lange Medical Publications, 1976, pp. 727-747.

37. ————. Disturbances of lipid metabolism. *Ibid.*, pp. 747-753.

38. Kolb, F. O. Endocrine disorders. In Krupp, Marcus A. and Chatton, Milton J. *Current Medical Diagnosis & Treatment*, 15th ed. Los Altos, California: Lange Medical Publications, 1976, pp. 645-649.

39. ————. Diseases of the hypothalamus and of the pituitary gland. *Ibid.*, pp. 649-656.

40. ————. Diseases of the thyroid gland — The parathyroids. *Ibid.*, pp. 656-679.

41. ————. Diseases of the adrenal cortex — Diseases of the adrenal medulla. *Ibid.*, pp. 686-721.

42. Kraft, J. R. Detection of diabetes mellitus in situ (occult diabetes). *Laboratory Medicine*, 6: 10-22, February, 1975.

43. Lai, C. C. Trisomy 8 syndrome. *Clinical Orthopaedics and Related Research*, 110: 239-243, July-August, 1975.

44. Lanier, V. C. The surgical treatment of exophthalmos. *Plastic and Reconstructive Surgery*, 55: 56-64, January, 1975.

45. Leaf, A. Posterior pituitary. In Beeson, Paul B. and McDermott, Walsh (eds.). *Textbook of Medicine*, 14th ed. Philadelphia: W. B. Saunders Co., 1975, pp. 1699-1700.

46. Levy, R. I. The meaning of lipid profiles. *Postgraduate Medicine*, 57: 34-38, April, 1975.

47. Lewandowski, R. et al. New chromosomal syndromes. *American Journal of Diseases of Children*, 129: 515-529, April, 1975.

48. Liddle, G. W. Adrenal cortex. In Beeson, Paul B. and McDermott, Walsh (eds.). *Textbook of Medicine*, 14th ed. Philadelphia: W. B. Saunders Co., 1975, pp. 1733-1751.

49. McKusick, V. A. Inheritance and growth. In Wintrobe, Maxwell M. (ed.). *Harrison's Principles of Internal Medicine*, 7th ed. New York: McGraw-Hill Book Co., 1974, pp. 323-341.

50. Miskin, M. et al. Ultrasonography of the thyroid gland. *Radiologic Clinics of North America*, 13: 479-492, December, 1975.

51. Monteleone, Patricia L., M.D. Personal communications.

52. New, Paul F. and Scott, William R. Pineal area tumors — Pituitary adenomas and craniopharyngiomas. *Computed Tomography of the Brain and Orbit*. Baltimore: Williams and Wilkins Co., 1975, pp. 178-208.

53. Paris Conference (1971), Supplement (1975). Birth defects. *Original Article Series*. New York: The National Foundation, Vol. XI, No. 9, 1975, pp. 14-33.

54. Pearson, C. M. Muscle and hormones. In Williams, Robert H. (ed.). *Textbook of Endocrinology*, 5th ed. Philadelphia: W. B. Saunders Co., 1974, pp. 994-1003.

55. Pilla, Lawrence A., M.D. Personal communications.

56. Pozefsky, T. et al. Studies with glucagon. *Diabetes*, 25: 128-135, February, 1976.

57. Rasmussen, H. Parathyroid hormone, calcitonin and the calciferols. In Williams, Robert H. (ed.). *Textbook of Endocrinology*, 5th ed. Philadelphia: W. B. Saunders Co., 1974, pp. 660-773.

58. Robbins, Stanley L. Adrenal cortex — Adrenal medulla. *Pathologic Basis of Disease*. Philadelphia: W. B. Saunders Co., 1974, pp. 1297-1320.

59. ————. Thyroid gland — Parathyroid glands. *Ibid.*, pp. 1346-1354.

60. ————. Pituitary — Thymus. *Ibid.*, pp. 1354-1370.

61. ————. Systemic diseases. *Ibid.*, pp. 259-313.

62. ————. Pancreas. *Ibid.*, pp. 1056-1077.

63. Rosen, I. B. et al. The application of ultrasound to the study of thyroid enlargement — Management of 450 cases. *Archives of Surgery*, 110: 940-944, August, 1975.

64. Salger, W. R. et al. Thymoma — A clinical and pathological study of 65 cases. *Cancer*, 37: 229-249, January, 1976.

65. Schimke, R. N. Multiple endocrine adenomatosis syndromes. In Stollerman, Gene H. *Advances in Internal Medicine*, Vol. XXI. Chicago: Year Book Medical Publications, 1976, pp. 249-265.

66. Schmid, R. Porphyria. In Beeson, Paul B. and McDermott, Walsh (eds.). *Textbook of Medicine*, 14th ed. Philadelphia: W. B. Saunders Co., 1975, pp. 1873-1876.

67. Sherwin, R. S. et al. Hyperglucagonemia and blood glucose regulation in normal, obese and diabetic patients. *New England Journal of Medicine*, 294: 455-461, February 26, 1976.

68. Snyder, S. M. Acromegaly and primary hypogonadism. *Annals of Internal Medicine*, 82: 542-543, April, 1975.

69. *Specialized Diagnostic Laboratory Tests*, 11th ed. Van Nuys, California: Bio-Science Laboratories, 1976, pp. 29-140.

70. ————. Chromosome analysis. *Ibid.*, pp. 174-177.

71. Taylor, S. Surgery of the thyroid gland. In De Groot, Leslie J. and Stanbury, John B. *The Thyroid and Its Diseases*, 4th ed. New York: John Wiley & Sons, 1975, pp. 776-799.

72. Uchida, I. Chromosomal abnormalities in man. In Vaughan, Victor C. III and McKay, R. James. *Nelson Textbook of Pediatrics*, 10th ed. Philadelphia: W. B. Saunders Co., 1975, pp. 289-310.

73. Valenta, L. H. Hyperparathyroidism due to parathyroid adenoma and carpal tunnel syndrome. *Annals of Internal Medicine*, 82: 541-542, April, 1975.

74. Van Gilder, J. C. et al. Hypophysectomy in metastatic breast cancer. *Archives of Surgery*, 110: 293-295, March, 1975.

75. Vaughan, Daniel and Taylor, Asbury. Genetic aspects. *General Ophthalmology*, 7th ed. Los Altos, California: Lange Medical Publications, 1974, pp. 252-257.

76. Volk, Sister Leo Rita, M. in MT. Personal communications.

77. Wertelecki, W. et al. The clinical syndrome of triploidy. *Obstetrics and Gynecology*, 47: 69-76, January, 1976.

78. Wurster-Hill, D. et al. Cytogenic studies of polycythemia vera. *Seminars in Hematology*, 13: 13-32, January, 1976.

Chapter XIII
The Sense Organ of Vision

EYE

A. Origin of Terms:

1. choroid (G) — skin-like
2. converge (L) — to come together
3. cornea (L) — horny
4. crystal (G) — clear ice
5. cyclo- (G) — circle
6. enucleate (L) — to remove kernel
7. iris (G) — rainbow
8. kerato- (G) — horny
9. nystagmus (G) — nod
10. oculus (L) — eye
11. ophthalmo- (G) — eye
12. opsis (G) — sight
13. opto- (G) — vision
14. phakos (G) — lens
15. pyon (G) — pus
16. schisis (G) — division
17. sclera (G) — hard
18. uva (L) — grape
19. vitreous (L) — glassy
20. zonule (L) — tiny band

B. Anatomic Terms:[73]

1. bulb of the eye — the globe or eyeball.
2. chambers of the eye:
   a. anterior chamber — space in front of the iris and back of the cornea.
   b. posterior chamber — space in back of the iris and in front of the lens.
3. coats of the eye:
   a. cornea — anterior transparent part of the outer tunic of the eye. The sclera is the posterior opaque part of the outer tunic. It is composed of dense fibrous tissue which has a protective function.[34, 60]
   b. retina — innermost light perceiving tunic, perceives and transmits the sensory impulses of light to the optic nerve.[57, 64]
   c. uvea, uveal tract — intermediate vascular tunic composed of the
      (1) choroid — which contains a layer of blood vessels and provides nutrition for part of the retina, lens and vitreous.
      (2) ciliary body — thickened part of the vascular tunic of the eye. Its circularly arranged processes secrete aqueous humor. The ciliary muscle helps to regulate the shape of the lens.
      (3) iris — anterior highly pigmented part of the uvea. The pupil is an opening in the center of the iris. Its size is controlled by a sphincter muscle and dilator muscle.[61]
4. ciliary zonule — suspensory ligament of the lens attaching the ciliary body and contiguous retina to the lens capsule.
5. fovea — small depression in the macula adapted for most acute vision.[57, 64]
6. fundus oculi — inner posterior portion of the eye which can be seen with an ophthalmoscope.
7. lens, crystalline lens — a transparent, biconvex body enclosed in a capsule and lying directly in back of the iris. It is a powerful refracting component of the visual system and focusing structure capable of changing its shape.[7, 31, 65]
8. macula lutea — small avascular area of the retina around the fovea.[64]
9. orbit — bony cavity of the skull in which lies the eyeball.[73]
10. trabeculae (sing. trabecula) — loosely arranged grayish-white fibrous strands in the filtration angle of the anterior chamber through which the aqueous escapes.[7, 73]
11. vitreous body — a jelly-like, transparent mass which occupies the space behind the lens and is normally in contact with the retina.[58]

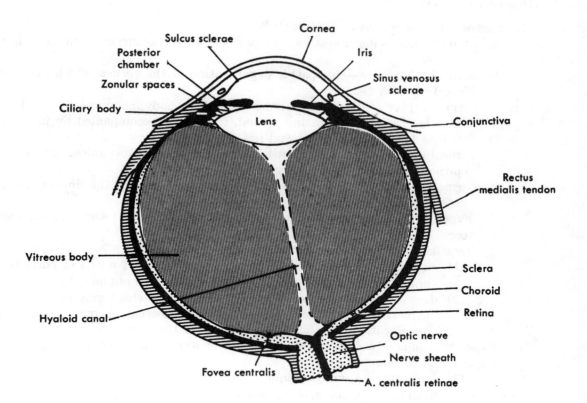

Fig. 69 — Horizontal section of eyeball through optic nerve.

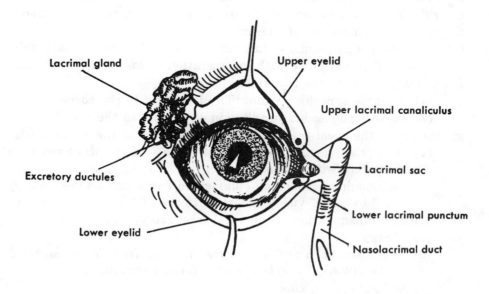

Fig. 70 — Lacrimal apparatus.

C. Diagnostic Terms:

1. disorders of the cornea and sclera:[34, 60]
   a. arcus senilis — degenerative change in the cornea occurring commonly in persons past 50.
   b. corneal dystrophy — idiopathic degeneration of the cornea which may seriously interfere with vision.
   c. corneal injury — damage to cornea by foreign body, chemical, thermal or radiation burn, laceration, penetrating wound, frequently accompanied by intraocular damage such as traumatic cataract and iris prolapse.
   d. corneal ulcer — a form of keratitis due to pathogenic organism entering the corneal epithelium. The stroma may also break down.[7]
   e. dermoid — a skin-like tumor or cyst generally located at the limbus and involving both cornea and sclera.
   f. hypopyon — pus in anterior chamber in back of cornea; sometimes associated with corneal ulcer.
   g. keratitis — inflammation of the cornea.
      (1) superficial — inflammatory reaction consisting of a loss of corneal epithelium and ulcer formation due to infection from the outside.
      (2) deep — invasion of deep layers of the cornea which may result in its perforation. Interstitial keratitis due to syphilis or tuberculosis may cause permanent opacification (loss of transparency) of the cornea.
   h. keratoconus — a conical bulging of the center of the cornea.
   i. scars of cornea:
      (1) leukoma — a white opaque cornea.
      (2) macula — opaque spot seen on cornea.
      (3) nebula — grayish opacity of cornea.
   j. scleritis — inflammation of the sclera.
2. disorders of the uveal tract:[61]
   a. choroidal hemorrhage — local bleeding of choroid which may be associated with vascular disorder, trauma, choroiditis, diabetes or other diseases.
   b. iridocyclitis — inflammation of the iris and ciliary body.
   c. iridodialysis — detachment of outer margin of iris from ciliary body.
   d. iritis — inflammation of the iris.
   e. sympathetic ophthalmia — inflammation of uveal tract usually following perforating wound of opposite eye with incarceration or loss of uveal tissue.[39]
   f. synechia — there are two kinds:
      (1) anterior synechia — adhesion of the iris to the cornea.
      (2) posterior synechia — adhesion of the iris to the lens.[39]
   g. tumors of the uveal tract — intraocular tumors of the choroid, iris or ciliary body.
      (1) nevi (sing. nevus), benign melanomas — pigmental lesions which usually do not interfere with vision.
      (2) malignant melanomas — pigmented cancerous lesions, usually unilateral, which lead to loss of vision and occur in the fifth or sixth decade of life.[11]
   h. uveitis — inflammation of the uveal tract caused by:
      (1) allergy
      (2) organisms such as *Coccidioides immitis, Histoplasma capsulatum, Mycobacterium tuberculosis, Toxoplasma gondii,* other organisms
      (3) irritants and toxins
      (4) connective tissue diseases.
3. disorders of the vitreous:[58, 62]
   a. vitreoretinal degeneration, Wagner disease — hereditary disorder of vitreous and retina characterized by marked liquefaction of central vitreous, reduced vision,

vitreous floaters, vitreous traction on retina resulting in retinal tears and breaks leading to retinal detachment.[58, 62]

   b. vitreous detachment — vitreous detached from retina in one or both eyes. It may lead to retinal tear.[62]

   c. vitreous hemorrhage — rare but serious disorder, usually caused by rupture of a retinal vessel and followed by sudden loss of vision.[62]

   d. vitreous infections — bacterial, fungal or parasitic infections resulting in liquefaction, opacification and shrinkage of vitreous.[58, 62]

4. disorders of the lens and intraocular pressure:

   a. aphakia — absence of the lens, congenital or acquired due to surgical removal; binocular or monocular in both eyes or in one eye.

   b. cataract — an opacity in the lens, congenital or acquired.[7] Lenticular opacity is usually linked with the process of aging. Insoluble proteins form in the lens and eventually lead to dehydration, lowered metabolism and tissue necrosis. In the cataractous lens sodium and calcium content tend to be increased and potassium, protein and ascorbic acid content decreased. Visual impairment is slowly progressive.[31, 42, 65]

   c. ectopia lentis — displacement of the lens seen primarily in Marfan's syndrome in its congenital form. It also may be due to trauma.[42]

   d. glaucoma — increased intraocular pressure which, untreated, leads to blindness. Some types of glaucoma are:

     (1) acute glaucoma — severe obstruction of aqueous humor drainage, sharp rise of intraocular tension, agonizing eye pain, dilated pupil, steamy cornea and ciliary injection.

     (2) chronic glaucoma

       (a) closed angle glaucoma — intermittent attacks of angle closure of anterior chamber, formation of adhesions in angle with attacks and gradual obliteration of angle requiring peripheral iridectomy, if unresponsive to medical therapy.

       (b) open angle glaucoma — interference with aqueous outflow creating an elevated intraocular pressure. The open type is bilateral and, if untreated, leads slowly to visual impairment and cupping of optic disk.[3, 8, 43, 66, 70]

     (3) malignant glaucoma — a distinct type of angle closure with a forward movement of the lens and direct closure of the angle occurring with or without glaucoma surgery (Levens' definition).[36, 51]

5. disorders of the retina:

   a. atrophy and degeneration of retina — a reduction of visual acuity due to degenerative processes seen in the elderly.

   b. Coats disease — eye condition characterized by abnormalities of the retinal vasculature, retinal microaneurysms in areas of destruction of small vessels, retinal hemorrhage and exudation.[10]

   c. detachment of the retina — separation of the retina from the choroid resulting in blindness if not relieved.[1, 57, 64]

   d. edema of the retina — condition due to active hyperemia, generally resulting from trauma.

   e. diabetic retinopathy — condition characterized by pinpoint aneurysms, which may be caused by dilatation of the retinal capillaries in diabetes mellitus.[57, 63]

   f. hypertensive retinopathy — retinal changes resulting from persistently high diastolic blood pressure. This condition may occur in essential hypertension, renal arteriolar sclerosis, glomerulonephritis and toxemias of pregnancy.[57, 63]

   g. macular degenerations — a group of degenerative disorders of the retina:[48, 54, 64, 77]

     (1) circinate degeneration — rather common macular retinopathy, seen in older age groups. It is usually bilateral and characterized by a girdle of yellow white

spots surrounding the macular area.   The peripheral vision may be retained but the central vision is lost.

    (2) cystic degeneration of macula — sharply delineated red, round cystic defect in macula.   The wall of the fluid-filled cyst may rupture and a macular hole may result.   If the fovea is involved, central vision is blurred.[48]

    (3) disciform macular degeneration, Kuhnt Junius disease — a dark dome-shaped elevation in the macular area apparently containing extravasated blood from a retinal hemorrhage.   Central vision is impaired or lost.[48]

    (4) retinoschisis — a separation of the sensory retina into two layers appearing as a shallow elevation of the peripheral retina.   Defect may not be progressive but vision in the involved area is affected.[7, 38, 48]

  h. occlusion of central retinal artery — rare unilateral disorder due to thrombus, embolus or atheromatous plaque suddenly causing total loss of sight in the affected eye.   It may occur in advanced age or during oral contraceptive therapy.[63]

  i. occlusion of central retinal vein — thrombosis of the central retinal vein leading to sudden, painless loss of sight.[63]

  j. retinal arteriolar sclerosis — a form of sclerosis due to hypertension characterized by copper-wire arterioles in the retina.   In the advanced stage of the sclerotic process the arterioles resemble silver wire.[63]

  k. retinal atherosclerosis — obstructive changes in retinal vessels which may cause a sudden vascular accident in the retina.[63]

  l. retinal hemorrhage — moderate or massive bleeding from the retina.[76]

  m. retinal tears — small holes or tears which unrepaired may enlarge and lead to retinal detachment and blindness.

  n. retinitis pigmentosa — hereditary degenerative disease principally affecting the rod and cone layer of the retina.   Ophthalmologic examination reveals spider-shaped pigment spots on the retina.   Night blindness is the dominant feature.[7, 57, 64]

  o. retrolental fibroplasia — bilateral, retinal disease in premature infants associated with high oxygen concentration in the infant's environment.[7, 59, 64]

  p. von Hippel-Lindau disease — retinal angioma usually associated with cerebellar angioma and polycystic kidneys.[2, 18, 74]

6. disorders of the optic nerve:

  a. optic atrophy — a destruction of the fibers of the optic nerve associated with loss of visual acuity.[56]

  b. optic coloboma — congenital defect in optic nerve resulting from imperfect closure of fetal cleft.   Defects in choroid and retina may coexist.   Visual impairment is common.[57]

  c. optic neuritis — inflammation of the optic nerve; may involve the sheaths of the nerve (optic perineuritis) or its main body.[57]

  d. papilledema, choked disk — edema of the papilla or optic nerve head usually due to increased intracranial pressure.[56, 57]

  e. papillitis — inflammation of the papilla or head of the optic nerve.

  f. retrobulbar neuritis — optic neuritis in which nerve involvement occurs behind the optic disk and cannot be seen ophthalmoscopically.   Visual acuity is seriously affected or entirely lost.   One of its most common causes is multiple sclerosis.

7. ocular infections:

  a. endophthalmitis — intraocular infection due to various etiologic agents. Early treatment may salvage the eye.[70]

  b. panophthalmitis — extensive ocular infection, usually resulting from eye injury and leading to corneal ulceration and total destruction of the eyeball.[70]

8. ocular tumors:[11, 14, 21, 59]

  a. melanomas of choroid or iris — malignant neoplasms derived from cells which form melanin, a black pigment.[11]

  b. optic nerve tumors

      (1) gliomas — glial tumors which may be derived from astrocytes of the optic nerve and are either solitary tumors or occur in von Recklinghausen's neurofibromatosis.[23]

      (2) meningiomas — usually orbital tumors arising in the sheath of the optic nerve.[21, 22]

   c. retinoblastomas — malignant tumors arising from the retina. They are hereditary, unilateral or bilateral, and readily metastasize to the optic nerve and brain.[11, 57, 59, 64]

Other common tumors are hemangiomas and orbital lymphomas.[7, 59]

D. Operative Terms:

1. cataract operations — various procedures for the removal of an opaque lens.[42, 65]

   a. aspiration and irrigation procedure — removal of a cataract by suction through a small limbal incision and simultaneous irrigation of the anterior chamber with normal saline solution through another limbal incision. The effective use of the operating microscope virtually permits aspiration of the entire opaque lens. Discission of the posterior capsule completes the procedure which is used for patients below the age of thirty.[42, 65]

   b. cryoextraction of cataract — application of the tip of the cryoextractor to the anterior surface of the lens until the cataract firmly adheres to the instrument. When the freezing process has extended for 2 to 3 mm into the lens substance, the probe with the lens frozen to it is lifted out.[42]

   c. enzymatic zonulysis (or zonulolysis) — instillation of alpha-chymotrypsin, a fibrinolytic enzyme, into the anterior chamber to dissolve the ciliary zonules and thus facilitate the removal of the cataractous lens. The procedure is used in the 20-50 year age group in whom the zonules are tough, making cataract extraction difficult.[42]

   d. extracapsular cataract extraction — incision into anterior capsule in order to express the opaque nucleus of the lens and some of the cortical material.[7]

   e. intracapsular cataract extraction — removal of entire lens in its capsule, a method of choice especially for senescent (senile) cataracts.[42, 65]

   f. phacoemulsification, Kelman technique — cataract removal by inserting a phacoemulsifier through a 2 to 3 mm incision and breaking up the sclerotic portion of the lens by ultrasonic vibration followed by aspiration of the lens fragments and irrigation of the eye.[30, 31, 42, 53, 65]

2. corneal operations:

   a. keratocentesis — puncture of the cornea.

   b. keratoplasty, corneal graft, corneal transplant — surgical replacement of a section of an opaque cornea with normal, transparent cornea to restore vision.

      (1) lamellar keratoplasty — using part thickness corneal transplant.

      (2) penetrating keratoplasty — using full thickness corneal transplant.[29, 34]

   c. thermokeratoplasty — new procedure based on the fact that the proper application of heat shrinks corneal collagen and thus prevents corneal scarring. A well controlled temperature probe flattens the keratoconus and makes the cornea more spherical. This operation is not indicated when scarring has already developed or the cornea is very thin.[29]

3. enucleation — removal of the eyeball indicated in penetrating injuries, malignant tumors of the eye and as an emergency measure in threatened sympathetic ophthalmia.[55]

4. evisceration — removal of contents of eyeball but leaving the sclera and cornea.

5. glaucoma operations — surgical procedures for highly increased intraocular pressure, irreducible by miotics or other medical treatment.[3, 7, 66]

   a. cyclocryosurgery — direct application of the cryoprobe to the conjunctiva over different locations in back of the limbus. The intense vascular response reduces ciliary body function and aqueous production. No incision is necessary.

   b. cyclodialysis — a filtering procedure allowing aqueous to drain into the suprachoroidal space in order to lower intraocular tension.[3, 66]

   c. iridencleisis — a filtering technique permitting aqueous to escape into the space below the conjunctiva where it is reabsorbed by the circulating blood and diffused into the tear film.[3, 43, 66]

   d. goniotomy — incision across anterior chamber for establishing normal aqueous outflow through regular channels in congenital and infantile glaucoma.[3, 43, 66]

   e. microsurgery in glaucoma — use of the operating microscope to facilitate direct surgery on the Schlemm's canal and trabecular meshwork in treating glaucoma.

       (1) trabeculectomy — elevation of a conjunctival flap to expose the sclera at the limbus and excision of a scleral portion including the trabecular meshwork. The appearance of a filtering bleb achieves ocular pressure control. Trabeculectomies have been successfully performed in adult phakic eyes with open-angle glaucoma.[3, 52, 66]

       (2) trabeculotomy — surgical fashioning of a scleral flap, meticulous dissection to locate the Schlemm's canal and insertion of a small probe into the canal and anterior chamber to relieve block to aqueous outflow, prone to be present in the trabecular meshwork.[3, 43, 52, 66]

   f. peripheral iridectomy — raising a small conjunctival flap at the limbus and entering the anterior chamber through a 4 mm incision to prevent pupillary block. This technique frees the filtration angle from the iris root and permits the aqueous to escape by the normal channel.[66, 72]

   g. thermal sclerostomy, Scheie's operation — a filtering procedure for severe glaucoma. Anterior chamber is entered through limbal incision and posterior portion of incision is cauterized, resulting in tissue shrinkage. This is followed by a peripheral iridectomy, repositioning of conjunctival flap at the limbus and wound closure. The use of the operating microscope is optional.[7, 43]

6. photocoagulation, ocular — use of light of appropriate intensity and wave length at a given distance to cause the coagulation of tissue. Photocoagulation techniques are used in the treatment of retinal vascular diseases, maculopathies, and peripheral chorioretinal disorders.

   a. argon laser beam — a blue-green light which is effectively absorbed by red hemoglobin choroid and pigment epithelium and has been used with success in the treatment of diabetic retinopathy and tried in senescent (senile) macular degeneration.[1, 2, 16, 18]

   b. xenon arc beam — emission of a white light which includes all wave lengths in the visible spectrum and may be used in most ocular diseases and lesions for which argon laser is recommended.[2, 10, 44, 45, 77]

7. repair of retinal holes or tears and retinal detachment — surgical reattachment of minor or major separations of the retina from the choroid.[13, 20, 26, 64] This can be accomplished by

   a. cryopexy of sclera — application of a supercooled probe to the sclera to produce a chorioretinal scar with minimal damage to the sclera.[57]

   b. laser photocoagulation — procedure for mending small retinal tears. A laser beam is directed through the dilated pupil to produce a chorioretinal inflammatory reaction which seals the small tear.[44, 57]

   c. scleral buckling operation — removal of strip of sclera near the retinal separation, drainage of subretinal fluid, placement of implant and tightening of sutures around implant to buckle the sclera.[20, 57]

8. vitrectomy, subtotal — partial removal of the vitreous for vitreous opacity in severe retinopathy with vitreous hemorrhage or for the control of fibrotic overgrowth in severe intraocular trauma. Vitreous surgery is rare and preferably performed with the operating microscope and slit illumination.[58]

E. Symptomatic Terms:[59,69]

1. amaurosis fugax — fleeting blindness manifested by transient monocular blindness. It may result from transient embolization of retinal arterioles and suggest pending stroke.

2. amblyopia — dimness of vision in one eye that is normal on ophthalmoscopic examination.

3. amblyopia ex anopsia — diminished visual acuity in one eye not due to organic eye disease. It is known as the "lazy eye".

4. ametropia — optic defect or refractive error which does not permit parallel light rays to fall exactly on the retina.

5. anisometropia — inequality in refractive power of right and left eye.

6. Argyll-Robertson pupil — absence of light reflex without change in the contractile power of the pupil, a reliable sign of syphilis of the central nervous system.

7. astigmatism — images are warped and distorted due to irregular corneal curvature which prevents clear focusing of light.

8. binocular blindness — blind in both eyes.

9. binocular vision — ability to focus both eyes on one object and fuse the two images produced into one.

10. color blindness — reduced ability to distinguish between colors.

11. cystoid maculopathy, cystoid macular edema — a vascular abnormality which may develop after cataract extraction and reduces the vision at variable degrees (20/40 to 20/200). Fluorescein angiography reveals typical star-shaped staining of the macular area.[32, 42, 69]

12. diplopia — double vision.

13. Elschnig pearls — clusters of transparent vacuoles, remnants of lenticular epithelium, seen in the eye after incomplete cataract removal.[42]

14. emmetropia — normal vision, no refractive error.

15. enophthalmos — recession of the eyeball into the orbit.

16. exophthalmos, exophthalmus — protrusion of the eyeball in hyperthyroidism and orbital space-taking lesions.[25]

17. hypermetropia, hyperopia — farsightedness, parallel rays of light from a distant object are focused behind the retina; a refractive error.[7]

18. hyphemia — blood in the anterior chamber in front of the iris.

19. leukokoria, white pupil — white pupillary reflex referred to as amaurotic cat's eye, suggesting the presence of a sight destroying condition such as a retinoblastoma, curable in its early phase.[59]

20. malignant exophthalmos, progressive proptosis — increasing forward displacement of the eyeball in Graves' disease causing severe ocular symptoms such as fullness of eyelids, lacrimation, epiphora, corneal ulcerations, chemosis and edema of conjunctiva.[25]

21. monocular blindness — blind in one eye.

22. myopia — nearsightedness; parallel rays from a distant object are focused in front of the retina; a refractive error.

23. nyctalopia — night blindness.

24. nystagmus — constant involuntary movement of the eyeballs. It may be due to a disease of the central nervous system.[56]

25. photophobia — marked intolerance to light.

26. presbyopia — gradual loss of accommodation, a common condition in persons past middle age.

27. scotoma — a blind spot in the vision.

28. vitreous floaters — dark opacities within the vitreous which are perceived as moving spots by the retina.[42, 58]

29. vitreous loss — leakage of vitreous into the anterior chamber which disrupts the normal contact of the vitreous with the retina, exerts traction on the retina and predisposes to the formation of retinal holes and tears.[42, 58]

ACCESSORY ORGANS OF VISION

A. **Origin of Terms:**

1. blepharo- (G) — eyelid
2. canaliculus (L) — small canal
3. cantho- (G) — angle
4. cilia (L) — eyelashes
5. dacryo- (G) — tear
6. dacryoaden (G) — tear gland

7. dacryocyst (G) — tear sac
8. fissure, fissura (L) — cleft, slit
9. fornix (L) — arch
10. junctus (L) — joined

11. lacrima (L) — tear
12. oblique (L) — slanting
13. palpebra (L) — eyelid
14. rectus (L) — straight

B. Anatomic Terms:[73]

1. canthus (pl. canthi) — the lateral or medial angles at both ends of the palpebral fissures (slits between the eyelids).
2. cilia, eyelashes — rows of hairs at the free margin of the eyelids.
3. conjunctiva (pl. conjunctivae) — mucous membrane that lines the deep surface of the eyelid and is reflected over the front of the eyeball. It is divided into a
    a. bulbar conjunctiva — colorless, transparent portion covering the anterior part of the globe.
    b. palpebral conjunctiva — lining the posterior or deep surface of the lids.
4. fornix (pl. fornices) conjunctivae — angle between palpebral and bulbar conjunctivae.
5. lacrimal apparatus:
    a. lacrimal gland — tear gland; its orbital part lies in the lacrimal fossa of the upper, outer part of the orbit, its palpebral part in the upper eyelid.
    b. lacrimal ducts — tear ducts extending from gland to superior conjunctival fornix.
    c. lacrimal canaliculi — one canaliculus (canal) for each eyelid to conduct tears from lacrimal punctum to lacrimal sac.
    d. lacrimal puncta (sing. punctum) — minute openings, the beginning of the canaliculi.
    e. lacrimal sac — tear sac situated in lacrimal groove or medial wall of orbit.
    f. nasolacrimal duct — duct draining lacrimal sac and opening into inferior nasal meatus.
6. ocular muscles — muscles controlling the movements of the eyeball.
    a. two oblique muscles (two obliqui).
    b. four rectus muscles (four recti).
7. palpebral fissure — opening between the eyelids.
8. tarsal glands — secretory follicles in the tarsal plate.
9. tarsal plate — supporting connective tissue of the eyelid.

C. Diagnostic Terms:

1. disorders of the eyelid.[67]
    a. blepharitis — inflammation of the eyelid.
    b. blepharoptosis — drooping of the upper eyelid, congenital or acquired.[12]
    c. chalazion (pl. chalazia) — a true granuloma of the eye appearing as a painless swelling at the tarsus.
    d. ectropion — outward turning of the margin of the eyelid.
    e. entropion — inward turning of the margin of the eyelid.
    f. hordeolum (pl. hordeola)
        (1) external hordeolum — pyogenic infection of a sebaceous gland at the margin of the lid.
        (2) internal hordeolum — purulent infection of a sebaceous gland embedded in the conjunctiva of the eyelid.
    g. tumors of the lid — congenital or acquired: dermoids, fibromas, hemangiomas and carcinomas.[6, 11, 14]
2. disorders of the conjunctiva:[67]
    a. conjunctivitis — inflammation of the conjunctiva associated with pain, edema, hyperemia, exudation and infiltration. There are many forms of conjunctivitis.
    b. keratoconjunctivitis sicca (KCS), dry eye syndrome — ocular dryness due to deficiency of one or more components of the tear film: mucin, aqueous or liquid. This results in the appearance of dry spots on the conjunctival and corneal epithelium.[49, 67]

    c. ophthalmia neonatorum, gonococcal conjunctivitis of the newborn — the conjunctival sac of the infant is filled with pus containing gonococci.

    d. pterygium — a membrane of conjunctival tissue which extends like a wing from the limbus toward the center of the cornea.

    e. trachoma — chronic inflammation of the conjunctivae followed by granulation, capillary infiltration of the cornea (pannus) and blindness.

3. disorders of the lacrimal apparatus:[49, 67]

    a. acute dacryoadenitis — unilateral or bilateral inflammation of the lacrimal gland. It is frequently seen in children as a complication of measles and parotitis (mumps).

    b. chronic dacryoadenitis — a chronic, painless swelling of the lacrimal glands showing no signs of acute inflammation.

    c. dacryocystitis — an acute or chronic inflammation of the lacrimal sac, usually due to nasolacrimal stenosis.

    d. lacrimal abscess — localized accumulation of pus in lacrimal gland.

4. disorders of ocular motility:

    a. ophthalmoplegia externa, external ophthalmoplegia — paralysis of extraocular muscles causing restriction or loss of eye movements.

    b. ophthalmoplegia interna, internal ophthalmoplegia — paralysis of the fibers of the third nerve causing paralysis of the iris sphincter and ciliary muscle.[56]

    c. strabismus, squint — condition in which the optic axes fail to be directed toward the same object.[68]

      (1) convergent squint or esotropia — the eyes are directed toward the medial line.

      (2) divergent squint or exotropia — the eyes are turned laterally (outwards).[68]

D. Operative Terms:

1. blepharectomy — excision of an eyelid.
2. blepharoplasty — plastic repair of an eyelid.[15]
3. blepharorrhaphy — suture of a lacerated or injured eyelid.
4. dacryoadenectomy — removal of a lacrimal gland.[49]
5. dacryocystectomy — removal of the lacrimal sac.
6. dacryocystorhinostomy — surgical creation of an opening into the nose for the tears.
7. repair of strabismus — surgical correction by advancement, recession, resection, tucking or tenotomy of any one or more of the ocular muscles.[68]
8. tarsorrhaphy — surgical closure of an eyelid.

E. Symptomatic Terms:

1. blepharedema — puffy, swollen, edematous eyelids.
2. chemosis — conjunctival swelling near the cornea.
3. epiphora — overflow of tears, often due to lacrimal duct obstruction.
4. hyperemia — congestion.
5. lacrimation — secretion of tears.
6. limbal damage — injury at the corneoscleral junction which may be due to the destruction of perilimbal blood supply interfering with the nutrition of the cornea.[34]
7. pannus — newly formed capillaries covering the cornea like a film.
8. symblepharon — adhesion between the palpebral and bulbar conjunctiva.
9. xerophthalmia — excessive dryness of the eye resulting from the destruction of mucin-producing goblet cells, lacrimal ducts and glands or other causes.[34]

RADIOLOGY

A. Terms Related to Diagnostic Radiology:

1. angiography of ophthalmic artery — radiographic visualization of the ophthalmic artery for the detection of primary and metastatic tumors of the orbit, extraorbital neoplasms, vascular malformations and occlusions and aneurysms of the ophthalmic artery.[24]

2. distention dacryocystography — forceful injection of contrast medium into canaliculus during x-ray exposure to outline the nasolacrimal duct system in distended state. Direct x-ray magnification aids in the detection of the obstructive lesion.[44]

3. orbital arteriography — serial angiograms of the orbital arteries primarily via the ophthalmic branch of the internal carotid artery and secondarily via branches of the external carotid artery. The technique is used to detect arterial malformation or arteriovenous fistula of orbital vessels.[71]

4. orbital tomography — tomographic sections of the orbit delineating its extent, size and relation to adjoining structures.[22]

5. orbital venography — procedure of choice in the diagnosis of space-occupying lesions. The frontal vein approach is preferred.[9, 22]

6. orbitography — useful diagnostic procedure for localization of retrobulbar tumors before visual damage has become irreparable.[12, 21, 23, 46]

    a. negative contrast orbitography, orbital pneumotomography — radiographic visualization of the orbit using air or oxygen as contrast medium. It is indicated primarily when tumors of the optic nerve are suspected.

    b. positive contrast orbitography — radiographic visualization of the orbit using water soluble preparations as contrast media. Retrobulbar lesions may be found in the muscle cone of the superior rectus.

B. Terms Related to Special Radiologic Procedures:

1. computed tomography in ophthalmology — use of an automatic electronic machine which provides scans of tissue planes at a given thickness. In ophthalmology scans are made of the orbit including the lateral and third ventricles to detect orbital disease or tumors as well as intracranial lesions: optic glioma, metastasis or brain injury.[4, 17, 33, 35, 41]

2. echo-ophthalmography, orbital echography, orbital ultrasonography, contact B-scan ultrasonography — important diagnostic aid in differentiating between intraocular and orbital diseases or tumors. Ultrasound can reliably demonstrate defects in orbital fat echoes produced by the invasion of an orbital neoplasm into the orbital fat.[25, 50, 69]

3. xeroradiography in orbital surgery — an electrostatic imaging device using selenium covered aluminum plates for x-ray exposure. It provides stereo effect, graphic visualization of facial bones and soft tissues and shows relationships of grafts, wires and bones.[37]

C. Terms Related to Therapeutic Radiology:[75]

1. irradiation in bilateral retinoblastoma — enucleation of the more affected eye; radiotherapy to the less affected eye to preserve some degree of vision.

2. irradiation in unilateral retinoblastoma — enucleation of eye and part of optic nerve; postoperative radiotherapy determined by histologic study.

3. irradiation in early epidermoid carcinoma of the conjunctiva — radium therapy may be able to eradicate the lesion.

CLINICAL LABORATORY

A. Terms Related to Bacteriologic Studies[69]

1. epithelial inclusion bodies — bodies found in conjunctival disease, such as inclusion blennorrhea of the newborn, some adult forms of diffuse, follicular conjunctivitis and in trachoma. Epithelial scrapings stained with Giemsa's or Wright's stain reveal the inclusion bodies.

2. epithelial scrapings from the cornea or conjunctiva — procedure used for identifying the etiologic organism of bacterial conjunctivitis or keratitis. A thin layer of epithelial cells is removed with a spatula or scalpel. The scrapings are transferred to two or more slides and stained; one by Gram's method, the other with Giemsa's or Wright's

stain. These methods permit the identification of the predominant organism as well as eosinophils and epithelial inclusion bodies. Since pathogenic organisms are freely present in epithelial cells before they appear in secretions, the study of scrapings offers a valuable aid to early diagnosis.

3. etiologic organisms in conjunctival disease, commonly seen
   a. *Diplococcus pneumoniae*
   b. *Neisseria gonorrhoeae*
   c. Staphylococcus
   d. Streptococcus
   e. Chlamydia (formerly virus of trachoma)

B. Terms Related Primarily to Functional Testing:[69]

1. accommodation — ability to see at various distances due to the contraction and relaxation of the ciliary muscle. The focusing power is measurable.
2. contact lenses — small corneal lenses which fit directly on the eyeball under the eyelids, medically used to correct vision in keratoconus (cone-shaped cornea) and other eye conditions.
3. corneal sensitivity — the examiner touches the corneas with a cotton fiber to determine whether each cornea is normally sensitive.
4. dark adaptation — ability of retina to adjust to low levels of illumination.
5. diopter — unit of measurement of refractive power or strength of lenses.
6. electroretinography — the recording of retinal action currents. Procedure aids in the detection of degenerative disorders of the retina.[21]
7. electrotonography — aqueous outflow study based on change in intraocular pressure following the application of an electronic tonometer to the eye for four minute period. Low pressure reading obtained from an electronic scale and recorded by an automatic writer suggest the presence of glaucoma.[69]
8. fluorescein angiography — intravenous injection of fluorescein followed by ophthalmoscopy or fundoscopy and rapid serial photography. Fluorescence of the vasculature aids in the detection of normal and abnormal states of the retinal and choroidal vessels including microaneurysms, neovascularization, atriovenous shunts, vascular leakage, retinal hemorrhage and subtle vascular conditions of the macula.[32, 69]
9. gonioscopy — examination of the iris angle of the eye using an optical instrument. Obstruction of the filtration angle may occur in glaucoma.[43, 69]
10. keratometry — measurement of the curves of the cornea with a keratometer.
11. major amblyoscopy — test for evaluating the sensory status of the eyes. Procedure is also used in orthoptic study before and after strabismus surgery.[69]
12. ocular stereophotography — three dimensional photographing to detect fundus lesions of the eye by means of the indirect ophthalmoscopic principle. Photographing is done at a known magnification, exposure and depth effect to determine progression or retrogression of lesions over a period of time.[69]
13. ophthalmodynamometry — measurement of the pressure in the central retinal arteries for indirectly evaluating the blood flow in the carotid arteries.[69]
14. ophthalmoscopy — examination of the eye grounds (fundi) with an ophthalmoscope.
15. orthoptic training — a program of scientifically planned exercises for promoting or restoring the normal coordination of the eyes.[69]
16. perimetry — instrumental measurement of field of vision.
17. probing of lacrimal drainage system — establishing drainage of obstructed system after unsuccessful irrigation. A metal probe is passed through the upper or lower punctum and canaliculus, into the lacrimal (tear) sac, nasolacrimal duct and nose.[69]
18. retinoscopy — light beam test for detecting refractive errors.
19. scotometry — examining the central visual field for areas of decreased sensitivity and mapping out blind spots (scotomas) on a special chart.[69]
20. slit lamp biomicroscopy — use of a combination of slit lamp and biomicroscope for intense illumination and high magnification of the eyeball or lids. Layers of cornea and lens are

clearly visualized and pathologic processes such as opacities are detected with accuracy.[69]

21. tonometry — determination of intraocular pressure by a tonometer; e.g. that of Schiotz.

22. visual acuity — determination of the minimum cognizable under standard conditions of illumination using the Snellen chart or one of its modifications.[20, 56]

ABBREVIATIONS

A. General:

A, Acc — accommodation

anisometr. — anisometropia

$AgNO_3$ — silver nitrate

Astigm. — astigmatism

CF — counting finger

C gl — with correction (with glasses)

C, Cyl — cylindric lens

cx — cylinder axis

D — diopter (lens strength)

Em — emmetropia

EOM — extraocular muscles

EPF — exophthalmos producing factor

EPS — exophthalmos producing substance

ET — esotropia

HM — hand motion

IOP — intraocular pressure

KW — Keith Wagner (ophthalmoscopic findings)

LP, PL — light perception

L proj. — light projection

LR — light reaction

Mix. Astig. — mixed astigmatism

Myop. — myopia

NPC — near point of convergence

OD, RE — right eye (oculus dexter)

ODM — ophthalmodynamometry

Ophth, Oph. — ophthalmology

OS, LE — left eye (oculus sinister)

OU — each eye (oculus uterque)

PD — interpupillary distance

Pr — presbyopia

PRRE — pupils round, regular and equal

s gl — without correction (without glasses)

S, Sph — spherical lens

Tn, T — intraocular tension

VA — visual acuity

VE — visual efficiency

XT — exotropia

B. Organizations:

NINDB — National Institute of Neurological Diseases and Blindness

NSPB — National Society for the Prevention of Blindness

ORAL READING PRACTICE

Glaucoma

Glaucoma is a disease of the eye characterized by an elevated intraocular pressure. Normally, the internal pressure of the eye is about 18-22mm Hg, a pressure higher than that of the other organs. The maintenance of a normal intraocular pressure depends primarily on the amount of **aqueous humor** present in the eye. The formation of aqueous humor and its elimination is a continuous process. If the production and absorption are in perfect balance, all is well, but if there is a disturbance of balance, the eye is seriously affected.

The **ciliary** processes form the aqueous humor which passes through the pupil space to the anterior chamber. It leaves through the **canal of Schlemm** and is picked up by the aqueous veins which contain a mixture of blood and aqueous. In most cases of glaucoma the elevated intraocular pressure results from interference with the elimination of aqueous humor, although increased rate of production may be the source of the imbalance.

Ophthalmologists distinguish two main types: primary and secondary glaucoma. Secondary glaucoma is related to various eye conditions which bring about marked fluctuations and elevations in the intraocular pressure; for example, **iritis** and **iridocyclitis, intraocular neoplasms,** dislocation of the lens, central **vein occlusion** and trauma.

The clinical picture is variable depending on the degree of elevation and gradual or abrupt onset. The patient with acute glaucoma may experience a sudden increase in pain which tends to be extreme and associated with nausea and vomiting. The cornea may look steamy and the conjunctiva **edematous.**

In chronic simple glaucoma no pain is present and visual loss proceeds insidiously. Treatment consists of the judicious use of drugs, e.g. miotics which sometimes constrict the pupil so effectively that the aqueous humor can escape. If no alleviation can be achieved, operative intervention becomes imperative. Various forms of surgical aqueous drainage are indicated depending on the kind of glaucoma and the presence or absence of **anterior synechias.** Traditionally, **peripheral iridectomy, iridencleisis, sclerectomy, cyclodialysis** or **goniotomy** were and, in selected cases, are still procedures of choice.[3, 43, 66] Currently **cyclocryosurgery** takes precedence over **cyclodiathermy** and **trabeculectomies** using **microsurgical** instrumentation are gaining wide acceptance.[3, 43, 52, 66] **Laser iridotomy** for **aphakic pupillary block** is another method to promote aqueous drainage and restore normal ocular tension.[44]

In secondary glaucoma resulting from obstruction of the **central retinal vein, enucleation** of the eye may be necessary.[43]

Table 28

SOME EYE CONDITIONS AMENABLE TO SURGERY

Organs Involved	Diagnoses	Operations	Operative Procedures
Eyeball	Penetrating wound of eyeball	Enucleation of eyeball	Removal of eyeball
Eyeball	Graves disease with malignant exophthalmos and corneal ulceration	Orbital decompression of the proptosed globe Krönlein orbitotomy[a]	Lateral opening of the orbit Krönlein approach allowing the orbital contents to overflow into the temporal fossa[a]
Retina Uvea Iris Conjunctiva	Retinoblastoma Malignant melanoma Epidermoid carcinoma	Enucleation of eyeball	Removal of the eyeball and as much as possible of the optic nerve in retinoblastoma[a]
Retina Choroid Sclera	Detachment of retina	Scleral buckling operation	Diathermy to sclera and choroid; release of subretinal fluid Inward buckling of treated area and insertion of silicone implant; firm contact of choroid with retina reestablished
Retina Choroid Sclera	Detachment of retina	Cryopexy	Application of freezing probe to sclera to promote formation of chorioretinal scar and thus fusion
Cornea	Corneal scar Keratoconus	Keratoplasty lamellar transplant or penetrating transplant	Replacement of opaque cornea with transparent cornea using part thickness or full thickness corneal graft

Organs Involved	Diagnoses	Operations	Operative Procedures

Vitreous
Cornea
	Small foreign
	  body in
	  vitreous
		Haab giant magnet
		  technique
		Keratotomy
			Foreign body dislodged by magnet
			  and removed through corneal
			  incision

Cornea
Iris
Vitreous
	Glaucoma
	  acute,
	  primary
		Keratocentesis
		Peripheral iridectomy
		
		Cyclodialysis
			Paracentesis of cornea
			Surgical removal of part of iris
			
			Surgical communication between
			  the anterior chamber and
			  suprachoroidal space

Cornea
Sclera
Trabeculum
	Glaucoma
	  open angle or
	  narrow angle
		Trabeculectomy[b]	Positioning the operating
			  microscope appropriately
			Raising a conjunctival
			  flap to expose the sclera
			Removing part of the sclera
			  together with the
			  trabecular meshwork

Crystalline
  lens
Iris
	Cataract
	  congenital
	  senescent
	  (senile)
		Discission
		Peripheral iridectomy
		
		Intracapsular extraction
		  of cataract
			Needling of lens
			Approach to cataract by removal
			  of part of iris
			Excision of cataract within its
			  capsule

Crystalline
  lens
	Cataract
	  infantile
	  juvenile
	  young adult
		Aspiration-irrigation
		  method of cataract
		  removal[c]
			Use of the operating microscope
			Two limbal incisions, one for
			  the insertion of a needle
			  knife into the lens to
			  aspirate the cataract, the
			  other for the insertion of a
			  hollow bore needle to irrigate
			  the anterior chamber with
			  saline

Crystalline
  lens
 	
Iris
	Cataract
	  congenital
	  infantile
	  senescent
		Microsurgical
		  phacoemulsifica-
		  tion
		  Kelman technique[c]
		
		Peripheral
		  iridectomy
			Operating microscope in position
			Tiny limbal incision followed
			  by:
			Excision of small capsular
			  portion to prolapse the lens
			  into the anterior chamber
			Insertion of phacoemulsifier
			  into lens using ultrasound
			  for its emulsification
			Aspiration of lens fragments
			  and irrigation of eye
			
			Removal of small radial
			  section between minor
			  circle and periphery to
			  prevent glaucoma after
			  cataract surgery

Crystalline
  lens
	Cataract	Intracapsular
		  cryoextraction
		  of cataract
			Tip of cryoextractor applied to
			  anterior surface of lens
			Freezing of lens substance
			Frozen lens lifted out
			  on cryoextractor

Iris	Cyst of iris	Electrolysis	Insertion of an electrolysis needle
			  in the center of cyst to induce
			  shrinkage

Organs Involved	Diagnoses	Operations	Operative Procedures
Ocular muscle	Strabismus	Recession of ocular muscle	Correction of defect by drawing muscle backward

Canthus Eyelid Lacrimal sac	Basal cell carcinoma medial canthal region-eyelid	Surgical ablation of entire malignant lesion
		
		Reconstruction of canthal region and lid[d]
			Excision of tumor
			  lacrimal sac
			  canaliculi
			  medial half of lid
			Surgical creation of a midline forehead flap covering the lid

Eyelid	Laceration of eyelid Hordeolum Blepharoptosis	Blepharorrhaphy Blepharotomy Repair of eyelid	Suture of eyelid Incision with drainage of meibomian gland Surgical correction of ptosis
Lacrimal sac	Abscess of lacrimal sac	Dacryocystotomy	Incision and drainage of tear duct
Lacrimal gland	Retention cyst of lacrimal gland	Dacryoadenectomy	Removal of tear gland
Lacrimonasal duct	Stenosis of lacrimonasal duct	Dacryocystorhinostomy	Fistulization of lacrimal sac into nasal cavity

[a] Stephen F. Bowen, M.D. Personal communications.

[b] A. L. Schwartz, et al. Trabecular surgery. *Archives of Ophthalmology*, 92: 134-138, August, 1974.

[c] D. Paton et al. Cataracts: Development, diagnoses and management. *Clinical Symposia*, 26: 2-32, No. 3, 1974.

[d] J. Bostwick et al. Basal cell carcinoma of the medial canthal area. *Plastic and Reconstructive Surgery*, 55: 667-675, June, 1975.

REFERENCES AND BIBLIOGRAPHY

1. Adams, S. T. Retinal detachment. *Archives of Ophthalmology*, 94: 569-570, April, 1976.

2. Apple, D. J. et al. Argon laser treatment of von Hippel-Lindau retinal angiomas. II. Histopathology of treated lesions. *Archives of Ophthalmology*, 92: 126-130, August, 1974.

3. Armaly, M. F. Glaucoma. *Archives of Ophthalmology*, 93: 146-162, February, 1975.

4. Baker, H. L. et al. Computerized transaxial tomography in neuro-ophthalmology. *American Journal of Ophthalmology*, 78: 285-294, August, 1974.

5. Benson, W. E. et al. Aphakic retinal detachment. *Archives of Ophthalmology*, 93: 245-249, April, 1975.

6. Bostwick, J. et al. Basal cell carcinoma of the medial canthal area. *Plastic and Reconstructive Surgery*, 55: 667-675, June, 1975.

7. Bowen, Stephen F., M.D. Personal communications.

8. Diamond, J. G. Open-angle glaucoma. *Archives of Ophthalmology*, 94: 41-47, January, 1976.

9. De Jong, Russell N. and Sugar, Oscar. Neurophthalmology. *Neurology and Neurosurgery*. Chicago: Year Book Medical Publishers, 1976, pp. 57-66.

10. Egerer, Ido et al. Coats disease. *Archives of Ophthalmology*, 92: 109-112, August, 1974.

11. Ellsworth, R. M. Tumors of the eye. In Holland, James F. and Frei, Emil. *Cancer Medicine*. Philadelphia: Lea & Febiger, 1973, pp. 1425-1436.

12. Erkonen, W. and Dolan, K. D. Ocular foreign body localization. *Radiologic Clinics of North America*, 10: 101-114, April, 1972.

13. Feeney, L. et al. Human subretinal fluid. *Archives of Ophthalmology*, 93: 62-69, January, 1975.

14. Ferry, A. P. et al. Carcinoma metastatic to the eye and orbit. *Archives of Ophthalmology*, 93: 472-482, July, 1975.

15. Fox, S. A. Upper lid reconstruction. *Archives of Ophthalmology*, 88: 46-48, July, 1972.

16. Galinos, S. O. et al. Choroidovitreal neovascularization after argon laser photocoagulation. *Archives of Ophthalmology*, 93: 524-530, July, 1975.

17. Ganler, J. S. et al. Computer assisted tomography in orbital disease. *British Journal of Ophthalmology*, 58: 571-587, June, 1974.

18. Goldberg, M. F. et al. Argon laser treatment of von Hippel-Lindau retinal angiomas. *Archives of Ophthalmology*, 92: 121-125, August, 1974.

19. Grayston, E. T. Viral diseases of the eye. In Wintrobe, Maxwell M. (ed.). *Harrison's Princi-*

280

ples of Internal Medicine, 7th ed. New York: McGraw-Hill Book Co., 1974, pp. 979-981.

20. Grupposo, S. S. Visual acuity following surgery for retinal detachment. *Archives of Ophthalmology*, 93: 327-330, May, 1975.

21. Gunkel, D. R. *et al.* A Ganzfeld stimulator for electroretinography. *Archives of Ophthalmology*, 94: 669-670, April, 1976.

22. Hanafee, W. N. Clinical diagnosis of orbital tumors. *Radiologic Clinics of North America*, 10: 3-83, April, 1972.

23. Harwood, N. D. C. Optic gliomas and pediatric neuroradiology, *Radiologic Clinics of North America*, 10: 83-100, April, 1972.

24. Hayreh, S. S. The ophthalmic artery. In Newton, Thomas H. and Potts, D. Gordon. *Radiology of the Skull and Brain Angiography*, Vol. II, Book 2. St. Louis: The C. V. Mosby Co., 1974, pp. 1333-1390.

25. Hodes, B. L. Eye signs of Graves' disease. *Postgraduate Medicine*, 57: 135-140, April, 1975.

26. Huamonte, F. *et al.* Expandable silicone implants for scleral buckling. *Archives of Ophthalmology*, 93: 354-356, May, 1975.

27. Iliff, W. J. *et al.* Invasive squamous cell carcinoma of the conjunctiva. *Archives of Ophthalmology*, 93: 119-122, February, 1975.

28. Jawetz, E. Trachoma and inclusion conjunctivitis. In Beeson, Paul B. and McDermott, Walsh (eds.). *Textbook of Medicine*, 14th ed. Philadelphia: W. B. Saunders Co., 1975, pp. 264-267.

29. Kaufman, H. E. Progress in corneal transplantation. *Southern Medical Journal*, 68: 671-673, June, 1975.

30. Kelman, C. D. Symposium: Phacoemulsification. History of emulsification and aspiration of senile cataracts. *Transactions of American Academy of Ophthalmology and Otolaryngology*, 78: OP-7-9, January-February, 1974.

31. Kirsch, R. E. The lens. *Archives of Ophthalmology*, 93: 284-314, April, 1975.

32. Kottow, M. *et al.* Iris angiography in cystoid macular edema after cataract extraction. *Archives of Ophthalmology*, 93: 487-493, July, 1975.

33. Lampert, V. L. *et al.* Computed tomography of the orbits. *Radiology*, 113: 351-354, November, 1974.

34. Lemp, M. A. Cornea and sclera. *Archives of Ophthalmology*, 92: 158-170, August, 1974 and 94: 473-490, March, 1976.

35. Lessel, S. Neuro-ophthalmology. *Archives of Ophthalmology*, 93: 434-464, June, 1975.

36. Levene, R. A new concept of malignant glaucoma. *Archives of Ophthalmology*, 87: 497-506, May, 1972.

37. Maillard, G. F. *et al.* Xeroradiography examinations in orbitonasal surgery. *Plastic and Reconstructive Surgery*, 55: 664-666, June, 1975.

38. Manschot, W. A. Pathology of hereditary juvenile retinoschisis. *Archives of Ophthalmology*, 88: 131-138, August, 1972.

39. Mattis, Robert D., M.D. Personal communications.

40. Mc Coy, D. A. Removal of nonmagnetic and magnetic intraocular foreign bodies with constant visualization. *Southern Medical Journal*, 68: 591-594, May, 1975.

41. Momose, K. J. *et al.* The use of computed tomography in ophthalmology. *Radiology*, 115: 361-368, May, 1975.

42. Paton, D. *et al.* Cataracts development, diagnosis and management. *Clinical Symposia*, 26: 2-32, August, 1974.

43. Paton, D. *et al.* Glaucomas. *Clinical Symposia*, 28: 3-47, June, 1976.

44. Patti, J. C. *et al.* Iris photocoagulation therapy of aphakic pupillary block. *Archives of Ophthalmology*, 93: 347-348, May, 1975.

45. Peyman, G. A. *et al.* Optical radiation and Zeiss short-pulsed xenon photocoagulators. *Archives of Ophthalmology*, 92: 341-347, October, 1974.

46. Saari, Matti *et al.* Acquired toxoplasmic chorioretinitis. *Archives of Ophthalmology*, 94: 1485-1488, September, 1976.

47. Sand, B. J. *et al.* Ophthalmic arterial blood pressures measured by ocular plethysmodynamography. *Archives of Surgery*, 110: 813-818, July, 1975.

48. Scheie, Harold G. and Albert, Daniel M. *Adler's Textbook of Ophthalmology*, 9th ed. Philadelphia: W. B. Saunders Co., 1977.

49. Scherz, W. *et al.* Is the lacrimal gland dispensible? Keratoconjunctivitis sicca after lacrimal gland removal. *Archives of Ophthalmology*, 93: 281-283, April, 1975.

50. Schutz, J. S. Ophthalmic contact B-scan ultrasonography. *Archives of Ophthalmology*, 92: 291-296, October, 1974.

51. Schwartz, A. L. Malignant glaucoma in an eye with no antecedent operation or miotics. *Archives of Ophthalmology*, 93: 379-381, May, 1975.

52. Schwartz, A. L. *et al.* Trabecular surgery. *Archives of Ophthalmology*, 92: 134-138, August, 1974.

53. Sigler, B. and Pilgrim, M. Phacoemulsification of cataracts. *American Journal of Nursing*, 75: 976-977, June, 1975.

54. Small, M. L. *et al.* Senile macular degeneration. *Archives of Ophthalmology*, 94: 601-611, April, 1976.

55. Soll, D. B. Enucleation surgery. *Archives of Ophthalmology*, 87: 196-197, February, 1972.

56. *Symposium of Neuro-Ophthalmology-Transactions of the New Orleans Academy of Ophthalmology*. St. Louis: The C. V. Mosby Co., 1976.

57. Tasman, W. The retina and optic nerve. *Archives of Ophthalmology*, 94: 1201-1224, July, 1976.

58. Tolentino, F. I. The vitreous. *Archives of Ophthalmology*, 92: 350-358, October, 1974.

59. Vaughan, Victor C. and Mc Kay, R. James. Pediatric ophthalmology. *Nelson Textbook of Pediatrics*, 10th ed. Philadelphia: W. B. Saunders Co., 1975, pp. 1569-1599.

60. Vaughan, Daniel and Asbury, Taylor. Cornea and sclera. *General Ophthalmology*, 7th ed. Los Altos, California: Lange Medical Publications, 1974, pp. 70-90.

61. _____. Uveal tract — specific types of uveitis. *Ibid.*, pp. 87-96.

62. _____. Vitreous detachment — vitreous hemorrhage, others. *Ibid.*, pp. 125-133.

63. _____. Ocular disorders associated with systemic disorders. *Ibid.*, pp. 227-251.

64. _____. Diseases of the retina — The macula. *Ibid.*, pp. 97-115.

65. _____. Lens — Cataract surgery. *Ibid.*, pp. 116-124.

66. _____. Glaucoma — Surgical procedures used in the treatment of glaucoma. *Ibid.*, pp. 192-209.

67. _____. Lids and lacrimal apparatus — Conjunctiva. *Ibid.*, pp. 40-69.

68. _____. Strabismus — Surgical treatment. *Ibid.*, pp. 171-191.

69. _____. Examination — Bacteriologic and microscopic examination — Appendix. *Ibid.*, pp. 13-32 and 316-318.

70. Vaughan D. Eye. In Krupp, Marcus A. and Chatton, Milton, *Current Medical Diagnosis and Treatment.* Los Altos, California: Lange Medical Publications, 1976, pp. 75-87.

71. Vignaud, J. *et al.* Orbital arteriography. *Radiologic Clinics of North America*, 10: 39-61, April, 1972.

72. Viswanathan, B. *et al.* Peripheral iridectomy with scleral cautery for glaucoma. *Archives of Ophthalmology*, 93: 34-35, January, 1975.

73. Warwick, R. Anatomy. In Sorsby, Arnold (ed.). *Modern Ophthalmology — Basic Concepts*, 2d ed., Vol. I. Philadelphia: J. B. Lippincott Co., 1972, pp. 37-201.

74. Watzke, R. C. Cryotherapy for retinal angiomatosis. *Archives of Ophthalmology*, 92: 399-401, November, 1974.

75. Weir, Don C., M.D. Personal communications.

76. Wiedman, M. High altitude retinal hemorrhage. *Archives of Ophthalmology*, 93: 401-403, June, 1975.

77. Wilkinson, C. P. Treatment of macular diseases. *Southern Medical Journal*, 68: 914-918, July, 1975.

Chapter XIV

The Sense Organ of Hearing

EAR

A. Origin of Terms:

1. acoustic (G) — hearing
2. aditus (L) — approach, entrance
3. auditio (L) — hearing
4. auricle (L) — ear
5. cochlea (G) — snail
6. labyrinth (G) — maze

7. myringa (L) — eardrum
8. ossicle (L) — little bone
9. ot, oto (G) — ear
10. salpingo (G) — tube, trumpet
11. tympano (G) — eardrum
12. vestibule (L) — antechamber

B. Anatomic Terms:[13]

1. external ear — division of ear consisting of the auricle and the external auditory canal or meatus.
   a. auricle, pinna — the external ear, made up chiefly of elastic fibrocartilage which is shaped to catch the sound waves.
   b. cerumen — ear wax, formed by the ceruminous glands of the skin lining the meatus.
   c. external auditory meatus — ear passage, composed of a cartilaginous and a bony part.
   d. helix — outer folded margin of the auricle.
2. middle ear, tympanic cavity — division of ear containing the ossicles for the conduction of air-borne sound waves.
   a. auditory tube, eustachian tube, pharyngotympanic tube — channel of communication between pharynx and middle ear.
   b. orifices of the tympanic cavity:
      (1) aditus ad antrum — opening to the mastoid antrum.
      (2) fenestra cochleae, fenestra rotunda — round window facing the internal ear.
      (3) fenestra vestibuli, fenestra ovalis — oval window in which the stapes lodges.
      (4) orifice from the external auditory meatus into the middle ear. It is closed by the tympanic membrane or eardrum.
      (5) opening into auditory tube.
   c. ossicles of the tympanic cavity — three tiny bones: malleus (hammer), incus (anvil) and stapes (stirrup). They transmit vibrations to the internal ear.
3. inner ear[13] — division of ear composed of a number of fluid-filled spaces and the membranous labyrinth which lies within the bony (osseous) labyrinth. The perilymphatic space of the bony labyrinth contains the cochlea, vestibule and semicircular canals. Because of the complexity of the structures, only a few basic facts are given here.
   a. cochlea — spiral tube possessing a bony core, the modiolus which contains the spiral ganglion and transmits the cochlear nerve. It is the essential organ of hearing.
   b. vestibular apparatus — the utricle and semicircular ducts which are concerned with the maintenance of the equilibrium.
   c. vestibulocochlear nerve, eighth cranial nerve, formerly acoustic or auditory nerve — nerve comprising two distinct fiber sets.
      (1) cochlear branch — fibers distributed to the hair cells of the spiral organ. They are concerned with hearing.
      (2) vestibular branch — fibers distributed to portions of the utricle, saccule, and semicircular ducts. They aid in maintaining body balance.[13]

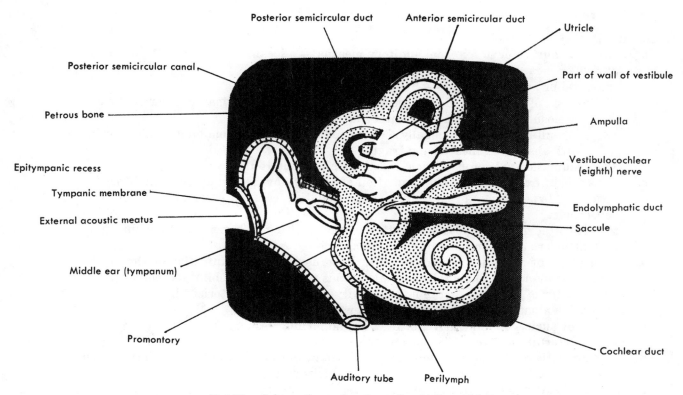

Posterior semicircular duct

Anterior semicircular duct

Utricle

Posterior semicircular canal

Part of wall of vestibule

Petrous bone

Ampulla

Epitympanic recess

Vestibulocochlear (eighth) nerve

Tympanic membrane

Endolymphatic duct

External acoustic meatus

Saccule

Middle ear (tympanum)

Promontory

Cochlear duct

Auditory tube

Perilymph

Fig. 71 — Schematic section through middle and internal ear.

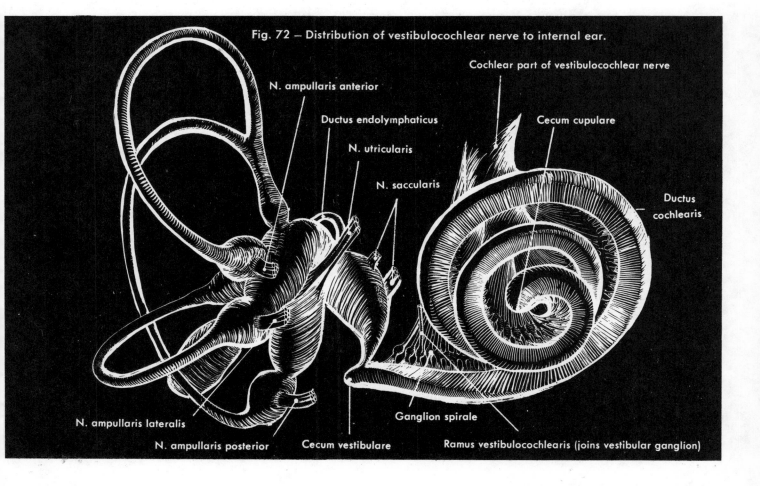

Fig. 72 — Distribution of vestibulocochlear nerve to internal ear.

N. ampullaris anterior

Cochlear part of vestibulocochlear nerve

Ductus endolymphaticus

Cecum cupulare

N. utricularis

Ductus cochlearis

N. saccularis

N. ampullaris lateralis

Ganglion spirale

N. ampullaris posterior

Cecum vestibulare

Ramus vestibulocochlearis (joins vestibular ganglion)

C. Diagnostic Terms:

1. conditions of the external ear:[11, 17]
    a. abscess of auricle or of external auditory meatus — a localized collection of pus of auricle or meatus.
    b. congenital or acquired defects —
        (1) atresia of external auditory meatus — absence of the normal opening of the ear or closure of the external auditory meatus.[28, 46]
        (2) congenital microtia — usually a deformed or misplaced, small aural tag associated with absence of meatus and tragus.[28]
        (3) traumatic avulsion of auricle — loss of pinna due to injury.
    c. dermatitis of external ear — inflammation of skin of auricle and external auditory meatus. Types encountered: dry, moist, exfoliative, contact, eczematous, allergic, seborrheic.
    d. frostbite of auricle — exposure to extreme cold resulting in hyperemia, blanching and, in severe cases, in ulceration and gangrene.
    e. furunculosis of the external auditory meatus — usually a mild infection of the sebaceous glands and hair follicles which tends to develop in debilitated persons.
    f. herpes zoster of auricle — acute inflammatory condition characterized by blister formation along the distribution of the sensory nerve.
    g. leprosy of auricle — infiltrative, ulcerative and nodular lesions of ear due to *Mycobacterium leprae.* The lobe of the auricle is the site of predilection.
    h. perichondritis of auricle — inflammation of the membrane of fibrous connective tissue around the cartilage marked by exudation, thickening and shriveling.
    i. tumors of external auditory canal
        (1) adenocarcinoma of cerumen gland — malignant tumor originating in ceruminous glands characterized by a tendency to invade soft tissues and bones and to recur after surgical removal.
        (2) aural polyp — benign tumor on a pedicle which may occlude the external auditory canal and thus interfere with sound conduction.
        (3) cerumen gland adenoma — benign tumor originating in ceruminous glands.
2. conditions of the tympanic membrane:[17]
    a. injury of tympanic membrane, for example, blow on the ear, violent sneezing with closed nostrils.
    b. myringitis, tympanitis — inflammation of the eardrum.
    c. perforation of tympanic membrane — hole in eardrum, if small will heal without treatment, if large may require tympanoplasty.
    d. rupture of tympanic membrane — condition usually due to trauma, for example, direct injury to ear.
    e. tumors — rare disorders which may be endotheliomatous, fibromatous, angiomatous or show other histologic patterns.
    f. tympanosclerosis — involvement of mucous membrane of middle ear or drum by sclerosis of exudate with fixation of the ossicles and drum, diffuse calcification and thickening of the mucosa lining the cavity.[3, 53]
3. conditions of the middle ear:
    a. aerotitis media, barotitis media, aural barotrauma — painful condition caused by atmospheric pressure changes in middle ear chiefly during ascent and descent of air travel or experienced on descent by navy divers.[14, 21]
    b. cholesteatoma — a globular pearly mass covered with a thin shell of epidermis and connective tissue. It usually forms following middle ear infection and is nature's way of arresting suppuration. Pseudocholesteatomas are common.[14, 43]
    c. congenital ossicular malformation — abnormality of ossicles which causes impaired hearing of the conductive type and may respond to surgical correction.[29, 43]
    d. dislocation of ossicles — condition usually due to head injury which damages the

eardrum, dislocates the ossicular chain thus causing a conductive type of hearing loss. Surgical repair is recommended.[58]

e. fracture of temporal bone — usually concurrent middle ear involvement signaled by the presence of blood and cerebrospinal fluid, vertigo, sensorineural or conductive hearing loss and paralysis of the facial nerve.[58]

f. glomus tumors, chemodectomas — common neoplasms of the head and neck:
   (1) glomus tympanicum — tumor originates in the middle ear and can usually be surgically removed.[6, 14, 49]
   (2) glomus jugulare — tumor containing chemoceptor cells arises from the jugular bulb in the middle ear. It may cause episodes of dizziness, nystagmus, blackouts and facial paralysis. Labyrinthine and cochlear invasion by the glomus leads to deafness. Complete surgical excision depends on the location and size of the tumor.[3, 6, 49, 50, 51]
   (3) glomus vagale — tumor arises along the course of the vagus nerve and is relatively uncommon.[14, 51]

g. mastoiditis — infection of the middle ear which has extended to the antrum and mastoid cells. Mastoiditis may be acute, subacute, chronic and recurrent.[11, 14]

h. middle ear effusion — acute or chronic presence of fluid in middle ear generally without infection.
   (1) secretory otitis media, mucoid otitis media, glucotitis — thick, cloudy, viscous exudate in middle ear containing cells and mucous strands.[14, 37]
   (2) serous otitis media — thin, clear amber fluid in middle ear.[11, 14]
   (3) serous otitis media with hemotympanum — serum and blood in middle ear space resulting from temporal bone fracture, tumor or blood disorder.

i. otitis media — inflammation of the middle ear. Common types encountered are:
   (1) acute suppurative otitis media — marked by intense congestion of mucosa of middle ear, blockage of eustachian tube, serous exudate which becomes infected and rupture of the eardrum. Bacterial invaders are *Staphylococcus aureus*, *Diplococcus pneumoniae*, *Streptococcus pyogenes*, *Hemophilus influenzae* and others.[11, 14]
   (2) chronic, suppurative otitis media — characterized by continuation of middle ear infection resulting in protracted suppuration.[11, 14, 37]

j. salpingitis of eustachian tube — inflammation of the auditory tube. It may be acute or chronic.

4. conditions of the inner ear:
   a. acoustic neuroma — benign tumor of the eighth cranial nerve affecting the vestibular branch more than the cochlear branch of the nerve and causing vertigo, tinnitus and hearing impairment.[12, 23]
   b. labyrinthitis — inflammation of the labyrinth, usually secondary to acute or chronic suppurative otitis media with or without cholesteatoma or to acute upper respiratory infection.[12, 16, 19]
   c. Menière's disease, endolymphatic hydrops — neurologic disorder in its classic form exhibiting a triad symptom complex:
      (1) explosive attacks of true vertigo
      (2) fluctuating hearing loss of the sensorineural type
      (3) tinnitus.
      Dizziness, ataxia and a feeling of fullness in the ear are usually present. Remissions may last years.[5, 12, 16, 19]
   d. objective tinnitus — hissing, ringing or roaring noise heard by the patient and perceived by the physician as an auscultative bruit. It is currently considered a nosologic entity or classified disease. Arteriovenous fistulae or abnormalities are common causes.[55]
      (1) arterial tinnitus — a pulsatile tinnitus or body sounds of vascular pulsations,

often associated with headache and papilledema in the presence of an intracranial lesion which may be visualized by cerebral angiography.

(2) venous tinnitus — a venous hum, formerly termed cephalic bruit or essential objective tinnitus. It is elicited by light pressure and position of the head related to the involved area.[55]

e. otosclerosis recently termed otospongiosis — newly formed spongy bone replacing the hard bone of the labyrinth. It may result in conduction deafness with fixation of the stapes and stapedial footplate followed later by nerve degeneration resulting in mixed deafness.[44]

f. vestibular neuronitis — sudden vestibular failure in one ear without hearing impairment or tinnitus, apparently due to viral infection or a demyelinating reaction to infection.[19]

5. hearing loss:

a. Two basic types are recognized.

(1) conductive hearing loss — impairment of hearing resulting from obstruction of sound waves which do not reach the inner ear. The interference may be due to impacted cerumen, exudate, blockage of external auditory canal or eustachian tube, otosclerosis or other causes. Otitis media of some type is the most common cause of conductive hearing loss.[3, 10, 15, 36]

(2) sensorineural hearing loss — inability of the cochlear division of the eighth cranial nerve to transmit electric impulses to the brain or of the hair cells of the organ of Corti to change sound to electric energy. Dysfunction may be due to neural degeneration of the organ of Corti, alterations in endolymph, cochlear conductive disorder or other causes.[3, 10, 15, 32, 33, 36, 39]

b. Conductive or sensorineural hearing loss or both may be found in the following types:[10]

(1) congenital deafness — loss of hearing from birth.

(2) hysteric deafness — simulated hearing loss associated with neurotic behavior and emotional instability, thus psychogenic in nature.

(3) Mondini's deafness — genetic deafness due to aplastic changes in the osseous and membranous labyrinth.[40]

(4) noise deafness, industrial hearing loss, occupational hearing loss — impairment or loss of hearing induced by constant noise, explosions or blows to the head. It disappears in a quiet environment if neural damage is in its early phase.

(5) sudden hearing loss, spontaneous hearing loss — usually an abrupt onset of sensorineural loss of hearing in one ear due to viral infection, vascular accident, trauma, shrinkage of organ of Corti or other causes. Bilateral sudden hearing loss is uncommon.

6. otogenic complications:[11, 14, 19, 50]

a. brain abscess — a sequela of chronic suppuration of the ear, often an otitis media.

b. lateral sinus phlebitis or thrombosis — usually the result of direct contact with infected mastoid cells. In thrombosis the clot may occlude the sinus.

c. otitic meningitis — inflammation of meninges following ear infection.

d. petrositis — inflammation of the petrous portion of the temporal bone.

D. Operative Terms:

1. microsurgery of ear — the use of a high power binocular dissecting microscope with built-in illumination in ear operations.[15]

2. the external ear:

a. amputation of the aural deformity (microtia) — excision of microtia, proper surgical revision of existing malformation as a foundation for a prosthesis and prosthetic reconstruction of pinna.[7, 17]

b. correction of meatal atresia — most difficult reconstructive procedure of the ear performed under high power magnification using a binocular dissecting microscope. It should only be attempted in the presence of bilateral atresia.[46]

c. otoplasty — correction of deformed pinna.[3]

d. otoscopy with magnification — inspection of the auditory canal and eardrum for diagnosis or for removal of polyp or granulation tissue followed by microscopic study.

e. pneumatic otoscopy — inspection of the ear using an otoscope with an attachment for stimulating variations in air pressure that put the eardrum in motion. It provides a valuable aid in the differential diagnosis of fluid ear, cholesteatoma, labyrinthine fistula and other ear conditions.[14]

3. the middle ear:

a. catheterization of auditory tube — removing exudate with catheter and inflating middle ear.

b. mastoid antrotomy — surgical opening of mastoid antrum, usually done for children with middle ear infection.

c. mastoidectomy, complete, Schwartze operation — mastoid air cells completely exenterated, antrum drained and myringotomy performed to promote escape of drainage in the presence of a subperiosteal abscess.[48]

d. mastoidectomy, radical — removal of all diseased tissue in mastoid antrum and tympanic cavity and conversion of both into one dry cavity which communicates with the external ear. An operating microscope is used.[14]

e. mastoidectomy, simple — postaural or endaural incision and removal of mastoid cells. In the presence of fluid in the middle ear a myringotomy is performed to establish drainage.

f. myringotomy, tympanotomy — opening of the eardrum in area which tends to heal readily, to avoid spontaneous rupture at a site which rarely closes.[14]

g. myringoplasty — surgical repair of tympanic membrane by tissue grafts.[47]

h. paracentesis tympani — surgical puncture of the eardrum for evacuation of fluid from middle ear.

i. stapedectomy — removal of stapes, reestablishing connection between incus and oval window by interposition of prosthesis and tissue or inert cover over oval window.[48, 56]

j. tympanoplasty — repair of perforated tympanic membrane with erosion of malleus by closing tympanum with graft against incus or remnant of malleus.
Several tympanoplastic procedures have been devised.[15, 18, 41, 42, 48]

k. tympanotomy, exploratory — exploration of middle ear through tympanomeatal approach.

4. the inner ear:

a. cochlear implant, cochlear prosthesis — electronic device designed to initiate motion in the ossicular chain and cochlear fluid and depolarize peripheral neurons thus producing auditory sensations.[4] By generating electric stimulation of various segments of the cochlear branch of the eighth cranial nerve, the cochlear prosthesis promises to become a functional implantable hearing aid which enhances the speech rehabilitation of the totally deaf.[34]

b. decompression of endolymphatic sac — removal of bone around the sac for improvement of vascularization so that endolymph can escape to cerebrospinal fluid system.[3, 16]

c. labyrinthectomy — total destruction of labyrinth with or without removal of Scarpa's ganglion for intractable vertigo.[3, 16]

d. ligation of internal jugular vein — tying of the internal jugular vein to relieve objective venous tinnitus, formerly known as cephalic bruit.[55]

e. surgery of internal auditory canal — transvestibular approach to canal

(1) for relief of disabling vertigo and tinnitus by section of the vestibular nerve or excision of acoustic neuroma.

(2) for facial paralysis by decompression of the facial nerve and facial nerve grafting.[2, 8]

E. Symptomatic Terms:

1. anacusis — sound perception as such completely lost.

2. auditory agnosia — sound perception at end organ intact, but comprehension of sound lost centrally.
3. aural discharge — drainage from ear.
4. impacted cerumen — dried ear wax.
5. nystagmus — involuntary rhythmic movements in one eye or both which may be horizontal, rotary, vertical, circulatory, oblique or mixed type. They commonly occur in vestibular disease.
6. otalgia — pains in ear, severe earache.
7. otorrhagia — bleeding from the ear.
8. otorrhea — purulent drainage from the ear.
9. paracusis of Willis — ability of person with conductive hearing loss to hear better in the presence of noise.
10. presbycusis — impaired hearing which is part of the aging process.
11. tinnitus — ringing in the ears.[15]
12. vertigo — illusion of movement of individual in relation to his environment. The patient feels that he himself is spinning (subjective type) or the objects are whirling about him (objective type).[15, 19]
    a. central vertigo — present in disorders of vestibular nuclei, cerebellum or brainstem, characterized by slow onset, prolonged duration and absence of hearing impairment or tinnitus.[19]
    b. peripheral vertigo — present in disorders of vestibular nerve and semicircular canals. It is episodic and explosive, marked by sudden, violent attack, lasting minutes to hours and usually accompanied by tinnitus and impaired hearing.[19]

RADIOLOGY

A. Terms Related to Diagnostic Radiology:

1. polytomography, tomography, otic — multiple serial section views of the ear which are of diagnostic value in middle and inner ear disorders such as pure cochlear otosclerosis, Menière's disease and others. It is also helpful in detecting the site of facial nerve injury by cholesteatoma or glomus jugulare, intracranial extension of glomus tumor, translucent areas of temporal bone, malformations of the middle and inner ear and ossicular chain injury.[24, 35, 50, 58]
2. posterior fossa myelography — radiologic procedure which aids in the detection of space occupying lesions particularly acoustic neuroma, meningioma and primary cholesteatoma.[20]
3. radiogram of skull — x-ray examination to detect temporal bone or basal skull fractures which cause cochlear or vestibular damage or to locate brain tumors which encroach on the auditory center or interfere with neural pathway of the 8th cranial nerve.[26, 29]
4. retrograde jugular venography — a venogram which demonstrates either a normal jugular vein, or venous narrowing due to external pressure, or partial or total occlusion of the jugular vein within the jugular fossa. The procedure is indicated when a glomus jugular tumor is suspected.[6]
5. ultrasonography — use of ultrasonic technique for detecting the presence of fluid in the middle ear space. No echo returns in the absence of fluid in normal ears; but echoes do return in fluid-filled ears.[1]

B. Terms Related to Therapeutic Radiology:

1. radiotherapy of glomus jugulare — irradiation of tumor to promote shrinkage; complete or permanent eradication of neoplasm, rarely, if ever achieved; a combination of surgical excision and radiotherapy advocated to prevent recurrence of glomus.[14, 51]
2. ultrasonic irradiation — ultrasound energy for round window irradiation in the treatment of Menière's disease.[1]

CLINICAL LABORATORY

A. Basic Terms Related to Audiology:[13]

1. air conduction — aerotympanic route or aerial transmission of sound waves across the tympanic cavity (middle ear) and through the round window into the inner ear.[13]
2. bone conduction — ossicular route or transmission of sound waves across the ossicles and through the oval window into the inner ear.[13]
   The mechanical force of air and bone conduction is transformed in the inner ear into electric energy which travels along the cochlear branch of the eighth cranial nerve to the brain where it is perceived as speech.[13]
3. decibel — unit expressing intensity of sound.
4. discrimination — ability to distinguish accurately between similarly sounding words.
5. displacusis — the same sound perceived differently by each ear. The subject hears two sounds.
6. frequency — the number of regularly recurrent sound vibrations emanating from a source and expressed in cycles per second.
7. intensity of sound — pressure exerted by sound and measured in decibels.
8. loudness — sound heard by person with normal hearing differing from that perceived by person with defective hearing while the intensity remains the same.
9. phonetically balanced — in speech audiometry one syllable words e.g. fish, cook, hair.
10. pure tone — tone produced by simple sound waves as those of a tuning fork.
11. recruitment — abnormal condition of the inner ear characterized by an extremely rapid increase in loudness.
12. sensitivity to sound — acuteness of hearing.
13. spondee words — in speech audiometry bisyllabic words, e.g. nosebleed, headache, eardrum.
14. threshold — the lowest limit of initial sound perception, 50% of words heard correctly.
15. tone decay — the tone becomes inaudible.

B. Terms Related to the Laboratory Diagnosis of Ear Conditions:

1. direct smears and cultures from middle ear secretions — tests to determine predominating organisms. Common bacterial invaders are in
   a. aural furunculosis — Staphylococcus of low virulence.
   b. suppurative otitis media:
      (1) *Diplococcus pneumoniae*
      (2) *Staphylococcus, albus* or *aureus*
      (3) *Streptococcus pyogenes,* others.
2. spinal fluid examination and blood cultures — tests detect complications such as otitic meningitis or bacteremia.

C. Terms Related to Functional Tests of Cochlear Apparatus:

1. audiometry — measurement of hearing for the purpose of accurately evaluating the extent and nature of hearing impairment.[16, 25]
2. audiometric test — a quantitative measurement of hearing loss. Results are plotted according to an established normal on an audiogram which is a graphic representation of patient's threshold of hearing at different frequencies and intensities.[10, 16, 30]
3. Bekesy audiometric test — test automatically presenting continuous pure tones and interrupted tones at different frequencies. The subject controls the intensity of the testing signal and a needle plots the audiogram on a record form.[16, 36]
4. electrocochleography — new method of testing hearing particularly in infants one to six months old. Electrodes are positioned on or near the cochlea and computer records low voltage electric potentials obtained from the inner ear.[9]
5. pure tone audiometry — use of an electric instrument for quantitatively measuring pure tones both by air conduction and bone conduction at threshold levels. Test detects the type of hearing loss.[10, 16]

6. short increment sensitivity index — test presenting continuous pure tone to subject and superimposing short pips of one decibel increments on constant pure tone. Subjects with cochlear impairment experience no difficulty in perceiving the pips, while those with normal hearing do so.[16, 36]

7. speech audiometry — valuable aid in clinical audiology. The patient's functioning in his environment is estimated by a speech discrimination score.

8. stereoaudiometry — term refers to audiometric procedures which seek to determine the efficiency of binaural hearing.

9. tone decay test — valuable special auditory test which demonstrates the phenomenon of tone becoming inaudible.[27]

10. tuning fork tests — means for determining the type of hearing impairment in relation to sound conduction and sound perception. The Rinne test, Bing test and Weber test are commonly used.[10, 16, 57]

D. Terms Related to Functional Tests of the Vestibular Apparatus:

1. caloric test — procedure which conveys information of the functional capacity of each labyrinth and the presence of horizontal and rotary nystagmus.[10, 16, 19]

2. electronystagmogram — a record of eye movements by electric tracing induced by caloric or positional stimulation.[3, 10, 16, 19, 45, 52]

3. Romberg test — procedure which tests body balance when eyes are closed and feet together side by side.

ABBREVIATIONS

ABLB — alternate binaural loudness balance
AC — air conduction
AC and BC — air and bone conduction
AD — right ear (auris dextra)
as — left ear (auris sinistra)
BC — bone conduction
CM — cochlear microphonics
CP — cochlear potentials
cps — cycles per second
db — decibel
ECoch — electrocochleography
ENG — electronystagmogram
ENT — ear, nose and throat
EP — endocochlear potential
ERA — evoked response audiometry

ETF — eustachian tubal function
HD — hearing distance
MACS — mastoid air cell system
Oto. — otology
P-B — phonetically balanced
PGSR — psychogalvanic skin resistance audiometry
PTS — permanent threshold shift
Sal — sensorineural acuity level
SDT — speech detection threshold
SISI — short increment sensitivity index
TDT — tone decay test
TTS — temporary threshold shift
VASC — visual-auditory screening test for children

ORAL READING PRACTICE

Otitic Meningitis

Acute or chronic suppurative otitis media may be followed by **intracranial** complications such as **thrombophlebitis** of the **lateral sinus, extra** or **intradural** abscess, **labyrinthitis,** facial paralysis and others.

Meningitis is one of the most serious **sequelae** of ear infections. Its incidence is higher in small children than in adults because of the intimate relation of the middle ear to the middle cranial fossa in early life. Symptoms may develop slowly or there may be an abrupt onset of the disease without **prodromal** manifestations. A chill occasionally signals the beginning of the acute phase. With the cerebral invasion of **pathogenic** organisms the cardinal symptoms make their appearance: a constantly high fever, a headache progressively becoming worse to the point of being excruciating, and vertigo, particularly in the presence of **labyrinthine** involvement.

As the disease progresses **prostration** increases, convulsions occur, particularly in children, and the patient becomes very irritable, exhibiting marked personality changes. **Delirium** simulates **maniacal** attacks in extreme cases. In infants the large fontanelle is bulging, but there is no pulsation. The Kernig's sign is positive as evidenced by pain and reflex contraction in the hamstring muscles when the examiner attempts to extend the leg after flexing the thigh upon the body. Muscular rigidity of back and neck and retraction of the head are characteristic manifestations. In addition, the patient suffers from **photophobia, hyperesthesia** at touch and **opisthotonos.** If treatment remains ineffectual, progressive drowsiness and coma develop, the deep reflexes disappear and the prognosis is poor.

Spinal fluid findings clinch the diagnosis. The fluid appears cloudy and purulent and the pressure is increased. The cell count is high in **lymphocytes** and **polymorphonuclear** leukocytes. The protein content of the spinal fluid markedly rises while the sugar drops. An excessively high protein is usually associated with **ventricular blockage** and signals a fatal outcome.

Smear and culture findings generally indicate that the bacterial invaders, causing the ear infection, are the same as those of the **otogenic** complication in the brain.

The *Streptococcus pyogenes* and *Diplococcus pneumoniae* are the common etiologic agents of diffuse purulent mennigitis, while *Neisseria meningitidis,* a very pyogenic diplococcus, provokes epidemic cerebrospinal meningitis.

The best treatment is prophylactic. Antibiotic therapy and the establishment of adequate drainage of the suppurative focus in the ear have lowered the incidence of otitic meningitis within the last two decades. Once the disease has developed, vigorous treatment must be instituted to combat the infection, prevent ventricular blocking and maintain electrolyte balance and nutrition.[11, 14, 19, 20, 50]

Table 29

SOME EAR CONDITIONS AMENABLE TO SURGERY

Organs Involved	Diagnoses	Operations	Operative Procedures
Ear	Carcinoma of ear	Amputation of ear Otoplasty	Removal of ear Plastic repair of ear
External auditory meatus	Foreign body in external auditory meatus Papilloma	Otoscopy with removal of foreign body Excision of papilloma	Endoscopic examination of external auditory meatus for removal of foreign body or lesion
Middle ear	Otitis media acute serous	Paracentesis tympani Myringotomy	Puncture of eardrum and evacuation of fluid from middle ear Incision of eardrum and drainage of middle ear
Middle ear	Perforation of eardrum chronic	Myringoplasty	Reconstruction of eardrum
Middle ear Mastoid	Otitis media acute Mastoiditis acute	Complete mastoidectomy	Scooping out and obliterating of infected air cells Removal of diseased mastoid process

Organs Involved	Diagnoses	Operations	Operative Procedures

Middle ear
 	
Mastoid
	Otitis media
	  chronic
	    suppurative
	Mastoiditis
	  chronic
	    suppurative
	    or
	    recurrent
		Radical mastoidectomy
		  or modified radical
		  mastoidectomy
		Repair of middle ear
		
		Tympanoplasty
			Endaural approach to temporal
			  bone and thorough removal of
			  diseased tissues
			Surgical creation of a new cavity
			  composed of healthy mastoid
			  tissue, the tympanum and
			  external auditory canal

Mastoid	Mastoiditis
	  chronic
	  perforation
	  of pars tensa
		Tympanoplasty with or
		  without mastoidectomy
			Closure of perforation by skin graft
			  or vein or fascia or perichondrium

Middle ear	Otosclerosis
	  conductive deafness
	  with fixation of
	  stapes
		Stapedectomy
		Stapedioplasty
			Removal of stapes
			Insertion of delicate
			  prosthesis to replace stapes

Middle ear
Tympanum
Mastoid
	Tympanomastoiditis
	Cholesteatoma
		Tympanomastoidectomy
		Tympanoplasty
			Postauricular incision
			Removal of necrotic incus
			Malleus and stapes freed by
			  dissection — tympanosclerosis
			  removed
			Complete enucleation of
			  diseased mastoid
			Fascial graft placed on
			  canal wall
			Tympanomeatal flap
			  positioned and secured
			  with gelfoam and silastic
			  sponge

Internal ear	Menière's disease
	  1. unilateral
	
	  2. bilateral
		Labyrinthectomy
		
		Exenteration of air cells
		Avulsion of endolymphatic
		  labyrinth
		
		Ultrasonic surgery
			Endaural or postaural approach
			  to inner ear
			Removal of air cells
			Destruction of membranous
			  labyrinth
			
			Selective destruction of osseous
			  vestibular labyrinth by ultrasonic
			  waves avoiding bombardment of
			  cochlea

Vestibulococh-
lear nerve
	Acoustic neuroma	Excision of neoplasm	Removal of neoplasm which involved
			  some area of the neural passage-
			  way of hearing

REFERENCES AND BIBLIOGRAPHY

1. Abramson, D. H. *et al.* Ultrasonics in otolaryngology. *Archives of Otolaryngology*, 96: 146-150, August, 1972.
2. Antoli-Candela, F. *et al.* Transvestibular approach to the internal auditory canal. *Annals of Otology Rhinology & Laryngology*, 84: 145-151, March-April, 1975.
3. Aylward, Howard J., M.D. Personal communications.
4. Bailey, B. J. What is new in surgery: Otolaryngology. *Surgery Gynecology & Obstetrics*, 140: 206-207, February, 1975.
5. Boles, R. *et al.* Conservative management of Menière's disease: Furstenberg regimen revisited. *Annals of Otology Rhinology & Laryngology*, 84: 513-517, July-August, 1975.
6. Britton, B. H. Glomus tympanicum and glomus jugulare tumors. *Radiologic Clinics of North America*, 12: 543-551, December, 1974.
7. Bulbulian, A. H. Prosthesis for microtia and other deformities of the ear. In Paparella, Michael M., Hohmann, Albert and Huff, John S. *Clinical Otology. An International Symposium.* St. Louis: The C. V. Mosby Co., 1971, pp. 83-93.

8. Cozar, F. A. *et al.* Transvestibular approach to the internal auditory canal. *Annals of Otology, Rhinology & Laryngology,* 84: 145-152, March-April, 1975.

9. Crowley, D. E. *et al.* Survey of the clinical use of electrocochleography. *Annals of Otology Rhinology & Laryngology,* 84: 297-307, May-June, 1975.

10. Deatsch, W. W. Hearing loss. In Krupp, Marcus A. and Chatton, Milton. *Current Medical Diagnosis and Treatment,* 15th ed. Los Altos, California: Lange Medical Publications, 1976, pp. 88-90.

11. _____. Diseases of the external ear — Diseases of the middle ear. *Ibid.,* pp. 90-94.

12. _____. Diseases of the inner ear. *Ibid.,* pp. 94-95.

13. De Weese, David D. and Saunders, William H. Anatomy of the ear — Physiology of hearing. *Textbook of Otolaryngology,* 4th ed. St. Louis: The C. V. Mosby Co., 1973, pp. 271-278.

14. _____. Diseases of the middle ear and mastoid. *Ibid.,* pp. 350-367.

15. _____. Hearing losses — Tinnitus — Dizziness and vertigo. *Ibid.,* pp. 350-435.

16. _____. Modern audiometry — The labyrinth. *Ibid.,* pp. 299-323.

17. _____. Diseases and abnormalities of the external ear — The tympanic membrane. *Ibid.,* pp. 324-349.

18. Don, A. *et al.* The fate of cartilage grafts for ossicular reconstruction in tympanoplasty. *Annals of Otology Rhinology & Laryngology,* 84: 187-191, March-April, 1975.

19. Drachman, D. A. Dizziness and vertigo. In Beeson, Paul B. and McDermott, Walsh (eds.). *Textbook of Medicine,* 14th ed. Philadelphia: W. B. Saunders Co., 1975, pp. 621-626.

20. Fisch, U. P. *et al.* Diagnostic value of meatocisternography. *Archives of Otolaryngology,* 101: 339-343, June, 1975.

21. Freeman, P. *et al.* Inner ear barotrauma. *Archives of Otolaryngology,* 95: 556-563, June, 1972.

22. Gardner, G. Shunt surgery in Menière's disease. *Southern Medical Journal,* 68: 611-614, May, 1975.

23. Glasscock, M. E. Complications in acoustic neuroma surgery. *Annals of Otology Rhinology & Laryngology,* 84: 518-526, July-August, 1975.

24. Guinto, F. C. Tomographic anatomy of the ear. *Radiologic Clinics of North America,* 12: 405-417, December, 1974.

25. Istre, C. O. *et al.* Variables in objective audiometry. *Southern Medical Journal,* 68: 844-848, July, 1975.

26. Jensen, J. Congenital anomalies of the inner ear. *Radiologic Clinics of North America,* 12: 473-482, December, 1974.

27. Jerger, J. A simplified tone decay test. *Archives of Otolaryngology,* 101: 403-407, July, 1975.

28. Konigsmark, B. W. *et al.* Recessive microtia, meatal atresia and hearing loss. *Archives of Otolaryngology,* 96: 105-109, August, 1972.

29. Lapayowker, M. S. Congenital anomalies of the middle ear. *Radiologic Clinics of North America,* 12: 463-471, December, 1974.

30. Lescouflair, G. Critical view of audiometric screening in schools. *Archives of Otolaryngology,* 101: 469-473, August, 1975.

31. Lin, Y. S. *et al.* Chronic middle ear effusions. *Archives of Otolaryngology,* 101: 278-286, May, 1975.

32. Linthicum, F. H. *et al.* Sensorineural hearing loss due to cochlear otospongiosis. *Annals of Otology Rhinology & Laryngology,* 84: 544-551, July-August, 1975.

33. Makishima, K. *et al.* Pathogenesis of hearing loss in head injury. *Archives of Otolaryngology,* 101: 426-432, July, 1975.

34. Michelson, R. *et al.* Present status and future development of the cochlear prosthesis. *Annals of Otology Rhinology & Laryngology,* 84: 494-498, July-August, 1975.

35. Mundnich, K. Dysplasias of the middle and the inner ear in different types of malformation. *Proceedings of Royal Society of Medicine,* 67: 1197, 1974.

36. Nelson, J. R. Hearing loss. In Beeson, Paul B. and McDermott, Walsh (eds.). *Textbook of Medicine,* 14th ed. Philadelphia: W. B. Saunders Co., 1975, pp. 619-621.

37. Palva, T. *et al.* Middle ear mucosa and chronic ear disease. *Archives of Otolaryngology,* 101: 380-384, June, 1975.

38. _____. Staged surgery in ears with excessive disease of tympanum. *Archives of Otolaryngology,* 101: 211-216, April, 1975.

39. Paparella, M. M. *et al.* Genetic sensorineural deafness in adults. *Annals of Otology Rhinology & Laryngology,* 84: 459-472, July-August, 1975.

40. Paparella, M. M. *et al.* Mondini's deafness. *Archives of Otolaryngology,* 95: 134-140, February, 1972.

41. Perkins, R. Grafting materials in reconstructive ear surgery. *Annals of Otology Rhinology & Laryngology,* 84: 518-526, July-August, 1975.

42. _____. Otologic homograft indications, techniques and anatomic and functional results. *Transactions of American Academy of Ophthalmology and Otolaryngology,* 80: 41-46, 1975.

43. Peron, D. L. *et al.* Congenital cholesteatomata with other anomalies. *Archives of Otolaryngology,* 101: 498-505, August, 1975.

44. Rovsing, Hans. Otosclerosis: Fenestral and cochlear. *Radiologic Clinics of North America,* 12: 505-515, December, 1974.

45. Rubin, W. *et al.* Electronystagmography: A review of 17 years experience. *Annals of Otology Rhinology & Laryngology,* 84: 541-543, July-August, 1975.

46. Schuknecht, H. F. Reconstructive procedures for congenital aural atresia. *Archives of Otolaryngology,* 101: 170-172, March, 1975.

47. Siedentop, K. H. Heterograft myringoplasty. *Archives of Otolaryngology,* 101: 229-231, April, 1975.

48. Snow, J. B. The ears. In Sabiston, David C. (ed.).

294

Davis — *Christopher Textbook of Surgery*, 10th ed. Philadelphia: W. B. Saunders Co., 1972, pp. 1204-1215.

49. Spector, G. J. Glomus tumors in the head and neck. *Annals of Otolaryngology Rhinology & Laryngology*, 84: 73-79, January-February, 1975.

50. Spector, G. J. *et al.* Neurologic implications of glomus tumors in the head and neck. *The Laryngoscope*, 85: 1387-1395, August, 1975.

51. Spector, G. J. *et al.* Glomus jugulare tumors: Effects of radiotherapy. *Cancer*, 35: 1316-1321, May, 1975.

52. Spector, M. Electronystagmographic findings in CNS disease. *Annals of Otology Rhinology & Laryngology*, 84: 374-378, May-June, 1975.

53. Teatini, G. Dealing with tympanosclerosis. In Paparella, Michael M., Hohmann, Albert and

Huff, John S. *Clinical Otology. An International Symposium.* St. Louis: The C. V. Mosby Co., 1971, pp. 140-143.

54. _____. Stereoaudiometry. *Ibid.*, pp. 34-39.

55. Ward, P. H. Operative treatment of surgical lesions with objective tinnitus. *Annals of Otology Rhinology & Laryngology*, 84: 473-482, July-August, 1975.

56. Willis, R. *et al.* A method of stapedectomy in the fenestrated ear. *Archives of Otolaryngology*, 101: 320-322, May, 1975.

57. Wilson, W. R. *et al.* Accuracy of the Bing and Rinne tuning fork tests. *Archives of Otolaryngology*, 101: 81-85, February, 1975.

58. Wright, J. William and Taylor, Clifford C. *Polytomography of the Temporal Bone.* St. Louis: Warren H. Green, Inc. 1973, pp. 68-87.

Chapter XV
Systemic Disorders

INFECTIOUS DISEASES

A. Origin of Terms:

1. ameba (G) — change
2. bacillus (L) — rod
3. coccus (G) — berry
4. gono (G) — seed
5. helminth (G) — worm
6. inoculate (L) — to engraft
7. lympha (L) — clear water
8. myco (G) — fungus
9. platy (G) — flat, broad
10. protozoon (G) — first animal
11. pseudopod (G) — false foot
12. saprophyte (G) — rotten plant
13. spirochete (G) — flowing hair
14. staphyl (G) — bunch of grapes
15. strepto (G) — curved
16. treponema (G) — turned thread
17. trich (G) — hair
18. vector (L) — carrier
19. virus (L) — poison
20. zoster (G) — girdle

B. Some Basic Terms:

1. acid-fast bacilli — organisms that resist acid-alcohol decolorization after they have been stained with a special dye (carbofuchsin).
2. aerobes — organisms requiring oxygen for growth.
3. agglutination — clumping of bacteria (or blood cells) following mixture with antisera.
4. allergen — substance capable of bringing about a hypersensitive state when introduced into the body.
5. allergy — state of hypersensitivity in which a person experiences certain symptoms upon coming in contact with an allergen.
6. anaerobes — organisms capable of growing in the absence of atmospheric oxygen.
7. antiseptic — substance that prevents bacterial growth.
8. antitoxin — immune serum that prevents the deleterious action of a toxin.
9. contagious — communicable.
10. culture medium — a milieu which promotes the growth of bacteria.
11. direct contact — spread of disease from person to person.
12. exudate — fluid or blood elements that have escaped into body cavities or tissues.
13. fungus (pl. fungi) — a vegetable, unicellular organism that feeds upon organic matter.
14. gram-negative — pertaining to bacteria which do not retain the Gram stain (crystal violet) following suitable decolorization.
15. gram-positive — pertaining to bacteria which retain the Gram stain after suitable decolorization.
16. immunity — resistance to disease, either natural or acquired.
17. inoculation — the process of introducing pathogenic organisms.
18. microorganism — a plant or animal only recognized under microscopic vision.
19. molds — plants belonging to a division of organisms known as fungi.
20. mycology — the study or science of fungi.
21. nosocomial infections — hospital acquired infections usually occurring in patients with defective host resistance or in recipients of cytotoxic drugs for malignancies, or of organ transplants treated with immunosuppressive therapy. Infective agents may be aspergillus, candida, nocardia, *Pneumocystis carini,* cytomegalovirus and other pathogenic microorganisms.[47, 52]
22. nosology — the science or study of classification of diseases.
23. nucleus — functional center of a cell.

24. parasite — a plant or animal that lives within or upon another and derives nourishment from its host.   Medical parasitology studies parasites in man, their life cycle in their hosts, pathogenic effect, prevention and control.   It deals with 2 major Phyla:[37, 39, 48]
   a.   Metazoa — multicellular parasites, for example:
      (1) helminthic infection — infestation by worms.
      (2) platyhelminthic infection — infestation by flatworms: tapeworms or flukes.
      (3) polyhelminthism — infestation of one individual by several species of worms.[20, 39, 55]
   b.   Protozoa — unicellular parasites, for example:
      (1) *Leishmania donovani* — etiologic agent of visceral leishmaniasis or kala-azar causing splenomegaly, bleeding, edema and emaciation.[39, 54]
      (2) *Trypanosoma* — protozoal parasites causing sleeping sickness in Africa and Chagas disease in America.   The latter affecting primarily children is characterized by intermittent parasitemia, fever, acute lymphadenitis and eyelid edema.[19, 39, 54]

25. pathogenic — disease producing.

26. putrefaction — decomposition of organic material.

27. pyogenic — pus forming.

28. saprophyte — an organism which grows on dead matter.

29. sensitivity (drug related) — ability of infective organism to respond to the bacteriostatic or bacteriocidal action of an antibiotic or other agent.

30. susceptibility — ability to acquire an infection following exposure to pathogenic organisms.

31. taxonomy — the classification of organisms of the plant or animal kingdom including the following categories in a descending order:
Phyla, Classes, Orders, Families, Genera, Species and Varieties.   The scientific names of organisms are binomial composed of a genus which is capitalized and a species which is given in small letters.
   a.   genus (pl. genera) — the division between family and species.
   b.   species (pl. species) — the division between genus and variety.[69]

32. virus (pl. viruses) — infectious agent of protein-coated nucleic acid and submicroscopic size, depending completely on the cells of its host.   Current research efforts focus on viruses as possible causes of cancer.   Trentin and others have shown that several serotypes of adenovirus are oncogenic producing sarcoma in hamsters.[40]

33. yeast — unicellular organism which usually reproduces by budding.

C.   Terms Pertaining to Infections Due to Viruses:[8, 24, 26, 30, 40, 46, 77]

1.   adenoviral infections — 31 serotypes of DNA bearing adenovirus, transmitted by person-to-person contact and capable of latency in lymphoid tissue.   Adenoviruses may cause epidemic outbreaks of
   a.   acute respiratory disease (ARD) — severe grippe-like respiratory infection involving the pharynx, larynx, bronchi and nasal mucosa and characterized by fever, sore throat, hoarseness, cough, headache and malaise.
   b.   febrile pharyngitis — inflammation of pharynx with exudate, enlarged cervical lymph nodes and fever.[31]
   c.   keratoconjunctivitis, epidemic (EKC) — serious eye infection with corneal infiltrates and follicular conjunctival lesions.   Epidemics may be initiated in clinics by contaminated eye drops.[22]
   d.   pharyngoconjunctival fever — severe type of pharyngitis associated with acute follicular conjunctivitis, usually lasting 5 days.[22]
   e.   pneumonia, adenoviral — highly fatal bronchopneumonia in infants, with sore throat, cough, prostration and high fever.[31, 77]

2.   arboviral infections — arthropod-borne viral infections which are usually transmitted to man by the bite of a blood sucking (hemaphagous) insect.   The viruses multiply in susceptible arthropods without producing the disease.   The arthropod vector acquires a lifelong

infection by ingesting vertebrate blood from a viremic host and maintains a complex vertebrate-arthropod-vertebrate cycle.[32, 64]

3. arbovirus encephalitides — various types of encephalitis, each having a specific host and viral vector according to its geographic distribution.[32, 63, 64] Those prevalent in the Americas are

    a. eastern equine encephalitis (EEE) in eastern and southern United States.

    b. St. Louis encephalitis (SLE) in nearly all the states of USA.

    c. Venezuelan equine encephalitis (VEE) in Central and South America and southern United States.

    d. western equine encephalitis (WEE) chiefly in Canada and western United States. The encephalitogenic arbovirus attacks man's neural tissues of the central nervous system especially those of the brain, the cerebral cortex, meninges, cerebellum, the neurons and supportive structures.[32, 63, 64]

4. chicken pox, varicella — acute infectious disease, characterized by sudden onset, mild fever and skin eruption. The prognosis is good.[31, 78]

5. cytomegalovirus infections — common viral infections occurring congenitally or in acquired forms in newborn, child or adult, with or without symptoms, as local or systemic disorders. Infected cells are oversize and contain intranuclear and cytoplasmic inclusion bodies. Viremia and viruria clinch the diagnosis.[31, 59, 67]

    a. congenital cytomegalic inclusion disease — infection developing in utero and primarily affecting premature infants. Lungs, kidneys, liver, spleen, pancreas, thymus, adenoids, parotid glands and other organs are infiltrated by viral foci in fatal disease of the neonate.[31, 59]

    b. cytomegalic inclusion disease, salivary gland virus disease — systemic disorder with cytomegalovirus present in salivary glands, liver, spleen and other viscera. In adults the disease is usually associated with the terminal phase of leukemia, malignancy or other chronic debilitating diseases.[31, 40, 67]

6. German measles, rubella — mildly contagious disease with catarrhal symptoms and a rash resembling measles.[33, 78]

7. herpes simplex, herpes febrilis, fever blisters — acute infectious condition of the skin or mucous membranes, marked by vesicular lesions which may become infected. Condition is primary or recurrent.[31]

8. herpes zoster — a viral disease affecting primarily one or more dorsal root ganglia or extramedullary cranial nerve ganglia. It is characterized by a vesicular eruption in the skin or mucous membrane along the course of the peripheral nerves which arise in the affected ganglia.[31, 78]

9. infectious mononucleosis — usually a benign infection due to Epstein-Barr virus. It exhibits a characteristic lymphocytosis and irregular clinical pattern. Glandular swelling (lymph node enlargement) throat symptoms, fever and splenomegaly are common manifestations. The disease occurs chiefly in adolescents and young adults.[31, 51]

10. influenza — acute febrile disease due to the influenza virus, A, B or C. It is generally characterized by respiratory symptoms and joint pains. It may occur in epidemic or even pandemic form.[33, 45]

11. measles, rubeola — highly communicable disease, clinically manifested by Koplik spots of the buccal mucosa, a rash and catarrhal symptoms.[33, 40, 78]

12. mumps, infectious parotitis — virus disease of the salivary glands, which tends to involve other organs, especially the testes and ovaries.[33]

13. rabies, hydrophobia — acute encephalitis which causes paralysis, delirium and convulsions.

14. smallpox, variola — communicable disease, characterized by a rash which changes from macules, papules, vesicles, pustules to scabs.

15. viral hepatitis, acute — disease associated with jaundice, liver damage resulting from hepatic cell necrosis followed by hepatomegaly, splenomegaly and viremia. Two forms, immunologically distinct, but clinically similar, are recognized.[41]

    a. hepatitis A — incubation period 15-50 days; infective agent: hepatitis virus A, transmitted orally or parenterally; virus present in feces; early symptoms: cough, pharyngitis and muscle pains.[21, 41]

 b. hepatitis B — incubation period 50-80 days, infective agent: hepatitis virus B; transmitted parenterally; virus rarely found in feces; a circulating antigen HB Ag present in early phase of hepatitis B.[41, 50, 71]

16. viral hepatitis, chronic active — long-term infection characterized by progressive destruction of liver cells and fibrotic changes followed by terminal cirrhosis.[42]

D. Terms Pertaining to Infections due to Chlamydiae:

1. chlamydiae (sing. chlamydia) — non-motile, gram negative microorganisms, restricted to an intracellular parasitic existence. They possess antigens and are inhibited by selected antimicrobial agents.[24, 36]

2. lymphogranuloma venereum (LGV) — venereal disease which evokes a painful suppurative inguinal adenitis and in its advanced course exhibits systemic manifestations such as fever, skin rashes, gastric upset, back pain, headache and meningeal irritation. Chlamydiae are the pathogenic microorganisms.[24, 36]

3. psittacosis, ornithosis, parrot fever — infectious disease characterized by variable symptoms from mild to acute fever, headache, lung involvement, cough, delirium and prostration. Chlamydiae are transmitted through contact with infected birds or with the sputum from chlamydial pneumonia patients.[24, 36]

4. trachoma and inclusion conjunctivitis (TRIC) — chronic infectious diseases of the conjunctiva which tend to be associated with infections of the urogenital tract. The etiologic agents, chlamydiae, are transmitted by human contact or flies. If left untreated, TRIC infections persist for years and produce corneal scarring and blindness.[24, 36]

E. Terms Pertaining to Infections Due to Cocci:*[24, 34, 72, 29]

1. erysipelas — acute febrile, inflammatory disease marked by localized skin lesions which tend to migrate. The infection is due to the *Streptococcus pyogenes*.

2. furunculosis — a condition resulting from boils generally caused by *Staphylococcus aureus*.[34]

3. gonorrhea — a specific infection which usually has its inception in the urethra and attacks the genital mucous membrane. The infection may also affect the conjunctiva and joints. The etiologic agent is *Neisseria gonorrhoeae* (gonococcus).

4. meningitis — inflammation of meninges. The epidemic form is caused by *Neisseria meningitidis*.

5. staphylococcal food intoxication — food poisoning due to staphylococcus associated with more or less violent and abrupt onset of nausea, vomiting and prostration. Severe diarrhea may occur.

F. Terms Pertaining to Infections Due to Bacilli:[24, 35]

1. bacillary dysentery, shigellosis — acute infection marked by diarrhea, tenesmus, fever and, in severe cases, mucus and blood in stool. Prognosis tends to be serious in infants and debilitated aged individuals. The disease is caused by various species of Shigella.[35]

2. diphtheria — an acute infection, generally associated with fever and the formation of a grayish membrane in the throat from which the Klebs-Loeffler bacillus can be cultured.[76]

3. food poisoning — disease characterized by an abrupt onset of gastrointestinal symptoms caused by food intoxication or infection.[34]

 a. botulism — true food poisoning, a fatal, afebrile condition, marked by weakness, constipation, headache and forms of paralysis. The intoxication is due to the botulinus bacillus (*Clostridium botulinum*).[34, 76]

---

* Infections due to cocci are so numerous that it has only been possible to give one example of the most important pathogenic organisms.

b. Salmonella infection, salmonellosis — condition causing typhoid and paratyphoid fevers.[35]

4. undulant fever, brucellosis — a general infection characterized by intermittent or continuous fever, headache, chills and profuse perspiration. The etiologic agents are three species of Brucella.[35]

G. Terms Pertaining to Infections Due to Fungi and Yeasts:[3, 18, 25, 80]

1. actinomycosis — chronic ray fungus disease characterized by multiple abscesses which form draining sinuses. Lesions occur in face, neck, lungs, abdomen, the latter being highly fatal.[18]

2. aspergillosis — infection with Aspergillus which attacks the lungs, skin, external ear, nasal sinuses, meninges and bones. It is mainly found among agricultural workers and pigeon feeders.[3, 18]

3. blastomycosis — mycotic infection either limited to subcutaneous tissue or disseminated throughout the lungs or multiple body systems. It is prevalent in Illinois, Tennessee, Louisiana and North Carolina.[3, 18]

4. candidiasis — acute or subacute fungus infection which causes thrush, glossitis, vaginitis, onychia and pneumonitis. It is also seen in patients receiving chemotherapy.[3, 18]

5. coccidioidomycosis — either a primary, acute infection of the lungs, lymph nodes or skin with a favorable prognosis or a generalized infection including the meninges that is prone to be fatal. It is prevalent in southwestern United States.[3, 18]

6. crytococcosis — a very serious mycotic infection forming multiple abscesses and lesions of skin, subcutaneous tissue, lungs and meninges. The etiologic agent is the *Crytococcus neoformans*.[3, 18]

7. histoplasmosis — mycotic disease caused by *Histoplasma capsulatum* which produces benign pulmonary lesions and rarely attacks the reticuloendothelial system. It is prevalent in Missouri, central Mississippi, and other parts of the United States.[3, 18]

8. mycosis (pl. mycoses) — any fungus disease.

9. nocardiosis — infection chiefly caused by *Nocardia asteroides*, either localized in the lungs or disseminated through multiple systems: skin, subcutaneous tissue, brain and others.[18]

H. Terms Pertaining to Infections Due to Spirochetes:[36, 75, 80]

1. leptospirosis — acute infection by one of the *Leptospira* species, transmitted to man by the ingestion of food which has been contaminated by the excretions of a reservoir animal: dog, rat, cattle or swine. Clinical manifestations include sudden onset of fever, chills, abdominal and muscular pains, intense headache, a palpable liver, jaundice, conjunctival redness, purpura and erythema of skin and in severe cases meningeal irritation.[10, 36, 65]

2. relapsing fever — acute spirochetal infection by *Borrelia recurrentis*, transmitted to man by insect vectors (lice) or infected insects (tics). Relapses of fever occur abruptly every week or two and gradually decrease in severity. They are accompanied by nausea and vomiting, joint and muscle pains, tachycardia, psychic, neurologic and hemorrhagic manifestations. Relapsing fever is endemic in western USA and many other countries.[36]

3. venereal syphilis — infectious, relapsing disease which is characterized by a primary lesion or hard chancre. It is followed by a secondary skin eruption with typical reddish brown, coppery spots, periods of latency and systemic late lesions in the central nervous and cardiovascular systems.[36]

I. Terms Pertaining to Infections Due to Protozoa:[19, 39, 53, 54]

1. amebic dysentery, amebiasis — a parasitic infection marked by diarrhea, pain and fever. It is caused by the protozoan *Entamoeba histolytica*.[54]

2. malaria — disease due to the presence and multiplication of parasites in the blood. It is manifested by splenomegaly, anemia and sweating.

There are four types:

   a. quotidian — paroxysms occur every 24 hours due to daily sporulation.

   b. tertian — paroxysms occur every 48 hours.

   c. quartan — paroxysms occur every 72 hours and are accompanied by seizures.

   d. falciparum — paroxysms usually occur between 24 - 48 hours; causes cerebral vascular occlusion. It has highest mortality of malaria.[54]

3. pneumocystis pneumonia — lung infection by *Pneumocystis carini* which produces an interstitial plasma cell pneumonitis. Outbreaks may occur in nurseries, particularly among premature and marasmic infants. Adults receiving antibiotic, cytotoxic or corticosteroid therapy over a prolonged period are likely to develop this disease.[19, 68]

J. Terms Pertaining to Infections Due to Metazoa:[20, 39, 55, 61]

1. cestodes — tapeworms[55]

   a. cestodiasis — infestation of the intestinal tract with a tapeworm.

   b. echinococcosis, hydatid disease — hydatid cyst of liver or lung caused by larvae of *Echinococcus granulosa,* a small tapeworm which has been sporadically endemic in Alaska, Canada, California and Utah. Man is usually infected hand-to-mouth by a host dog that harbors eggs in its fur. Ingested eggs deliver larvae that penetrate the intestinal wall and are carried by the circulating blood to the liver and sometimes to the lungs where they form a hydatid cyst. The cysts are asymptomatic unless rupture occurs.

   c. taenia, tapeworm infection — human parasitic infestation by the beef or pork or fish tapeworm caused by the ingestion of poorly cooked, infected meat or fish.[20, 55]

A tapeworm has 3 distinct parts, the head or scolex, the neck and the segments or proglottids. Its length may exceed 10 feet. Single segments are prone to detach themselves from the entire chain and to be eliminated in the feces. A rupture of a gravid (pregnant) segment delivers a huge number of eggs which may be eaten by cattle, develop into embryos in their animal host and lodge in muscles as cysticerci. When infected meat is consumed by man a cysticercus grows into an adult tapeworm.

Larvae of the pork tapeworm in man are disseminated to all organs of the body. In

   (1) cerebral cysticercosis — larval invasion of the brain results in epilepsy, mental decline, internal hydrocephalus, headache, nerve palsies and personality disorders.

   (2) muscle cysticercosis — larval invasion of muscles is followed by calcification of cysticerci after prolonged infestation as confirmed by radiographic studies.

2. nematodes — roundworms[20, 39, 55]

   a. ascariasis — human infestation with the giant intestinal roundworm, *Ascaris lumbricoides,* and in the past endemic in the southern states of USA. Larvae of the roundworm may severely damage the lungs causing an Ascaris pneumonitis prevalent in children. Adult ascarids may be expelled in vomitus or feces.[39]

   b. enterobiasis — pinworm infection usually found in children, dormitory groups and mental hospitals. The gravid (pregnant) female migrates from the lower intestine to lay her eggs on the perianal skin where they cause intense itching.[20, 56]

   c. filariasis — filarial roundworm infection transmitted to man by the bite of certain mosquitoes that are the hosts of infective larvae. These larvae grow into adult worms near or in lymph nodes of the human host. The adults release numerous motile larvae, the microfilariae which usually circulate in the blood during the night. In advanced filariasis obstruction of the lymph flow leads to elephantiasis, lymphedema, hydrocele, skin and other problems.[20, 39, 55]

   d. hookworm disease — infection by *Necator americanus,* the American hookworm of the southern states, 1 cm in length, its head curved backward and attached to the intestinal mucosa.   Tarry, viscous stools associated with poor digestion, malnutrition, anemia and moderate heart failure suggest heavy intestinal infection. The initial reaction to larval invasion is ground itch.   There may be a creeping eruption, tortuous and raised, caused by the larvae's subcutaneous tunnels.[20, 39]

    e. onchocerciasis — disease caused by microfilariae, infective larvae of a roundworm which are transmitted to man by the bite of a black fly. Intense pruritus and skin eruptions are early symptoms.   Painful nodules which form around dead and living worms and serious ocular lesions occur late in the disease.[20, 39]

    f. strongyloidiasis — threadworm infection, prevalent in southern United States. It is characterized by a high degree of toxemia, urticaria and prolonged mucous diarrhea indicative of intestinal invasion.[39]

    g. trichiniasis, trichinosis — infection acquired by man by the ingestion of encysted larvae of *Trichinella spiralis* in poorly cooked pork.[20, 55]

    h. trichuriasis — whipworm infection producing serious toxic reactions in the host such as marked emaciation, anemia, diarrhea and bloody stools.

  3. trematodes — flukes.[20, 39, 55]

    a. fasciolopsiasis — infection with large intestinal fluke by eating uncooked infected water plants.   The flukes may cause severe cramping pain, nausea, anorexia, diarrhea, finally edema, ascites, cachexia and death.

    b. schistosomiasis, bilharziasis — Schistosoma infection by fluke invasion causing several trematode diseases in Asia, Africa and South America.[20, 39, 55]

      (1) intestinal schistosomiasis — cercariae, infective larvae, pierce the human skin or mucous membranes where they are in contact with water.   Maturation, mating and delivery of eggs takes place in the veins of the intestinal wall.   Eggs may be eliminated in feces or reach the liver provoking cirrhosis, portal hypertension and ascites in the advanced stage.

      (2) vesical or urinary schistosomiasis — maturation of the fluke occurs in the venous networks of the prostate, bladder and uterus leading to cystitis, pyelonephritis and later to terminal hematuria, uremia and death.[20, 55]

K. Terms Pertaining to Conditions of Undetermined Cause:

1. cystic fibrosis — a systemic hereditary disease of unknown etiology seen in children and adolescents.   It is characterized by a more or less extensive involvement of the exocrine glands, especially those secreting mucus and sweat.   It may include a variety of clinical conditions:

    a. meconium ileus causing intestinal obstruction in the newborn

    b. chronic pulmonary disease often leading to fatal complications

    c. pancreatic insufficiency resulting in malnutrition

    d. abnormally raised levels of sweat electrolytes causing salt depletion and cardiac collapse in hot weather.[82]

2. fever of unknown origin — persistent elevated body temperature, unexplained by serologic and bacteriologic studies or other diagnostic measures.

3. sarcoidosis — a systemic granulomatous disease of undetermined etiology and pathogenesis. Mediastinal and peripheral lymph nodes, lungs, liver, spleen, skin, eyes, phalangeal bones and parotid glands are most often involved but other organs and tissues may be affected.   (Definition by the International Conference of Sarcoidosis).[38, 60]

IMMUNOLOGIC DISEASES

A. Origin of Terms:

1. ana (G) — without
2. auto (G) — self
3. fluorescent (L) — to flow
4. histos (G) — tissue, web

5. immune (L) — safe, exempt
6. lysis (G) — dissolution
7. phoresis (G) — a carrying in
8. phylaxis (G) — protection

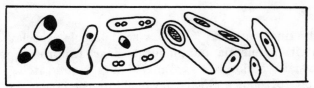

Fig. 73 — Bacilli. Rod-shaped or club-shaped organisms.

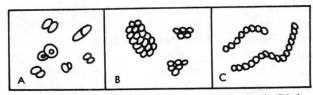

Fig. 74 — Cocci. Spherical or oval organisms. A. Diplococci (in pairs); B. Staphylococci (in clusters); C. Streptococci (in chains).

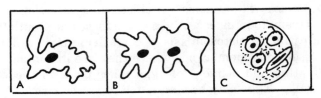

Fig. 75 — Amebae. Unicellular animal organisms, capable of changing form by throwing out foot-like processes (pseudopodia) which help them to move about and obtain nourishment. A. Ameba; B. Ameba dividing; C. Cyst of *Entamoeba histolytica*.

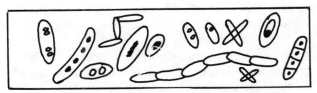

Fig. 76 — Salmonella and Shigella. Simple, non-spore forming rods, often joined end-to-end.

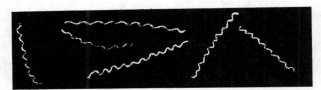

Fig. 77 — *Treponema pallidum.* Coiled, virulent organisms containing 8 to 14 spirals.

B. Some Basic Terms:

1. anaphylaxis — excessive hypersensitivity to foreign protein or other substance, clinically manifested by edema of the larynx, hypoxia, respiratory distress, hypotension and vascular collapse.[1, 28]

2. antibodies — specialized proteins or immunoglobulins, formed in response to an antigen.[27, 73]

3. antigens — substances that will cause the body to form antibodies.[27, 73]

4. autoantibodies — antibodies elicited by an individual's own antigens.[27]

5. autohemolysins — antibodies acting on the corpuscles of an individual's own blood.

6. autoimmunization — the production of antibodies or other immunologic responses to antigens in an individual without any artificial intervention.[1]

7. cytopathic effect (of viruses) — biologic changes produced by the multiplication of viruses in cell culture.[30]

8. cytotoxicity — the destruction of cells by autoantibodies as seen in acquired hemolytic anemia and other diseases.

9. fluorescein — a red crystalline powder used for diagnostic purposes.

10. fluorescence — luminescence of a substance when exposed to short wave rays.

11. histocompatibility — tissue compatibility between a recipient and donor based on immunologic identity or similarity of tissues necessary for successful transplantation.

12. hypersensitivity — exaggerated sensitivity to an infective, chemical or other agent, such as an extreme allergic reaction to a foreign protein.[1, 28] Hypersensitivity may be of the
    a. immediate type — occurring within 1 to 30 minutes, e.g. anaphylactic shock.
    b. cell-mediated, delayed type — developing gradually within 24 to 48 hours or longer, e.g. a tuberculin reaction.
    c. subacute delayed type, Arthus reaction, developing within 4 to 10 hours, characterized by a marked infiltration of small vessels with polymorphonuclear leukocytes, local edema and bleeding without thrombus formation.[1, 28]

13. immune response — formation of antibodies due to a specific stimulus.[1]

14. immunohematology — branch of hematology dealing with antigen-antibody reactions and their effects on the blood.

15. immunoelectrophoresis — procedure employed to separate and identify multiple protein components. In the test use is made of physiochemical and immunologic specificity.[73]

16. immunogen — one of a group of substances capable of stimulating an immune response or initiating a certain degree of active immunity under favorable conditions. Its effects may be detrimental or beneficial.[1]

17. immunogenicity — the ability of an immunogen to evoke an immune response, or the ability of an antigen to stimulate antibody formation.
    Immunogenicity is the same as antigenicity.[73]

18. immunoglobulins (Igs) — antibodies capable of reacting specifically with the antigen which caused their formation. They are similar in structure but diverse antigenically.[15, 27]
    Molecules of immunoglobulins are composed of
    a. heavy (H) chains — large polypeptide chains. Each of the 5 classes of immunoglobulins are antigenetically distinct, namely:
        γ in IgG — Immunoglobulin G
        α in IgA — Immunoglobulin A
        μ in IgM — Immunoglobulin M
        δ in IgD — Immunoglobulin D
        ξ in IgE — Immunoglobulin E.
    Molecular weights are 50,000 to 70,000.[27]
    b. light (L) chains — small polypeptide chains, either of the kappa (k) or lambda (λ) type. Molecular weight is 25,000.[27]

19. immunoglobulin concentration — the amount of serum protein components determined by immunoelectrophoresis for establishing the presence or absence of elevated or depressed immunoglobulin levels. Thus an exaggerated susceptibility to infection or antibody deficiency may be detected.

304

20. immunology — the medical science which is concerned primarily with immunity or resistance to disease of the human being. In its practical aspects it deals with methods of diagnosing or preventing disease or influencing its course by serotherapy and vaccination.
21. immunopathology — the study of disorders or diseases resulting from antigen-antibody reactions or alterations produced by immunologic responses.[73]
22. immunosuppressive therapy — treatment instituted to suppress all immune responses and thus prevent the rejection of the graft.[66, 73]
23. lymphocytes — white blood cells originating in lymphoid tissue and capable of responding to immunologic stimulation. There are two types of cells:
   a. B-lymphocytes — about 20% of lymphocytes in the circulating blood.
      They are short-lived, capable of proliferating, differentiating and maturing into plasma cells, functioning independently of the thymus and responsible for a specific immunoglobulin or serum antibodies.[1, 27, 70]
   b. T-lymphocytes — about 65 to 80% of lymphocytes in the circulating blood.
      They are long-lived, have few immunoglobulin molecules, depend on a functioning thymus and are cytotoxic to grafted cells thus causing graft rejection, a graft versus host reaction.[1, 27, 70]
24. rejection phenomenon — reaction to graft based on the formation of antibodies directed against the donated tissue or organ.[73]
25. transplantation immunity — immune responses to transplanting organs depending on the histocompatibility of the type of graft.[49, 62]
   a. allograft, homograft — tissue or organ from one individual is transferred to another individual of the same species.
   b. autograft — tissue or organ is transplanted from one part of the body to another in the same individual.
   c. isograft — tissue or organ is transplanted from one identical twin to another. Histocompatibility exists in its most complete form.
   d. xenograft, heterograft — tissue or organ from donor from one species is implanted in recipient from another species. Grafts between species are subject to intense medical research.[49, 63]

C. Diagnostic Terms:

1. autoimmune diseases — immunologic disorders in which the patient's own tissues produce antigenic stimuli. By using the fluorescein antibody technique, the presence of autoimmunity has been detected in certain cases of chronic thyroiditis, disseminated lupus erythematosus, poliomyelitis, rheumatoid arthritis, viral hepatitis and other diseases.[9, 28]
   a autoimmune hemolytic anemia — clinical syndrome of uncompensated hemolytic anemia due to an aberrant immune response initiated by a host and directed against the host's normal red cell antigens.[9, 57]
   b. secondary autoimmune hemolytic anemia — hemolytic anemia characterized by the presence of autoantibodies and a coexisting disease which constitutes the basic ailment, e.g. anemia caused by chronic infection or neoplasm.[9, 57]
2. heavy-chain diseases — disorders demonstrating a typical heavy-chain immunoglobin fragment in urine or serum or in both.[17, 81]
   a. alpha (α) heavy chain disease — a lymphocyte dyscrasia usually associated with malignant lymphoma of intestine resulting in nutritional malabsorption. The diagnosis is based on the detection of an abnormal protein in urine and serum which reacts with antiserums to alpha chains.[81]
   b. gamma (γ) heavy-chain disease — disorder primarily seen in the elderly, clinically manifested by weight loss, weakness, enlarged liver, recurrent infections, involvement of lymph glands, lymphocytosis, anemia and platelet deficiency.[81]
3. immunologic deficiency states — disorders reflecting defective cellular immunity or decreased antibody production or both resulting in increased susceptibility to infection.[15, 70]

a. Bruton's agammaglobulinemia — severe familial X-linked deficiency of gammaglobulins in the blood, marked deficiency of all classes of immunoglobulins and absence of plasma cells.[15]

b. Wiskott-Aldrich syndrome — severe immunodeficiency disease of a familial type, characterized by eczema, low platelet count and frequent infections associated with abnormal immunoglobulins, lymphopenia, delayed hypersensitivity and impaired immune response.[14, 15]

4. plasma cell and lymphocyte dyscrasias — disorders manifesting uncontrolled proliferation of cells usually active in antibody synthesis and homogenous immunoglobulin synthesis. Typical protein abnormalities in serum and urine clinch the diagnosis.[81]

a. macroglobulinemia, Waldenström's macroglobulinemia — dyscrasia including several clinical disorders in which the common denominator is the presence of monoclonal macroglobulin formed by cells involved in immunoglobulin M synthesis (IgM). Clinical features are anemia, bleeding, lymph gland involvement, enlarged spleen and liver.[16, 81]

b. multiple myeloma — severe plasma cell dyscrasia associated with decreased antibody synthesis and low immunoglobulin levels resulting in recurrent infections. There is considerable infiltration of the bone marrow by neoplastic plasma cells which in advanced disease proliferate, cause osteoporosis, typical punched-out skeletal lesions and pathologic fractures, especially of the ribs and vertebrae. Renal disease and anemia are usually present. Multiple myeloma runs a progressive course extending over one or more decades.[16, 44]

DISEASES OF CONNECTIVE TISSUE

A. Origin of Terms:

1. colla (G) — glue
2. erythema (G) — redness
3. lupus (L) — wolf, meaning destructive
4. sclera, sclero (G) — hard

B. Anatomic Terms:

1. collagen — a substance present between the fibers of connective tissue throughout the body.
2. collagen diseases — a group of diseases in which the connective tissues have undergone pathologic changes. The prognosis is fatal.
3. connective tissue — a variety of tissues composed of widely spaced cells between which intercellular material is deposited. This intercellular substance offers the distinguishing mark of the specific connective tissue; for example, mineral salts are located in the interspaces of bone and are responsible for its hardness, while for blood the intercellular substance is liquid. Other variations of connective tissue are areolar, adipose, fibrous, cartilage and lymphoid tissues.

C. Diagnostic Terms:

1. dermatomyositis — a disease of unknown etiology. It is characterized by an insidious onset, and subsequent dermatitis and widespread degeneration of the skeletal muscles.[13, 43]
2. disseminated lupus erythematosus — collagenous disease which affects the synovial and serous membranes and vascular system. It is clinically recognized by a typical butterfly lesion on the bridge of the nose and on the cheeks. The prognosis is usually fatal.[11, 12]
3. Marfan's syndrome, arachnodactyly — hereditary disorder of a conective tissue element resulting in skeletal, ocular and cardiovascular abnormalities. Clinical features are spidery fingers, disproportionately long limbs, funnel chest, lax, redundant ligaments, ectopia lentis (displaced lens) with impaired vision. Hemodynamic stress on the media of the aorta may lead to dissecting aortic aneurysm. Other disorders may be present.[4, 6]
4. polyarteritis, periarteritis nodosa — a systemic disease, characterized by the presence of nodules along the course of the muscular arteries.[13]

5. scleroderma — chronic disease causing a leathery induration of the skin, progressive atrophy and pigmentation. Systemic involvement of the mucous membranes, musculoskeletal, vascular and digestive systems may lead to a fatal prognosis.[13, 23, 83]

Table 30

IMPORTANT LABORATORY TESTS FOR INFECTIOUS DISEASES

A. VIRAL DISEASES[a,b,c]

Diseases	Etiologic Agent	Tests for Diagnosis
Acute respiratory disease Conjunctivitis Keratoconjunc- tivitis Pharyngitis	Adenovirus type 4 and 7, others type 3, others type 8, also 3 and 7a	Virus isolation from throat and conjunctival swabs or washings Complement fixation Neutralization Hemagglutination-inhibition
Classic influenza	Orthomyxovirus Influenza A,B,C	Virus isolation from nasal swabs and throat washings Hemagglutination-inhibition Complement-fixation Neutralization
Laryngotrache- itis Bronchitis Bronchiolitis Pneumonitis Croup	Paramyxovirus Parainfluenza 1, 2, 3, 4	Hemagglutination-inhibition Complement fixation Neutralization
Bronchitis Bronchiolitis Pneumonia Coryza	Respiratory syncytial virus RSV	Complement fixation
Measles (rubeola)	Measles virus	Virus isolation from blood and nasopharynx Hemagglutination-inhibition Complement fixation Neutralization
German measles (rubella)	Rubella virus	Virus isolation from cell culture
Congenital rubella syndrome		Virus isolation from throat, nasopharynx, urine, blood
Mumps (epidemic parotitis)	Mumps virus	Virus isolation from saliva, urine, cerebrospinal fluid Complement fixation Hemagglutination-inhibition Skin test antigen

Diseases	Etiologic Agent	Tests for Diagnosis
Common cold	Picornavirus Rhinovirus	Virus isolation from nose and throat
Herpangina Common cold	Coxsackie virus A	Virus isolation from nasal secretions

Pleurodynia
Aseptic
  meningitis
Myocardiopathy
Neonatal
  disease
	Coxsackie
	virus B
		Virus isolation from CSF
		Neutralization
		Complement fixation

Infant diarrhea
Febrile
  illnesses
  with or
  without rash
Aseptic
  meningitis
	Echovirus
	30 types
		Virus isolation from body fluids or lesions, feces, throat, cerebrospinal fluid

Poliomyelitis
  abortive
  nonparalytic
  paralytic
	Poliovirus	Cytology of CSF
		Virus isolation from throat, feces, rarely from CSF
		Complement fixation
		Neutralization

Acute hemorrhagic
  conjunctivitis
  AHC
  (epidemic
  pandemic)
Meningitis
Encephalitis
	New enterovirus
	types 68, 70,
	71
		Virus isolation in human cell culture
		
		Virus isolation from brain (postmortem)

Viral
  hepatitis A
Viral
  hepatitis B
	Hepatitis virus
	Hepatitis A virus
	  HAV
	Hepatitis B virus
	  HBV
		Tissue from liver biopsy
		Liver function tests:
		  Transaminase increased
		    SGPT and SGOT
		Immune electron microscopy
		Others

Herpes simplex
Aphthous
  stomatitis
Keratocon-
  junctivitis
Meningoen-
  cephalitis
	Herpesvirus
	Herpesvirus
	  type 1
		Virus isolation from herpetic lesions of skin, cornea of eye, brain, throat, saliva, feces

Genital herpes
Neonatal
  herpes
	Herpesvirus
	  type 2
		Passive hemagglutination
		Sheep cell agglutination
		Others

Varicella
  (chickenpox)
 	
Zoster
  (herpes zoster
  shingles)
	Varicella-zoster
	virus
		Virus isolation from vesicle fluid of skin lesion
		Complement fixation
		Neutralization
		Antibodies in human serum by immunofluorescence

Diseases	Etiologic Agent	Tests for Diagnosis
Cytomegalic inclusion disease (salivary gland virus disease)	Cytomegalovirus CMV	Virus isolation from mouth, adenoids, urine, kidneys, liver, peripheral leukocytes Neutralization tests to measure antibodies in tissue culture Immunofluorescence to detect antibodies in human sera
Infectious mononucleosis (glandular fever) Burkitt's lymphoma Nasopharyngeal cancer	EB herpesvirus or Epstein-Barr virus EBV	Heterophil antibodies agglutinating sheep red cells Antibodies against EBV measured by immunofluorescence with virus-containing cells

B. BACTERIAL DISEASES[d]

Diseases	Etiologic Agent	Tests for Diagnosis
Abscesses	*Staphylococcus aureus*	Microscopic: Smears and cultures from infected lesions
Bacterial endocarditis	Streptococcus various kinds	Microscopic: Blood culture
Erysipelas	*Streptococcus pyogenes* (hemolyticus)	Microscopic: Smears and cultures of material obtained from nasal orifices
Gonococcal infections	*Neisseria gonorrhoeae* (gonococcus)	Microscopic: Smears and cultures from secretions Kolmer complement fixation test for gonorrhea
Meningococcal meningitis	*Neisseria meningi-tidis* (meningococcus)	Microscopic: Smears and cultures from nasopharynx, spinal fluid and blood
Pneumonia	*Diplococcus pneumoniae*	Microscopic: Typing and culturing of sputum; blood culture Animal inoculation of sputum
Scarlet fever	*Streptococcus pyogenes* (hemolyticus)	Skin tests: Dick test: Intradermal injection of dilute scarlet fever streptococcus toxin Schultz-Charlton test, the Rash Extinction Test for Scarlet Fever: Intradermal injection of convalescent scarlet fever serum
Genitourinary infections	*Streptococcus faecalis* (enterococci)	Microscopic: Smears and cultures
Genitourinary infections Enteric infections	Enterobacter group Escherichia group Klebsiella Proteus group *Pseudomonas aeruginosa*	Microscopic: Smears and cultures

Diseases	Etiologic Agent	Tests for Diagnosis or Susceptibility
Bacillary dysentery	*Shigella dysenteriae* *Shigella flexneri*	Serologic: Agglutination test Microscopic: Culture from stool
Diphtheria	*Corynebacterium diphtheriae* (Klebs-Loeffler bacillus)	Microscopic: Culture from throat or larynx Schick test: Intradermal injection of diluted diphtheria toxin
Food poisoning (botulism)	*Clostridium botulinum*	Animal inoculation for toxin in suspected food
Gas gangrene	*Clostridium perfringens* (Welchii)	Microscopic: Anaerobic culture from lesion
Influenzal meningitis in children	*Hemophilus influenzae* usually type B	Microscopic: Cultures from mouth or nose Typing of organism
Leprosy (Hansen's disease)	*Mycobacterium leprae* (leprosy or Hansen's bacillus)	Microscopic: Smear and culture from cutaneous skin lesions — nodules, plaques, ulcers Animal inoculation
Tuberculosis, pulmonary and extrapulmonary	*Mycobacterium tuberculosis* (tubercle bacillus)	Microscopic: Smear and culture from sputum, gastric, and bronchial washings, drainage and tuberculous lesions from organs Animal inoculation of material Tuberculin tests — Mantoux, Tine, Heaf
Tularemia	*Pasteurella tularensis* (bacterium tularense)	Serologic: Agglutination test Animal inoculation of material Skin test for tularemia
Typhoid fever Paratyphoid fever Food infection	*Salmonella typhi* *Salmonella paratyphi* - A, B or C	Microscopic: Culture from stool and urine Serologic: Widal reaction agglutination of bacilli
Undulant fever (brucellosis)	*Brucella melitensis abortus suis*	Serologic: Agglutination test for undulant fever
Whooping cough (pertussis)	*Bordetella pertussis* (pertussis bacillus)	Microscopic: Culture on cough plate Skin test

C. MYCOTIC DISEASES[e]

Diseases	Etiologic Agent	Tests for Diagnosis
Actinomycosis	Actinomyces	Microscopic: Direct smears or cultures from sinuses, sputum Animal inoculation
Blastomycosis	Blastomyces	Microscopic: Direct smears or culture from abscesses, sputum Animal inoculation

Diseases	Etiologic Agent	Tests for Diagnosis
Candidiasis	Candida albicans (Monilia)	Microscopic: Direct smears and cultures from skin and nail scrapings, sputum, material from vagina
Coccidioido-mycosis	Coccidioides immitis	Microscopic: Direct smears or culture from sputum, gastric content, pleural fluid, abscesses Animal inoculation Skin test
Histoplasmosis	Histoplasma capsulatum	Microscopic: Direct smears or culture of bone marrow, lymph nodes Animal inoculation Skin tests — Tine and intradermal
Nocardiosis	Nocardia asteroides and related species	Microscopic: Cultures from sputum, lung abscesses, brain abscesses, skin or other lesions

D. SPIROCHETAL AND PROTOZOAL DISEASES[f]

Diseases	Etiologic Agent	Tests for Diagnosis
Leptospirosis	Leptospira species: Lept canicola (of dogs) Lept ictero-haemorrhagiae (of rats) Lept pomona (of cattle and swine)	Urine culture Dark-field examination of patient's blood Culture on Korthof's medium Specific agglutination titers Specific serologic tests of anicteric form of leptospirosis
Syphilis	Treponema pallidum	Serologic: Wasserman, Kahn, Kolmer, VDRL and RPCF Dark field examination of scraping from chancre and TPI
Amebic dysentery	Entamoeba histolytica	Microscopic: Examination of fresh stools
Malaria Malignant cerebral malaria	Plasmodium vivax malariae falciparum	Microscopic: Examination of blood smears
Pneumocystis pneumonia	Pneumocystis carini	Lung puncture biopsy
Toxoplasmosis	Toxoplasma gondii	Serologic: Sabin-Feldman dye test Complement fixation Agglutination Fluorescence Skin test

E. METAZOAL DISEASES⁸

Diseases	Etiologic Agent	Tests for Diagnosis
Ascariasis	**Nematodes** Ascaris lumbricoides (large intestinal roundworm)	Stool specimen containing characteristic ova (eggs) Sputum occasionally containing larvae
Enterobiasis	Enterobius vermicularis (pinworm)	Stool specimen containing adult worms Microscopic: Smears from pressure sensitive tape to perianal skin
Filariasis In advanced stage: Elephantiasis	Brugia malayi Wuchereia bancrofti (and other infective larvae)	Day and night blood specimens for identification of microfilariae (motile larvae) Complement fixation Skin test for microfilariae
Hookworm disease	Ancylostoma duodenale (European hookworm) Necator americanus (American hookworm)	Stool specimen containing characteristic eggs — guaiac positive Microscopic: thick fecal smear placed in tube held clear of 1 cm of water in bottom of tube Eggs hatch and larvae migrate to water
Onchocerciasis	Onchocerca volvulus (filarial roundworm)	Aspiration of nodules for detection of eggs Excision of nodules for demonstrating larvae and adult worms Microscopic: skin shavings and conjunctival snips Slitlamp examination for ocular onchocerciasis
Strongyloidiasis	Strongyloides stercoralis (threadworm)	Stool specimen containing larvae or adult worms Duodenal aspiration if not found in stool
Trichinelliasis Trichiniasis Trichinosis	Trichinella spiralis (pork roundworm)	Skin test Precipitation and complement-fixation tests Muscle biopsy for encysted larvae
Trichuriasis Trichocephaliasis	Trichuris trichiura (whipworm)	Stool specimen containing ova of whipworm Concentration by centrifugation if eggs not found in direct fecal smear

Diseases	Etiologic Agent	Tests for Diagnosis
Echinococcosis Hydatid disease	**Cestodes** *Echinococcus granulosis* (small tapeworm)	Microscopic: Examination of cyst contents of hydatid tumor in liver or other organs
Taenia infestation	*Taenia lata Diphyllobothrium latum* (fish tapeworm) *Taenia saginata* (beef tapeworm) *Taenia solium* (pork tapeworm) (3 large tape worms)	Stool specimens containing eggs and segments Microscopic: Examination of segment Skin and complement-fixation tests if cerebral cysticercosis is suspected.
Fasciolopsiasis	**Trematodes** *Fasciolopsis buski* (large intestinal fluke)	Stool specimen containing eggs and occasionally flukes
Schistosomiasis Bilharzias	*Schistosoma haematobium* (vesical or urinary fluke) *Schistosoma japonicum* (intestinal fluke) *Schistosoma mansoni* (intestinal fluke)	Urine specimens containing eggs Cystoscopic biopsy Stool specimen containing eggs Serologic: positive Stool specimen containing eggs Rectal biopsy Serologic: positive

a E. Jawetz, J. L. Melnich and E. A. Adelberg. Adenovirus family — Orthomyxovirus family. *Review of Medical Microbiology*, 12th ed. Los Altos, California: Lange Medical Publications, 1976, pp. 436-441 and 404-413.

b _____. Paramyxovirus family — Picornavirus family. *Ibid.*, pp. 414-424 and 368-380.

c _____. Hepatitis viruses — Herpesvirus family. *Ibid.*, pp. 381-391 and 442-453.

d _____. Pyogenic cocci — Gram-positive bacilli — Mycobacteria — Gram-negative bacilli — Spirochetes and other spiral microorganisms. *Ibid.*, pp. 169-236.

e G. L. Baum. Diagnosis and treatment of systemic mycoses. *Medical Clinics of North America*, 58: 661-681, May, 1975.

f R. S. Goldsmith. Infectious diseases: Protozoal. In Krupp, Marcus A. and Chatton, Milton. *Current Medical Diagnosis and Treatment*, 15th ed. Los Altos, California: Lange Medical Publications, 1976, pp. 850-862.

g _____. Infectious diseases: Metazoal. *Ibid.*, pp. 863-882.

CLINICAL LABORATORY

A. Terms Related to Hematologic and Serologic Tests:

1. infectious mononucleosis
   a. sheep cell differential test — a specific and qualitative test based on the fact that anti-sheep agglutinins in infectious mononucleosis are completely removed with beef cells and are incompletely or not removed with Forssman antigen (guinea pig or horse kidney).[29]

    b. spot test for infectious mononucleosis, Monospot — a complete one-minute differential slide test for the detection of the specific heterophile antibodies associated with infectious mononucleosis.

      Negative test — the agglutination pattern is stronger on the right side of the slide (II).

      Positive test — the agglutination pattern is stronger on the left side of the slide (I). If no agglutination appears on either side of the slide or if agglutination is equal on both sides of the slide (I-II), the test is negative.

      The basic principles of absorption in the Monospot slide test are comparable to those laid down by Davidsohn in the sheep agglutinin differential test.

2. lupus erythematosus

    a. anti-DNP, antinucleoprotein — the most typical antinuclear antibody (ANA) which causes the LE-cell phenomenon and is present in untreated systemic lupus erythematosus (SLE). Antinuclear factors may also be found in rheumatoid arthritis, other connective tissue diseases and disseminated malignancies.

    b. LE-cell — large granulocyte containing purplish stainable inclusions (Wright stain) thinly rimmed with cytoplasm. The nucleus is pushed aside.

    c. LE-cell factor, LE-serum factor — one of several autoantibodies reacting against nucleoprotein to transform nuclei into homogenous globular bodies which are then phagocytized by intact granulocytes to form typical LE-cells.

    d. LE-cell phenomenon — the presence of the LE serum factor (antinucleoprotein factor) causing an agglutination reaction between antigen-treated particles and the serum containing antinuclear globulins.

    e. LE-test — rapid slide test for antinucleoprotein factors associated with systemic lupus erythematosus. The test specimen is compared with control serums.

      Negative test — no agglutination

      Positive test — any degree of agglutination of the latex particles.

3. rheumatoid arthritis

    a. rheumatoid factor — protein belonging to a family of antibodies which evolved in response to antigenic stimulation by an altered immunoglobulin. Consequently they are antiglobulins.[29, 74]

    b. tests for rheumatoid factor — they utilize the ability of antiglobulins to agglutinate cells coated with 7S immunoglobulin. Examples are:

      (1) bentonite flocculation test — pooled human gammaglobulin is used as antigen for coating particles.

      (2) latex fixation test — pooled human gammaglobulin is adsorbed to standard latex particles.

      (3) Rheumanosticon — a rapid slide test for the detection of the rheumatoid factor, performed on serum or whole blood. The rheumatoid factor reacts with the coating material causing a visual agglutination of the inert latex particles.

      Negative end point — the mixture remains milky with no visible flocculation as demonstrated by the negative control.

      Positive end point — coarse agglutinated flocs are present as demonstrated by the positive control.

B. Terms Related to Serologic and Immunologic Tests:

1. antibody labeling with fluorescein — a histochemical technique for identifying antigen and antibody within tissues.

    a. direct immunofluorescent staining — sensitive serologic test in which the specific antibody is labeled with fluorescein and the fluorescing antigen-antibody complex viewed in the tissues.

    b. indirect immunofluorescent method — procedure in which fluorescein-labeled anti-human globulin is employed in the detection of unlabeled antibody in human tissues. Since plasma cells show marked fluorescence, they are thought to be antibody-producing cells.

Examples: Immunofluorescent skin test in systemic lupus erythematosus and rheumatoid factor by indirect immunofluorescence.[5, 7, 27, 74]

2. complement fixation (CF) test — antigen-antibody reaction requiring a complement for the union of antigen and antibody.[2, 27, 30]

3. hemagglutination inhibition (HI) test — the detection of the presence of specific antibodies capable of inhibiting agglutination of red cells by agents such as viruses.[3, 30]

4. immunofluorescence — the tagging of antibodies with a fluorescent dye in order to detect or localize antigen-antibody combinations.[73]

5. neutralization test — detection of the presence of antibodies capable of inactivating an infective agent, thus rendering it noninfective or neutral.[3, 27, 30]

C. Terms Related to Tests for Syphilis:[29, 75]

1. dark-field illumination — test of choice for the detection of primary or secondary syphilis by identifying *Treponema pallidum* in a smear of a suspected lesion.

2. fluorescent treponemal antibody (FTA) test — indirect immunologic test based on a reaction between a treponemal antigen and the specific antispirochetal antibody in the syphilitic serum of the patient. Treponemas coated with fluorescent antibodies are seen under the ultraviolet microscope.

3. fluorescent treponemal antibody-absorption test — of greater sensitivity and specificity for syphilis than the FTA test. Fluorescein tagged antihuman globulin is used as the reaction indicator and the reaction is visualized with an ultraviolet microscope.

4. Kahn test — a flocculation test for syphilis, using a nontreponemal antigen, usually cardiolipin, an extract of beef heart.

5. Kolmer test — a modification of the Wasserman complement fixation test. The antigen used is nonspecific, that is, not derived from *Treponema pallidum*.

6. Reiter protein complement-fixation test (RPCF) — a new reliable test for syphilis. It is essentially Kolmer's technique using Reiter's protein antigen prepared from *Treponema pallidum*.

7. Venereal Disease Research Laboratory — a flocculation test for syphilis which is widely accepted.[73]

8. Wasserman test — original complement fixation test for syphilis, a rather complex procedure. The antigen used is nontreponemal.

ABBREVIATIONS

AD — adenovirus
ALG — antilymphocytic globulin
ALS — antilymphocytic serum
ANA — antinuclear antibodies
APC — adenoidal-pharyngeal-
conjunctival
Arbo — arthropod-borne
ARD — acute respiratory disease
BFP — biologic false positive
(reaction)
CF — complement fixation
CID — cytomegalic inclusion disease
CPE — cytopathic effect
FA — fluorescent antibody
FTA — fluorescent treponemal
antibody
FTA-ABS — fluorescent treponemal
antibody absorption
FUO — fever of unknown origin

GvH — graft versus host
(reactivity)
HI — hemagglutination-inhibition
LE — lupus erythematosus
MHA — microhemagglutination
(test for syphilis)
Nt — neutralization
RPCF — Reiter protein complement fixation
RPR — rapid plasma reagin
RSV — respiratory syncytial virus
SLE — St. Louis encephalitis
SLE — systemic lupus erythematosus
STS — serologic test for syphilis
TPI — *Treponema pallidum* immobilization
va — variety
VD — venereal disease
VDG — venereal disease gonorrhea
VDRL — venereal disease research
laboratory

ORAL READING PRACTICE

Herpes Zoster

Herpes zoster, zoster or shingles is an infectious disease caused by the zoster virus. It is characterized by vesicular lesions which follow the course of a **peripheral nerve** in a band-like fashion. Prior to the eruption, the patient may experience pain for several days without other symptoms. Once the **erythema** and **vesicles** appear in a typical **zoniform** distribution, the diagnosis is readily made. In the beginning, the eruption exhibits slightly **edematous,** fairly well-defined **erythematous,** oval or round areas on which vesicles form in groups. Generally, sensory changes along the path of the affected **neural zones** are associated with the eruption. Pain precedes, accompanies and follows the appearance of the skin lesion. It varies in duration and intensity from slight, brief **hyperesthesia** to **paroxysmal** attacks of pain or persistent, excruciating **neuralgia.** Similar to other nerve root involvements, the pain is especially agonizing at night and is intensified by motion. In rare cases it has led to drug addiction and even suicide. **Paresthesia** of the skin may be brought on by touching the affected area or it may develop spontaneously. In addition, the patient may develop tender, enlarged lymph nodes, rheumatic pains and general **malaise.**

Although the characteristic feature of the disease is the skin eruption, herpes zoster is essentially an inflammation of one or more posterior root ganglia. The rash is confined to the **dermal segment** supplied by the sensory nerve arising from the involved **posterior (sensory) root ganglion.** The **neurotropic virus** destroys the ganglion cells and fibers. These changes result in a degeneration of the corresponding peripheral nerve.

One of the most painful forms of herpes is Zoster ophthalmicus, caused by a viral infection of the **trigeminal nerve.** This may lead to corneal ulceration, keratitis, iritis, conjunctivitis and edema of the eyelids.

Zoster oticus results from an inflammation of the **vestibulocochlear** nerve and is associated with deafness, **vertigo, tinnitus** and severe pain.[78]

REFERENCES AND BIBLIOGRAPHY

1. Austen, K. F. Disorders due to hypersensitivity and altered immune response. In Wintrobe, Maxwell M (ed.). *Harrison's Principles of Internal Medicine,* 7th ed. New York: McGraw-Hill Book Co., 1974, pp. 342-348.

2. Banks, P. M. *et al.* American Burkitt's lymphoma. *American Journal of Medicine,* 58: 322-329, March, 1975.

3. Baum, G. L. Diagnosis and treatment of systemic mycoses. *Medical Clinics of North America,* 58: 661-681, May, 1974.

4. Bearn, A. G. The Marfan syndrome. In Beeson, P. B. and McDermott, W. (eds.). *Textbook of Medicine,* 14th ed. Philadelphia: W. B. Saunders Co., 1975, pp. 1869-1870.

5. Caperton, E. M. *et al.* Immunofluorescent skin test in systemic lupus erythematosus. *Journal of American Medical Association,* 222: 935-937, November 20, 1972.

6. Chatton, M. J. *et al.* Marfan's syndrome. In Krupp, Marcus A. and Chatton, Milton J. *Current Medical Diagnosis and Treatment,* 15th ed. Los Altos, California: Lange Medical Publications, 1976, pp. 781-782.

7. Cooperative Study. Uses for immunofluorescence tests of skin and sera: Utilization of immunofluorescence in the diagnosis of bullous diseases, lupus erythematosus and certain other dermatoses. *Archives of Dermatology,* 111: 371-381, March, 1975.

8. Coronavirus: Newly found in victims of chronic bronchitis. *Infectious Diseases,* 4: 3-23, December, 1974.

9. Davidsohn, Israel *et al.* Immunohematology. In *Todd-Sanford Clinical Diagnosis by Laboratory Methods,* 15th ed. Philadelphia: W. B. Saunders Co., 1974, pp. 223-236.

10. Davis, Bernard D, Renato Dulbecco, Herman N. Eisen, Harold S. Ginsberg and W. Barry Wood. *Microbiology Including Immunology and Molecular Genetics,* 2d ed. New York: Harper & Row, Publishers, Inc. 1973, pp. 894-896.

11. Dubois, E. L. (ed.). *Lupus Erythematosus.* Los Angeles: University of Southern California Press, 1974.

12. Engleman, E. P. *et al.* Systemic lupus erythematosus. In Krupp, Marcus A. and Chatton, Milton. *Current Medical Diagnosis and Treatment,* 15th ed. Los Altos, California: Lange Medical Publications, 1976, pp. 483-486.

13. _____. Dermatomyositis, polyarteritis, diffuse scleroderma, *Ibid.,* pp. 486-488.

14. Faraci, R. P. Malignant lymphoma of the jejunum in a patient with Wiskott-Aldrich syndrome. *Archives of Surgery,* 110: 218-220, February, 1975.

15. Franklin, E. C. Immunoglobulins and immunologic deficiency states. In Wintrobe, Maxwell M. (ed.). *Harrison's Principles of Internal Medicine,* 7th ed. New York: McGraw-Hill Book Co., 1974, pp. 348-353.

16. ————. Multiple myeloma and other plasma cell and lymphocytic dyscrasias. *Ibid.*, pp. 354-359.

17. ————. μ-Chain disease (Micron chain disease) *Archives of Internal Medicine*, 135: 71-72, January, 1975.

18. Goldin, M. Medical mycology. In Davidsohn, Israel and Henry, John B. (eds.). *Todd-Sanford Clinical Diagnosis by Laboratory Methods*, 15th ed. Philadelphia: W. B. Saunders Co., 1974, pp. 1118-1150.

19. Goldsmith, R. S. Infectious diseases: Protozoal. In Krupp, Marcus and Chatton, Milton. *Current Medical Diagnosis and Treatment*, 15th ed. Los Altos, California: Lange Medical Publications, 1976, pp. 850-862.

20. ————. Infectious diseases: Metazoal. *Ibid.*, pp. 863-882.

21. Graville, R. *et al.* Hepatitis A: Report of a common source outbreak with recovery of a possible etiologic agent. *Journal of Infectious Diseases*, 131: 167-171, February, 1975.

22. Grayston, J. T. *et al.* Viral diseases of the eye. In Wintrobe, Maxwell M. (ed.). *Harrison's Principles of Internal Medicine*, 7th ed. New York: McGraw-Hill Book Co., 1974, pp. 979-981.

23. Gregor, R. E. Familial progressive systemic scleroderma. *Archives of Dermatology*, 111: 81-85, January, 1975.

24. Grossman, M. *et al.* Infectious diseases: Viral and rickettsial — Bacterial. In Krupp, Marcus A. and Chatton, Milton. *Current Medical Diagnosis and Treatment*, 15th ed. Los Altos, California: Lange Medical Publications, 1976, pp. 791-840.

25. Halde, C. Infectious diseases: Mycotic. In Krupp, Marcus A. and Chatton, Milton. *Current Medical Diagnosis and Treatment*, 15th ed. Los Altos, California: Lange Medical Publications, 1976, pp. 883-890.

26. Hall, C. B. *et al.* Clinically useful method for the isolation of respiratory syncytial virus. *Journal of Infectious Diseases*, 131: 1-5, January, 1975.

27. Jawetz, Ernest, Melnick, Joseph L. and Adelberg, Edward A. Immunology I. Antigens and antibodies. *Review of Medical Microbiology*, 12th ed. Los Altos, California: Lange Medical Publications, 1976, pp. 137-155.

28. ————. Immunology: II. Antibody-mediated and cell-mediated (hypersensitivity and immunity) reactions. *Ibid.*, pp. 156-168.

29. ————. Principles of diagnostic medical microbiology. *Ibid.*, pp. 272-288.

30. ————. Isolation of viruses from clinical specimens — Serologic diagnosis of virus infections. *Ibid.*, pp. 329-335.

31. ————. Adenovirus family — Herpesvirus family. *Ibid.*, pp. 436-453.

32. ————. Arthropod-borne (Arbo) viral diseases. *Ibid.*, pp. 352-367.

33. ————. Orthomyxovirus family — Paramyxovirus family and rubella virus. *Ibid.*, pp. 404-424.

34. ————. Pyogenic cocci — Gram-positive bacilli. *Ibid.*, pp. 169-191.

35. ————. Mycobacteria — Gram-negative organisms. *Ibid.*, pp. 196-224.

36. ————. Spirochetes and other spiral microorganisms — Chlamydiae. *Ibid.*, pp. 225-244.

37. ————. Medical parasitology. *Ibid.*, pp. 492-523.

38. Johns, C. J. Sarcoidosis. In Wintrobe, Maxwell M. (ed.). *Harrison's Principles of Internal Medicine*, 7th ed. New York: McGraw-Hill Book Co., 1974, pp. 1058-1063.

39. Joklik, Wolfgang K. and Willet, Hilda P. (eds.). *Zinsser Microbiology*, 16th ed. New York: Appleton-Century-Crofts, 1976, pp. 1115-1165.

40. Kilbourne, E. E. Introduction to viral diseases — Measles — Rubella. In Beeson, P. B. and McDermott, W. (eds.). *Textbook of Medicine*, 14th ed. Philadelphia: W. B. Saunders Co., 1975, pp. 182-205.

41. Koff, R. S. *et al.* Acute hepatitis. In Wintrobe, Maxwell M. (ed.). *Harrison's Principles of Internal Medicine*, 7th ed. New York: McGraw-Hill Book Co., 1974, pp. 1528-1537.

42. ————. Chronic active hepatitis. *Ibid.*, pp. 1537-1540.

43. Krain, L. S. Dermatomyositis in six patients without initial muscle involvement. *Archives of Dermatology*, 111: 241-245, February, 1975.

44. Levin, W. C. Multiple myeloma. *Archives of Internal Medicine*, 135: 27-28, January, 1975.

45. Marymont, J. H. Influenza — Parainfluenza (PI) viruses — Rhinoviruses. In Davidsohn, Israel and Henry, John B. (eds.). *Clinical Diagnosis by Laboratory Methods*, 15th ed. Philadelphia: W. B. Saunders Co., 1974, pp. 1183-1190.

46. McCabe, W. R. *et al.* The relation of K-antigen to virulence of *Escherichia coli*. *Journal of Infectious Diseases*, 131: 6-10, January, 1975.

47. McHenry, M. C. *et al.* Hospital-acquired pneumonia. *Medical Clinics of North America*, 58: 565-580, May, 1974.

48. McQuay, R. M. Medical parasitology. In Davidsohn, Israel and Henry, John B. (eds.). *Todd-Sanford Clinical Diagnosis by Laboratory Methods*, 15th ed. Philadelphia: W. B. Saunders Co., 1974, pp. 1020-1117.

49. Merrill, J. P. *et al.* Transplantation — immunologic considerations. In Wintrobe, Maxwell M. (ed.). *Harrison's Principles of Internal Medicine*, 7th ed. New York: McGraw-Hill Book Co., 1974, pp. 359-368.

50. Neurath, A. R. *et al.* Thyroxine binding by hepatitis B surface antigen. *Journal of Infectious Diseases*, 131: 172-175, February, 1975.

51. Niederman, J. C. Infectious mononucleosis. In Wintrobe, Maxwell M. (ed.). *Harrison's Principles of Internal Medicine*, 7th ed. New York: McGraw-Hill Book Co., 1974, pp. 1063-1068.

52. Petersdorf, R. G. Nosocomial infections. In Wintrobe, Maxwell M. (ed.). *Harrison's Principles of Internal Medicine*, 7th ed. New York: McGraw-Hill Book Co., 1974, pp. 730-734.

53. Peterson, D. R. *et al.* Prevalence of antibody to Toxoplasma among Alaskan natives. *Journal of Infectious Diseases*, 130: 557-563, December, 1974.

54. Plorde, J. J. *et al.* Diseases caused by protozoa. In Wintrobe, Maxwell M. (ed.). *Harrison's Principles of Internal Medicine*, 7th ed. New York: McGraw-Hill Book Co., 1974, pp. 1014-1029.

55. _____. Diseases caused by worms. *Ibid.*, pp. 1035-1058.

56. Pinworm infestations rampant in children. *Infectious Diseases*, 4: 1-9, December, 1974.

57. Pirofsky, B. Immune haemolytic disease: The autoimmune haemolytic anemias. *Clinics in Haematology*, 4: 167-180, February, 1975.

58. Ritzmann, S. E. *et al.* Idiopathic (asymptomatic) monoclonal gammopathies. *Archives of Internal Medicine*, 135: 95-108, January, 1975.

59. Robbins, Stanley L. Cytomegalic inclusion disease. *Pathologic Basis of Disease*. Philadelphia: W. B. Saunders Co., 1974, pp. 560-563.

60. _____. Sarcoidosis — Cystic fibrosis. *Ibid.*, pp. 467-470 and 560-563.

61. _____. Diseases caused by helminths. *Ibid.*, pp. 456-466.

62. _____. Diseases of immunity. *Ibid.*, pp. 194-258.

63. Rosenthal, M. S. Viral infections of the central nervous system. *Medical Clinics of North America*, 58: 593-604, May, 1974.

64. Sanford, J. P. Arbovirus and adenovirus infections. In Wintrobe, Maxwell M. (ed.). *Harrison's Principles of Internal Medicine*, 7th ed. New York: McGraw-Hill Book Co., 1974, pp. 990-1012.

65. _____. Leptospirosis. In Beeson, Paul B. and McDermott, Walsh, (eds.). *Textbook of Medicine*, 14th ed. Philadelphia: W. B. Saunders Co., 1975, pp. 438-442.

66. Santos, G. W. Immunosuppression in clinical marrow transplantation. *Seminars in Hematology*, 11: 341-351, July, 1974.

67. Sheldon, W. H. Cytomegalic inclusion disease (salivary gland virus disease). In Wintrobe, Maxwell M. (ed.). *Harrison's Principles of Internal Medicine*, 7th ed. New York: McGraw-Hill Book Co., 1974, pp. 989-990.

68. _____. *Pneumocystis carini* pneumonia (pneumocystis interstitial plasma cell pneumonia). *Ibid.*, pp. 1031-1033.

69. *Stedman's Medical Dictionary*, 23rd ed. Baltimore: The Williams and Wilkins Co., 1976, p. 1306.

70. Strober, S. *et al.* Immunologic disorders. In Krupp, Marcus A. and Chatton, Milton. *Current Medical Diagnosis and Treatment*, 15th ed. Los Altos, California: Lange Medical Publications, 1976, pp. 987-998.

71. Symuness, W. *et al.* Hepatitis B surface antigen in blood donors. *Journal of Infectious Diseases*, 131: 111-118, February, 1975.

72. Tager, Ira *et al.* Role of infection in chronic bronchitis. *New England Journal of Medicine*, 292: 563-569, March 13, 1975.

73. Tucker, Eugene, M.D. Personal communications.

74. Vardiman, J. *et al.* Localization of rheumatoid factor by direct immunofluorescence. *Laboratory Medicine*, 3: 39-40, November, 1972.

75. Varmus, H. Infectious diseases: Spirochetal. In Krupp, Marcus A. and Chatton, Milton. *Current Medical Diagnosis and Treatment*, 15th ed. Los Altos, California: Lange Medical Publications, 1976, pp. 841-849.

76. Weinstein, L. Diseases caused by toxin-producing bacteria. In Wintrobe, Maxwell M. (ed.). *Harrison's Principles of Internal Medicine*, 7th ed. New York: McGraw-Hill Book Co., 1974, pp. 841-855.

77. Wintrobe, Maxwell M. Viral diseases of the respiratory tract. *Harrison's Principles of Internal Medicine*, 7th ed. New York: McGraw-Hill Book Co., 1974, pp. 928-942.

78. _____. Diseases with lesions of skin or mucous membrane. *Ibid.*, pp. 961-979.

79. _____. Diseases caused by gram-positive cocci, gram-negative cocci, gram-negative bacilli. *Ibid.*, pp. 766-834.

80. _____. Diseases caused by fungi — Spirochetal diseases, *Ibid.*, pp. 876-907.

81. Wintrobe, Maxwell M. *et al.* Macroglobulinemia, heavy chain diseases and other lymphocyte and plasma cell dyscrasias. *Clinical Hematology*, 7th ed. Philadelphia: Lea and Febiger, 1974, pp. 1624-1648.

82. Woodruff, C. *et al.* The challenge of cystic fibrosis. *Missouri Medicine*, 72: 129-133, March, 1975.

83. Wuthrich, R. C. *et al.* Localized scleroderma. *Archives of Dermatology*, 111: 98-100, January, 1975.

Chapter XVI
Geriatrics and Psychogeriatrics

ORIENTATION

A. Origin of Terms:

1. arcus (L) — bow, arch
2. asthenia (G) — weakness
3. chalasis (G) — a slackening
4. geras (G) — old age
5. geron (G) — old man
6. presbys (G) — old
7. rhytis (G) — wrinkle
8. senilis (L) — old
9. senium (L) — old age
10. senescere (L) — to grow old

B. General Terms:

1. geriatrician — specialist in diseases of old age.
2. geriatrics — branch of medical science concerned with the diseases of old age and their treatment.
3. gerontologist — scientist who studies the process of aging in its biologic, mental and socioeconomic implications.
4. gerontology — the scientific study of all facets of aging including branches of science which contribute to an understanding of older adults such as physiology, psychology, sociology and public health.[17, 18, 19]
5. podiatrist — specialist concerned with the diagnosis and treatment of defects, injuries and diseases of the feet. Older adults are in particular need of the services of a podiatrist.
6. presbyatrics, presbytiatrics — the medical treatment of the aging.
7. psychogerontology — science that deals with the mental and emotional life of older persons, their ideation, memory and level of consciousness.[25, 26]
8. senescence — the declining years of life or a normal process of growing old.[17, 18, 19]
9. senility — old age with its mental and physical infirmities.

SOME PHYSICAL DISORDERS OF OLDER ADULTS*

A. Diagnostic Terms:

1. cranial arteritis, giant cell arteritis, arteritis of the aged — a panarteritis of older adults primarily involving the temporal arteries, ophthalmic and retinal arteries and clinically noted for a boring headache, scalp tenderness; pain, blanching and occasionally gangrene of the tongue probably due to lingual arteritis; peripheral neuropathy and sudden blindness.[23]
2. osteitis deformans, Paget's disease of bone — a skeletal disorder characterized by decalcification, marked bone destruction and rapid bone repair, architectural abnormality of new bone, increased vascularity and fibrosis. Striking features are its intensification with advancing years, fracture proneness and the frequency of a coexisting osteogenic sarcoma.[10, 14, 20]
3. polymyalgia rheumatica — a special type of muscular rheumatism seen more frequently

---

*These disorders of the aging belong to the large group of physical infirmities which afflict the elderly, but may also be found in younger age groups.

Since the adjective "senile" has a connotation, unacceptable and disconcerting to those older individuals who possess their cognitive faculties, it is advisable to delete it in relation to physical illness and to use it rarely if ever in reference to irreversible dementia. Even as the finality of life is imminent the aged person still needs a wholesome degree of self-esteem to sustain his mental health.

in older women than men, clinically manifested by pain and stiffness in back, shoulder, neck and occasionally in pelvic girdle.[11]

4. senescent (senile) macular degeneration* — a degenerative process initially noted by a disturbance of pigmentation in the macula, associated with abnormal foveal reflex and leading to visual loss in the aging.[20]

5. senescent (senile) osteoporosis* — a disorder of protein metabolism seen in the aging marked by increased porosity of bone which is especially pronounced in the spine and pelvis and leads to spontaneous fractures, deformities and collapse of vertebrae with reduction of the person's height.[20, 23]

6. senescent (senile) purpura* — hemorrhagic disorder characterized by easy bruising and purple extravasations chiefly on arms and legs of aging skin.

7. senescent (senile) sebaceous adenomas* — benign lesions, typically appearing on the face of elderly persons as pearly oval papules with a central depression.

B. Operative Terms:

1. blepharoplasty for blepharochalasis — plastic repair of redundant eyelids.[13]
2. dermabrasion and excision of
   a. furrowed brows — application of dermabrader to frown furrows and removal of skin over furrowed area.
   b. perioral wrinkles — application of dermabrader to each vertical lip line for elimination of wrinkles around the mouth.[22]
3. face-lift operation — reconstructive plastic surgery of the face, the art of surgical sculpture applied to the human face to restore function, remove the marks of time and correct defects.[22, 27]
4. rhytidectomy — surgical removal of subcutaneous fat pads and superfluous skin to eliminate wrinkles.[2, 16, 22]
5. rhytidoplasty — surgical elimination of wrinkles achieved by removal of excess skin and tightening of remaining skin to restore youthful appearance. A dermal fat graft is inserted in the following forms of repair:
   a. glabellar rhytidoplasty — operative procedure for removing the vertical furrows between the eyebrows.
   b. cervicofacial rhytidoplasty — surgical correction of wrinkles of the neck and face.[22, 28]

C. Symptomatic Terms:

1. arcus senilis, gerontoxon — white or grayish opaque ring just within the sclerocorneal junction of the eye, seen in elderly persons.
2. blepharochalasis — relaxed, baggy eyelids; redundancy may interfere with vision.
3. geroderma — atrophic, thinned and wrinkled skin of old age.
4. gerontopia, senopia — second sight.
5. presbyacusia, presbycusis — impaired perception and discrimination of sounds seen in the aging.
6. presbyopia — defective vision resulting from changes in accommodation in the aging process.
7. progeria of adult — premature aging including early graying, baldness, sparse eyebrows, fine wrinkles around the mouth, others.
8. senescent (senile) pruritus* — itching of brittle, dry skin of the aged leading to scratching followed by excoriations and eczematoid changes.
9. senescent (senile) tremor* — in the aged this is usually an intention tremor of variable etiology, rarely a constant tremor.

SOME MENTAL DISORDERS OF OLDER ADULTS

A. Diagnostic Terms:

1. Alzheimer's disease — a degenerative disorder beginning in the fifth or sixth decade of life, pathologically characterized by cortical atrophy, loss of nerve cells, senile plaques in

*See footnote p. 318.

gray matter and neurofibrillar degeneration. The onset of the dementia is insidious. The patient loses interest in social contacts, becomes anxious, depressed, disoriented; aphasia, agnosia and apraxia develop; the gait shows a hesitant shuffle and incapacitating flexion contractures mark the terminal decerebrate phase of life.[4, 21, 29]

2. organic brain syndrome — permanent damage to brain tissue leading to cerebral insufficiency and deterioration of cognitive faculties. It is usually associated with advanced cerebral atherosclerosis in the aging.[4, 21, 29]

3. Pick's disease — progressive dementia due to severe cortical atrophy of frontal and/or temporal lobes. The presence of Pick bodies in cortical neurons clinches the diagnosis. Characteristically there is relative retention of concrete learned material and of personal orientation.[4, 21, 29]

4. senescent (senile) psychoses — inclusive term concerned with a variety of states from mild senescent mental disorders to the extreme deterioration of senile dementia. Kolb refers to the following clinical types.

    a. delirium and confusion — a psychotic reaction to fever, dehydration, surgery and other somatic states. The aged is disoriented, bewildered, hallucinating and wandering about aimlessly.

    b. depression and agitation — psychotic state characterized by egocentric behavior, melancholy, intense agitation, defective memory and mental decline.

    c. paranoia — a common psychotic reaction of senescence in which delusions of persecution tend to predominate.

    d. presbyophrenia — mental disorder found in older individuals who previously had a dynamic personality. The presbyophrenic patient is constantly busy in an unproductive or destructive way, he is out of touch with reality, very forgetful, covering up his memory lapses with confabulations.

    e. senile dementia — irreversible deterioration of cognitive faculties.[4, 21]

B. Symptomatic Terms:

1. agnosia — sensory inability to recognize objects.
2. alienation — estrangement felt by the (aged) individual in a cultural environment that he considers undesirable, unpredictable, and detrimental to his way of life.
3. aloneness — a feeling of being forsaken or left alone due to the loss of family members and friends.[29]
4. apraxia — total disability to execute purposeful movements although muscle strength, coordination and sensibility appear intact.
5. confabulation — making up tales to fill in memory gaps. The patient is not construing deliberate falsehoods but believes his fantasies to be true.
6. disengagement — a term used by Cumming and Henry in reference to an inevitable mutual withdrawal of the aging individual resulting in decreased social interaction. Multiple factors precipitate disengagement: sensory deficits, especially loss of hearing and sight, retirement, reduced income, declining physical and mental capacities and progressive isolation due to the death of friends and relations. Disengagement is only unhealthy in its extreme form.[4, 7, 29]
7. grief reaction — a bereavement by the death of, or separation from a significant person which may be first expressed by a feeling of numbness and later by profound yearning for the lost one, restlessness and psychophysiologic responses. It may also be related to matters of importance such as enforced retirement or loss of home.[21]
8. depression — morbid sadness, melancholy, dejection out of proportion with loss or injury endured; frequently observed in the aged.
9. regression — return to infantile patterns of reacting, seen in psychosis, severe illness and under other circumstances.
10. rigidity — an abnormal resistance to change.

ABBBREVIATIONS

AAHA — American Association of Homes
for the Aging

AARP — American Association of
Retired Persons

ANHA — American Nursing Home
Association

AOA — Administration on Aging

HUD — Housing and Urban Development

NCOA — National Council on the
Aging

VISTA — Volunteers in Service
to America

WHCoA — White House Conference
on Aging

ORAL READING PRACTICE
ATHEROSCLEROTIC OCCLUSIVE DISEASE OF THE DESCENDING
AORTA AND ITS MAIN BRANCHES

Despite variable pathologic features **atherosclerotic occlusive** disease exhibits a distinctive pattern especially as to the extent and location of the occlusion. No matter where the **obliterative** process occurs the lesion is generally **segmental** in nature and well localized.[9] It is significant that a comparatively normal **patent lumen** exists **proximal** and **distal** to the obstructed segment. Confirmatory evidence of these characteristic findings is provided by **arteriography** which is of primary importance in diagnostic evaluation.

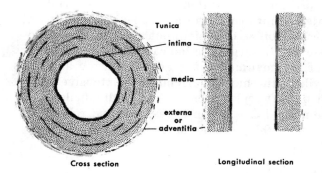

Cross section   Longitudinal section

Fig. 78 — Normal artery, arterial coats and lumen.

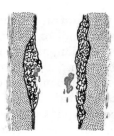

Fig. 81 — Atheromatous plaques in intima, capillary bleeding and early mural thrombosis.

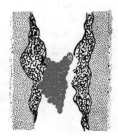

Fig. 83 — Rupture of ulcerated, intimal plaque, mural thrombosis and occlusion.

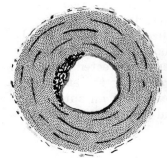

Fig. 79 — Early atherosclerosis.

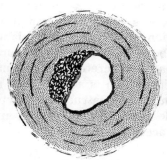

Fig. 80 — Advanced atherosclerosis.

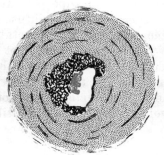

Fig. 82 — Far advanced atherosclerosis.

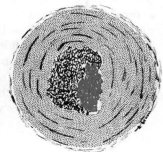

Fig. 84 — Thrombosis and occlusion.

As in occlusive vascular disease of the heart and brain the pathologic lesions consist of **intimal atheromatous plaques** with or without **thrombus** formation.[23] Their typical location is the bifurcation of arteries where they produce arterial obstruction followed by **arterial** insufficiency of the parts distal to the occlusive process. The segmental localization of the **atheromatous** lesions permits a direct surgical attack for restoring the circulation in the major blood vessels. Three basic operative procedures are currently advocated: **thromboendarterectomy, excision** and

graft replacement and graft bypass.[9]   Severe coexisting **cardiac** and **cerebral** disease as well as far advanced senescence are considered contraindications, but elderly persons, otherwise in fair health, are thought to be good candidates for surgical intervention.   Low risk patients with **compensated heart disease, diabetes mellitus** and **hypertension** are also advised to undergo surgery.

The most common types of **atherosclerotic vascular** disease apart from **coronary** or cerebral involvement are **aortoiliac** and **femoropopliteal** occusions and occlusions of the **renal** artery.

Aortoiliac Occlusions

The **aortic bifurcation occlusion syndrome** or Leriche's syndrome is also known as chronic **aortoiliac thrombosis.**   This progressive atheromatous occlusive disease of the abdominal aorta is seen chiefly in males of middle age or advancing years.[9]

Symptoms are those of **ischemia** including coldness, intermittent **claudication, paresthesias** and muscular **atrophy** of the lower extremities.   **Peripheral** pulses of the **femoral, popliteal** and **pedal** regions tend to be markedly decreased to the point of being barely palpable or completely absent. **Ischemic** changes may eventually produce **pregangrenous** or gangrenous lesions of the feet. Another significant feature is a soft blowing **systolic murmur** heard over the abdomen.

The **pathologic** picture usually reveals atheromatous mural lesions of considerable extent with relatively uninvolved proximal and distal arterial segments adjoining the occlusion.

Angiographic studies are imperative, since they provide **visualization** of the entire arterial tree below the area where the **contrast medium** is injected into the aorta at the level of the twelfth **lumbar vertebra.**   This method not only demonstrates aortoiliac occlusion, but also an associated superficial **femoral** artery occlusion, should it be present.   If surgery is indicated both occlusions can be corrected in one operation.   In the presence of minimal **medial** and **adventitial** mural lesions which are well localized, a thromboendarterectomy will be the method of choice.   Extensive obstructive lesions are usually treated by excision with graft replacement.   Aged individuals seem to get best results from **bypass** grafts.[9]   Since normal circulation is restored and followed by symptomatic relief, surgical intervention has proven highly satisfactory.

Femoropopliteal Occlusions

The atherosclerotic obstruction in the femoropopliteal region tends to be discrete, locally confined to a segment and framed on either side by comparatively normal arterial lumen.   There may be extensive involvement of the superficial femoral artery with **patency** of the popliteal artery.   Sometimes the occlusive lesion is diffuse and spreads to the small arteries of the calf making surgery impossible.   Principal manifestations are intermittent **claudication** and **peripheral** ischemia.   **Radiographic** visualization should not be restricted to the femoropopliteal arteries but include the iliacs and abdominal aorta to insure that no discrete lesions remain undetected.   The operation of choice is femoropopliteal reconstruction which is achieved by removing the **saphenous** vein from the knee to the **saphenofemoral junction.**   The obstruction is bypassed by an **autogenous** graft of the saphenous vein.   Since distal **pulsatile** blood flow is restored and symptoms are relieved, the objectives of the surgical attack are accomplished.[1, 8, 9]

Occlusions of the Renal Artery

When atherosclerotic renal artery occlusion is associated with hypertension it requires **antihypertensive** therapy.   The occlusive process may occur **unilaterally** or **bilaterally.**   **Aortography** permits visualization of the renal arteries and their occlusive lesions.   The normal circulation to the kidney may be restored by a bypass graft.

Results of Vascular Surgery

De Bakey and Crawford, prominent **cardiovascular** surgeons, reported gratifying results in 1221 patients who had undergone surgery for aortoiliac and femoropopliteal occlusions despite the fact that many if not most of them were of advanced age.[9]   Recent reports by Barker and Cutler show similar success.[1, 8]

Vascular occlusion presents a major health problem in senescence.   Its onset and insidious continuance is part of physiologic aging.   It assumes pathologic dimensions only after months or years of undetected progress.   It must be emphasized that modern vascular surgery can provide relief for aging patients with atherosclerotic occlusive disease.

REFERENCES AND BIBLIOGRAPHY

1. Barker, W. F. et al. The current status of femoropopliteal bypass for arteriosclerotic occlusive disease. *Surgery*, 79: 30-36, January, 1976.
2. Berner, R. E. et al. Hematoma after rhytidectomy. *Plastic and Reconstructive Surgery*, 57: 314-319, March, 1976.
3. Beverly, E. V. Raising the retiree's level of safety consciousness. *Geriatrics*, 31: 119-125, June, 1976.
4. Brophy, J. J. Psychiatric disorders — Geriatric disorders. In Krupp, Marcus A. and Chatton, Milton J. *Current Medical Diagnosis & Treatment*, 15th ed. Los Altos, California: Lange Medical Publications, 1976, pp. 638-644.
5. Burch, G. E. Interesting aspects of geriatric cardiology. *American Heart Journal*, 89: 99-113, January, 1975.
6. Caldwell, J. R. (ed.). Symposium: Perspectives in hypertension — 1976. *Geriatrics*, 31: 46-130, January, 1976.
7. Cumming, E. and Henry, W. E. *Growing Old*. New York: Basic Books, 1961, pp. 293-296.
8. Cutler, B. S. et al. Autologous saphenous vein femoropopliteal bypass: Analysis of 298 cases. *Surgery*, 79: 325-331, March, 1976.
9. DeBakey, M. E. and Crawford, E. S. Atherosclerotic occlusive vascular disease. *Modern Concepts of Cardiovascular Disease*, 29: 571-576, January, 1960.
10. Duvoisin, R. Parkinsonism. *Clinical Symposia*, 28: 3-29, March, 1976.
11. Engleman, E. P. et al. Arthritis & allied rheumatic disorders. In Krupp, Marcus A. and Chatton, Milton J. *Current Medical Diagnosis and Treatment*, 15th ed. Los Altos, California: Lange Medical Publications, 1976, pp. 488-501.
12. Frenay, Sr. Agnes Clare and Pierce, Gloria. The climate of care for a geriatric patient. *American Journal of Nursing*, 71: 1747-1750, September, 1971.
13. Graham, W. P. et al. Blepharoplasty. *Plastic and Reconstructive Surgery*, 57: 57-61, January, 1976.
14. Greer, M. Achieving maximum benefit in Parkinson's disease. *Geriatrics*, 31: 89-96, April, 1976.
15. Gutman, E. et al. Fast and slow motor units in aging. *Gerontology — International Journal*, 22: 280-300, 1976.
16. Juri, J. et al. Reconstruction of the sideburn for alopecia after rhytidectomy. *Plastic and Reconstructive Surgery*, 57: 304-307, March, 1976.
17. Kent, S. Structural changes in the brain may short-circuit transfer of information. *Geriatrics*, 31: 128-131, June, 1976.
18. _____. Scientists count brain cells to figure theory of aging. *Ibid.*, 31: 114-122, April, 1976.
19. _____. Why do we grow old. *Ibid.*, 31: 135-138, February, 1976.
20. Kolb, F. O. Metabolic bone disease — Non-metabolic bone disease. *Current Medical Diagnosis & Treatment*, 15th ed. Los Altos, California: Lange Medical Publications, 1976, pp. 679-686.
21. Kolb, Lawrence C. Bereavement — Senile and presenile psychoses. *Modern Clinical Psychiatry*, 8th ed. Philadelphia: W. B. Saunders Co., 1973, pp. 142-195.
22. Pickrell, K. L. Reconstructive plastic surgery of the face. *Clinical Symposia*, 19: 71-99, July-August-September, 1967.
23. Robbins, Stanley L. Diseases of aging. *Pathologic Basis of Disease*, Philadelphia: W. B. Saunders Co., 1974, pp. 571-607.
24. Small, M. L. et al. Senile macular degeneration. *Archives of Ophthalmology*, 94: 601-611, April, 1976.
25. Steger, H. G. Understanding the psychologic factors of rehabilitation. *Geriatrics*, 31: 68-76, May, 1976.
26. Storandt, M. Psychologic aspects. In Steinberg, F. U. *Cowdry's The Care of the Geriatric Patient*, 5th ed. St. Louis: The C. V. Mosby Co., 1976, pp. 321-333.
27. Sturman, M. J. Sideburn relationship in the male face lift. *Plastic and Reconstructive Surgery*, 57: 248-250, February, 1976.
28. Vinas, J. C. et al. Forehead rhytidoplasty and brow lifting. *Plastic and Reconstructive Surgery*, 57: 445-454, April, 1976.
29. Weinberg, J. Geriatric psychiatry. In Freedman, Alfred M., Kaplan, Harold I., Sadock, Benjamin J. *Comprehensive Textbook of Psychiatry*, 2d ed. Baltimore: Williams & Wilkins Co., 1975, pp. 2405-2420.

PART II

SUPPLEMENTARY TERMS

Chapter XVII
Selected Terms Pertaining to Oncology
ORIENTATION

A. Origin of Terms:

1. astro- (G) — star
2. benign (L) — mild
3. carcino- (G) — cancer
4. ependyma (G) — wrap
5. glia (G) — glue
6. kerato- (G) — horny
7. malignant (L) — of bad kind
8. medulla (L) — marrow
9. oma (G) — tumor
10. onco (G) — mass
11. plakia (G) — plate
12. plasia (G) — a molding
13. proliferate (L) — to bear offspring
14. sarco (G) — flesh
15. scirrhous (G) — hard
16. tumor (G) — swelling

B. Terms Used in Oncology:

1. anaplasia — undifferentation in tissue cells frequently accompanied by malignant behavior.[26]
2. autonomy — disregard by the malignant tumor for normal limitations of growth.
3. behavior of tumor — a biologic interpretation indicating the potentialities of a new growth; for example, its ability to spread its histologic appearance, cellular proliferation (rapid cell division) and others.[21]
4. benign — mild, not malignant, not recurrent.
5. cachexia — a progressive state of malnutrition, emaciation, debilitation and anemia.
6. cancer — a group of malignant diseases characterized by uncontrolled cell growth.
7. cancer cell — a cell which has lost its control mechanism as seen in cell culture. A new antigen emerges from the transformed cell.[21]
8. carcinogenic agent — an agent capable of inducing a carcinoma.
9. carcinoid, argentaffinoma — tumor, chiefly found in intestine and derived from argentaffin cells. Contains a large amount of serotonin and may metastasize.[26]
10. carcinolysis — destruction of cancer cells.
11. carcinoma — malignant neoplasm which arises from epithelial tissue.
12. carcinoma in situ — a true malignant tumor of squamous or glandular epithelium in which no invasion of underlying or adjacent structures has occurred. Lesions may remain in situ (position) for an indefinite period, even years, before they become invasive.
13. dedifferentiation — alterations toward decreased specialization of tissue.[21]
14. differentiation — specialization of a tissue or organ to perform a particular function. It is accompanied by characteristic morphologic alterations simulating parent tissue.[21]
15. dyskeratosis — premature keratinization of epidermal cells due to a defect in keratin formation. It may be benign or malignant.
16. embryonal, embryonic — pertaining to an embryo, also to marked immaturity.
17. erythroplakia — well defined red patches with a velvety appearance and often tiny ulcers which may signal a malignant change in the mucous membrane.
18. functioning tumor — term usually refers to neoplasm of endocrine derivation which synthesizes and releases hormones into the bloodstream and may cause some endocrine dysfunction. In a broader sense any well-differentiated neoplasm capable of forming the product of the normal parent cell, may be considered a functional tumor.
19. hyperplasia — abnormal increase in number of cells or, expressed differently, cellular proliferation in excess of normal, not progressive (as in neoplasia) but reaching an equilibrium.[26]
20. implantation — the spontaneous passage of tumor cells to a new site with subsequent growth.

21. invasion — the act of invading or infiltrating and destroying the surrounding tissue.
22. leukoplakia — condition of the mucous membrane showing dyskeratosis and characterized by well-defined white patches which may be precancerous or cancerous lesions.[26]
23. malignant — virulent, pertaining to the invasive, metastatic properties of a new growth.
24. medullary — marrow-like; term used in oncology in reference to soft tumors.
25. metastasis formation — development of secondary centers of neoplastic growth at some distance from the primary tumor.
26. metastasize — to disseminate or spread via lymphatics or blood stream; term used in relation to malignant tumors.
27. neoplasm — an actively growing tissue composed of cells which have undergone an abnormal type of irreversible differentiation. The new growth is useless and progressive.
28. papilloma — benign growth which resembles in its histologic structure that of the parent epithelium from which it is derived. Some skin papillomas are wart-like growths derived from squamous epithelium. Papillomas arising from the larynx, tongue, urinary bladder or ureter are usually composed of transitional epithelium and tend to undergo malignant changes.[4, 21]
29. papillomatosis — the presence of multiple papillomata.
30. polyp — a nonspecific term signifying a tissue growth of mucous membrane which may be an inflammatory lesion or a true tumor. There are two kinds:
    a. pedunculated polyp — a mass of tissue attached to an organ by a freely movable, narrow stalk or pedicle.
    b. sessile polyp — a mass of tissue attached by a broad base.
31. polyposis — the presence of multiple polyps usually in the gastrointestinal tract. Multiple polyps show a definite tendency to undergo malignant transformation.[5, 23]
32. sarcoma — a malignant connective tissue tumor.[4, 21]
33. scirrhous — hard; term used in oncology to designate a hard tumor.
34. specific viral oncogenes — tumor producing hereditary units of viral origin which have their locus on chromosomes and are capable of reproduction. They may be included in the tissue of a healthy host in a state of repression in which they cause no harm. The period of repression may last months, years or a lifetime. For no apparent reason or for a known possible cause these embryonal genes may undergo malignant transformation and multiply rapidly. Excessive proliferation and disorderly cell growth are indicative of the process of derepression resulting in active oncogenesis or tumor formation.[10, 13]
35. staging of cancer — classification or grading of cancer, considered applicable to all neoplasms according to a system, e.g. the TNM system. T refers to the primary tumor, N to regional lymph node involvement and M to metastatic spread.[21]

C. Some Terms Related to Immunologic Studies in Cancer:

1. alpha$_1$ (α_1) fetoprotein, fetal α_1 globulin (AFP) — alpha$_1$ globulin, synthesized by the embryo in the liver cell, normally present in serum and cord blood of the fetus and absent in the normal infant. If α_1 fetoprotein is found in child or adult a hepatoma or embryonal teratoblastoma are suspected.[24, 27]
2. bacille Calmette Guérin (BCG) — immunotherapeutic agent used to destroy tumors or to prevent new or recurrent tumorigenesis (tumor formation). BCG is directly injected into metastatic skin lesions (nodules) or into unaffected areas by scarification. For maximal results BCG injections are given. The immunopotentiating effect of BCG is increased by the simultaneous use of antineoplastic agents at regular intervals.[5, 30]
3. carcinoembryonic antigen (CEA) — nonspecific test and glycoprotein, found in malignant entodermal layers of tissue including colorectal, pancreatic, gastric and pulmonary carcinomas as well as in nonmalignant disorders and nonentodermal carcinomas. The CEA test aids in evaluating the patient's response to treatment. Its lack of specificity limits its usefulness.[2, 18, 24]
4. estradiol receptor assay (ERA) — test predicting the effectiveness of hormone therapy or hormone deprivation (endocrine ablation therapy) in particular breast cancers.[24]

5. tumor associated antigens (TAA) — antigens absent in normal tissues, but found in leukemia, lymphoma, myeloma, melanoma, meningioma, neuroblastoma, hepatoma, osteogenic sarcoma and tumors of the urogenital organs.[16, 30]

6. tumor immunity — the presence of tumor antibodies toward the specific tumor as detected by immunofluorescence, complement fixation tests and cytotoxicity tests.[21, 26]

Table 31

CLASSIFICATION OF COMMON NEOPLASMS

Histologic Derivation	Benign Neoplasms	Malignant Neoplasms[a]	Site of Predilection
Epithelial tissue (a) Covering epithelium	Squamous cell papilloma — a benign neoplasm composed of squamous epithelial cells, flat and pavement-like in appearance	Carcinomas:[a,b] Epidermoid carcinoma Squamous cell carcinoma — a malignant neoplasm of squamous epithelial cells	Skin, buccal mucosa, tongue, salivary gland, lip, larynx, lung, bladder, others
		Oatcell carcinoma — a very malignant undifferentiated, small cell tumor	Lung
		Basal cell carcinoma — a malignant neoplasm, frequently forming a rodent ulcer and destructive by invasion, rarely by metastasis	Skin, especially face: canthus of eye, tip of nose, chin, lip, others
(b) Glandular epithelium	Adenoma — a benign neoplasm arising from glands	Adenocarcinoma — a malignant neoplasm composed of glandular epithelium and characterized by many variations of anaplasia and metastases	Breast, bronchi, digestive tract, especially stomach and rectosigmoid, endocrine glands, others
	Cystadenoma — a cystic neoplasm arising from glandular epithelium (a) serous type — uni or multilocular serous cyst composed of epithelial and connective tissue (b) pseudomucinous type — a cystic neoplasm in which the lining epithelium produces mucus	Cystadenocarcinoma — a cystic, malignant new growth of glandular epithelium (a) serous type — (rare) frequently bilateral loculations characteristic; cyst containing a transudate (b) pseudomucinous type — malignant changes, cells undergoing stratification; implants on peritoneal surface characteristic of neoplasm: fluid of cyst viscid in nature	Ovary, salivary gland, breast, thyroid Ovary Ovary
Embryonal tissue		Choriocarcinoma — a highly malignant tumor of chorionic epithelium; early metastasis common	Uterus, testes, mediastinum

Histologic Derivation	Benign Neoplasms	Malignant Neoplasms[a]	Site of Predilection
Embryonal tissue	Testicular adenoma — a glandular tumor derived from germinal epithelium, extremely rare[c]	Embryonal carcinoma of testis — a malignant new growth of germinal epithelium[e]	Testes
		Seminoma — a testicular neoplasm of distinctive seminoma cells and lymphocytic stroma[e]	Testes, epididymis, pelvic and paraaortic lymph nodes, others
	Teratoma, mature — a mixed tumor composed of any type of embryonic and adult tissue, as teeth, hair, bone, cartilage, others	Malignant teratoma, immature — a mixed tumor malignant in one or the other tissue elements	Testes, ovaries, retroperitoneal and sacrococcygeal regions
Connective tissue	Chondroma — a benign neoplasm composed of cartilaginous elements	Sarcomas: Chondrosarcoma — a malignant neoplasm of cartilaginous elements usually arising from the end of long bones	Bones: femur, humerus, endolarynx, maxillary sinus, nasal fossa, others
	Lipoma — a benign neoplasm composed of adipose tissue (fat)	Liposarcoma — a sarcoma composed of adipose tissue	Neck, shoulder, back, gluteal region, thigh, others
	Fibroma — a benign mass or firm nodule of fibroblasts or fibrocytes	Fibrosarcoma — variable degrees of anaplasia and growth rate of tumor in subcutaneous or deeper structures[f]	Extremities, head, neck, breast, others
	Leiomyoma — a benign neoplasm of smooth muscle tissue	Leiomyosarcoma — a malignant neoplasm of smooth muscle tissue	Uterus, endometrium, vulva, bladder, small intestine, esophagus, stomach, others
	Rhabdomyoma — a benign tumor arising in skeletal muscle	Rhabdomyosarcoma — a malignant, poorly differentiated, bizzare mass in striated muscle[b,f]	Any skeletal muscles especially of lower extremities as the adductors, biceps and quadriceps
	Osteoid osteoma — benign tumor derived from osteoblastic tissue	Osteosarcoma, Osteogenic sarcoma — a malignant tumor of osteoblastic or osseous tissue	Long bones, especially femur, humerus, fibula, also bones of pelvis, others
Reticuloendothelial tissue		Ewing's sarcoma — a malignant tumor of reticuloendothelial tissue; early and wide metastases to other bones[b]	Femur, tibia, fibula, humerus, mandible, pelvic bones, others
		Multiple myeloma, Plasma cell myeloma — malignant tumors derived from plasma cells of bone marrow[f]	Flat bones, ribs, vertebrae, pelvis, skull, others

Histologic Derivation	Benign Neoplasms	Malignant Neoplasms[d,e]	Site of Predilection
Hematopoietic or hemato-logic tissue		Leukemias — stem cell, undifferentiated or differentiated forms[g]	Blood
Lymph forming or lymphoid tissue		Lymphomas — stem cell or histiocytic, poorly or well differentiated forms[g]	Lymph nodes, spleen, liver, other viscera
		Hodgkin's lymphoma — lymphocytic predominance or depletion, mixed cellularity or nodular sclerosis[g]	Lymph nodes, spleen, liver, bones, other viscera
Vascular tissue	Angioma Hemangioma — a tumor of blood vessels	Angiosarcoma Hemangiosarcoma — a malignant blood vessel tumor	Blood vessels, subcutaneous tissues, muscles, others
	Lymphangioma — a tumor of the lymphatic vessels	Lymphangiosarcoma — a sarcoma of the lymphatic vessels	Lymphatic vessels, neck, others
Nerve tissue or other tissue found in nervous system		Glioma group — primary intracranial tumors composed of glial tissues. Various types of cells are present[b,f]	Brain
		(a) Astrocytoma — a neoplasm of glial tissue containing star-shaped cells or astrocytes[b,f]	Cerebral hemisphere, brain stem
		(b) Ependymoma — a neoplasm of the lining of the ventricles	Ventricles of the brain
		(c) Glioblastoma multiforme — most malignant form of gliomas, highly invasive and destructive	Cerebrum, cerebellum, brain stem, spinal cord
		(d) Oligodendroglioma — a relatively rare, slowly growing glioma with areas of calcification[b,f]	White matter of the frontal lobe
		Medulloblastoma — a malignant tumor composed of medullary or neuroepithelial tissue	Cerebellum
	Meningioma — a benign tumor arising from the meninges; a common tumor		Meninges, cerebral hemisphere, optic chiasm

Histologic Derivation	Benign Neoplasms	Malignant Neoplasms	Site of Predilection
Nerve tissue		Neuroblastoma — a highly malignant, lethal tumor of neuroblasts occurring in children[f]	Adrenal gland, sympathetic nerve chains, jaw, lip, nose, abdominal viscera, others
	Ganglioneuroma	Ganglioneuroblastoma — malignant ganglioneuroma composed of ganglionic cells and neuroblasts	Mediastinum, retroperitoneum
	Neurilemoma — a benign encapsulated tumor usually arising from peripheral nerve[b]		Peripheral or sympathetic nerves, eighth cranial nerve
	Neurofibroma — a tumor of peripheral nerve sheaths	Neurofibrosarcoma — a malignant neoplasm of peripheral nerve sheath	Peripheral nerves, hand, mediastinum, ureter, others
Pigment-forming tissue	Nevus — pigmented mole of developmental origin	Malignant melanoma — a malignant pigmented tumor[i]	Skin, eye, extremities

[a] Juan A. del Regato, et al. Cancer — Diagnosis Treatment and Prognosis, 5th ed. St. Louis: The C. V. Mosby Co., 1977.

[b] Eugene F. Tucker, M.D. Personal communications.

[c] H. B. Hornback, et al. Oat cell carcinoma of the lung. Cancer, 37: 2658-2664, June, 1976.

[d] Edmund R. Novak, et al. Benign tumors of the ovary — Malignant tumors of the ovary. Novak's Textbook of Gynecology, 9th ed. Baltimore: Williams and Wilkins, Co., 1975, pp. 444-541.

[e] Stanley L. Robbins. Testicular tumors. Pathologic Basis of Disease. Philadelphia: W. B. Saunders Co., 1974, pp. 1183-1189.

[f] _____. The musculoskeletal system — The nervous system. Ibid., pp. 1420-1545.

[g] _____. Disorders of the white cells — Lymph nodes and spleen. Ibid., pp. 726-781.

[h] Russell N. De Jong and Oscar Sugar (eds.) Tumors. Neurology and Neurosurgery, Chicago: Year Book Medical Publishers, Inc., 1976, pp. 435-540.

[i] H. W. Southwick. Malignant melanoma. Cancer, 37: 202-205, January, 1976.

ORAL READING PRACTICE

Neoplasms

Oncology is the science or study of tumors. A **neoplasm** or tumor is a new growth of tissue which may distort the size and appearance of the organ. It serves no useful purpose since it adds nothing to the further development or repair of the organ.

Tumors may be divided into **benign** and **malignant** neoplasms. Typical benign tumors are generally encapsulated by connective tissue, not invasive, and slow-growing. They never metastasize. However, they may cause serious dysfunctions if they encroach on vital organs, obstruct the circulation or air passages and compress nerves. Microscopically, the pattern of benign neoplasms is orderly and well organized.[4, 21]

In contradistinction, typical malignant tumors have no capsule, are **invasive,** progressively growing, metastasize and endanger physical well-being and even life. Their microscopic pattern exhibits disorder. Benign tumors may persist for years and then, without apparent cause, undergo malignant changes.

Another method of classifying tumors is based on their histologic derivation. The majority of tumors arise from **epithelial** and **connective** tissues, others from **hemopoietic, vascular** and nerve tissue and still others are of mixed origin.[4, 21]

The actual cause of tumor formation is unknown although experimental investigations have established a few theories which merit attention.

The **embryonic theory** maintains that cells which should have produced tissue cease to develop prematurely in the embryo and are included in the growing tissue after birth. Such embryonic remnants are responsible for malignancies, especially the sarcomas. According to this theory, the classification of neoplasms is related to the degree of maturity of the tumor cells. Benign tumors are composed of mature cells, while malignant tumors approach more closely the embryonic character of tissue.

Convincing as the embryonic theory seems to be, it is no longer tenable. The differences of the histologic components of tumors outweigh the similarities to embryonic tissue in neoplasms. Most authorities in **pathology** accept the view that tumors arise from adult cells and in the **neoplastic** process develop characteristics which differ considerably from those of the embryonic stage of tissue development.

The **biochemical theory** assumes that certain biophysical and biochemical changes in the environment of the cells cause the cells to develop neoplastic properties.

The **virus theory** asserts that **viruses** are an integral part of the malignant transformation of cells. This concept has met with disfavor on the ground that cancer is not of infectious origin. Opponents argue that tumors cannot be transmitted from person to person or other contact infection. Despite opposition the **viral etiology** of cancer continues to be the subject of intensive research.[28]

A working **hypothesis** is expressed by Gross who assumes that **latent oncogenic viruses** may be present in normal healthy hosts. Prompted by certain **trigger stimuli** these inactive, but potentially **oncogenic viruses** may change into **formidable pathogens,** accelerate the multiplication of cells and develop malignant tumors, lymphomas or leukemia.[10]

Gross further comments that an inactive **oncogenic virus** could be suspected on the basis of the individual's family history of tumors or leukemia among grandparents, parents and siblings. This assumption does not imply that all descendants would necessarily harbor an oncogenic agent nor would it mean that all who carry oncogenic viruses would develop cancer or leukemia. Tumor producing viruses appear to be well adapted to their **carrier hosts** and become activated only on occasions.[10]

A new view of cancer viruses has gained wide acceptance within the past decade. Temin of the University of Wisconsin presented convincing evidence that in cells invaded by **cancer-inducing RNA viruses, DNA is synthesized** from the **viral RNA template.** The discovery of an enzyme, the **RNA dependent polymerase,** gives further support to the presence of viruses in cancer cells.[15, 29]

Robert Huebner of the **viral carcinogenesis** group of the National Cancer Institute at Bethesda, Maryland, confirms the presence of the RNA dependent polymerase in oncogenic viruses.[13]

The Huebner-Todaro **hypothesis** implies that "the occurrence of most cancer is a natural biologic event determined by **spontaneous** and/or **induced derepression** of an **endogenous specific viral oncogene.** Viewed in this way ultimate control of cancer will therefore very likely depend on delineation of the factors responsible for **derepression** of virus expression and of the nature of the **repressors** involved."[13]

Presently, the tumor antigens of oncogenic adenoviruses are widely studied in relation to malignancy in man.

Tumorigenesis in animals induced by **onconaviruses** have shown some similarities to human cells and plasma as detected by **electron microscopy** in patients with leukemia, lymphoma, certain sarcomas and solid tumors. No conclusive evidence is available.[15, 20, 22]

Seroepidemiologic studies shed light on oncogenic **herpesviruses** and related antibody production. Herpesvirus simplex type 2, found in cervical cancer enters the human body by **venereal** transmission. The Epstein-Barr herpesvirus is an etiologic factor in **nasopharyngeal** carcinoma and Burkitt's lymphoma.[6, 8, 9, 15, 19, 20, 29]

Reports from the Virus Cancer Program of the National Cancer Institute indicate that the immunologic control of virus-associated tumors in man may be realized in the near future.[12, 14, 28]

The **genetic theory** which offers evidence that heredity influences susceptibility to neoplastic reactions, is linked to the viral theory through extensive research confirming the possible transmission of the C-type RNA virus from parent to offspring.[10, 13]

For several decades the familial occurrence of cancer has been sporadically pointed up in medical literature. It may well be that current advances in viral carcinogenesis provide the answer.[1, 7, 17, 23]

Genetic analysis has drawn attention to familial predisposition to cancer as gleaned from the concurrence of leukemia in identical twins or aggregations of neuroblastoma, Wilms' tumor, carcinoma of the liver and adrenal cortex in families. In addition Mendelian inheritance patterns are found in retinoblastoma, Gardner's syndrome and familial polyposis of the colon to mention but a few.[21]

The unraveling of further **genetic data** and their implications in the clinical field should prove to be a most fascinating adventure and become a major benefit to mankind.

It is an established fact that malignant neoplasms may be induced by hormones such as human **chorionic gonadotropin** found regularly in large amounts in **gestational choriocarcinoma** as well as in about 50% of **testicular** tumors and 25% of gastrointestinal cancers.[2, 24]

Estrogens are associated with pelvic malignancy, especially endometrial adenocarcinoma in the middle and older age groups. In granulosa cell carcinoma of the ovary increased estrogen secretion by this functional tumor is blamed for inducing endometrial adenocarcinoma. Another evidence is clear cell carcinoma of the cervix or vagina in adolescent girls whose mothers had taken diethylstilbestrol. There is no doubt that the oncogenic potentials of hormones are multiple and highly problematic, defying any solution.[20, 26]

Ionizing radiation and carcinogenic chemicals have been incriminated in causing cancer. **Leukemogenic** agents as phenylbutazone are reported to have induced leukemia. The epidemiologic approach to carcinogenesis has led to the conclusion that human cancer has a multiple factorial etiology.[11, 21, 23]

A new cancer theory developed by Szent-Gyögyi assumes that **electronic biology** may solve the cancer mystery. Since every cell has the capacity to proliferate it is the primary task of the cancer researcher to suppress this innate capacity of malignant cells.[25]

REFERENCES AND BIBLIOGRAPHY

1. Anderson, D. E. Familial susceptibility to cancer. *Ca — A Cancer Journal for Clinicians*, 26: 143-149, May-June, 1976.
2. Berlin, N. I. An overview of research in cancer diagnosis. *Mayo Clinic Proceedings*, 50: 249-254, May, 1975.
3. Chan, R. C. Carcinoma of the prostate. *Cancer*, 37: 2749-2754, June, 1976.
4. del Regato, Juan A. and Spjut, Harlan. *Cancer*, 5th ed. St. Louis: C. V. Mosby Co., 1977.
5. Eilber, F. R. Immunotherapy with BCG for lymph node metastases from malignant melanoma. *New England Journal of Medicine*, 294: 237-240, January 29, 1976.
6. Epstein, M. A. Epstein-Barr virus — Is it time to develop a vaccine program? *Journal of the National Cancer Institute*, 56: 697-700, April, 1976.
7. Fraumeni, J. F. *et al.* Six families prone to ovarian cancer. *Cancer*, 36: 364-369, August, 1975.
8. Goldberg, R. J. *et al.* Herpes simplex virus type-2 markers in cervical carcinoma. *Cancer Research*, 36: 795-799, February, 1976.
9. Gravell, M. *et al.* Epstein-Barr virus in Burkitt's lymphoma. *Journal of the National Cancer Institute*, 56: 701-704, April, 1976.
10. Gross, L. Viral etiology of cancer, leukemia and allied diseases. *Ca — A Cancer Journal for Clinicians*, 20: 242-247, July-August, 1970.
11. Hammond, E. C. The epidemiologic approach to

the etiology of cancer. *Cancer,* 35: 652-654, March, 1975.

12. Hilleman, M. R. Herpex simplex vaccines. *Cancer Research,* 36: 857-858, February, 1976.

13. Huebner, R. J. and Todaro, G. J. Oncogenes of RNA tumor viruses as determinants of cancer. *Proceedings of the National Academy of Science,* 64: 1087-1092, November, 1969.

14. Huebner, R. J. *et al.* Suppression of murine type C RNA virogenes by type-specific oncornavirus vaccines: Prospects for prevention of cancer. *Proceedings of the National Academy of Science — USA,* 73: 620-624, February, 1976.

15. Jawetz, Ernest, Melnick, Joseph L. and Adelberg, Edward A. Oncogenic viruses. *Review of Medical Microbiology,* 12th ed. Los Altos, California: Lange Medical Publications, 1976, pp. 461-491.

16. Krueger, R. G. *et al.* Tumor associated antigens in human myeloma. *Journal of the National Cancer Institute,* 56: 711-715, April, 1976.

17. Leklem, J. E. *et al.* A family with a history of bladder cancer. *Journal of the National Cancer Institute,* 56: 1001-1004, June, 1976.

18. Macdonald, J. S. *et al.* Pancreatic carcinoma. *Journal of the National Cancer Institute,* 56: 1093-1099, June, 1976.

19. Melnick, J. L. *et al.* Studies on Herpes simplex virus and cancer. *Cancer Research,* 36: 845-856, February, 1976.

20. Piver, M. S. Estrogens in gynecologic cancer. *Ca — A Cancer Journal for Clinicians,* 25: 291, September-October, 1975.

21. Robbins, Stanley L. Neoplasia — Clinical aspects of neoplasia. *Pathologic Basis of Disease.* Philadelphia: W. B. Saunders Co., 1974, pp. 106-165.

22. Sakurai, M. *et al.* Prognostic value of chromosomal findings in Ph^1 — positive chronic myelocytic leukemia. *Cancer Research,* 36: 313-318, February, 1976.

23. Sherlock, P. Etiology of gastrointestinal cancer: Heredity vs. environment. *Digestive Diseases,* 21: 68-70, January, 1976.

24. *Specialized Diagnostic Laboratory Tests,* 11th ed. Van Nuys, California: Bio-Science Laboratories, 1976, pp. 164-170.

25. Szent-Györgyi, Albert. *Electronic Biology and Cancer — A New Theory of Cancer.* New York: Marcel Dekker, Inc., 1976.

26. Tucker, Eugene F., M.D. Personal communications.

27. Vaughan, Victor C. and McKay, R. James. *Nelson Textbook of Pediatrics,* 10th ed. Philadelphia: W. B. Saunders Co., 1975, p. 876.

28. Virus Cancer Program — National Cancer Institute Symposium. Immunologic control of virus associated tumors in man. Part II. *Cancer Research,* 36: 559-869, February, 1976.

29. Watson, James D. The viral origins of cancer. *Molecular Biology of the Gene,* 3rd ed. Menlo Park, California: W. A. Benjamin, Inc., 1976, pp. 641-689.

30. Wells, J. V. *et al.* Immunology of genito-urinary tumors. In Smith, Donald R. *General Urology,* 8th ed. Los Altos, California: Lange Medical Publications, 1975, pp. 239-246.

Chapter XVIII
Selected Terms Pertaining to Anesthesiology

GENERAL ANESTHESIA

A. Origin of Terms:

1. algesia (G) — sense of pain
2. basis (G) — base
3. conscious (L) — aware
4. esthesia (G) — sensation
5. ether (G) — air
6. ignis (L) — fire
7. narcose (G) — stupor
8. sedation (L) — quieting, calming

B. General Terms:

1. analeptics — stimulants of central nervous system, for example, coramine and caffeine.
2. analgesia — loss of normal sense of pain.
3. analgesics — drugs which relieve pain.
4. anesthesia — inability to feel.
   a. general anesthesia — state of unconsciousness accompanied by varying degrees of muscular relaxation and freedom from physical pain.
   b. local anesthesia — absence of sensation and, consequently, of pain in a part of the body; consciousness retained.
5. anesthesiologist — a physician who specializes in anesthesiology.
6. anesthesiology — the science and study of anesthesia.
7. anesthetic — an agent producing insensibility to pain.
8. anesthetist — a professional person, not necessarily a physician, who is qualified to administer anesthesia.
9. ataractics, ataraxics, tranquilizers — drugs exerting a calming effect and frequently an antiemetic action. They are used for premedication as antianxiety agents.[8]
10. basal anesthesia — anesthesia providing a state of unconsciousness (narcosis) which usually lacks sufficient depth to permit major surgery.[28]
11. controlled breathing — respiratory rate and depth regulated by the intermittent pressure on a reservoir bag of the anesthetic machine or by a device known as ventilator or respirator.[8]
12. deliberate hypertension — induced, controlled hypertension permitting improved oxygenation of the brain resulting from increased perfusion during general anesthesia.[6, 8]
13. deliberate hypotension — technique used to diminish blood loss, create a relatively dry surgical field and prevent the risk of hypertension. After obtaining a stable anesthetic level with halothane or enflurane it is safe to use a short-acting hypotensive to lower the blood pressure.[12]
14. eyelash reflex — touching the eyelashes to evoke lid movement. The eyelash reflex is a guide to determine the depth of anesthesia.
15. hypercarbia, hypercapnia — excess of carbon dioxide in the blood.
16. hyperventilation — excessive respiration (or movement of air in and out of the lungs) causing an abnormal loss of carbon dioxide from the blood.
17. hypoxia — a reduction of oxygen supply to the body tissues.
18. inhalational therapy — administration of inhalant gases such as oxygen or carbon dioxide to relieve oxygen want or stimulate respiration.
19. lid reflex — tapping of the eyelid to evoke its immediate closure; the lid reflex is a guide to determine the depth of anesthesia. It is lost in the stage of surgical anesthesia.
20. malignant hyperthermia — an inherited, life-threatening syndrome usually characterized by a quick rise in body temperature, tachycardia, metabolic acidosis, increased CPK (creatine phosphokinase) and decreased Ca^{++} (calcium). It may be initiated by

potent anesthetic inhalants as enflurane or halothane or neuromuscular blocking agents as succinylcholine.[9]

21. neuroleptanalgesics — potent analgesics and tranquilizers producing detached quiescence and somnolence, used for premedication and general anesthesia or as adjuncts to other anesthetic agents.

22. neuromuscular blocking agents, skeletal muscle relaxants — drugs which serve as adjuncts to general anesthesia by producing muscular relaxation thus reducing the need for deep levels of anesthesia.
    a. depolarizing agents — relaxants which block motor nerve impulses at the myoneural junction, e.g. succinylcholine chloride (Anectine Chloride) and decamethonium bromide (Syncurine). Depolarizing agents mimic the action of acetylcholine at the nerve-muscle junction causing a discharge of the end-plate potential.[25, 26, 28, 32]
    b. nondepolarizing agents — relaxants which inhibit transmission of motor nerve impulses at the myoneural junction, e.g. gallamine triethiodide (Flaxedil Triethiodide). Pancuronium bromide (Pavulon) is a competitive blocking neuromuscular agent which is longer acting and does not possess histamine or ganglionic blocking properties.[5, 26, 28, 32]

23. preanesthetic medication, premedication — a combination of drugs including opium derivatives, barbiturates, tranquilizers, ataraxics, neuroleptanalgesics and the belladonna group in the preanesthetic preparation. Their function is:
    a. to induce psychic depression and tranquilization
    b. to reduce reflex activity and metabolic rate
    c. to decrease nausea and vomiting
    d. to protect cardiovascular stability
    e. to minimize mucus production
    f. to prevent convulsive reactions.
    Less anesthetic is needed and anesthesia is achieved more rapidly. Type and dosage of premedicants must be tailored to the individual patient's needs.[28, 41]

24. transient global amnesia — syndrome characterized by an abrupt loss of memory which is self-limited, not recurrent nor associated with severe damage of the central nervous system. It occurs in the postanesthetic period and lasts less than 24 hours.[11]

25. vasoconstrictors — drugs causing a constriction of the blood vessels. They are used in combination with local anesthetics to produce a vasoconstriction locally, thus preventing the anesthetic from being carried away from the site of injection.

C. Terms Related to Stages of Anesthesia:

1. stage of analgesia — period from first inhalations of anesthetic to beginning of loss of consciousness. The patient is awake, his sensorium is clear, his reflexes continue to be active, but he is insensitive to surface pain.

2. stage of delirium — period from loss of consciousness to beginning of surgical anesthesia. There is depression of the cerebral cortex and loss of control of higher centers. Reflexes tend to be exaggerated, struggling, excitement, incoordination and disorientation may occur. This stage is often absent in children.

3. stage of surgical anesthesia — period from second stage to cessation of spontaneous respiration. This stage is subdivided into 4 planes.
    a. the first plane — muscle tone is unchanged and eyeball movements continue when the lids are raised The pupil reacts to light.
    b. the second plane — smaller muscles throughout the body lose their tone and ocular movements cease. The pupils are centrally fixed.
    c. the third plane — muscular relaxation throughout the body includes large muscles. The corneal reflexes are abolished. Respiration becomes diaphragmatic.
    d. the fourth plane — the relaxation of large muscles and loss of reflexes are complete. The pupils are widely dilated. Diaphragmatic activity is decreased.

4. stage of toxicity — period from onset of apnea to circulatory failure. Respiratory move-

ment ceases, the depression of the cardiovascular system increases and the blood pressure drops rapidly. If artificial respiration is instituted, the condition may be reversible.[28]

D. Terms Related to Methods of General Anesthesia:

1. endotracheal anesthesia — introduction of a catheter into the trachea for the purpose of conducting the anesthetic mixture directly from the apparatus to the lungs. This may be achieved by oral or nasal intubation. The catheter is then attached to a closed or semiclosed inhaler. In present day practice this form of inhalation anesthesia is the method of choice for most major operations since it permits a patent airway, aspiration of secretions, use of positive pressure, controlled breathing, adequate ventilation and isolation of the respiratory tract from the gastrointestinal tract.[8, 23, 28, 37]

2. hypercarbic anesthesia — excess carbon dioxide content of the blood and controlled hypertension causing improved oxygenation and decreased oxygen consumption during general anesthesia. The increased cerebral blood flow results from a vasodilation of hypercarbia and the increased cerebral perfusion of induced hypertension.[6]

3. hypocarbic anesthesia — low carbon dioxide content and deliberate hypertension as an adjunct to general anesthesia.[6]

4. inhalation anesthesia — general anesthesia produced by the inhalation of vaporized liquids or gases.[33] Several methods are used.

   a. the closed method — a technic in which the patient rebreathes the anesthetic mixture, contained in a special apparatus. This apparatus is composed of a tight fitting mouth or nose mask or tube, a rebreathing bag and a device permitting the absorption of carbon dioxide.

   b. the open method — a liquid anesthetic drug dropped on a gauze mask which covers the patient's nose and mouth and permits the inhalation of the vaporized drug.

   c. the semiclosed method — a technic which differs from the closed method by the use of an exhalation valve which allows partial rebreathing and carbon dioxide removal with soda lime.[28, 35, 37]

5. intravenous anesthesia — the intravenous administration of drugs for basal narcosis. A stage of unconsciousness is produced, but analgesia and muscular relaxation may prove unsatisfactory.[10, 28, 35]

6. rectal anesthesia — the rectal administration of drugs to produce basal anesthesia. The reflexes are partially abolished and a hypnotic state is present. Pentothal, Avertin and Ether have been used for this purpose.

E. Terms Related to Dissociative Anesthesia:

1. dissociative anesthesia — selective blocking of pain conduction and perception, leaving those parts of the central nervous system which do not participate in pain transmission and perception, free from the depressant effects of drugs. The profound analgesia induced by this type of anesthesia is associated with somnolence in which the patient appears to be disconnected from his environment.[8]

2. neuroleptanalgesia, neuroleptanesthesia — a balanced highly effective anesthetic state for control of well-defined pain during surgery resulting from the depression of certain corticothalamic systems. It may be used as sole anesthesia or as adjunct to local, regional or general anesthesia. Neuroleptanalgesia is a type of dissociative anesthesia.[2, 4, 7, 10, 16, 41]

LOCAL AND REGIONAL ANESTHESIA

A. Origin of Terms:

1. acus (L) — needle
2. cauda (L) — tail
3. conduct (L) — to lead
4. dura (L) — hard
5. filter (L) — to strain through
6. hypno (G) — sleep
7. segment (L) — portion
8. pressor (L) — to press
9. punctura (L) — puncture
10. vas, vaso (L) — vessel

B. Terms Related to Methods of Local Anesthesia:

1. acupuncture anesthesia — insertion of stainless steel acupuncture needles at carefully selected points identified as the most effective for anesthesia of a particular operation. The needles are connected to a direct current battery source for electric stimulation. Instead of electricity the acupuncturist may manipulate the needles in an up-and-down, plus twirling motion, for twenty minutes to produce anesthesia. The advantages of Chinese acupuncture are:
   a. absolute safety of the anesthesia
   b. effective anesthetic for debilitated patients
   c. patient conscious and alert during entire procedure
   d. adequate anesthesia for prolonged surgery
   e. no interruption of food and fluid intake
   f. no postoperative nausea, vomiting, low blood pressure or respiratory complications.[18, 20, 22, 24]

2. block anesthesia — procedure seeks to interrupt conduction in the autonomic and somatic nervous systems by using local anesthetics. This may involve a block of a single nerve or of a nerve complex.[38, 39]

3. caudal or sacral anesthesia — a method of epidural anesthesia in which the anesthetic solution is injected into the sacral canal.[1, 29]

4. conduction anesthesia — term including various forms of local anesthesia: direct nerve block, epidural block, spinal anesthesia and infiltration anesthesia.[29]

5. epidural block — spinal nerves blocked as they pass through the epidural space.[15, 29]

6. infiltration anesthesia — injection of a dilute anesthetic agent under the skin to anesthetize the nerve endings and nerve fibers.[29, 38]

7. intravenous regional anesthesia — a method of producing analgesia in the extremities using lidocaine (or other drug) as regional anesthetic to act at the main nerve trunks.[14, 21]

8. nerve and field block — insensibility of a local area achieved by:
   a. direct nerve block — injection of an anesthetic solution into easily accessible nerves, as those of the extremities.
   b. field block — anesthetic solution deposited around the nerve at the point of its terminal branches.[38]

9. spinal anesthesia — anesthesia produced by the injection of a local anesthetic solution into the subarachnoid space of the lumbar region to block the roots of the spinal nerves. Tetracaine, procaine and lidocaine are frequently used.[21, 29]

10. subarachnoid alcohol block — injection of absolute ethyl alcohol (hypobaric alcohol about 0.8 ml) in any interspace of the spinal cord. The alcohol floats to the top, bathes the nerve roots and destroys the pain fibers.

11. surface or topical anesthesia — direct application of an anesthetic drug to a mucous membrane to produce insensibility to the nerve endings. Cocaine and viscous lidocaine are used for surface anesthetics.[38]

ABBREVIATIONS

A. General:

ACh — acetylcholine
Anes. — anesthesiology
$CHCl_3$ — chloroform
C_{10} — decamethonium
C_3H_6 — cyclopropane
C_2H_4 — ethylene
C_2H_5Cl — ethylchloride
C_2HCl_3 — trichloroethylene (Trilene)
CO_2 — carbon dioxide
dTC — d-tubocurarine
HCl — hydrochloride

He — helium
NLA — neuroleptanalgesia
N_2O — nitrous oxide
NR — non-rebreathing
NT — nasotracheal
O_2 — oxygen
OD — open drop
OT — orotracheal
Pent. — pentothal
SC — semiclosed
Vin. — vinyl ether (Vinethene)

B. Standard Pharmacology Texts:

ADI — American Drug Index
NF — The National Formulary
PDR — Physicians' Desk Reference

USD — The Dispensary of the
　　　United States of America
USP — United States Pharmacopeia

ORAL READING PRACTICE

Induced Hypothermia

The value of local **hypothermia** was recognized a century ago by Larrey, surgeon general of Napoleon's army. It was his custom to pack the soldiers' injured extremities in ice to control shock and pain. In 1939 Temple Fay used hypothermia as a **palliative** measure for patients suffering from **malignancies.** This treatment he abandoned since it proved to be no cure for cancer.[13]

Interest in hypothermia was revived when Bigelow and his associates published their investigation. They found that progressive body cooling lowers the **metabolic** requirements of the patient. They also found that shivering neutralizes the benefit obtained by hypothermia since it increases the oxygen requirement.

Further research led from the application of these physiologic findings to the regime of anesthesia used during **intracardiac** surgery. Prior to 1950 the high oxygen requirement of the heart and brain and the continuous flow of blood through the cardiac chambers had presented insurmountable barriers to direct vision surgery of the heart. The development of safe techniques employing hypothermia and **extracorporeal circulation** removed these barriers and opened a new era in the correction of **cardiovascular** defects.[40]

The **anesthesiologist** who uses hypothermia is primarily concerned with reducing the patient's oxygen requirement, for it results in **hypometabolism** and a diminished need for anesthesia. In the past decades several methods of hypothermia have been developed some of which are now obsolete.

Zeavin, Virtue and Swan of the University of Colorado advocate **immersion cooling,** a form of surface cooling, to lower the temperature of the body surface. Following the **induction** of anesthesia, the patient is immersed in ice water. His temperature continues to fall an additional 50% after he is removed from the ice bath. For example, if during the immersion his temperature was lowered 10°C (centigrade), it will fall another 5° after immersion has been discontinued.

At present surface cooling and blood cooling are methods of choice. A widely accepted technique is surface cooling which can be used under controlled conditions. After the patient is anesthetized and an **endotracheal** tube has been inserted, it is possible to lower his body temperature gradually by wrapping the patient in an ice cold blanket or placing him on a water mattress through which ice water circulates. Continuous recording of the **esophageal** temperature by a special recorder keeps the anesthesiologist informed of changes in body temperature. Light anesthesia is generally an adequate means of preventing shivering. **Muscle relaxants** and tranquilizers have also been used as **adjuncts.**[40]

With hypothermia of the body to 28°C, it is possible to perform **inflow occlusion** by obstructing the **inferior** and **superior venae cavae** and to operate within the heart for a period of eight minutes.

The limitations with respect to time prevented the repair of many acquired and **congenital cardiac defects** and led to the development of the heart-lung machine which extends this time to several hours. The temperature of the patient is controlled during **cardiopulmonary bypass** by the use of a heat **exchanger** in the **extracorporeal circuit** allowing body temperature to be varied as needed by surgical requirements.[40, 42]

In the past the heart-lung machine was usually primed with cold blood which induced body cooling. Presently cold intravenous fluids are used for priming and lowering the body temperature. Simultaneously, fluid replacement with balanced **electrolyte** solution is made possible.

Hypothermia frequently results in **ventricular fibrillation** at a temperature below 25°C. This ineffective type of muscular contraction of the heart must be converted by **electric defibrillation** to a state of cardiac **asystole** whereupon the normal **pacemaker** will usually become operative and restore an effective output of blood from the heart.

Cardiac massage is employed to propel blood to the vital organs during **ventricular asystole** (arrest) or ventricular fibrillation until conversion to an effectively beating heart is accomplished.

With the use of the **pump oxygenator** cardiac massage is unnecessary as the vital organs are being perfused.   In all other situations of **cardiac arrest** or ventricular fibrillation cardiac massage is a life-supporting emergency measure.[40]

In the late sixties induced hypothermia fell into disrepute because of the risk of **cardiac arrhythmias** complicating the extreme lowering of body temperature.   Many anesthesiologists abandoned the procedure in favor of **normothermia**.[42]   By introducing effective safety measures in the anesthetic program, Mohri and colleagues stimulated renewed interest in hypothermia in the early seventies.   They advocated surface cooling with ice bags, a short period of cardiopulmonary bypass before **circulatory arrest** and **bypass resuscitation** and rewarming for cardiac surgery in neonates and infants.[30]

There is ample evidence that surface-induced profound hypothermia is capable of producing a quiet, flaccid, bloodless heart which permits adequate surgical exposure and correction of complex cardiac **anomalies**.   Since the period of extracorporeal circulation is markedly reduced, **cellular** damage is minimized.[3, 31, 42]

Cardiac hypothermia may be achieved by **cor** (coronary) **perfusion** or by iced normal saline solution used topically on the **myocardium**.   Whatever the technique may be, hypothermia is recognized today as an invaluable component of cardiac anesthesia.[3, 17, 31, 42]

Table 32

CLASSIFICATION OF GENERAL ANESTHETICS

Anesthetic Agents	Systemic Effects

A. Volatile substances, administered by inhalation
  1. *Liquids* producing vapors:
    Chloroform ....USP
    Enflurane (Ethrane) ....Experimental
    Ether ....USP
    Ethyl chloride ....USP
    Halothane (Fluothane) ....USP
    Methoxyflurane (Penthrane) ....ND
    Trichloroethylene (Trilene) ....USP
    Vinyl ether (Vinethene) ....USP
 	
  2. *Gases:*
    Cyclopropane ....USP
    Ethylene ....USP
    Nitrous oxide ....USP
	A. Chemical substances and depressants of central nervous system; surgically useful because they are complete anesthetics providing
	
	  1. analgesia
	
	  2. suppression of reflex activity
	
	  3. muscular relaxation
	
	  4. loss of consciousness

B. Nonvolatile substances administered intravenously or rectally
  1. Ultrashort acting Barbiturates
    Methohexital (Brevital) ....USP
    Thiamylal (Surital) ....USP
    Thiopental (Pentothal) ....USP
 	
  2. Derivative of Ethyl Alcohol
    Tribromoethanol (Avertin) ....USP
    Solution Avertin in Amylene hydrate
	B. Basal narcotics, medullary depressants and incomplete anesthetics; surgically useful as adjuncts to other anesthetics. They produce
	  1. unconsciousness
	
	  2. inadequate control of reflex activity
	
	  3. unsatisfactory muscular relaxation
	
	  4. hypnosis and amnesia (following Avertin)

Anesthetic Agents	Systemic Effects

C. Nonvolatile substances administered intravenously or intramuscularly
 	
  1. Neuroleptics and Nonbarbiturates
     Ketamine (Ketalar)
     Droperidol (Inapsine)
 	
  2. Neuroleptic and Potent Narcotic Analgesic
     Innovar (Droperidol and Fentanyl)
	C. Shortacting anesthetics, depressants of certain corticothalamic systems; useful as sole anesthetic and as adjunct to conventional anesthesia. They produce
	  1. profound analgesia
	
	  2. amnesia
	
	  3. increased cardiovascular activity
	
	  4. unsatisfactory muscular relaxation

REFERENCES AND BIBLIOGRAPHY

1. Abouleish, E. Caudal analgesia for quadruplet delivery. *Anesthesia and Analgesia . . . Current Researches*, 55: 61-66, January-February, 1976.
2. Amberg, H. L. *et al.* Low-dose intramuscular ketamine for pediatric radiotherapy. *Anesthesia and Analgesia . . . Current Researches*, 55: 92-94, January-February, 1976.
3. Bailey, L. L. *et al.* Surgical management of congenital cardiovascular anomalies with the use of profound hypothermia and circulatory arrest. *Thoracic and Cardiovascular Surgery*, 71: 485-492, April, 1976.
4. Becker, L. D. *et al.* Biphasic respiratory depression after fentanyl-droperidol or fentanyl alone to supplement nitrous oxide anesthesia. *Anesthesiology*, 44: 291-296, April, 1976.
5. Bentz, E. W. *et al.* Prolonged response to succinylcholine following pancuronium. *Anesthesiology*, 44: 258-260, March, 1976.
6. Beven, E. G. Carotid endarterectomy. *Surgical Clinics of North America*, 55: 1111-1124, October, 1975.
7. Bidwai, A. V. *et al.* Reversal of innovar-induced postanesthetic somnolence and disorientation with physostigmine. *Anesthesiology*, 44: 249-252, March, 1976.
8. Brielmaier, Charles R., M.D. Personal communications.
9. Caropreso, P. R. *et al.* Malignant hyperthermia associated with enflurane anesthesia. *Archives of Surgery*, 110: 1491-1493, December, 1975.
10. Conahan, T. J. New intravenous anesthetics. *Surgical Clinics of North America*, 55: 851-859, August, 1975.
11. Dykes, M. H. *et al.* Transient global amnesia following spinal anesthesia. *Anesthesiology*, 36: 615-617, June, 1972.
12. Edwards, M. W. *et al.* Deliberate hypotension. *Surgical Clinics of North America*, 55: 947-957, August, 1975.
13. Frenay, Sr. Agnes Clare. Balanced anesthesia and induced hypothermia. *American Journal of Nursing*, 55: 1245-1247, October, 1955.
14. Iwane, T. *et al.* Management of intractable pain in adiposis dolorosa with intravenous administration of lidocaine. *Anesthesia and Analgesia . . . Current Researches*, 55: 257-259, March-April, 1976.
15. James, F. M. Bacteriologic aspects of epidural analgesia. *Anesthesia and Analgesia . . . Current Researches*, 55: 187-190, March-April, 1976.
16. Jobes, D. R. Anesthesia for cardiac surgery. *Surgical Clinics of North America*, 55: 893-902, August, 1975.
17. Lamberti, J. J. *et al.* Local cardiac hypothermia for myocardial protection during correction of congenital heart disease. *Annals of Thoracic Surgery*, 20: 446-455, October, 1975.
18. Lee, P. K. *et al.* Incidence of prolonged pain relief following acupuncture. *Anesthesia and Analgesia . . . Current Researches*, 55: 229-231, March-April, 1976.
19. Lemole, G. M. Improved technique of double valve replacement. *Thoracic and Cardiovascular Surgery*, 71: 759-764, May, 1976.
20. Levitt, E. E. *et al.* Evaluation of acupuncture in the treatment of chronic pain. *Journal of Chronic Diseases*, 28: 311-316, June, 1975.
21. Linke, C. L. *et al.* A regional anesthetic approach for renal transplantation. *Anesthesia and Analgesia . . . Current Researches*, 55: 69-73, January-February, 1976.
22. Lloyd, M. A. *et al.* Acupuncture analgesia and radiant-heat pain. *Anesthesiology*, 44: 147-151, February, 1976.
23. Loehning, R. W. *et al.* Lidocaine and increased respiratory resistance produced by ultrasonic aerosols. *Anesthesiology*, 44: 306-310, April, 1976.
24. Melzak, R. How acupuncture works. *Psychology Today*, 10: 28-37, June, 1973.
25. Miller, R. D. *et al.* Duration of halothane anesthesia and neuromuscular blockade with d-tubocurarine. *Anesthesiology*, 44: 206-210, March, 1976.
26. Miller, R. D. Early and late relative potencies of pancuronium and d-tubocurarine in man. *Anesthesiology*, 44: 297-300, April, 1976.
27. _____. Antagonism of neuromuscular blockade. *Ibid.*, pp. 318-329.
28. Model, Walter, Schild, Heinz O. and Wilson, Andrew. General anesthesia. *Applied Pharmacology*. Philadelphia: W. B. Saunders Co., 1976, pp. 409-433.
29. _____. Local anesthesia. *Ibid.*, pp. 434-450.

30. Mohri, H. *et al.* Deep hypothermia combined with cardiopulmonary bypass for cardiac surgery in neonates and infants. *Thoracic and Cardiovascular Surgery,* 64: 422-429, September, 1972.

31. Mohri, H. *et al.* Heparinless, oxygenatorless perfusion rewarming following surface-induced deep hypothermia for open heart surgery. *Thoracic and Cardiovascular Surgery,* 71: 792-799, May, 1976.

32. Neigh, J. L. Neuromuscular blockade. *Surgical Clinics of North America,* 55: 837-850, August, 1975.

33. Nozomu, Y. *et al.* Metabolism of methoxylflurane in man. *Anesthesiology,* 44: 372-379, May, 1976.

34. Oglietti, J. *et al.* Myocardial revascularization: Early and late results after reoperation. *Thoracic and Cardiovascular Surgery,* 71: 736-740, May, 1976.

35. Price, H. L. General anesthetics. In Goodman, Louis S. and Gilman, Alfred. *The Pharmacological Basis of Therapeutics,* 5th ed. New York: Macmillan Publishing Co. Inc., 1975, pp. 81-101.

36. Price, H. L. Myocardial depression by nitrous oxide and its reversal by Ca++. *Anesthesiology,* 44: 211-215, March, 1976.

37. Rehder, K. *et al.* General anesthesia and the lung. *Respiratory Disease,* 112: 541-563, October, 1975.

38. Ritchie, J. M. *et al.* Local anesthetics. In Goodman, Louis S. and Gilman, Alfred. *The Pharmacologic Basis of Therapeutics,* 5th ed. New York: Macmillan Publishing Co. Inc., 1975, pp. 379-403.

39. Schurman, D. J. Ankle-block anesthesia for foot surgery. *Anesthesiology,* 44: 348-352, April, 1976.

40. Schweiss, John F., M.D. Personal communications.

41. Sloan, J. B. Innovar as a preoperative medication. *Southern Medical Journal,* 68: 1407-1409, November, 1975.

42. Tyson, K. R. T. Congenital heart disease in children. *Clinical Symposia,* 27: 2-36, November, 1975.

43. Viljoen, J. K. Anesthesia and monitoring techniques for open heart surgery in the adult. *Surgical Clinics of North America,* 55: 1217-1241, October, 1975.

Chapter XIX
Selected Terms Pertaining to Physical Therapy

ORIENTATION

A. Origin of Terms:

1. kine, kineto (G) — motion
2. manus (L) — hand
3. physical (L) — natural
4. therapy (G) — treatment

B. General Terms:

1. kinesiology — the science of human motion.[10, 14]
2. kinesthesia — sensory perception (awareness) of movement.
3. orthosis — correction of defects.
4. pathokinesiology — the study of kinesiology as related to abnormal human motion.[21]
5. physiatrist — a physician who specializes in physical medicine and rehabilitaton.
6. physical agents — active forces such as water, radiant energy, massage, exercise, electricity and ultrasound energy.
7. physical medicine — that branch of medical science which uses physical agents in the diagnosis and management of disease.
8. physical therapist — a professional person qualified to provide physical therapy in areas such as: direct patient care, consultation, supervision, teaching, administration, research and community service.[29]
9. physical therapist assistant — a skilled technical worker who administers physical therapy treatments under the supervision of a physical therapist.[29]
10. physical therapy — a profession which uses knowledge and skills pertaining to physical therapy in caring for individuals disabled by disease and injury. The primary focus is on the functional restoration of patients affected with skeletal, neuromuscular, cardiovascular and pulmonary disorders.
11. prosthetics — the designing and fitting of an artificial part, e.g. to replace a limb.
12. rehabilitation — a treatment process designed to help physically handicapped individuals make maximal use of residual capacities and to enable them to obtain optimal satisfaction and usefulness in terms of themselves, their families and their community.[24]

PHYSICAL THERAPY PROCEDURES AND RELATED TESTS

A. Origin of Terms:

1. actino (G) — ray
2. cryo, crymo (G) — cold
3. electro (G) — amber
4. helio (G) — sun
5. hydro (G) — water
6. insulate (L) — to make
7. ion (G) — going
8. mechano (G) — machine
9. meter (G) — measure
10. ortho (G) — correct, straight
11. oscillation (L) — swinging
12. phono (G) — voice, sound
13. phoresis (G) — to carry, to bear
14. photo (G) — light
15. polar (G) — axis, pole
16. radio (L) — ray
17. thermo (G) — heat

B. Terms Related to Physical Therapy Procedures:

1. electrotherapy — the use of electric currents in the treatment of disease. Included are general terms and terms related to procedures:
   a. biofeedback — a process by which physiologic activity of a patient can be translated into electric signals of a visual or auditory system. Myofeedback is a type of biofeedback where the physiologic process is muscular activity.[19, 22, 27, 35]

    b. diathermy — the therapeutic use of high frequency currents to generate deep heat within parts of the body. Types of diathermy include the microwave and shortwave units.[33]

    c. electric current — a stream of electrons flowing along a conductor.
        (1) alternating current — an intermittent, asymmetric current obtained from the secondary winding of an induction coil, also known as faradic current.
        (2) direct current — a unidirectional current with distinct polarity, also called constant or galvanic current.[31, 33]

    d. iontophoresis — the introduction of medicinal ions into the tissues by means of a direct current.[31, 33]

    e. low intensity direct current (LIDC) — any current less than one milliampere in intensity. It may be used therapeutically to heal indolent ulcers.[18]

    f. transcutaneous electric nerve stimulation (TENS) — the use of low voltage or low amperage current to produce sensory modulation for control of pain.[28]

    g. ultrasonics — the use of sound waves, considerably above the range of hearing, for therapeutic purposes.
        (1) phonophoresis — the introduction of medicinal ions, as hydrocortisone, into the tissues by means of ultrasound.[23]
        (2) ultrasound — a form of acoustic vibration occurring at frequencies too high to be perceived by the human ear.[23, 33]

    h. vibratory stimulation — the use of a high frequency, low amplitude vibrator for stimulation of skeletal muscles to produce reflex effects in the treatment of motor disorders.[5]

2. hydrotherapy — the use of water in its various forms: liquid, solid and vapor. Included are terms related to the use of heat and cold.
    a. Archimedes' principle — a body fully or partially immersed in a liquid experiences an upward thrust equal to the weight of the liquid which it displaces.[31]
    b. conduction — heat transferred from a warmer object to a cooler one when both objects are in contact.
    c. contrast bath — the use of hot and cold water alternately.
    d. convection — heat exchange between a surface and a fluid moving adjacent to the surface.
    e. cryotherapy, crymotherapy — the use of cold, especially cold packs, immersion in ice water, or ice massage.[11, 26]
    f. hydrocollator packs — local hot packs which employ silica gel as the heat-retaining agent.
    g. paraffin packs — the use of hot paraffin for therapeutic purposes.
    h. sauna — a form of dry or wet heat.[16, 32]
    i. thermotherapy — the treatment of disease using various forms of heat.
    j. underwater exercise — immersion of the patient in water, tank or pool, to permit free active motion, relaxation and full abduction of the extremities, and sometimes gait training.
    k. whirlpool — a treatment which offers temperature control in combination with the mechanical effects of water in motion.

3. massage — manipulation of the soft tissues of the body most effectively performed with the hands, and administered to produce effects on the nervous and muscular systems and the local and general circulation of the blood and lymph.[38]
    a. acupressure — application of pressure to acupuncture sites to relieve pain.[36]
    b. cryokinetics — ice massage.[11, 26]
    c. effleurage — superficial or deep stroking movements.
    d. friction — deep circular or rolling movements.
    e. percussion — repeated taps or blows differing in force.
    f. petrissage — kneading or compression or compression movements.
    g. shiatsu — a pressure form of massage.[36]

    h. tapotement — percussion movements including cupping, hacking, clapping, tapping and beating.

    i. vibratory massage — frequently performed with a mechanical device especially to increase bronchial drainage.

4. radiation therapy — the therapeutic use of radiant energy, especially infrared and ultraviolet rays.

    a. infrared — an invisible form of radiant energy, ranging from about 760 mμ to 15000 mμ in the electromagnetic spectrum, and producing heat on absorption.

    b. ultraviolet — an invisible form of radiant energy ranging from about 180mμ to 400mμ and producing chemical actions on absorption.[33]

        Related terms are:

      (1) cold quartz — a type of ultraviolet lamp used for local irradiation.[33]

      (2) cosine angle law — a law which indicates that the intensity is greatest when the surface to be treated is at a right angle to the lamp.[33]

      (3) electromagnetic spectrum (EMS) — a graphic representation of the various waves of radiant energy in ascending order of length.[33]

      (4) erythema — a latent inflammatory reaction caused by a chemical action which takes place in the skin.

      (5) heliotherapy — exposure of the body to sunlight or solar radiation.

      (6) inverse square law — a law which states that the intensity of radiation from any source varies inversely with the square of the distance from the source.[33]

      (7) minimal erythema dose — irradiation sufficient to cause slight reddening of the skin.[33]

      (8) suberythema dose — irradiation insufficient to cause slight reddening of the skin.[33]

      (9) third-degree erythema dose — irradiation sufficient to cause edema and blister formation.[33]

5. therapeutic exercise

    a. terms related to muscle action

      (1) agonist, prime mover — a muscle which is considered the principal one in a specific movement.[10, 17]

      (2) antagonist — a muscle which acts on a joint in the opposite direction of the agonist.[2, 17]

      (3) concentric — muscle contraction in which the external length of the muscle is decreased; the muscle tension overcomes the load.[14, 17]

      (4) eccentric — muscle contraction in which the muscle lengthens as the load overcomes the tension developed by the muscle.[14, 17]

      (5) isometric or static — muscle contraction in which the muscle is not allowed to shorten or lengthen.[14, 17]

      (6) isotonic or dynamic — muscle contraction in which invisible shortening or lengthening of the muscle occurs.[14, 17]

      (7) synergist — a muscle which contracts together with another muscle and has an action identical or nearly identical to the agonist.[10, 17]

    b. terms related to exercise[17]

      (1) active — exercise done with voluntary muscle contraction.

      (2) active assistive — exercise done with a combination of voluntary muscle contraction and assistance of an external force.[17, 34]

      (3) breathing — exercise to any of the muscles of breathing designed to decrease the work of breathing.

      (4) conditioning — exercises to improve the fitness of a system, e.g. the cardiovascular system.

      (5) facilitation — stimulation designed to increase muscle tone.[9, 17]

      (6) inhibition — stimulation designed to decrease muscle tone.

(7) mobilization — gentle passive motion used to reestablish joint play between moving parts of joints.[1, 17]

(8) passive — joint movements performed by an outside force, usually another person with the patient neither assisting or resisting the movements.

(9) resistive — an active exercise carried out by the patient working against resistance produced by either manual or mechanical means.[17, 30]

C. Terms Related to Evaluation and Measurements:

1. ADL testing — a test which serves to outline as accurately as possible how a patient functions in everyday life, how many daily activities he can perform in his own home and in connection with his work.

2. development testing — observing a child under five years of age and recording milestones in areas of: gross and fine motor reflexes, language, social, emotional, self-care, and cognitive development.[17]

3. electrotesting — the use of electric currents to test the reaction of muscles and motor nerves.[33] This includes:

    a. chronaxie — the minimum time required for a current twice the strength of rheobase to elicit a muscle contraction.[12]

    b. electromyography — the amplification and recording, both visually and audibly, of minute electric potentials generated by muscle contractions. Electromyograms are valuable in the study of neuromuscular disorders.[2, 12, 27, 31, 33]

    c. nerve conduction velocity — electric testing to determine the speed of nerve conduction and residual latency.[2]

    d. reaction of degeneration — the reaction of a muscle to galvanic but not faradic current.

    e. rheobase — the minimal intensity of current required to elicit muscle contraction.

    f. strength duration curve — the graphic representation of current strength and duration required to elicit a minimal muscle contraction.

    g. vibratory stimulation — the use of a high frequency low amplitude vibrator for stimulation of skeletal muscles in evaluating motor disorders.[6]

4. gait analysis — methods used to detect deviations in gait resulting from pain, weakness, incoordination or deformities.[7]

5. goniometry — testing the range of joint motion with the aid of a goniometer.[8]

6. manual muscle testing — an important tool used to determine the extent and degree of muscle weakness resulting from disuse, injury or disease.

7. perceptual motor testing — testing for perceptual motor skills: a response or family of responses in which receptor, effector and feedback processes show a high degree of spatial and temporal organization.

8. posture evaluation — evaluating the position in which various parts of the body are held while sitting, walking and lying.

9. reflex testing — a method by which the patient's involuntary response to a stimulus is tested to determine the status of the nervous system.[29]

10. sensory testing — using various tools and techniques to test the patient's responses to sensory stimuli.[29]

11. volumetric measurement — determining the volume of a limb by measuring the water displaced when the extremity is immersed in a container of water.[17]

ABBREVIATIONS

A° — angstrom unit

AC — alternating current

ACC — anode closing contraction

AD — abdominal diaphragmatic breathing

ADL — activities of daily living

AE — above elbow

AK — above knee

AKO — ankle knee orthoses

AOC — anode opening contraction

APRL — Army Prosthetic Research Laboratoy

APTA — American Physical Therapy Association

ATR — achillis tendon reflex

346

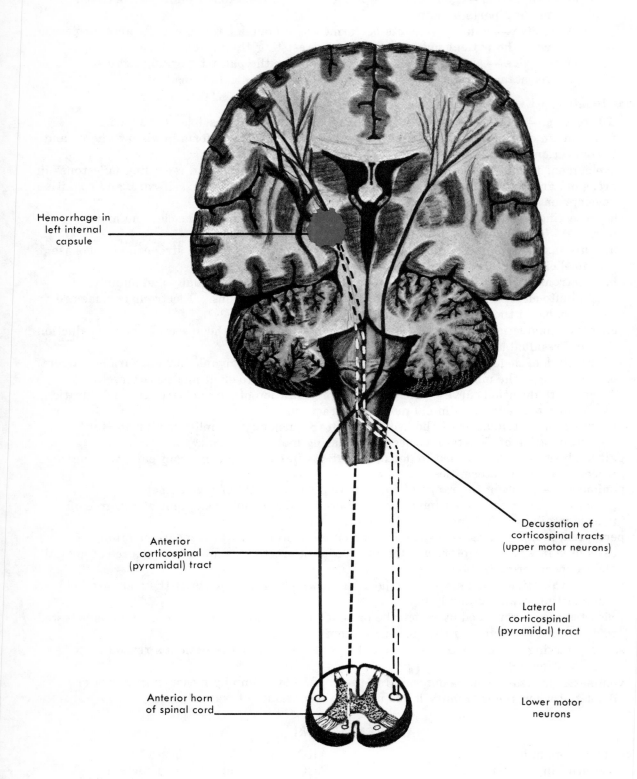

Hemorrhage in
left internal
capsule

Decussation of
corticospinal tracts
(upper motor neurons)

Anterior
corticospinal
(pyramidal) tract

Lateral
corticospinal
(pyramidal) tract

Anterior horn
of spinal cord

Lower motor
neurons

Fig. 85 — Cerebral hemorrhage in the left internal capsule resulting in right-sided hemiplegia because of the crossing (decussation) of the corticospinal (pyramidal) tracts in the medulla oblongata.

BE — below elbow
BK — below knee
BP — blood pressure
CNS — cutaneous nerve stimulation
CCC — cathode closing contraction
COC — cathode opening contraction
COLD — chronic obstructive lung disease
COPD — chronic obstructive pulmonary
disease
CPR — cardiac pulmonary resuscitation
DOE — dyspnea on exertion
DTR — deep tendon reflex
EIB — exercise-induced bronchospasm
EMG — electromyogram, electromyograph
EMS — electromagnetic spectrum
FAO — foot ankle orthoses
IR — infrared
KJ — knee jerk
LOM — limitation of motion
MA — milliampere
MBD — minimal brain dysfunction
MED — minimal erythema dose
MFT — muscle function test
MHz — megahertz

NCV — nerve conduction velocity
PFT — pulmonary function test
PNF — proprioceptive neuromuscular
facilitation
PR — pulse rate
PRE — progressive resistive exercise
PROM — passive range of motion
RD — reaction of degeneration
ROM — range of motion
SACH — solid ankle cushion heel
SCI — spinal cord injury
SCRAM — speed-controlled respirometer
for ambulation measurement
SED — suberythema dose
SES — subcutaneous electric stimulation
SOB — short of breath
TCP — time care profile
TENS — transcutaneous electric
nerve stimulation
TSW — toe off and heel strike swing phase
US — ultrasound
UV — ultraviolet
WCPT — World Confederation for
Physical Therapy

ORAL READING PRACTICE

Hemiplegia

Hemiplegia is one of the most common muscular disorders of central origin. When the paralysis occurs suddenly, it is referred to as stroke or **apoplexy.** The involvement affects the **corticobulbar** and **corticospinal fibers.** Motor neurons, with cell bodies located in the **cortex** and **axons** extending into the cord, are known as upper motor neurons in contradistinction to those in the **anterior horn** of the cord which extend toward the muscles and are called lower motor neurons. A similar division exists for the cranial nerves in regions where their nerve nuclei perform a function corresponding to that of the spinal cord.

A **cerebral thrombosis** tends to devitalize an upper motor neuron resulting in its degeneration all the way from the thrombotic lesion to the cord. The lower motor neuron remains uninvolved. Following the initial period of shock, the muscles respond to **reflex arcs** mediated by the cord. Since these reflexes tend to be exaggerated, the muscles of the hemiplegic patient become spastic. This **spasticity** may interfere seriously with the exercise of the **voluntary** muscle power that the patient has regained. Drugs and therapies have been tried to overcome the unfortunate handicap and, in extreme cases, surgical intervention has been imperative. It consists of a **transection** of the motor nerve to the extremity, resulting in **flaccid musculature,** which is preferred to the incapacitating spasticity.

Hemiplegia which occurs suddenly is usually due to involvement of the **internal capsule** resulting from a rupture of a small branch of the middle **cerebral artery.** An occlusion of the main trunk affects a large portion of the **cerebral hemisphere** and causes contralateral hemiplegia. Small infarcts may produce transient and permanent paralysis. Since the advent of **angiography,** there has been sufficient evidence that the **vascular occlusion** may involve the **cervical** segment of the internal **carotid** artery.

It is a well known fact that hemiplegia occurs on the side opposite to the brain injury. The reason for this is that about ninety per cent of upper motor neurons cross over to the contralateral side at the level of the medulla oblongata.

With adequate rehabilitation the majority of patients who survive a stroke can literally be put back on their feet and return to normal living with little or no **residual damage** depending on the extent of their **cerebrovascular accident.**[7, 15, 19, 20, 25]

Chapter edited by Sister Mary Imelda Pingel SS.M., professor and chairman of the Department of Physical Therapy, and faculty, St. Louis University.

REFERENCES AND BIBLIOGRAPHY

1. Anderson R. Active exercise and passive mobilization in the treatment of Colles' fracture. *Seventh International Congress.* London: World Confederation for Physical Therapy, 1974, pp. 437-442.
2. Basmajian, J. V. *Muscle Alive: Their functions revealed by electromyography,* 3rd ed. Baltimore: The Williams and Wilkins Co., 1974.
3. Beverly, E. V. The mechanics of putting those little used muscles in motion. *Geriatrics,* 31: 132-134, January, 1976.
4. _____. An assortment of fitness programs. *Ibid.,* 31: 122-131, February, 1976.
5. Bishop, G. Neurophysiology of motor responses evoked by vibratory stimulation. *Physical Therapy,* 54: 1273-1282, December, 1974.
6. _____. Vibratory stimulation as an evaluation tool. *Ibid.,* 55: 28-34, January, 1975.
7. Bogardh, E. *et al.* Gait analysis and relearning of gait control in hemiplegic patients. *Seventh International Congress.* London: World Confederation for Physical Therapy, 1974, pp. 443-453.
8. Brinkworth, K. E. Modified goniometer for the knee joint. *Physical Therapy,* 56: 189-190, February, 1976.
9. Brunkow, R. Facilitation of normal movement in patients of different age groups. *Seventh International Congress.* London: World Confederation for Physical Therapy, 1974, pp. 411-415.
10. Brunnstrom, Signe. *Clinical Kinesiology,* 3rd ed. Philadelphia: F. A. Davis Co., 1975, pp. 1-53.
11. Bugaj, R. The cooling analgesic and rewarming effects of ice massage on localized skin. *Physical Therapy,* 55: 11-19, January, 1975.
12. Chusid, Joseph. Electromyography. *Correlative Neuroanatomy and Functional Neurology,* 16th ed. Los Altos, California: Lange Medical Publications, 1976, pp. 235-244.
13. Coleman, L. Final goals of physical therapy. *Geriatrics,* 31: 91-95, May, 1976.
14. Cooper, John M. and Glasow, Ruth B. *Kinesiology,* 4th ed. St. Louis: The C. V. Mosby Co., 1976, pp. 3-108.
15. Currier, R. D. Acute stroke due to ischemic cerebrovascular disease. In Conn, Howard F. *Current Therapy 1976,* Philadelphia: W. B. Saunders Co., 1976, pp. 682-685.
16. Davies, H. Cardiovascular effects of the sauna. *American Journal of Physical Medicine,* 54: 178-185, August, 1975.
17. Dry, Victoria D., M.S. in PT. Personal communications.
18. Gault, W. R. Use of low intensity direct current in management of ischemic skin ulcers. *Physical Therapy,* 56: 265-267, March, 1976.
19. Grynbaum, B. B. Sensory feedback therapy for stroke patients. *Geriatrics,* 31: 43-50, June, 1976.
20. Hirschberg, G. G. Ambulation and self-care are goals of rehabilitation after stroke. *Geriatrics,* 31: 61-67, May, 1976.
21. Hislop, H. J. The not-so-impossible dream. *Physical Therapy,* 55: 1069-1080, October, 1975.
22. Johnson, R. *et al.* Myofeedback: A new method of teaching breathing exercises to emphysematous patients. *Physical Therapy,* 56: 826-829, July, 1976.
23. Kleinkort, J. *et al.* Phonophoresis. *Physical Therapy,* 55: 1320-1324, December, 1975.
24. Krusen, F. H. *et al. Handbook of Physical Medicine and Rehabilitation,* 2nd ed. Philadelphia: W. B. Saunders Co., 1971, pp. 1-13.
25. Lee, J. E. Rehabilitation of the patient with hemiplegia. In Conn, Howard F. *Current Therapy 1976,* Philadelphia: W. B. Saunders Co., 1976, pp. 682-685.
26. Lowdon, B. *et al.* Determinants and nature of intramuscular temperature changes during cold therapy. *American Journal of Physical Medicine,* 54: 223-233, October, 1975.
27. Nafpliotis, H. Electromyographic feedback to improve ankle dorsiflexion, wrist extension and hand grasp. *Physical Therapy,* 56: 821-825, July, 1976.
28. Picaza, J. A. *et al.* Pain suppression by peripheral nerve stimulation. *Surgical Neurology,* 4: 105-114, July, 1975.
29. Pingel, Sister Mary Imelda, B.S. in PT, Ed.M. Personal communications.
30. Pollock, D. Progressive resistive exercise device for quadriplegic patients. *Physical Therapy,* 55: 992-993, September, 1975.
31. Scott, Pauline M. *Clayton's Electrotherapy and Actinotherapy,* 7th ed. Baltimore: The Williams and Wilkins Co., 1975, pp. 378-390.
32. Shoenfeld, Y. *et al.* Heat stress in saunas. *Archives of Physical Medicine and Rehabilitation,* 57: 126-129, March, 1976.
33. Shriber, William J. *A Manual of Electrotherapy,* 4th ed. Philadelphia: Lea and Febiger, 1975, pp. 11-245.
34. Tigny, R. Device for assistive and resistive exercise for wrist and hand. *Physical Therapy,* 56: 426-427, April, 1976.
35. Teng, E. L. *et al.* Electrical stimulation and feedback training: Effects on the voluntary control of paretic muscles. *Archives of Physical Medicine and Rehabilitation,* 57: 228-233, May, 1976.
36. Vega, R. Shiatsu: A pressure technique. *Physical Therapy,* 55: 381-382, April, 1975.
37. Waylonis, G. W. Subcutaneous electrical stimulation (acupuncture) in the clinical practice of physical medicine. *Archives of Physical Medicine and Rehabilitation,* 57: 161-165, April, 1976.
38. Wood, Elizabeth. *Beard's Massage: Principles and Techniques,* 2nd ed. Philadelphia: W. B. Saunders Co., 1974, pp. 3-148.

Chapter XX
Selected Terms Pertaining to Nuclear Medicine

ORIENTATION

A. Origin of Terms:

1. atom (G) — indivisible
2. dense (L) — dense, compact
3. fission (L) — cleft, split
4. ion (G) — going
5. iso (G) — equal

6. kinetic (G) — movable
7. proto- (G) — first
8. tope (G) — place
9. tele- (G) — distant
10. scintilla (L) — spark

B. General Terms Related to Nuclear Medicine:

1. activated water — water contaminated by ionizing radiation.
2. activation analysis — a method for identifying and measuring the chemical elements in a sample to be analyzed. The sample is first made radioactive by bombardment with neutrons, charged particles, or other nuclear radiation. The newly radioactive atoms in the sample give off characteristic nuclear radiations that can identify the atoms and indicate their quantity. Activation analysis is frequently more sensitive than chemical analysis. It is being used more and more in research.[22]
3. acute exposure — a brief, intense radiation exposure in contradistinction to prolonged or chronic exposure.
4. alpha particle — a positively charged helium nucleus characterized by poorly penetrating but strongly ionizing radiation.
5. annihilation reaction — the rapid collision of a positron and electron resulting in a gamma ray.[17]
6. atom — smallest unit of any element which consists of a central nucleus and outer orbital electrons. The nucleus is composed of protons and neutrons except that of the hydrogen atom which has no neutrons.
   a. electrons — negatively charged particles revolving around the nucleus.
   b. neutrons — electrically neutral particles present in the nucleus of an atom.
   c. protons — positively charged particles present in the nucleus of an atom.
7. atomic weight — relative weight of an atom compared to that of one oxygen atom which is 16.
8. background radiation — the radiation of man's natural environment, consisting of that which comes from cosmic rays and from the naturally radioactive elements of the earth, including that from within man's body. The term may also mean radiation extraneous to an experiment.[22]
9. beta particle — nuclear particle either positively or negatively charged. When positively charged the positron is useful for its gamma ray produced at decay which is a form of annihilation reaction. When negatively charged the beta particle is essentially an electron, more penetrating and less ionizing than an alpha particle. The effect of beta particles is moderately destructive and usually limited to the first few millimeters of tissue.[17]
10. body burden — the amount of radioactive material present in the body of man or animal.[22]
11. bone seeker — a radionuclide that tends to lodge in the bones when it is introduced into the body. Example: strontium-90, which behaves chemically like calcium.[22]
12. byproduct material — in atomic energy law, any radioactive material (except source or fissionable material) obtained in the process of producing or using source or fissionable material. Includes fission products and many other radioisotopes produced in nuclear reactors.

13. contamination, radioactive — the spread of radioactivity to places where it can have adverse effects on persons, experiments and equipment.

14. counter — a device for making radiation measurements or counting ionizing events. The term is used loosely as a synonym of detector.

15. curie — the unit for measuring the activity of all radioactive substances, or the quantity of radioactive material which undergoes 3.7×10^{10} disintegrations per second.

16. cyclotron — a particle accelerator in which charged particles receive repeated synchronized accelerations of "kicks" by electric fields as the particles spiral outward from their source. The particles are kept in the spiral by a powerful magnet. Cyclotrons are a valuable source of radionuclides for medical diagnosis and research.

17. decay, radioactive — diminished activity of a radioactive substance in the course of time.[47]

18. decontamination — the removal of harmful radioactive material from persons, equipment, instruments, rooms and the like. Some articles may be decontaminated by thorough washing with detergents or other chemicals.[40]

19. dose (clinical radionuclides) — the amount of radionuclides for diagnostic evaluation known as tracer dose or for treatment referred to as therapeutic dose.[17]

20. dosimeter — an instrument for measuring the dose of radiation.[16]

21. external hazards — exposure to ionizing radiation from radioactive sources outside the body.

22. film badge — photographic, dental size x-ray film worn on the person for detecting radiation exposure.[16]

23. gamma ray — short wave length electromagnetic radiation of nuclear origin. Gamma rays are more penetrating than alpha and beta particles, are similar to x-rays and very useful in diagnostic nuclear medicine.[17]

24. Geiger-Müller counter — a sensitive radiation detector composed of a tube filled with gas and a scaler. It is used to detect nuclear radiation.[17]

25. half-life, biologic — the time required for a biologic system, such as a man or an animal, to eliminate, by natural processes, half the amount of a substance which has entered it.

26. half-life, radioactive — time required for a radioactive substance to lose 50 percent of its activity by decay.

    For example:

    Radiophosphorus — ^{32}P has a half-life of 14 days. This means that a quantity of ^{32}P having a radioactivity of

    250.0 mCi (millicuries) on a certain day will have an activity of

    125.0 mCi (millicuries) 14 days later and

    62.5 mCi (millicuries) 28 days later.

27. health physics (radiobiology) — a branch of physics which deals with the protection of personnel from the hazards of ionizing radiation.[22]

28. internal hazards — those caused by exposure to ionizing radiation from radioactive substances deposited inside the body.

29. ion — an atomic particle, charged atom or chemically bound group of atoms.

30. ionization — the process of producing ions.

31. isotopes — atoms having the same number of protons (atomic number) but differing by their atomic weight.

32. labeled compound — a compound composed in part of a radionuclide. For example:

    Sodium radioiodide .... $Na^{131}I$

    Radiocobalt B_{12} .... $^{60}CoB_{12}$

    Chromic radiophosphate .... $Cr^{32}PO_4$

33. mass number — the sum of the neutrons and protons in a nucleus. The mass number of uranium-235 is 235. It is the nearest whole number to the atom's actual atomic weight.

34. maximum permissible concentration — that amount of radioactive material in air, water, and foodstuffs which competent authorities have established as the maximum that would not create undue risk to human health. (See also radioactivity concentration guide.)[22]

35. maximum permissible dose — that dose of ionizing radiation which competent authorities have established as the maximum that can be absorbed without undue risk to human health. (See also radiation protection guide.)[16, 22]

36. median lethal dose (MLD, LD_{50}) — radiation dose which kills, in a given period, 50 per cent of a large group of animals or other organisms.[40]

37. microcurie (nuclear medicine) — unit for measuring the energy of a radionuclide in a tracer dose. One microcurie is one millionth of a curie.[40]

38. millicurie (nuclear medicine) — unit for measuring the energy of a radionuclide in a therapeutic dose. One millicurie equals a thousand microcuries.[40]

39. monitoring — area monitoring, a procedure for determining the amount of radioactive contamination present in a certain locality and at a given time. In personnel monitoring, individuals are monitored; namely, their breath, excreta, clothing and the like in order to detect health hazards and provide environmental safety.[17]

40. nuclear fission — the splitting of a heavy nucleus into two or more nuclei, resulting in nuclear conversion and the release of powerful energy.

41. nuclear numbers:[33]

Symbol

a. atomic number   Z — number of protons in the nucleus of an atom.

b. neutron number N — number of neutrons in the nucleus of an atom.

c. mass number   A — sum of neutrons and protons in the nucleus of an atom.
   $A = Z + N.$

42. nucleon — an essential part of a nucleus, synonym for protons or neutrons.

43. nucleus of an atom — central part of atom containing protons, or positively charged particles, and neutrons, or neutral particles.

44. nuclide — term denoting all nuclear species of chemical elements, both stable and unstable. It is used synonymously with isotope.

45. overexposure to radiation — excessive contamination by radiant energy which has deleterious effects on a person's health. In massive overexposure symptoms of radiation injury develop in hours, days or weeks; in chronic overexposure to small amounts of radiation, within months or years.

46. photon — a discrete quantity of electromagnetic energy. Photons have momentum but no mass or electric charge.[22]

47. positron — a positively charged nuclear electron.[17]

48. proton — an elementary particle with a single positive electric charge and a mass approximately 1847 times that of the electron. The atomic number of an atom is equal to the number of protons in its nucleus.

49. radiation — the propagation of energy through matter or space in the form of waves. In atomic physics the term has been extended to include fast-moving particles (alpha and beta rays, free neutrons, etc.). Gamma rays and x-rays, of particular interest in atomic physics, are electromagnetic radiation in which energy is propagated in packets called photons.

50. radiation protection guide — the total amounts of ionizing radiation dose over certain periods of time which may safely be permitted to exposed industrial groups. These standards, established by the Federal Radiation Council, are equivalent to what was formerly called the "maximum permissible exposure."

51. radiation protection procedures — techniques used to safeguard patients and personnel from external and internal exposure. Principles of safety are concerned with:

a. time — the shorter the period of exposure the less dangerous the radiation dose.

b. distance — the further away from the radioactive substance, the less radiation received. Distance is a more important factor than time, and it varies inversely as the square of the distance.

c. shielding — the denser the material between the individual and radioactive material, the less is the radiation hazard. Protection from internal exposure is achieved by avoiding ingestion, inhalation and direct contact with radioactive materials.

Monitoring records must be kept on all persons exposed to nuclear radiation in their employment.[17]

52. radioactive tracer — radionuclide used in minute amount in diagnostic testing.[17]

53. radioactivity — the spontaneous decay or disintegration of an unstable atomic nucleus, accompanied by the emission of radiation.

54. radioassay — quantitative analysis of substances using radionuclide tracer techniques to detect minute quantities not easily measured by other means.[17]

55. radioautograph, autoradiograph — record of radiation from radioactive material in an object, made by placing its surface in close proximity to a photographic emulsion.[40]
    By this technique differences in cell function are discernible.

56. radiobiology — a branch of biology dealing with the effects of radiation on biologic systems.

57. radioimmunoassay (RIA) — technique of measuring minute amounts of substances by employing antigens and or antibodies labeled with radioactive tracers.
    This technique has been applied to other biologically active substances including nonimmune systems. Commonly used radioassay procedures measure serum levels of
    a. cardiac glycosides such as digoxin
    b. cortisol
    c. folic acid
    d. triiodothyronine (T-3)
    e. thyrotoxine (T-4)
    f. vitamin B_{12}.
    Radioimmunoassays offer reliable data and excel in specificity and sensitivity.[5, 17, 26, 39]

58. radioisotopes — chemical elements that have been made radioactive by bombardment with neutrons in an atomic pile or cyclotron. Some occur in nature. By giving off radiation, they provide a valuable means for diagnosis and treatment. Radioisotopes differ from their nonradioactive partners by their atomic weight.
    For example:
    Potassium, the stable isotope has an atomic weight of 39.
    Radiopotassium, the unstable isotope has an atomic weight of 42.

59. radionuclides, radioactive nuclides — comprehensive terms including isobars, isomers, isotones and isotopes that exist for a measurable length of time and differ by atomic weight, atomic number and energy state. The term radioisotope has become obsolete and radionuclide is the accepted term.
    a. isobars — atoms have the same mass number (A), but have different atomic numbers (Z) and neutron numbers (N).
    b. isomers — atoms have the same atomic numbers (Z) and the same mass numbers (A) but differ in nuclear energy states.
    c. isotones — atoms have the same number of neutrons in the nucleus (N) but differ in atomic numbers (Z) and number of mass particles (A).
    d. isotopes — atoms have the same atomic numbers (Z), different numbers of mass particles (A) and therefore different number of nuclear neutrons (N).[33]

60. radionuclidic imaging devices — currently several instruments are in common use:
    a. Anger camera, scintillation camera, gamma camera — an instrument for presenting images of the distribution of radioactivity in any organ or part of the body.
       Its greatest assets are speed and sensitivity, which are of particular significance in dynamic function studies.[4, 6]
    b. Anger multiplane tomographic scanner — nuclear instrument which provides six complete synchronized images or readouts of variable depth or plane on a single scan (film).[4, 17, 41]
    c. autofluoroscope, digital autofluoroscope — a device for producing pictures of the distribution of gamma-emitting radionuclides within organs. It is capable of concentrating on areas of special importance, which increases the value of dynamic function studies.[6]
    d. PETT — device for positron emitting transaxial tomography.[17]
    e. rectilinear scanner — the conventional scanner and a moving detector of radioactivity in selected areas of the body which is useful for static studies.[4, 6, 42]

61. reactor — a device by means of which a fission chain reaction can be initiated, maintained and controlled. Its essential component is a core with fissionable fuel. It usually has a moderator, a reflector, shielding, and control mechanisms.[22]
62. relative biologic effectiveness (RBE) — the relative effectiveness of a given kind of ionizing radiation in producing a biologic response as compared with gamma rays.
63. scaler — an electronic instrument for counting radiation-induced pulses from Geiger counters and other radiation detectors.[22]
64. scan — image of the deposit of a radionuclide.
    a. photoscan — the pattern of radioactivity presented on x-ray film by a photorecorder.
    b. scintillation scan — image made by a scintillation counter to determine the size of a tumor, goiter or other involvement and to locate aberrant, metastatic lesions.
65. scanning (nuclear medicine) — method of mapping out the deposition of a radionuclide in an organ using a rectilinear or other scanning device.[17]
66. scintillation counter — a highly sensitive detector for measuring ionizing radiation capable of counting scintillations (light flashes) induced by radiation in certain materials.[4]
67. scintiphotography, gammaphotography — the use of the Anger scintillation camera for obtaining photographs of the distribution of gamma-emitting radionuclides in living subjects.[6]
    Scintiphotography may be employed for:
    a. dynamic studies portraying rapidly changing images as the visualization of blood flow, vascular filling, or of ventilation.
    b. static studies requiring highly technical performance of individual images (views) and comparability of tracer concentration in related organs, for example: the intensity of radioactivity concentration in the spleen and marrow compared with that in the liver, in order to demonstrate portal-systemic shunting of venous blood flow after surgery.[4, 6]
68. teletherapy with ^{60}Co — treatment using shielded units which emit radiocobalt gamma rays from a distance. An effective dose permits the internal bombardment of deep seated tumors, a small dose suffices for surface lesions, and rotation allows the selection of irradiation patterns.[17, 19, 22]
69. tracer — an element or compound that has been made radioactive so that it can be easily followed (traced) in biologic and industrial processes. Radiation emitted by the radioisotope pinpoints its location.[17]
70. waste, radioactive — equipment and materials (from nuclear operations) which are radioactive and for which there is no further use. Wastes are generally referred to as high-level (having radioactivity concentrations of hundreds to thousands of curies per gallon or cubic foot), low-level (in range of 1 microcurie per gallon or cubic foot) and intermediate (between these extremes).[22]
71. whole body counter — a device used to identify and measure the radiation in the body (body burden) of humans and animals; uses heavy shielding to keep out background radiation and ultrasensitive scintillation detectors and electronic equipment.[4]

NUCLEAR MEDICINE

A. Terms Related to Radionuclide Imaging:

1. blood flow imaging, perfusion studies — noninvasive, dynamic, nuclear uptake measurements to detect occlusive or stenotic vascular lesions or malformations of the brain, heart, lungs, kidneys, skeletal muscles, others.[8, 10, 17, 43, 44, 45]
2. bone marrow imaging — delineation of areas of active bone marrow to detect abnormal expansion of bone marrow and areas of bone marrow destruction.[21, 25]
3. bone imaging — scintillation imaging following the intravenous injection of a bone seeking radionuclide such as one of the technetium-99m phosphate complexes to detect metastases to osseous tissue and help determine the extent of pathologic bone lesions or healing processes.[17, 36, 38, 46]

4. brain imaging — radionuclide uptake studies, dynamic or static, to detect intracerebral space occupying lesions, malformations, trauma or cerebrovascular disease. Radionuclides such as technetium 99m bound to diethylenetriamine pentaacetic acid (DTPA) are often used as diagnostic tracers.[7, 14]   Included in these studies are

   a. cerebral circulation imaging — dynamic brain imaging to visualize cerebral blood flow, to compare values in different regions, to analyze cerebrovascular disease or other vascular abnormalities.   A series of images are taken at specific intervals.[43]

   b. radionuclide cisternography — intrathecal injection of a tracer for diagnostic evaluation.   Scans of cisterns are useful in delineating obstructive, nonobstructive or *ex vacuo* types of hydrocephalus.   They also aid in visualizing the point of leak in a cerebrospinal fluid (CSF) fistula, manifested by CSF otorrhea or rhinorrhea. This type of "flow" study is considered an integral part of the CNS diagnostic brain study.[15, 17]

   c. radionuclide ventriculography — a tagged albumin tracer is injected into both lateral ventricles or into a neurosurgical shunt to demonstrate the patency or blockage of the ventricular-vascular communication.[15, 17]
Nuclear cisternography and ventriculography aid in the diagnosis of subarachnoid hemorrhage or block, intraventricular tumor, obstructive hydrocephalus and in the evaluation of neurosurgical shunts.[14, 15, 17]

5. heart and circulation imaging

   a. dynamic cardiovascular studies

     (1) cardiac function by blood pool imaging and measurements, e.g. comparing systole with diastole, others

     (2) evaluation of myocardial perfusion

     (3) evaluation of myocardial damage, others.[1, 7, 17, 30, 31, 35, 44, 48]
In order to study heart function, a physiologic synchronizer such as the EKG triggered "gating" device is needed to help eliminate the artifacts inherent to myocardial contraction and relaxation.[17]

   b. static mediastinal studies — blood pool measurements of cardiac silhouette for mediastinal imaging to differentiate pericardial effusion from cardiac dilatation or other disorders.[7, 17, 44]

6. kidney imaging, renal imaging — nuclear tracer visualization of kidneys to study their structural and functional status and detect congenital abnormalities, perfusion defects, renovascular disease, obstructive lesions, kidney trauma or other renal disorders.[7, 10]

7. liver imaging, hepatic imaging — nuclear method of assessing liver damage, hepatomegaly, tumors, metastases, liver abscess, other.[7, 18, 34]

8. lung imaging — pulmonary imaging by

   a. technetium-99m aggregated human serum albumin injected into the pulmonary circulation for perfusion studies.   The particles lodge in the capillaries of the lung except in areas of embolic obstruction or other blockage (about 70% of emboli are multiple).[17, 45]

   b. xenon-133 (^{133}Xe) for ventilatory studies injected or inhaled to differentiate between emphysematous involvement or pulmonary emboli.
The diagnosis is based on the interpretation of blood flow through the lungs in serial scans.   Perfusion defects, seen in early nuclide image and cleared after 4 to 5 days of anticoagulation therapy, are presumptive evidence of recovery from embolic disease. No change in serial lung scans suggests the presence of obstructive lung disease as emphysema, carcinoma or other disorders.[2, 3, 17, 20, 23, 45]

B. Terms Related to Radionuclides in Diagnostic Tests:

1. blood studies:

   a. blood volume — sum total of red cell volume and plasma volume using chromium (^{51}Cr) labeled red cells or technetium-99m (^{99}Tc) labeled red cells for measuring the blood volume.

Normal ranges

total red cell volume........25-30 ml/kg
total plasma volume........30-45 ml/kg
total blood volume.........55-75 ml/kg

Findings are valuable in the diagnosis of polycythemia vera and management of fluid balance after surgery and severe burns.[17]

b. iron studies, ferrokinetic tests — they include:

   (1) incorporation of iron (^{59}Fe) into red blood cells which in normal subjects is 60 to 80 per cent of the dose administered in 7 to 10 days

   (2) plasma iron clearance — iron (^{59}Fe) disappearance half time in plasma which is normally 60 to 120 minutes

   (3) plasma iron pool (in milligrams) — determination by multiplying serum iron in milligrams per milliliter with plasma volume per milliliter.

Results may indicate iron deficiency anemias, polycythemias, others.[8, 24]

c. red cell sequestration, RBC sequestration — measurement of rate of accumulation of chromium-51 (^{51}Cr) tagged red cells in spleen, liver and precordium by scintillation counting. The test aids in the diagnosis of hypersplenism due to any cause.

d. red cell survival — determination of the rate of disappearance of labeled erythrocytes from the circulating blood. Chromium-51 (^{51}Cr) is usually the tagging agent. **Normal rate** of RBC disappearance from the circulation is 28 to 32 days. **Decreased rate** of cell survival is present in hemolytic anemias.[8, 24]

2. clot formation studies:

a. fibrinogen uptake test ^{125}I — detection of thrombi in their formative stage by locating the vascular lesion where fibrinogen is being utilized.

b. fibrinogen uptake test ^{131}I — (same as above except for the tracer ^{131}I).[17]

3. gastrointestinal studies:

a. fat absorption test, lipid absorption test — measurement of fat digestion and absorption with radioiodine labeled triolein and oleic acid, useful in distinguishing malabsorption syndromes.[34]

b. GI blood loss determination — measurement of gastrointestinal bleeding by using chromium-51 (^{51}Cr) tagged red cells. They are normally absorbed into the digestive tract and are almost completely recovered in a 6 day stool collection. The test is of value in the detection of chronic and intermittent GI bleeding.[24, 34]

c. GI protein loss determination — measurement of albumin leakage into the gastrointestinal tract using intravenous injection of chromium-51 (^{51}Cr) labeled albumin.[34]

d. vitamin B_{12} absorption test, method of Schilling — determination of vitamin B_{12} absorption as aid in diagnosis of pernicious anemia and malabsorption of B_{12} due to other causes. Using cobalt 57, 58 or 60 as a tracer, the amount of B_{12} absorbed is indirectly measured by determining the per cent of the test dose that is excreted in the urine in 24 hours. Since the pathophysiology of pernicious anemia is the inability to absorb vitamin B_{12}, the urinary excretion in these patients is low (less than 10 per cent). If a potent intrinsic factor is administered with the test dose B_{12}, it will permit absorption of B_{12} from the intestine in pernicious anemia, but will not increase the absorption of B_{12} in the presence of malabsorption due to diseases other than pernicious anemia.[17, 24, 34, 39]

4. renal clearance study — functional renal imaging based on the fact that different radionuclear tracers measure the physiologic ability of specific areas of the kidney such as
a. effective renal plasma flow (ERPF) through glomeruli and proximal tubules
b. glomerular filtration rate (GFR).[8, 10, 17]

5. renography — a graphic demonstration of both kidneys following the intravenous injection of a radioactive tracer and the placement of a sensitive detector over the kidneys. In the presence of unilateral disease the curve of the moving nuclear bolus reflects reduced or increased tracer uptake by the affected kidney.[8, 10, 13, 17]

6. thyroid studies (major tests):[8, 11, 17, 29, 32, 39]

WHAT ARE NUCLIDES?

NUCLIDES ARE ATOMS OF AN ELEMENT DISTINGUISHABLE BY THEIR WEIGHT

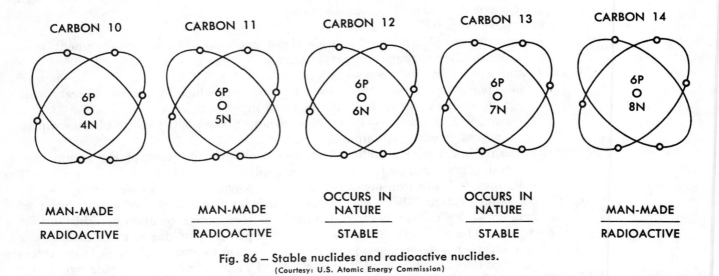

CARBON 10	CARBON 11	CARBON 12	CARBON 13	CARBON 14
6P O 4N	6P O 5N	6P O 6N	6P O 7N	6P O 8N
MAN-MADE	MAN-MADE	OCCURS IN NATURE	OCCURS IN NATURE	MAN-MADE
RADIOACTIVE	RADIOACTIVE	STABLE	STABLE	RADIOACTIVE

Fig. 86 — Stable nuclides and radioactive nuclides.
(Courtesy: U.S. Atomic Energy Commission)

RADIOACTIVE IODINE — ^{131}I

FOR DIAGNOSING AND TREATING THYROID GLAND DISORDERS

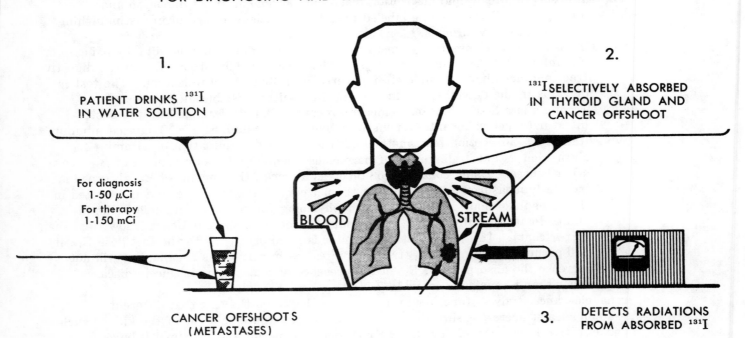

1.

PATIENT DRINKS ^{131}I
IN WATER SOLUTION

For diagnosis
1-50 μCi
For therapy
1-150 mCi

2.

^{131}I SELECTIVELY ABSORBED
IN THYROID GLAND AND
CANCER OFFSHOOT

BLOOD STREAM

CANCER OFFSHOOTS
(METASTASES)

3. DETECTS RADIATIONS
FROM ABSORBED ^{131}I

MEDICAL ACTION:

1. DIAGNOSIS AND TREATMENT OF HYPERTHYROIDISM
2. LOCATION OF THYROID CANCER OFFSHOOTS (METASTASES)
3. LOCATION OF THYROID CANCER AND METASTASES

Fig. 87 — Radioiodine and the thyroid gland.
(Courtesy: U.S. Atomic Energy Commission)

a. FTI, free thyroxine index, free T-4 index, FTE, free thyroxine estimate — a calculated result based on measuring the total thyroxine (T-4 MP or T-4 RIA) and TBI or similar test. The FTI eliminates errors of interpretation due to medication, pregnancy or other causes.[17]

    (1) competitive protein binding T-4, Murphy-Pattee technique, T-4 MP — determination of an unknown quantity of thyroxine by measuring the displacement of radionuclide-tagged thyroxine from its specific binding globulin. The tagged thyroxine will be released in proportion to the level of untagged thyroxine present.[17]

    (2) TBI, thyroxine binding index — a test of thyroid function based on thyroxine binding globulin levels in patient's serum. A major problem is that the use of the contraceptive pill has become so prevalent that it interferes with the clinical interpretation of the test by elevating the level of the thyroxine binding globulin (TBG) similar to pregnancy.[17]

b. RAIU, radioactive iodine uptake determination — test measures the ability of the thyroid gland to trap and organify the nuclide following the oral ingestion of a radioiodine tracer dose. A scintillation detector is used to determine the percentage of the thyroidal uptake of the radioiodine at some convenient time, usually 6 and 24 hours after the administration of the tracer dose.[8, 17, 39]

c. TBG, thyroxine binding globulin serum level — measurement of circulating levels of TBG. It is not to be confused with thyroxine binding index (TBI).[11, 17, 39]

d. TRF, thyrotropin releasing factor, TRH, thyrotropin releasing hormone serum level — measurement of TRF (or TRH) released from hypothalamus. It regulates release of thyrotropin from pituitary and is influenced by levels of serum thyroxine.[8, 11, 17]

e. TSH, thyroid stimulating hormone serum level — measurement of circulating levels of TSH. It is a valuable diagnostic aid in hypothyroidism in addition to the evaluation of pituitary function.[8, 11, 17]

f. TSH thyroid stimulation test — a radioiodine measurement of thyroid gland following the parenteral injection of thyroid stimulating hormone (TSH). The test aids in the differential diagnosis of primary hypothyroidism in which a diseased thyroid fails to respond to TSH. In secondary hypothyroidism the thyroid gland will begin to function after a TSH injection since the gland is simply dormant rather than diseased.

g. T-3 RIA serum level — measurement of triiodothyronine (T-3) in human serum by radioimmunoassay. An elevated T-3 serum level in the presence of normal T-4 (thyroxine) concentration may indicate T-3 toxicosis.[17]

h. T-3 or T-4 suppression test — measurement of the thyroidal uptake of radioiodine and scan following the oral administration of triiodothyronine (T-3) or thyroxine (T-4). In euthyroid patients there is usually a 50% suppression of the thyroidal uptake. In thyrotoxicosis it does not drop below the normal range. The test is useful in distinguishing neurotic individuals with borderline uptake from true hyperthyroidism.[17]

A summary of radionuclides used in diagnostic evaluation is presented.

Table 33
SOME RADIONUCLIDES IN DIAGNOSIS[a, b, c]

Radionuclide	Labeled Tracer	Diagnostic Procedures	Clinical Use
Iodine-131 or 123 ^{131}I ^{123}I	Sodium iodide	Thyroid scan and uptake RAIU	Thyroid carcinoma Thyroid adenoma Thyroid nodule Others
Iodine-125 ^{125}I	Thyroxine T-4	Thyroid function studies T-4 CPB (Thyroxine by competitive protein binding)	Thyroid disease T-4 toxicosis

Radionuclide	Labeled Tracer	Diagnostic Procedures	Clinical Use
	Triiodothyronine T-3	TBI (Thyroxine binding index) FTI (Free thyroxine index) T-3 (Triiodothyronine uptake test)	T-3 toxicosis
	Others	TSH (Thyroid stimulating hormone)	Others
	Fibrinogen	Clot formation study ^{125}I fibrinogen uptake	Detection of thrombi in formative stage
	Human serum albumin	Blood volume determination, cardiac output, circulation time	Vascular and cardiac disease
		Others	Others
Iodine-131 or 123 ^{131}I ^{123}I	Rose bengal	Liver scan Rate of clearance of labeled tracer	Patency of biliary system
Technetium-99m ^{99m}Tc	Diethylenetriamine pentaacetic acid DTPA or DTPA chelate	Brain scan Perfusion studies Nuclear cisternography Nuclear ventriculography	Brain lesion Vascular disorder Hydrocephalus Others
	DTPA or DTPA chelate	Measurement of renal function a. Effective renal plasma flow-ERPF b. Glomerular filtration rate-GFR	Renal clearance
	Pertechnetate	Renography or imaging	Renal disorder unilateral or bilateral obstructive renovascular hypertensive
		Perfusion studies	Transplanted kidney
	Pertechnetate	Cerebral circulation studies	Cerebrovascular disorders
	Human serum albumin	Nuclear cisternography Nuclear ventriculography	Hydrocephalus Others
	Aggregated human serum albumin	Nuclear cardiology Angiocardiographic studies	Congenital cardiac defects Myocardial infarction Ventricular aneurysm Others
	Aggregated human serum albumin	Lung perfusion studies	Pulmonary embolism Pulmonary venous hypertension Arteriovenous shunt Response to anti-coagulation therapy

Radionuclide	Labeled Tracer	Diagnostic Procedures	Clinical Use
	Phosphate complexes	Bone scan	Metastatic bone lesions Osteomyelitis
	Sulfur colloid	Liver and spleen scans	Primary or metastatic cancer Hepatic abscess Others

Chromium-51
^{51}Cr
	Human red cells
	Human serum albumin
		Blood volume determination
		Red cell survival
		Fecal analysis for
		  blood loss
		  protein loss
			Hemolytic disease
			
			Intestinal protein loss in hypoproteinemia

Iron-52 or 59
^{52}Fe
^{59}Fe
	Ferrous citrate	Determination of
		  plasma iron clearance
		  plasma iron turnover rate
		  plasma iron pool
			Aplastic anemia
			Hemolytic anemia
			Iron deficiency anemia
			Others

Cobalt-57 or 60 ^{57}Co ^{60}Co	Cyanocobalamine B$_{12}$	Determination of intestinal absorption of vitamin B$_{12}$	Pernicious anemia Sprue

aJohn A Gantz, M.D. Personal communications.

bM. D. Blaufox and L. M. Freeman. *Physicians' Desk Reference for Radiology and Nuclear Medicine*, 6th ed. Oradell, N.J.: Medical Economics, 1976-1977.

cHenry N. Wagner (ed.). *Nuclear Medicine.* New York: HP Publishing Co., Inc., 1975.

RADIOACTIVE PHOSPHORUS-32 THERAPY

In Form of

Colloidal ^{32}P Chromic Phosphate

Given by Intracavitary Injection (not absorbed by bone marrow)

Effective agent in

1. partial or complete suppression of formation of fluid

2. prevention and treatment of metastases

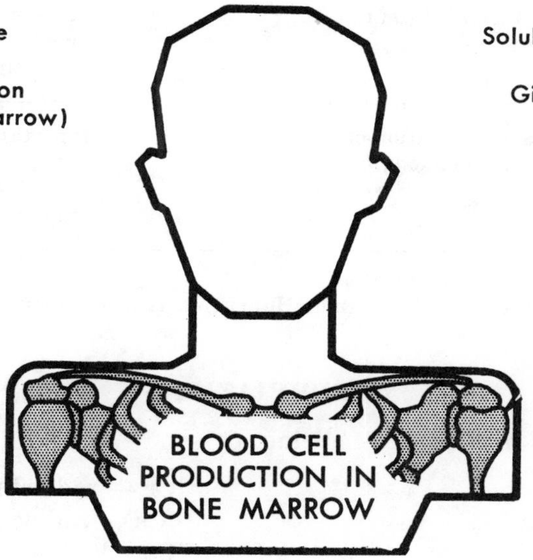

Soluble ^{32}P Disodium Phosphate

Given by Intravenous Injection (selectively absorbed by bone marrow)

Effective agent in

1. polycythemia vera to reduce the production of RBC

2. chronic leukemia to inhibit the production of WBC

BLOOD CELL PRODUCTION IN BONE MARROW

Fig. 88 — Important therapeutic uses of radioactive phosphorus.

C. Terms Related to Radionuclides in Therapy:

In nuclear medicine radionuclides are primarily used for tracer studies and their significance in diagnostic evaluation has been firmly established. In contradistinction the application of radionuclides to treatment is more restricted in its scope than it is in regard to diagnosis. In the past research efforts have been principally directed toward the conquest of malignancies. Experience proves that radionuclides in the treatment of carcinomas serve as palliative agents with potential for prolonging life and a low capacity for inhibiting or destroying malignancies other than certain thyroid and ovarian cancers.[17]

In addition, the possible carcinogenic properties of radioactive drugs constitute a limiting factor, particularly in the management of young patients. Current therapeutic uses of radionuclides are presented in Table 34.

Table 34

SOME RADIONUCLIDES IN THERAPY

Radionuclide	Method	Clinical Use

Cobalt-60
^{60}Cobalt
	Brachytherapy
	    Intracavity insertion of
	        radiocobalt rods, pellets,
	        beads
	    Interstitial use of
	        radiocobalt needles,
	        sutures or wires
	
	Teletherapy
	    External high energy
	        irradiation by telecobalt
	        unit
		Cancer of uterine cervix,
		    larynx, nasopharynx,
		    bladder
		
		Others
		
		Cancer of breast and
		    other malignancies

Phosphorus-32
^{32}P
	Intravenous administration
	    of disodium phosphate
	
	Intracavitary infusion
	    of colloidal chromic
	    phosphate
		Polycythemia vera and
		    selected cases of leukemia
		    or lymphoma
		
		Palliation of pain in some
		    bone metastases
		
		Therapeutic or palliative
		    treatment of pleural and
		    peritoneal malignancy or
		    resulting effusion

Iodine-131
^{131}I
	Oral administration of
	    sodium radioiodine
		Hyperthyroidism adenocarcinoma
		    of thyroid
		Selected cases of angina pectoris
		    and heart failure

aJohn A. Gantz, M.D. Personal communications.

bF. W. George. Radionuclide therapy. In Wagner, Henry N. *Nuclear Medicine.* New York: HP Publishing Co., Inc., 1975, pp. 215-224.

ABBREVIATIONS

A. Symbols of Radionuclides in Nuclear Medicine:

^{111}Ag — radiosilver

^{72}As, ^{74}As — radioarsenic

^{198}Au — radiogold

^{57}Co, ^{60}Co — radiocobalt

^{51}Cr — radiochromium

^{137}Cs — radiocesium

^{61}Cu, ^{64}Cu — radiocopper

^{18}F — radiofluorine

^{52}Fe, ^{59}Fe — radioiron
^{67}Ga — radiogallium
^{197}Hg, ^{203}Hg — radiomercury
^{113m}In — radioindium
^{125}I, ^{131}I — radioiodine
^{192}Ir — radioiridium
^{42}K — radiopotassium
^{52}Mn — radiomagnesium
^{24}Na — radiosodium

^{32}P — radiophosphorus
^{86}Rb — radiorubidium
^{35}S — radiosulfur
^{85}Sr, ^{87}Sr — radiostrontium
^{99m}Tc — radiotechnetium
^{169}Yb — radioytterbium
* — radioactive (*Au — radiogold)
^{90}Y — radioyttrium

B. Symbols of Tests and Miscellaneous:

A — mass number
B/K — bladder kidney (scan ratio)
^{57}Co or ^{60}Co B$_{12}$ — radiocobalt labeled vitamin B$_{12}$
CPB — competitive protein binding
CPM — count per minute
EOB — end of bombardment
FTI — free thyroxine index
FUT — fibrinogen uptake test
GM — Geiger-Müller (counter)
HEG — high energy gamma
IHSA — iodinated human serum albumin
^{131}IHSA — radioiodinated human serum albumin
LD$_{50}$ — median lethal dose
MAA — macroaggregated albumin
MHP — mercuryhydroxypropane
MLD — median lethal dose
MPC — maximum permissible concentration

MPL — maximum permissible level or limit
N — neutron
PBI-131 — protein bound radioiodine
PIT — plasma iron turnover rate
RAIU — radioactive iodine uptake
RBE — relative biologic effectiveness
REG — radiation exposure guide
RISA — radioiodinated human serum albumin
TBG — thyroxine binding globulin
TBI — thyroxine binding index
TBP — thyroxine binding protein
TBPA — thyroxine binding prealbumin
T-4 MP — T-4 Murphy-Pattee test
TRF — thyrotropin releasing factor
TRH — thyrotropin releasing hormone
TSH — thyrotropin, thyroid stimulating hormone
Z — atomic number

C. Scientific Organizations:

ABNM — American Board of Nuclear Medicine
ACR — American College of Radiology
AEC — Atomic Energy Commission (previous name, now NRC)
ARRS — American Roentgen Ray Society
ARRT — American Registry of Radiologic Technologists
ERDA — Energy Research and Development Agency
FASRT — Fellow of American Society of Radiologic Technologists
FRC — Federal Radiation Council

HP Soc. — Health Physics Society
ICRP — International Commission on Radiation Protection
ICRU — International Commission on Radiation Units
NCRP — National Commission on Radiation Protection
NRC — Nuclear Regulatory Commission (previously AEC)
RSNA — Radiological Society of North America
SNM — Society of Nuclear Medicine
UNSCEAR — United Nations Scientific Committee on the Effects of Atomic Radiation

D. Multiples of Curie Units:[17]

1 Ci	curie		1 curie
1 mCi	millicurie		10^{-3} curie
1 μCi	microcurie		10^{-6} curie
1 nCi	nanocurie		10^{-9} curie
1 pCi	picocurie		10^{-12} curie

E. Other Units of Measurements:

Bev — 1 billion electron volts
E — energy in ergs
erg — 1 unit of work
ev — 1 electron volt
Kev, keV — 1 thousand electron volts

Mev, MeV — 1 million electron volts
r — roentgen
RAD, rad — radiation absorbed dose, 100 ergs/gm tissue
REM, rem — roentgen equivalent, man
REP, rep — roentgen equivalent, physical

F. Symbols of Useful Landmarks:

AM — auditory meatus
CM — costal margin
G — glabella
I — inion
IC — iliac crest
N — nose

SN — sternal notch
SP — symphysis pubis
TC — thyroid cartilage
U — umbilicus
XP — xiphoid process

ORAL READING PRACTICE

The Thyroid Gland and Radioiodine

The avidity of the thyroid for iodine is an interesting and unique characteristic of this endocrine gland. It is the basis of many thyroid function studies and the medical treatment of many thyroid diseases.

With the development of nuclear reactors as a part of the atomic weapons program, radionuclides became abundantly available as byproducts. Investigations proved that many of these are useful in clinical medicine.

Nuclides are varieties of a chemical element that differ in their atomic weights, but possess the same chemical properties. Some elements are available as both stable and **radioactive nuclides,** for example:

Iodine-127, the stable element with an atomic weight of 127

Iodine-131, one of the **radionuclides** with an atomic weight of 131.

The latter is a widely used radionuclide of iodine and is generally the one implied by the term **radioiodine.**

The value of radioiodine (^{131}I) in the diagnosis and treatment of **hyperthyroidism** and in thyroid cancer therapy was established within the past decades. ^{131}I does not differ chemically from iodine, but differs physically in that it emits beta particles and gamma rays. Since the beta particles penetrate only 2 mm of tissue, they are almost all absorbed within the gland. On the other hand, about 90 per cent of the gamma rays escape and can be accurately measured outside the body with a radiation detector such as a **scintillation counter.**[17]

^{131}I has a half-life of eight days. This means that every eight days its radioactivity is reduced to half the intensity present eight days previously. The half-life is of clinical importance since the nuclide must exert its effect not too long, to avoid excessive radiation damage, nor too short to insure adequate results.

When a radioiodine uptake study is ordered, the patient receives a callibrated dose of ^{131}I either in a capsule or in a solution. The tracer dose ranges from 5-25 **microcuries** (μCi), while therapeutic doses are measured in millicuries (1mCi = 1000 μCi). After oral administration radioiodine is rapidly absorbed from the gastrointestinal tract and selectively picked up by thyroid tissue. Within 4 to 6 hours the gland has become the depot for about one-fourth of the nuclide ingested. In 24 hours thyroid function can be estimated by the amount of radioiodine retained. The thyroidal uptake of ^{131}I by the normal gland in 24 hours is 15-40 per cent of the tracer dose. In hyperthyroidism it is 50-100 per cent.

Currently T-4 **competitive protein binding,** Murphy-Pattee technique, together with thyroxine binding index and their calculated results, the free thyroxine index have gained wide acceptance and are thought to yield reliable evaluation of thyroid function.[17, 39]

REFERENCES AND BIBLIOGRAPHY

1. Ahmad, M. *et al.* Technetium 99m stannous pyrophosphate myocardial imaging in patients with and without left ventricular aneurysms. *Circulation*, 53: 833-838, May, 1976.
2. Alderson, P. O. *et al.* The role of ^{133}Xe ventilation studies in the scintigraphic detection of pulmonary embolism. *Radiology*, 120: 633-640, September, 1976.
3. Anderson, T. M. *et al.* Radionuclide perfusion lung studies. *Radiology*, 120: 125-130, July, 1976.
4. Anger, H. O. Instruments: Specific devices. In Wagner, Henry N. *Nuclear Medicine.* New York: HP Publishing Co. Inc., 1975, pp. 29-40.
5. Berson, S. A. and Yalow, R. S. Radioimmunoassay. In Wagner, Henry N. (ed.). *Nuclear Medicine.* New York: HP Publishing Co. Inc., 1975, pp. 225-243.
6. Blaufox, M. Donald and Freeman, Leonard M. (eds.). Instrumentation. *Physicians' Desk Reference for Radiology and Nuclear Medicine,* 6th ed. Oradell, New Jersey: Medical Economics Co., 1976-1977, pp. 1-3.
7. _____. Organ imaging procedures in diagnostic nuclear medicine. *Ibid.,* pp. 36-68.
8. _____. Radionuclide procedures which do not require imaging. *Ibid.,* pp. 4-35.
9. _____. Therapeutic uses of radionuclides. *Ibid.,* pp. 81-85.
10. Blaufox, M. D. The kidneys. In Wagner, Henry N. (ed.). *Nuclear Medicine.* New York: HP Publishing Co. Inc., 1975, pp. 161-169.
11. Braverman, L. E. *et al.* The thyroid. In Wagner, Henry N. (ed.). *Nuclear Medicine.* New York: HP Publishing Co., Inc., 1975, pp. 127-135.
12. Chiu, L. C. *et al.* Computed tomography and brain scintigraphy in ischemic stroke. *American Journal of Roentgenology,* 127: 481-486, September, 1976.
13. Cole, A. T. *et al.* Bone scan in diagnosis of renal cell carcinoma. *Journal of Urology,* 114: 364-365, September, 1975.
14. DeLand, F. The brain. In Wagner, Henry N. (ed.). *Nuclear Medicine.* New York: HP Publishing Co. Inc., 1975, pp. 84-93.
15. DiChiro, G. The third circulation. In Wagner, Henry N. (ed.). *Nuclear Medicine.* New York: HP Publishing Co. Inc., 1975, pp. 103-111.
16. Frankel, Robert. *Radiation Protection for Radiologic Technologists.* New York: McGraw-Hill Book Co., 1976, pp. 117-124.
17. Gantz, John A., M.D. Personal communications.
18. Gumerman, L. W. Nuclear medicine studies in the diagnosis of diseases of the liver, pancreas and spleen. *Surgical Clinics of North America,* 55: 427-447, April, 1975.
19. Halsted, James A. (ed.). Radioactive pharmaceuticals. *The Laboratory in Clinical Medicine.* Philadelphia: W. B. Saunders Co., 1976, pp. 815-816.
20. Kassner, E. G. *et al.* Persisting perfusion defects. *Radiology,* 121: 139-142, October, 1976.
21. Knospe, W. H. Bone marrow scanning with [52]Iron ([52]Fe). *Cancer,* 37: 1432-1442, March, 1976.
22. Lyman, James D. and Loeb, Benjamin, S. (eds.). *Nuclear Terms.* Washington, D.C.: U. S. Atomic Division, 1964, pp. 1-35.
23. McGinnis, E. J. *et al.* Bronchial adenoma causing unilateral absence of pulmonary perfusion. *Radiology,* 120: 367-368, August, 1976.
24. McIntyre, P. A. The blood and blood forming organs. In Wagner, Henry N. (ed.). *Nuclear Medicine.* New York: HP Publishing Co. Inc., 1975, pp. 185-204.
25. _____. The reticuloendothelial system. *Ibid.,* pp. 205-222.
26. Murphy, Pearson, B. E. Competitive protein binding. In Wagner, Henry N. (ed.). *Nuclear Medicine.* New York: HP Publishing Co. Inc., 1975, pp. 233-237.
27. National Council on Radiation and Measurements. *Precautions in the Management of Patients who have Received Therapeutic Amounts of Radionuclides — Report 36.* Washington, D.C.
28. National Council on Radiation Protection. *Review of the Current State of Radiation Protection — NCRP, Report 43.* Washington, D.C., 1975.
29. Osathanondh, R. *et al.* Total and free thyroxine and triiodothyronine in normal and complicated pregnancy. *Clinical Endocrinology and Metabolism,* 42: 98-104, January, 1976.
30. Pitt, B. *et al.* Myocardial imaging in the non-invasive evaluation of patients with suspected ischemic heart disease. *American Journal of Cardiology,* 37: 797-806, April, 1976.
31. Platt, M. R. *et al.* Technetium stannous pyrophosphate myocardial scintigrams in the recog-

nition of myocardial infarction in patients undergoing coronary artery revascularization. *Annals of Thoracic Surgery*, 21: 311-317, April, 1976.

32. Premachandra, B. N. *et al.* Increased free thyroxine in a euthyroid patient with thyroxine-binding globulin deficiency *Clinical Endocrinology and Metabolism,* 42: 309-329, February, 1976.

33. Quimby, Edith H., Feitelberg, Sergei and Gross, William. *Radioactive Nuclides in Medicine and Biology,* 3rd ed. Philadelphia: Lea & Febiger, 1970, pp. 7-16.

34. Quinn, J. L. The gastrointestinal tract. In Wagner, Henry N. (ed.). *Nuclear Medicine.* New York: HP Publishing Co. Inc., 1975, pp. 153-160.

35. Ritchie, J. L. *et al.* Myocardial imaging with radionuclide-labeled particles. *Radiology,* 121: 131-138, October, 1976.

36. Schechter, J. P. *et al.* Bone scanning in lymphoma. *Cancer,* 38: 1142-1148, September, 1976.

37. Shani, J. *et al.* Adverse reactions to radiopharmaceuticals. *Seminars in Nuclear Medicine,* 6: 305-328, July, 1976.

38. Siegel, B. A. *et al.* Skeletal uptake of ^{99m}Tc-diphosphate in relation to local bone blood flow. *Radiology,* 120: 121-123, July, 1976.

39. *Specialized Diagnostic Laboratory Tests,* 11th ed. Van Nuys, California: Bio-Science Laboratories, 1976, pp. 4-120.

40. Thoma, George E., M.D. *Glossary of Terms in Nuclear Medicine.* St. Louis University School of Medicine.

41. Turner, D. A. *et al.* Brain scanning with the Anger multiplane tomographic scanner. *Radiology,* 121: 115-124, October, 1976.

42. Wagner, Henry N. (ed.). Computers. *Nuclear Medicine.* New York: HP Publishing Co. Inc., 1975, pp. 41-53.

43. ———. The cerebral circulation. *Ibid.,* pp. 94-101.

44. ———. The heart and circulation. *Ibid.,* pp. 112-120.

45. ———. The pulmonary circulation. *Ibid.,* pp. 122-126.

46. Weber, D. A. Characteristics of ^{99m}Tc labeled complexes used for bone imaging. *Radiology,* 120: 615-621, September, 1976.

47. Winchell, H. S. Radiopharmaceuticals. In Wagner, Henry N. (ed.). *Nuclear Medicine.* New York: HP Publishing Co. Inc., 1975, pp. 61-72.

48. Wiseman, J. *et al.* Gallium-67 myocardial imaging for the detection of endocarditis. *Radiology,* 120: 135-138, July, 1976.

Index

Brush biopsy. See bronchial
brushing, 156
Bruton's agammaglobulinemia, 305
BS, 157
BSP, 180, 182
Buccal smear test, 260
Budd-Chiara syndrome, 172
Buerger's disease. See
thromboangiitis, 102
Bulb of eye, 264, 265
Bulimia, 167
BUN, 204, 206
Bundle branch block, 92
Bundle of His. See atrioventricular
bundle, 88, 91
Bunionectomy, 44
Burkitt's lymphoma, 131, 308
Burn, 20
first degree, 20
second degree, 21
third degree, 21
Bursa, 39
Bursitis, 40
Bypass graft,
autogenous, 103
Byproduct material, 349

— C —

C₁, 50
C₂, 50
CA, 80
Ca, 50
Cachexia, 325
Café au lait spots, 24
Calcaneous, 33
Calcification, 155
of tracheal rings, 148
Calcitonin, 257
Calculus, pl. calculi of
bladder, 196
ureter, 195
Caldwell-Luc operation, 147
Calendar rhythm, 228
Calices, sing. calyx, 190, 191
Callositas, 21
Callus, 38
Caloric test, 290
Cancellous bone, 33
Cancer, 325
cell, 325
Candidiasis, 161, 299, 310
Canthus, pl. canthi, 272
Capillary fragility
tourniquet test, 134, 136
Capsular laceration, 44
Caput
medusae, 176
succedaneum, 234
Carbohydrate tolerance tests, 257
glucose tolerance, 257
postprandial, 257
tolbutamide tolerance, 257
Carbon dioxide
capacity, 258
combining power, 257
Carbuncle, 21
Carcinoembryonic antigen, 326
Carcinogenic agent, 325
Carcinoid, 325
Carcinoid syndrome, carcinoidosis, 249
Carcinolysis, 325

Carcinoma, 4, 325
in situ, 325
Carcinoma of
breast. See breast cancer, 25
cervix uteri, 215
esophagus, 164
gallbladder, 173
lung, 151
salivary gland, 162
vagina, 212
vulva, 212
Carcinoma of cervix uteri, 215
adenocarcinoma, 215
epidermoid, 215
invasive, 215
microinvasive, 215
preinvasive, 215
squamous cell, 215
Cardia, 165
Cardiac, 7
Cardiac catheterization of left atrium
Radner method, 108
Ross method, 108
suprasternal, 108
transseptal, 108
Cardiac catheterization of left ventricle
direct puncture, 108
retrograde method, 108
Cardiac (diagnoses)
arrest, 90
arrhythmias, 90
dysrhythmias, 90
edema, 100
syncope, 100
tamponade, 93
Cardiac orifice, 165
Cardiac pacing,
electronic, 97
physiologic, 97
Cardiac (procedures)
biopsy, 94
index, 106
massage, 94
monitor, 96
pressures (intracardiac), 108, 109
transplantation, 95, 114
Cardiac (radiology)
fluoroscopy, 105
series with barium swallow, 105
tomography, 105
Cardiogenic shock, 100
Cardiopulmonary
arrest, 93
bypass, 97
resuscitation, 97
Cardiorrhexis, 4
Cardioversion, 97
Carditis, 4
Carina, 148
Carotid
artery ligation, 67
compression test, 80
endarterectomy, 67
occlusive disease, 101
pulse. See pulse analysis, 111
reconstruction, 67
sinus syncope, 100
Carotid-subclavian
anastomosis, 103
bypass, 103, 115
Carpal tunnel syndrome. See painful
shoulder, 41
Carpoptosia, 46
Cartilaginous joint. See articulation, 39

Castle's intrinsic factor. See intrinsic
factor, 168
Castration, 221
CAT, 81
Catalepsy, 74
Cataract, 267
operations, 269
Cataract extraction
extracapsular, 269
intracapsular, 269
Catecholamines
in urine, 256
Catharsis, 74
Catheterization, left atrium, 108
suprasternal, Radner, 108
transseptal, Ross, 108
modifications
Brockenbrough, 108
Shirey, 108
Catheterization of auditory tube, 287
Caudal. See inferior, 17, 18
Causalgia, 58
Cavities of heart, 88
Cavity of tooth, 161
CBC, 139
CBF, 80
CBI, 206
CBS, 80
CC, 28, 206
cc, 28
CCA, 111
CCC, 347
CCCR, 111
CCU, 111
C, Cyl, 276
CDC, 29, 239
CDH, 50
CEA, 182, 326
Cecectomy, 170
Cecostomy, 170, 185
Cecum, 168
Celiac disease, celiac sprue
adult, 169
childhood, 169
Cell body, 57, 59
Cellulitis, 21
Central, 17
venous pressure, 106
Centromere, 252
Cephalad, 7
Cephalic, 7. See superior, 17, 18
Cephalin cholesterol
flocculation, 181, 182
Cephalitis, 7
Cerebellum, 60, 62
Cerebral, 7
Cerebral
aneurysm, 63
atherosclerosis, 63
arteriovenous malformation, 63
concussion, 63
embolism, 63
hemorrhage, 234
infarction, 63
ischemia, 63
palsy, 63
thrombosis, 63, 347
Cerebral
angiography, 75
circulation imaging
(nuclear), 354, 358
Cerebral
aqueduct. See ventricles, 61, 62
cortex, 60